Acute Respiratory Care of the Neonate

3rd Edition

Edited by Debbie Fraser, MN, RNC-NIC

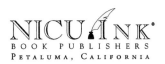
NICU Ink®
BOOK PUBLISHERS
PETALUMA, CALIFORNIA

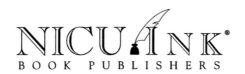

1425 North McDowell Blvd., Suite 105
Petaluma, CA 94954-6513
888-642-8465

Editor-in-Chief: Charles Rait, RN, MSEd, PNC
Managing Editor: Suzanne G. Rait, RN
Editorial Coordinator: Tabitha Parker
Editors: Beverley DeWitt., BA
Sylvia Stein-Wright, BA
Proofreader: Joanne Gosnell, BA
Indexer: Mary Coe, Potomac Indexing, LLC

Book design and composition:
Marsha Godfrey Graphics

LIBRARY OF CONGRESS CATALOGING-IN-PUBLICATION DATA
ISBN 978-1-887571-15-9

Library of Congress Cataloging-in-Publication Data

Acute respiratory care of the neonate / edited by Debbie Fraser. — 3rd ed.
  p. ; cm.
 Includes bibliographical references and index.
 ISBN 978-1-887571-15-9 (pbk.)
 I. Fraser, Debbie, 1959-
 [DNLM: 1. Intensive Care, Neonatal—methods. 2. Respiratory Distress Syndrome, Newborn—nursing. 3. Infant, Premature. WY 157.3]

 618.92'200428--dc23
                2012020793

TABLE OF CONTENTS

Contributing Authors

Ruben E. Alvaro, MD, FAAP
St. Boniface General Hospital
University of Manitoba

Susan Givens Bell, DNP, MABMH, RNC-NIC
All Children's Hospital
St. Petersburg, Florida

Debra Bingham, DrPH, RN
Association of Women's Health, Obstetric and
Neonatal Nurses (AWHONN)
Washington, District of Colombia

Bill Diehl-Jones, RN, PhD
University of Manitoba
Winnipeg, Manitoba

Debbie Fraser, MN, RNC-NIC
Athabasca University and
St. Boniface General Hospital
Winnipeg, Manitoba

Jay S. Greenspan, MD
Nemours Children's Clinic
Alfred I. duPont Hospital for Children
Wilmington, Delaware

Thomas R. Harris, MD (retired)
University of Arizona College of Nursing (1975–1980)
University of Utah College of Nursing (1981–1985)

Martin Keszler, MD
Brown University
Warren Alpert Medical School
Women and Infants Hospital
Providence, Rhode Island

Kathleen Koszarek, NNP-BC, MSN
Aurora BayCare Medical Center
Green Bay, Wisconsin

Gerry Matranga, MN, APRN, NNP-BC
Ochsner Health System
New Orleans, Louisiana

Susan Orlando, DNS, APRN, NNP-BC
LSU Health Sciences Center School of Nursing
New Orleans, Louisiana

Dawn Ricouard, RNC-NIC, BSN
Ochsner Health System
New Orleans, Louisiana

Kristine Strecker, APRN, NNP-BC
Ochsner Health System
New Orleans, Louisiana

ACKNOWLEDGMENT

I would like to acknowledge and thank the following people for their help and support:

the dedicated authors whose wealth of experience enrich the pages of this book; my colleagues at St. Boniface Hospital, especially Dr. Ruben Alvaro and Joe Miller for their review and suggestions, Chuck and Suzanne Rait, and Tabitha Parker for making this book possible; and special thanks to Bill and the CLAN, Cayly, Liam, Anna, and Nicole.

Dedicated to the NICU babies and their families from whom we've all learned.

INTRODUCTION

Since the first edition of "ARC" came off the press in 1991, newborn respiratory care has continued to evolve. In the third edition of this text we have updated information on synchronized and volume ventilation, nitric oxide, pulmonary function testing, and high-frequency ventilation. Noninvasive ventilation strategies have been emphasized in keeping with the renewed interest in these modes of ventilation. The remaining chapters have been updated and revised to reflect the continued growth in our understanding of the impact of respiratory disease on the newborn infant.

This text continues its commitment to provide that blend of the nursing art and science so critical to the care of high-risk infants. As never before, the challenge of providing care to our future leaders and their families lies before us. This book is dedicated to helping those that accept that challenge.

Debbie Fraser, MN, RNC-NIC
St. Boniface General Hospital
Athabasca University

1 Physiologic Principles of the Respiratory System

Bill Diehl-Jones, RN, PhD

A central issue in caring for ill or premature infants is the successful management of respiratory status. Management can be complicated by the relative lack of development of these infants' respiratory structures and the functional immaturity of their respiratory systems. This chapter therefore begins with a review of the developmental and functional anatomy of the lungs and associated structures. Subsequent sections address lung mechanics, the synthesis and roles of pulmonary surfactant, and the physiology of lung fluid and of fetal breathing. The events of transition and other elements of neonatal respiratory physiology are also discussed. Particular attention is given to those issues that are unique to the neonate, with the hope that this information will assist the clinician in understanding and optimally facilitating respiration in the newborn infant.

RESPIRATORY SYSTEM DEVELOPMENT

The organs of the lower respiratory system, which include the larynx, trachea, bronchi, and lungs, begin to develop during the embryonic period, in the fourth week following conception. Once the basic rudiments of the respiratory system have been established, they undergo considerable refinement during the subsequent fetal period of life. Even after parturition, respiratory structures, most notably the lungs, continue to mature and change both structurally and functionally. The focus of this section of the chapter is lung development during the embryonic, fetal, and postnatal periods. Various mechanical and biochemical signals control these developmental events.[1] These mediators are discussed later in the chapter.

EMBRYONIC LUNG DEVELOPMENT

Late in the embryonic period (four weeks postconception), the rudiments of the respiratory system are established. The lower respiratory structures, which include the larynx, trachea, bronchi, and lungs, begin to form in this period.[2] The anatomic precursor of the future respiratory system is the laryngotracheal groove, an outgrowth of the primordial pharynx, which is visible by approximately day 24 of embryonic development (Figure 1-1). This groove extends downward and is gradually separated from the future esophagus by a septum. Failure of the septum to develop completely results in a tracheoesophageal fistula. Several other congenital anomalies of the respiratory system can develop during the embryonic and/or early fetal periods; they are summarized in Table 1-1.

Most of the anatomic rudiments of the respiratory system are laid down during the eight weeks comprising the embryonic period. Between days 26 and 28 postconception, the first dichotomous branches of the lung (bronchial) buds can be seen (Figure 1-2). By 35 days of embryonic development, secondary bronchi are evident; at 56 days postconception, three divisions are distinguishable on the right and two on the left (lobar and segmental bronchi). While these buds are dividing, the trachea is forming through the elongation of the upper portion of the lung bud. By the end of the embryonic period, the conductive lung pathways have been formed and need only to lengthen and increase in diameter.[3,4] The portions of the lungs related to gas exchange have not yet been elaborated, however, and must develop before the fetus can survive.

FIGURE 1-1
Development of the larynx at (A) 4 weeks, (B) 5 weeks, (C) 6 weeks, and (D) 10 weeks.

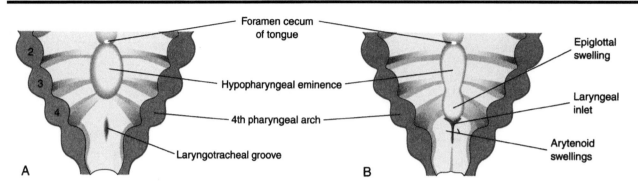

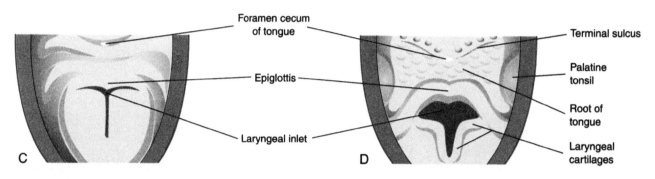

From: Moore KL, and Persaud TVN. 2008. *The Developing Human: Clinically Oriented Embryology,* 8th ed. Philadelphia: Saunders, 200. Reprinted by permission.

FETAL LUNG DEVELOPMENT

There are four stages in lung maturation, which span the end of the embryonic and all of the fetal period of development (weeks 6–40). These include the pseudoglandular, canalicular, terminal saccular, and alveolar stages. Lung maturity, both anatomic and functional, is key to successful transition to the extrauterine environment, and these stages are discussed in that context.

Pseudoglandular Stage (6–16 weeks)

From 5 to 17 weeks postconception, a tree of narrow tubules forms. New airway branches arise through a combination of cell multiplication and necrosis.[5] These tubules have thick epithelial walls composed of columnar or cuboidal cells. This morphology, along with the loose mesenchymal tissue surrounding the tree, gives the lungs the appearance of an exocrine gland. The ends

TABLE 1-1
Congenital Anomalies of the Respiratory System

Anomaly	Origin	Time Frame/Incidence
Pulmonary atresia (single lung or lobe)	Failure of primitive foregut branches to develop	Four to six weeks
Tracheoesophageal fistula	Failure of foregut (tracheoesophageal) septum to completely divide the esophagus and trachea	Four to five weeks Incidence: 1 in 2,500 births
Tracheal stenosis/atresia	Unequal division of foregut into trachea and esophagus	Four to five weeks Incidence: Rare
Diaphragmatic hernia	Failure of fusion of the septum transversum, pleuroperitoneal membranes, lateral body wall, and dorsal mesentery of esophagus	Six to ten weeks Incidence: 1 in 2,000 births

FIGURE 1-2
Development of the bronchial buds, bronchi, and lungs.

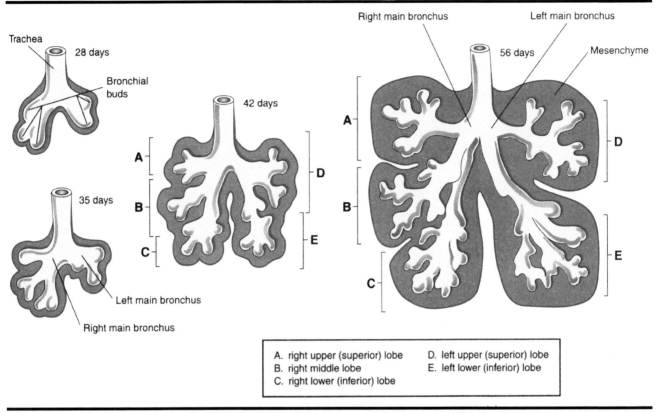

A. right upper (superior) lobe   D. left upper (superior) lobe
B. right middle lobe   E. left lower (inferior) lobe
C. right lower (inferior) lobe

From: Moore KL, and Persaud TVN. 2008. *The Developing Human: Clinically Oriented Embryology,* 8th ed. Philadelphia: Saunders, 203. Reprinted by permission.

of the tubules are terminal bronchioles (Figure 1-3A), which are too thick to permit gas exchange. Fetuses born during this period are therefore unable to survive. The conductive portion of the tracheobronchial tree (trachea to terminal bronchioles) is now well established, and rudimentary forms of cartilage, connective tissue, muscle, blood vessels, and lymphatics can be identified.[6] One of the primary developmental anomalies during this period is diaphragmatic hernia (see Table 1-1).

Canalicular Stage (16–26 weeks)

The canalicular stage overlaps the pseudoglandular stage because the superior lung segments develop before the inferior segments. The epithelial cells of the distal air spaces (future alveolar lining) flatten sometime between weeks 13 and 25, signaling the beginning of the canalicular stage (Figure 1-3B). A rich vascular supply begins to proliferate, and with the changes in mesenchymal tissue, the capillaries are brought closer to the airway epithelium. By week 24 of gestation, terminal bronchioles give rise to two or more respiratory bronchioles, which

in turn develop into alveolar ducts. Toward the end of this crucial developmental period, primitive alveoli called terminal saccules develop at the tips of the respiratory bronchioles. These structures are thin walled, thereby permitting gas exchange. The increased vascularity evident by this time, along with the development of the terminal saccules, makes it possible for infants born at the end of this stage to survive with intensive care, depending on the degree of saccular-capillary coupling.[7]

Terminal Saccular Stage (26 weeks–birth)

Two critical changes occur during the terminal saccular stage: Many more terminal saccules develop, and their epithelium becomes increasingly thin. Capillaries invade what are now developing alveoli, and the blood-air interface becomes more elaborate (Figure 1-3C). This involves a close physical association between thin alveolar epithelial cells and capillary endothelial cells, which in many regions share a fused basement membrane, greatly facilitating gas exchange. Early in this period, most cells lining the alveoli are squamous cells, called

FIGURE 1-3
Progressive stages of lung development (illustrated using histologic sections).

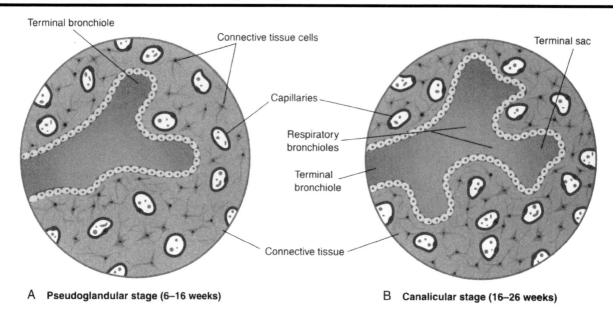

A Pseudoglandular stage (6–16 weeks)   B Canalicular stage (16–26 weeks)

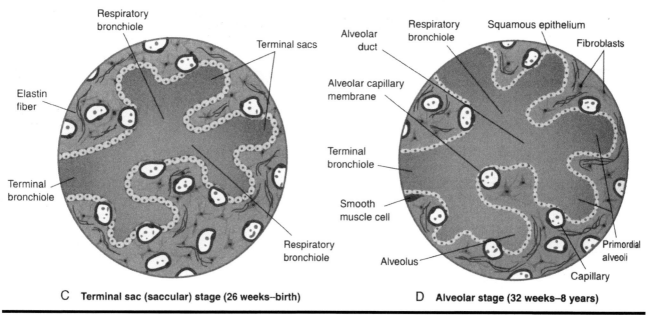

C Terminal sac (saccular) stage (26 weeks–birth)   D Alveolar stage (32 weeks–8 years)

From: Moore KL, and Persaud TVN. 2008. *The Developing Human: Clinically Oriented Embryology,* 8th ed. Philadelphia: Saunders, 204. Reprinted by permission.

type I alveolar cells, or pneumocytes. Increasingly, rounded pneumocytes, or type II cells, also populate the primitive alveoli. These cells secrete pulmonary surfactant, a complex mixture of phospholipids, which forms a monomolecular layer over the internal surface of the terminal saccules. The biochemistry of surfactant and its role in lung compliance are discussed later in this chapter. Birth during this phase may result in several conditions, including respiratory distress syndrome (RDS).

Alveolar Stage (32 weeks–8 years)

Structures resembling alveoli are usually present on the terminal saccules by 32 weeks gestation. At the beginning of this period, respiratory bronchioles end in several thin-walled saccules that are surrounded by connective tissue. The squamous epithelial cells lining the terminal sacs acquire a thin, stretched appearance, and adjacent capillaries encroach into the terminal saccules. These primitive alveoli are recognizable as small bulges on the walls of terminal saccules and respiratory bronchioles (Figure 1-3D). Mature alveoli typically do not form until after birth. At birth, primordial alveoli enlarge as the lungs expand. The main contributor to the increase in lung volume that is seen after birth, however, is a growth in the number of respiratory bronchioles and alveoli; approximately 95 percent of all alveoli develop after birth.

Genetic and Environmental Influences on Prenatal Lung Development

The four fetal development stages and their associated morphologic changes are tightly regulated. The developmental program that guides these events is complex, but we are now beginning to understand the molecular genetic control mechanisms, which include multiple tissue interactions, transcription factors that decode specific genes, and growth and signaling factors that are expressed or become active at specific time points. A detailed review of these genes and molecules is beyond the scope of this chapter. An overview of the subject is useful, however, in that knowledge of the molecular controls of lung development will likely yield treatment strategies for respiratory problems associated with premature birth or abnormal lung development.[8]

During the embryonic stage, when the trachea and lungs originate from endoderm, two key transcription factors are implicated: hepatocyte nuclear transcription factor (HNF-3β) and thyroid transcription factor (TTF-1). If the gene coding for HNF-3β is experimentally ablated in mice, the foregut does not form, which leads to the absence of lungs.[9] Furthermore, HNF-3β controls the expression of surfactant protein B and Clara-cell–specific protein.[10] As for TTF-1, mice lacking this gene exhibit tracheoesophageal fistulae and hypoplastic lungs.[11] Still other genes, such as sonic hedgehog (Shh), fibroblast growth factor-8, and N-cadherin, modulate the expression of the transforming growth factor-8 family of genes, resulting in left-right asymmetry of the lungs.[8] Many of these genes have multiple functions and are expressed at specific locations. For example, Shh is expressed at the tips of developing lung branches and appears to control pulmonary cell proliferation.[12]

During the pseudoglandular stage, when preacinar airways and blood vessels develop and the branching pattern of the bronchial tree is formed, two genes appear to be especially important: Gata-6 and N-myc.[13,14] Mutations in and/or knockouts of these genes result in reduced branching and lung hypoplasia. Many other gene products and receptors are implicated in this process, yet the essential question that underpins lung development in the fetus is "What specifies when and where these genes get 'turned on'?" The answer must, in part, lie in the physical environment of the lung.

During the pseudoglandular stage of development, fetal breathing, peristaltic airway contraction, and the beginning secretion of lung fluid exert physical forces on the lungs.[8] If these forces are disrupted through surgical or mechanical means, lung hypoplasia results. For example, chronic deflation of a lung results in hypoplasia, whereas chronic overexpansion produces hyperplasia.[15] Although the notion that mechanical forces playing a role in lung development may seem intuitive, it is important to remember that this process is regulated at the molecular level. The question then becomes "How do these mechanical forces generate molecular signals?" An emerging body of evidence suggests that physical stress can stimulate growth factor and growth factor receptor expression. The clinical relevance is that, as we understand more about these signals and forces, it may be possible to therapeutically enhance them through targeted gene expression.

In addition to the genetically programmed events of lung development discussed in the following sections, the environment of the uterus itself likely influences growth. Fetal hypoxemia, which has been studied extensively in sheep, is known to affect a variety of physiologic parameters, lung growth and development included. For example, moderate degrees of hypoxemia affect the hypothalamic-pituitary-adrenal axis in sheep, even when pH and arterial carbon dioxide tension ($PaCO_2$) level are controlled.[16] These effects of hypoxemia include increased plasma adrenocorticotrophic hormone (ACTH) and cortisol, the latter being critical for the structural and functional maturation of surfactant-secreting type II alveolar cells. Furthermore, surfactant protein A messenger RNA (mRNA) is increased in hypoxemic fetuses, whereas insulin-like growth factor-I and its binding protein-5 mRNA are decreased. Other work with fetal lung explants subjected to hypoxia has shown the suppression of several biochemical and morphologic markers of lung cell differentiation.[17] Other uterine environment (maternal) factors are also likely to elicit changes in prenatal lung development and may present opportunities for therapeutically modulating fetal lung maturation.

FIGURE 1-4
Development of the intra-acinar arteries.

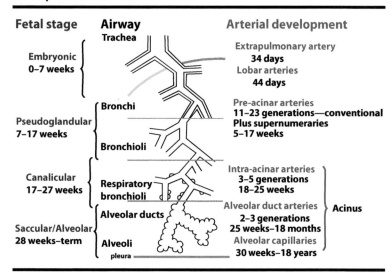

From: Hislop A. 2005. Developmental biology of the pulmonary circulation. *Paediatric Respiratory Reviews* 6(1): 35. Reprinted by permission.

POSTNATAL LUNG DEVELOPMENT: GENETIC AND ENVIRONMENTAL INFLUENCES

Lung development continues for a considerable time after birth; the developmental program spans not only embryonic and fetal life, but also infancy and early childhood. In addition to genetic factors, the extrauterine environment also comes into play, and exogenous factors help to shape lung growth and development. These forces may be classified as either mechanical or nonmechanical. With respect to the former, septal wall strain, which can be induced by growth of the thorax and/or hyperinflation, is known to influence lung growth and maturation.[18] Capillary distention and shear forces can also affect lung growth. Ligation of one pulmonary artery increases alveolar growth of the contralateral lung in newborn piglets.[19] We also know that pulmonary venous hypertension in humans can cause thickening of the endothelium and epithelium of the alveolar-capillary barrier.[20] Acute interstitial edema in the lungs increases the synthesis and deposition of collagen and glycosaminoglycans.[21]

How these mechanical signals are transduced into structural/biochemical alterations in lung tissue is a broader question. Without doubt, biochemical mediators are involved. Many nonmechanical mediators of lung growth have been identified. They include hormones, growth factors, and cytokines.

PULMONARY VASCULATURE

Pulmonary vasculature develops in conjunction with the branching of the bronchial tree.[22] This process involves both vasculogenesis, or new growth of blood vessels from embryonic angioblasts, and angiogenesis, or the "sprouting" of blood vessels from existing vessels.[1] As the preacinar airways develop, bronchial or systemic vessels also differentiate, dividing into the conventional and supernumerary tributaries that supply the peripheral acini. This development is complete by approximately 16 weeks of gestation, but the vasculature continues to grow in length and diameter to accommodate lung growth. Generally, if there is a decrease in the number of preacinar airways, there is a concomitant decrease in conventional and supernumerary arteries.[23]

As development progresses into the canalicular and terminal saccular stages, intra-acinar arteries appear; they will continue their development during the postnatal period (Figure 1-4). The conventional arteries continue their development for the first 18 months of life, and supernumerary arteries continue to be laid down for the first eight years.[24] These late-developing supernumerary vessels are smaller and more numerous than their precursors, servicing the alveoli directly.[25] If blood flow is reduced or blocked through the conventional arteries, the supernumerary arteries may serve as collateral circulation, maintaining lung function during periods of ischemia or increased pulmonary vascular resistance.[26] Postnatally, the intra-acinar vessels multiply rapidly as alveoli appear.[22]

The pulmonary veins develop more slowly. By 20 weeks gestation, however, preacinar veins are present.[24] The structural development of veins parallels that of the arteries and conducting airways, although supernumerary veins outnumber supernumerary arteries. Interestingly, both acinar and supernumerary veins appear simultaneously.[6] The development of additional veins, as well as the lengthening of existing veins, continues postnatally.

Further development of the pulmonary circulation is related to changes in muscle wall thickness and muscle extension into arterial walls. The pulmonary artery wall is relatively thick at birth, as a result of the low oxygen tension in the intrauterine environment. The wall thins as oxygen tension rises at birth, and the medial-layer

TABLE 1-2
Surfactant Composition

Composition by Weight (Percent)	
Phospholipids	85
Saturated phosphatidylcholine	60
Unsaturated phosphatidylcholine	20
Phosphatidylglycerol	8
Phosphatidylinositol	2
Phosphatidylethanolamine	5
Sphingomyelin	2
Others	3
Neutral lipids and cholesterol	5
Proteins	10
Contaminating serum proteins	8
Surfactant protein 35 (32–36,000 daltons)	~1
Lipophilic proteins (6–12,000 daltons)	~1

From: Jobe A. 1987. Questions about surfactant for respiratory distress syndrome (RDS). In *Mead Johnson Symposium on Perinatal and Developmental Medicine*. Evansville, Indiana: Mead Johnson, 43. Reprinted by permission.

FIGURE 1-5
Pathways for phosphatidylcholine synthesis.

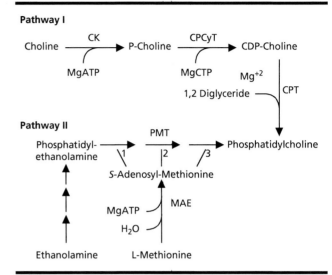

From: Farrell PM, and Ulane RE. 1981. The regulation of lung phospholipid metabolism. In *Physiological and Biochemical Basis for Perinatal Medicine*, Minkowski A, and Monset-Couchard M, eds. Basel, Switzerland: S. Karger AG, 31. Reprinted by permission.

elastic fibrils become less organized. The pulmonary vein is deficient in elastic fibers at parturition and progressively incorporates muscle and elastic tissue during the first two years of life.[24]

The intrapulmonary arteries also have relatively thick walls. The smaller arteries have increased muscularity and dilate actively as oxygen tension increases postnatally.[23] There is a concomitant fall in pulmonary vascular resistance.[6] Between 3 and 28 days postnatally, these vessels achieve their adult ratio of wall thickness to external diameter. The larger arteries take longer, increasing to adult thickness between 4 and 18 months postparturition.[24]

The systemic arteries of the fetus are also more muscular than those of the adult or child. The ratio between muscle thickness and external diameter of the systemic arteries decreases postnatally.[24] Muscle distribution changes following birth (with the muscle extending peripherally) and continues to change during the first 19 years of life.

ALVEOLAR EPITHELIUM

The respiratory portion of the lung has a continuous epithelial lining composed mainly of two cell types: type I and type II pneumocytes. The type I cells are squamous, or flattened, and cover approximately 95 percent of the alveolar surface via numerous interdigitating cytoplasmic extensions.[27,28] The thinnest area of the alveolus is composed of these extensions, and gas exchange occurs here most rapidly. The type II pneumocyte, although more numerous than the type I pneumocyte, occupies less than 5 percent of the alveolar surface.[27] Osmiophilic, lamellated bodies are characteristic of the type II cells, which are under the control of numerous hormonal axes and which will ultimately produce pulmonary surfactant. The first type II cells are seen in the fetus between 20 and 24 weeks gestation. Surfactant secretion is detectable between 25 and 30 weeks gestation, although the potential for alveolar stability is low.

PULMONARY SURFACTANT

As indicated previously, surfactant coats the inner surface of the alveoli and is a key determinant of inward-directed collapsing pressure in the lungs. It is therefore also important with respect to compliance. This section discusses both the composition and synthesis of surfactant, as well as the influence of hormones on surfactant biosynthesis and secretion.

COMPOSITION AND SYNTHESIS

The composition of pulmonary surfactant is shown in Table 1-2. Surfactant is a lipoprotein, with 90 percent of its dry weight composed of lipid.[29] The majority of this lipid (60 percent) is saturated phosphatidylcholine (PC), of which dipalmitoylphosphatidylcholine (DPPC) is the most abundant. DPPC is the component responsible for

FIGURE 1-6
Biosynthesis of phospholipids.

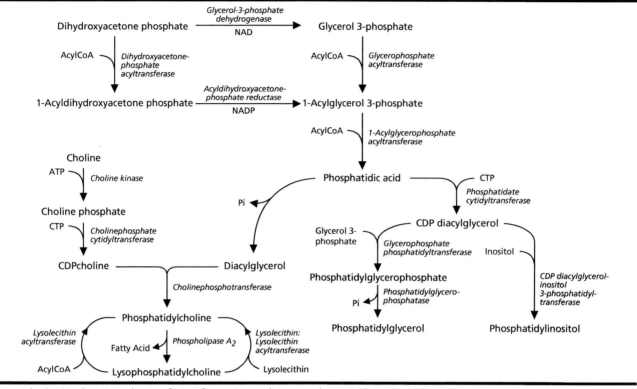

From: Jobe A. 1987. Questions about surfactant for respiratory distress syndrome (RDS). In *Mead Johnson Symposium on Perinatal and Developmental Medicine*. Evansville, Indiana: Mead Johnson, 13. Reprinted by permission.

decreasing the surface tension to almost zero when compressed at the surface during inspiration.

Phosphatidylglycerol (PG) accounts for another 8 percent of the phospholipid in surfactant, a ratio that is unique to lung cells. PG is the last phospholipid to develop in surfactant. Because fetal lung fluid flows into the amniotic cavity, the presence of PG in the amniotic fluid is a good marker for the presence of surfactant and, hence, lung maturity. The rest of the compound is involved in intracellular transport, storage, exocytosis, adsorption, and clearance at the alveolar lining.[27,29]

Surfactant synthesis involves a series of biochemical events that includes synthesis and integration of surfactant components in the membranes of the smooth and rough endoplasmic reticulum and multivesicular bodies of the type II pneumocyte.[27] Once assembled, surfactant is transported intracellularly to the Golgi apparatus and then on to the lamellar bodies.[30] The biosynthesis of surfactant is discussed in detail in several publications.[27,29] Chapter 11 also contains more information on surfactant.

Before it is biochemically functional, surfactant is transformed into a lattice-shaped structure known as tubular myelin. This transformation is influenced to a large extent by surfactant protein D.[31] This substance enhances surfactant spreadability and adsorption. Surfactant is then stored in the lamellar bodies of type II pneumocytes. Secretion occurs by exocytosis; however, surfactant must diffuse to the surface of the liquid layer to be physiologically functional.[27]

There are two major pathways for PC synthesis (Figure 1-5). Key precursors for PC synthesis include glycerol, fatty acids, choline, glucose, and ethanolamine.[32] The primary synthetic pathway for PC is the cytidine diphosphate choline system. The other biosynthetic pathway—the methyltransferase system—leads to phosphatidylethanolamine formation. The latter has minor significance in the adult lung and seems to play a relatively insignificant role in fetal lung development.[32]

The biosynthesis of PC, phosphatidylinositol, and PG is depicted in Figure 1-6. The schematic illustrates the importance of phosphatidic acid biosynthesis. The increased production of phospholipids seen in late gestation depends on the increased synthesis of this acid.

FIGURE 1-7
Biosyntheses and remodeling of phosphatidylcholine.

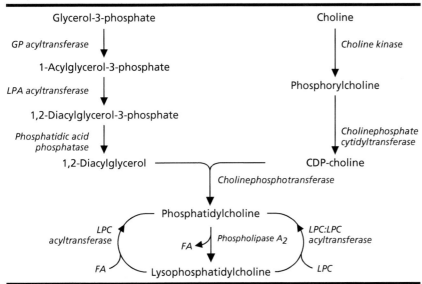

From: Farrell PM, and Ulane RE. 1981. The regulation of lung phospholipid metabolism. In *Physiological and Biochemical Basis for Perinatal Medicine*, Minkowski A, and Monset-Couchard M, eds. Basel, Switzerland: S. Karger AG, 33. Reprinted by permission.

The majority of phospholipid produced is PC; Figure 1-7 represents the biosynthesis and remodeling of this critical phospholipid.[29]

Figure 1-7 also demonstrates the interaction of the choline pathway and the diglyceride synthesis mechanisms that yield increased PC synthesis during late gestation. Although this interaction produces increased quantities of PC, the PC is not the highly saturated version identified in the final surfactant compound. The remodeling of PC that occurs in the phosphatidylcholine-lysophosphatidylcholine cycle provides the dipalmitoyl-PC required for surfactant.[32]

As gestation advances, alveolar phospholipid content and saturation increase. This is accompanied by a growth in the number of osmiophilic inclusion bodies within type II pneumocytes. Choline incorporation, which is low in early gestation, has been reported to rise abruptly in Rhesus monkeys when gestation is 90 percent complete.[33] This suggests that this particular pathway is upregulated in advance to meet postnatal needs.

Enzymatic changes in the phospholipid synthesis pathway are discussed in several review articles.[29,32,34] The correlation of these changes with the surge in saturated PC and increase in PG and the concomitant decrease in phosphatidylinositol is not yet understood. Whether it is a change in concentration of enzyme or substrate, adjustment in catalytic efficiency, change in substrate affinity, or activation of latent enzymes is not known.

HORMONAL INFLUENCES ON SURFACTANT SECRETION AND PRODUCTION

In addition to enzymes, hormones also regulate surfactant biosynthesis and secretion. Those hormones that have been implicated include glucocorticoids, ACTH, thyroid hormones, estrogens, prolactin, thyrotropin-releasing hormone, catecholamines, insulin, fibroblast pneumocyte factor, prostaglandins, and epidermal growth factor. Only glucocorticoids, thyroid hormones, catecholamines, and insulin are reviewed here because these endocrine factors are the primary axes affecting lung development.

Glucocorticoids

Glucocorticoids are probably the best known of the hormones affecting surfactant. Liggins' observations in 1969 set off a flurry of research in the area of hormonal control of fetal lung development that has continued to the present.[35] Glucocorticoids accelerate the normal pattern of fetal lung development by increasing the rate of glycogen depletion and phospholipid biosynthesis.

Depletion of glycogen leads to direct anatomic changes in alveolar structures, thinning the interalveolar septa while increasing the size of the alveoli. Other morphologic changes include increases in the numbers of type II pneumocytes and lamellar bodies within those cells. This occurs in conjunction with a functional maturation of these cells, leading to an accelerated synthesis of surfactant phospholipids.[29,36]

Glucocorticoids, like most steroid ligands, bind to intracellular receptors, forming a receptor-ligand complex that acts as a nuclear transcription factor. This ultimately results in the generation of a repertoire of new proteins, the identities of which are currently unknown. Dexamethasone and betamethasone have a higher affinity for the glucocorticoid receptor than do the natural corticoids (cortisol and cortisone), which favors the use of betamethasone to enhance lung maturation during preterm labor.[37]

The question of whether the triggering of protein synthesis accounts for the increase in fatty acid synthetase, phosphatidic acid phosphatase, and choline-phosphate cytidyltransferase activity is yet to be answered. Conflicting evidence suggests that glucocorticoids could promote the synthesis of an enzyme activator that may influence the production of the heavier of the surfactant apoproteins.[38]

Several other questions have yet to be answered as well. It is evident that glucocorticoid action is centered on surfactant synthesis, not secretion. It is also clear that it affects more than surfactant synthesis. Acting directly on lung tissue, glucocorticoids increase the number of β-adrenergic receptors and enhance elastin and collagen production, which improves lung compliance.[39]

What has until recently not been evident is whether glucocorticoids directly affect type II pneumocytes or whether they mediate their actions through other lung cells, such as fibroblasts. Smith suggested that, rather than having a direct impact on type II cells, glucocorticoids may act on fibroblasts (increasing the production of fibroblast pneumocyte factor), which then affects surfactant production.[40] More recently, however, experiments with cultured human type II pneumocytes have revealed that these cells produce at least two surfactant components in response to synthetic glucocorticoids. In experiments by Ramin and coworkers, type II cells were exposed to physiologic concentrations of either betamethasone or dexamethasone. Surfactant protein B mRNA production increased after 48 hours' exposure to steroids, as determined by quantitative reverse transcription-polymerase chain reaction.[41] This would imply that type II cells do not require the cooperation of other lung cells to respond to steroids. As determined by other researchers using cultured pneumocytes, this effect is likely limited to seven to eight days after exposure to dexamethasone.[42] Glucocorticoids also regulate the expression of at least one other surfactant gene in type II cells. Studies with a fetal rat type II cell line have established that glucocorticoids regulate the expression of the fatty acid synthase (FAS) gene.[43] The protein product of this gene is a key enzyme that is involved in *de novo* synthesis of fatty acids, which are integral components of pulmonary surfactant. Interestingly, glucocorticoids increased FAS activity, protein content, mRNA content, and rate of transcription in type II cells, but not in lung fibroblasts. Although these findings do not rule out positive cooperation between type II pneumocytes and other cells such as fibroblasts, they do suggest that type II cells can respond autonomously to glucocorticoids. Yet another gene, ABCA3, which is involved in membrane transport in type II cells, is also up-regulated by glucocorticoids.[44] Defects in this gene have been found in newborns with fatal surfactant deficiency.

Not only are glucocorticoids involved in the regulation of surfactant production; they also appear to regulate architectural changes in the newborn lung. During the canalicular stage of development (see **Canalicular Stage [16–26 weeks]**, earlier in this chapter), septal wall thickness decreases, in part as a result of a lessening in the amount of fibronectin, an extracellular matrix protein. In rats treated with dexamethasone, fibronectin expression falls, a finding congruent with the notion that dexamethasone promotes alveolar-wall thinning.[45] The cellular target in this case is unknown, although it seems likely that alveolar fibroblasts are involved.

In all research involving cell cultures, an important caveat is that cultured cells are genetically different from their cells of origin, and they are not in the same cellular milieu as cells *in vivo* or in intact lungs. Despite these limitations, cell culture studies have provided important information that may be generalized to the neonate. For example, prenatal (maternal) betamethasone administration changes the phospholipid profile in tracheal aspirates of very preterm infants.[46] It is also generally accepted that glucocorticoids enhance both biochemical and structural maturation of the neonatal lungs.[47] Cell culture work has enabled us to more specifically identify the likely effectors of glucocorticoids. There are, however, controversies related to the choice of glucocorticoid, number and timing of doses, as well as side effects.[48] These topics are addressed in Chapter 11.

Thyroid Hormones

The idea that hormones may work in conjunction with other compounds or hormones is reinforced by observations of the actions of thyroid hormones. Thyroxine (T_4) and triiodothyronine (T_3) have been shown to increase the rate of phospholipid synthesis.[29,49–51] As do glucocorticoids, thyroid hormones enhance production of PC through choline incorporation. They do not, however, increase PG synthesis or stimulate the production of surfactant-specific proteins.[52,53] Although glucocorticoids increase fatty acid synthetase activity, thyroid hormones seem to decrease it.[54] These disparities suggest different sites of action for these hormones, as well as their need to act in conjunction with other hormones.[52]

Low maternal T_3 and T_4 levels have been associated with RDS in the neonate, although exact mechanisms are unclear.[32,36,51,55] It has also been shown that the effects of thyroid hormones are mediated by a specific thyroid receptor that is a potent phospholipid-synthesis stimulator and to which T_3 has a higher affinity than T_4.[56]

Clinical application of this information is aimed at maximizing beneficial effects through the delivery of hormones or hormone-activating substances that cross the placenta. Naturally occurring thyroid hormones do not readily cross the placenta unless concentrations far exceeding normal levels are achieved. However, thyrotropin-releasing hormone does cross the placenta and stimulates the fetal pituitary gland to produce thyroid-stimulating hormone, resulting in increased production of PC.[36,57]

Continued investigation into the precise mechanisms of thyroid hormone action is essential. There seems to be little doubt that synergistic interaction between glucocorticoids and thyroid hormones occurs, apparently at the level of mRNA.[52] A significant increase in PC production occurs in a shortened period of time when these two hormones are used together prior to delivery.[50,51,56] These findings may have significant clinical implications, which may alter future therapeutic interventions. A review of the Cochrane database has shown, however, that antenatal coadministration of thyroid-releasing hormone with glucocorticoids does not improve any fetal, neonatal, or childhood outcomes.[58] Prenatal administration of TSH appears to have a number of adverse effects for both women and their infants, including increased likelihood of ventilation and lower five-minute Apgar scores for the neonate, and poorer outcomes when children are seen at follow-up.[58]

Catecholamines

Glucocorticoids and thyroid hormones play a role in enhancing the synthesis of phospholipids, whereas catecholamines stimulate the secretion of surfactant into the alveolar space. This appears to be a direct action of adrenergic compounds on type II cells.[59] The response is prompt, occurring in less than an hour.

Research has shown that catecholamines increase surfactant and saturated PC in the lung fluid and improve lung stability. This is demonstrated in an increased ratio of lecithin to sphingomyelin. An added benefit is a decrease in fetal lung fluid within the alveoli at the time of delivery. These two effects (increase in surfactant and decrease in lung fluid) work together to prepare the fetus for respiratory conversion.[36,60]

Insulin

Surfactant development appears to be inhibited in neonates born to diabetic mothers whose blood sugar levels are not well controlled. Whether this is caused by hyperglycemia, hyperinsulinemia, or both is unclear, and research continues to provide conflicting answers. Maturation of surfactant synthesis occurs at the same time glycogen is depleted from the lungs. Insulin inhibits glycogen breakdown, thereby decreasing the substrate available for PC synthesis as well as altering the natural anatomic changes that occur with glycogen depletion.[29,36] These alterations affect the ability of the lungs to perform respiratory functions.

Insulin also reduces the effect of cortisol on choline incorporation, even though it does not reduce cortisol effects on cell growth.[61] The biochemical interactions are complex; some researchers were unable to document evidence of an insulin influence or of any insulin antagonism of the usual dexamethasone response.[62] Others have reported a synergistic effect when cortisol and insulin were combined.[25]

Insulin may antagonize glucocorticoids at the fibroblast level, affecting the production of the fibroblast pneumocyte factor.[63] Miakotina and colleagues have shown that insulin directly inhibits surfactant-associated peptides A and B expression in lung epithelial cells.[64] Clinically, this likely predisposes infants of diabetic mothers to RDS, which argues for stricter monitoring and control of maternal glucose levels.

At present, surfactant synthesis appears to be controlled by a complex interaction of several hormones and factors. Normal lung function clearly depends on the presence of surfactant, which permits a decrease in surface tension at end-expiration and an increase in surface tension during lung expansion. This prevents atelectasis at end-expiration and facilitates elastic recoil on inspiration. Surfactant provides the lung with the stability required to maintain homeostatic blood gas pressures while decreasing the work of breathing. For the preterm infant, endotracheal administration of exogenous surfactant has been unequivically established as an efficacious treatment to minimize respiratory morbidity and mortality. Currently, there are studies that suggest that intrapartum administration of surfactant (before the first breath is drawn) may be safe and effective, although more studies are required.[65]

LUNG FLUID

In utero, the lung epithelium secretes fluid into the air spaces, a process necessary for development of the alveoli.[66] A delicate balance of secretion and reabsorption of fluids occurs during lung development. The relative

FIGURE 1-8
Switch from net fluid secretion (fetus) to fluid absorption (neonate) as part of transition from placental to atmospheric oxygen delivery.

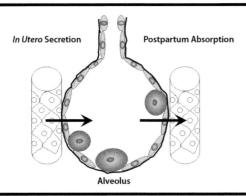

Courtesy of William Diehl-Jones.

FIGURE 1-9
Ion and water transport in production of alveolar fluid.

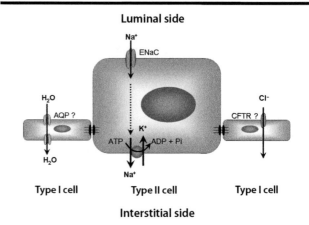

Key: ATP = adenosine triphosphate; ADP = adenosine diphosphate; AQP = aquaporin; CFTR = cystic fibrosis transmembrane conductance regulator; ENaC = epithelial sodium channel; Pi = inorganic phosphate.

Courtesy of William Diehl-Jones.

rates of these two processes shift between the prenatal and the postnatal periods. Alveolar fluid is secreted from the beginning of the canalicular stage until birth. In the newborn lamb at term, this fluid is continually secreted and reabsorbed, with complete turnover every ten hours. It is quite likely that lung fluid plays an important part in cell maturation and development, as well as in determining the formation, size, and shape of the developing air spaces. For example, alterations in fluid dynamics affect pulmonary cell proliferation and differentiation.[67]

At birth, however, the infant must make the transition from placental to atmospheric oxygen delivery. This necessitates a switch from net fluid secretion to absorption (Figure 1-8). As with secretion of many types of fluid, alveolar fluid production depends on sodium transport, which in turn drives osmotic water movement. To facilitate these fluxes, the appropriate ion and water transporters must be present. Lung fluid is believed to be derived from alveolar epithelial cells, and experimental evidence suggests that type II alveolar cells are the primary site of fluid secretion: They possess both amiloride-sensitive epithelial sodium channels (ENaCs) and water channels called aquaporins (AQPs).[67] The ENaC proteins allow vectorial transport of sodium ions, whereas AQPs facilitate water movement along the osmotic gradient established by sodium (Figure 1-9). A host of other ion channels, including potassium, chloride, and proton channels, are also found in types I and II alveolar cells; these permit the transport of ions that contribute to alveolar and tracheal fluid. Osmolarity, sodium, and chloride levels are lower in amniotic fluid than in tracheal fluid; pH, glucose, and protein are higher.[68] Some lung fluid is swallowed, and some moves into the amniotic fluid,

although lung fluid's contribution to the amniotic fluid is not significant when compared with the volume secreted by the kidneys. The lung fluid volume is approximately equal to the functional residual capacity (FRC) and must be either expelled or absorbed at birth.[69,70]

Animal fetuses whose tracheas have been ligated develop relatively large but immature lungs. Fetuses whose lungs have been drained have thick alveolar walls, smaller lungs, and more abundant type II cells.[71] This is consistent with the finding that human infants who have experienced amniotic fluid leakage have reduced numbers of alveoli.[72] These data together suggest that reduced lung fluid production or leakage of amniotic fluid places the fetus at risk for lung hypoplasia.[73] Chronic tracheal obstruction leads to hyperplasia, with an increase in the number of alveoli, although they are functionally immature.[26]

As indicated earlier, concomitant with the increase in alveolar absorption as birth approaches, there is a lessening in the rate of secretion. The administration of epinephrine to lambs leads to a decrease in fluid secretion. This effect is mediated by β-adrenergic receptors in the alveolar epithelium and may either suppress chloride transport or activate a second transport process (such as amiloride-sensitive sodium channels) that enhances the absorption process.[74] The absorption rate is known to grow as gestation progresses; this increase in absorption can be correlated with a gain in catecholamine levels.[75] During gestation, the fetal adrenal glands are probably not stimulated to produce sufficient amounts of catecholamines to trigger the absorption process; labor, however, provides sufficient stimulus to the glands to release enough epinephrine to prompt the switch from secretion to absorption.[76] The catecholamine surge that occurs at delivery is probably the final mechanism to assure that the change from secretion to absorption is completed.[68]

The drop in pulmonary vascular resistance with aeration and the rise in oxygen tension increase the number of alveolar capillaries perfused, enhancing blood removal capacity. Between the enlarged lymphatic flow and the dramatic change in pulmonary blood flow, lung fluid is dispersed within the first few hours following delivery.

FETAL BREATHING

Fetal breathing movements can be seen on ultrasound as early as 11 weeks gestation.[77] They are rapid (80–120 breaths per minute [bpm]) and irregular, occurring intermittently early in gestation. As gestation progresses, their strength and frequency increase, until they occur between 40 and 80 percent of the time, at a rate of 30–70 bpm.[60,78] Large movements (gasping) occur 5 percent of the total breathing time, one to four times per minute.[77]

This respiratory activity may contribute to lung fluid regulation, thereby influencing lung growth. The diaphragm seems to be the major structure involved, with minimal chest wall excursion (4–8 mm change in transverse diameter).[77] Movement of the diaphragm is necessary if the chest wall muscles and diaphragm are to gain adequate strength for the initial breath.[78]

Diaphragm movement also influences the course of lung cell differentiation and proliferation. Bilateral phrenectomy results in altered lung morphology, with an increase in type II over type I cells.[71] Presumably, the innervated diaphragm enlarges the thorax, thereby increasing mechanical tissue stress, which affects morphology. This idea is supported by numerous studies. For example, mechanical stretch *in vitro* increases fetal rat lung cell proliferation.[79] Several growth-associated genes, including c-fos, junB, fibroblast growth factor, and transforming growth factor, are all up-regulated by different forms of mechanical lung stress.[18] Furthermore, hypoplastic lungs are found in situations in which fetal breathing movements do not occur.[80–82]

Fetal breathing movements vary significantly from fetus to fetus. Initially, they are infrequent, increasing

with gestational age and becoming more organized and vigorous.[68] Even with these gestational changes, tracheal fluid shifts are negligible, the pressure generated being no more than 25 mmHg.[80–82] Fetal maturation leads to the appearance of cycles, with a growth in the number of fetal breathing movements during daytime hours.[77–83] Fetal breathing movements peak in late evening and reach their nadir in the early morning hours.[84]

Abnormal breathing patterns can be seen during periods of hypoxia. Mild hypoxemia decreases the incidence of fetal breathing movements; severe hypoxemia may cause them to cease for several hours. The onset of asphyxia leads to gasping that persists until death.[85] Interestingly, the onset of mild hypoxemia (as with umbilical artery occlusion of short duration) may lead to quiet sleep, which for the fetus decreases activity, energy expenditure, and oxygen consumption.[77] Although paradoxical in nature, this conservation mechanism may save the fetus until cardiac output is redistributed toward the placenta.

A reduction in fetal breathing movements before delivery coincides with the increase in prostaglandin E concentrations seen during the final days of gestation. These factors play a role in respiratory conversion at birth.[86] Furthermore, the placenta may be a key source of inhibitory prostaglandins. Infusion of the prostaglandin biosynthesis inhibitors aspirin and indomethacin with placental extracts significantly inhibits fetal breathing in sheep.[87] That finding further implicates prostaglandins as one of the factors regulating fetal breathing. Why irregular fetal breathing movements lead to the sustained respirations of postnatal life remains unknown.

TRANSITIONAL EVENTS

RESPIRATORY CONVERSION

At term, the acinar portion of the lung is well established, although "true" alveoli are only now beginning to develop. The pulmonary blood vessels are narrow; only 5–10 percent of the fetal cardiac output perfuses the lungs to meet cellular nutrition needs. This low-volume circulation results in part from the high pulmonary vascular resistance created by constricted arterioles.

At term, the lung holds approximately 20 mL/kg of fluid.[68] Lung aeration is complete when the liquid is replaced with an equal volume of air, and FRC is established. A substantial amount of air is retained with the early breaths. Within an hour of birth, 80–90 percent of the FRC is created. Surfactant and decreased surface tension facilitate the retention of air. Surfactant decreases the tendency toward atelectasis, promotes capillary circulation by increasing alveolar size (which indirectly dilates precapillary vessels), improves alveolar fluid clearance, and protects the airway.[27]

The gas tension levels that characterize the fetal state would result in significant hyperventilation postnatally; this indicates a diminished respiratory center responsiveness to chemical stimuli in the blood during intrauterine life. Postnatal breathing is responsive to stimuli from arterial and central chemoreceptors (oxygen and carbon dioxide tension in the blood), chest wall and lungs, musculoskeletal system, and skin, as well as emotions and behavior. The changes that take place at birth and the increase in aerobic metabolism are not only rapid, but irreversible. Within a few hours of birth, the neonate responds to hypoxia and hypercapnia in much the same manner as an adult.[88]

The actual mechanics of respiratory conversion begin with the passage of the fetus through the birth canal. The thorax is markedly squeezed during this passage, with external pressures of 160–200 cmH$_2$O being generated.[30,63,89] When the infant's face or nares are exposed to atmospheric pressure, variable amounts of lung fluid are expressed.[89] As much as 28 mL of fluid have been expelled during the second stage of labor, leading to the creation of a potential air space.[68] Recoil of the chest to predelivery proportions allows for passive "inspiration" of variable amounts of air. This initial step helps reduce viscous forces that must be overcome to establish an air-liquid interface in the alveoli.[86]

The forces that must be overcome during the first breaths include the viscosity of the lung fluid column, the tissue resistive forces (compliance), and the surface tension forces at the air-liquid interface. Surface tension results when the intermolecular attraction among liquid molecules exceeds the attraction between air and liquid and plays a major part in the lung's retractive forces. The viscosity of lung fluid, which provides resistance to movement of fluid in the airways, is at its maximum at the beginning of the first breath. The greatest displacement of fluid with the first breath occurs in the trachea.[89,90] The dissipation of tracheal fluid during the vaginal squeeze reduces the amount of pressure that must be generated to push the liquid column down the conducting airways.

As the column progresses down the conducting branches, the total surface area of the air-liquid interface increases as bronchiole diameter becomes smaller. The surface tension, however, increases.[68] Surface tension

forces are the hardest to overcome during first-breath events. Maximal forces are encountered where the airways are smallest (terminal bronchioles), and pressure is inversely proportional to the radius of the curvature in the airway.[68,89] In this vicinity, the intraluminal pressure must be at its peak to prevent closure of the airway by tension in the intraluminal walls.[73] If the airways were filled with fluid only (no air-liquid interface), the inspiratory pressures needed to move from being filled with liquid to being filled with air would be considerably less. This would, however, make alveolar expansion more difficult because surface tension forces would be very high and it is extremely difficult to move columns of fluid. Surface tension forces drop again once air enters the terminal air sacs.[68]

Tissue-resistive forces are unknown at birth. However, the small amount of fluid within the terminal air sacs enhances air introduction, possibly by modifying the configuration of the smaller units of the lung. The fluid enlarges the diameter of the alveolar ducts and terminal air sac, facilitating expansion. Lung fluid also likely reduces the possibility of cellular debris obstructing the small ducts.

Researchers have reported that the first diaphragmatic inspiration begins within nine seconds of delivery and generates very large negative intrathoracic pressures (mean of 70 cmH$_2$O). Air enters as soon as the intrathoracic pressure begins to drop, with mean inspiratory pressures of 30–35 cmH$_2$O.[3,68,91]

The large transpulmonary pressure generated by the diaphragm lasts only 0.5–1 second, pulling in 10–70 mL of air.[92] The layer of fluid at the alveolar lining becomes established after the first breath, allowing the molecules of surfactant to reduce the surface tension during expiration.[89] The first expiration is also active, leaving behind a residual volume of up to 30 mL. The magnitude of the expiratory pressure contributes to FRC formation, even distribution of air, and elimination of lung fluid.[68] The second and third breaths are similar to the first but require less pressure because the small airways are open and surface-active forces are diminished.[89] Lung expansion augments surfactant secretion, providing alveolar stability and FRC formation.

By 10 minutes of age, an infant's FRC is equal to 17 mL/kg; at 30 minutes, it is 25–35 mL/kg.[93] The relative hypoxia of birth results in a decrease in muscle tone; as muscle tone returns after the first breath, chest wall stability improves, helping to maintain FRC.[30,68]

Lung compliance increases by four to five times in the first 24 hours of extrauterine life and continues to increase gradually over the first week of life. Flow resistance decreases by one-half to one-fourth during this time, and the distribution of ventilation is as even after day 1 as it is on day 3 or 4.[68]

PULMONARY VASCULAR CHANGES

According to Haworth and colleagues, postnatal structural changes in the pulmonary circulation occur in three overlapping phases:[19]

1. Recruitment (progressive opening of arterial beds) of nonmuscular and partially muscular arteries occurs in the first 24 hours of life. The external diameter of these vessels increases, and the swollen endothelial-lining cells flatten. These endothelial cells may play a role in the relaxation of smooth muscle by metabolizing substances such as acetylcholine.
2. Reduced muscularity occurs during the first two weeks of life. During this time, partially muscular and wholly muscular vessels become nonmuscular and partially muscular, respectively.
3. A growth phase begins after the first two weeks of life. Muscle tissue begins to reappear in the acinus and continues to develop slowly during childhood. The initial two phases allowed for the functional adaptation necessary for extrauterine life; this third phase brings about structural remodeling. This growth creates the relationships seen in the mature system between the external vessel diameter and muscle wall thickness.

In conjunction with the local vascular changes in the pulmonary bed, there are major reorganizational changes within the cardiovascular system. The respiratory events and the cardiovascular events cannot be separated; they are interdependent, and both must occur for transition to be successful.

CARDIOVASCULAR CONVERSION

In the fetus, oxygenated blood returns from the placenta via the umbilical vein, with an arterial oxygen tension (PaO_2) of 35 mmHg. This blood enters the liver, where a small percentage feeds the liver microcirculation, and ends up in the inferior vena cava. The major portion of the returning blood is shunted directly into the inferior vena cava via the ductus venosus.

FIGURE 1-10
Fetal circulation.

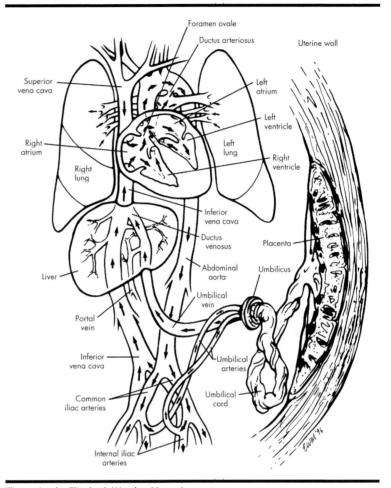

Illustration by Elizabeth Weadon Massari.

The inferior vena cava enters the right atrium, where the majority of its blood flow (approximately 60 percent) is deflected across the right atrium and through the foramen ovale into the left atrium. There it mixes with the unoxygenated blood returning from the fetal lungs, drops into the left ventricle, and is ejected into the ascending aorta to feed the cerebral arteries and upper extremities.

The remainder of the right atrium blood mixes with the unoxygenated superior vena cava blood returning from the upper body and enters the right ventricle. This mixed blood is ejected through the pulmonary arteries toward the lungs. The high pulmonary vascular resistance allows only 5–10 percent of the blood to enter the lungs, the majority being shunted across the ductus arteriosus into the thoracic aorta, which services the lower segments of the body (Figure 1-10).

With clamping of the umbilical cord, the placenta, which is a low-resistance organ (contributing to the low systemic vascular resistance found in the fetal state) is unavailable. The net result is an increase in pulmonary blood return to the heart and a decrease in systemic blood return. These changes modify the pressures within the atria. Left atrial pressure increases above the right, leading to functional closure of the foramen ovale. The increase in PaO_2 and decrease in prostaglandin levels facilitate functional closure of the ductus arteriosus. These modifications in blood flow and pressure indicate the change from "series" to "parallel" circulation and herald cardiovascular conversion.

Once the first breath is taken and cardiovascular conversion is initiated, the infant must be able to establish sustained rhythmic respirations. This requires that the central nervous system be "turned on" so that it can take over the regulation of respiratory activity.

LUNG MECHANICS

The primary role of the lungs is to permit gas exchange between the atmosphere and the blood. This activity is contingent on ventilation, or air movement into and out of the lungs. During inspiration, the combined actions of the external intercostal muscles and the diaphragm cause lung expansion and subsequent movement of air into the lungs. During expiration, the lung recoils, forcing air out, primarily through elastic recoil forces and surface tension. In any discussion of lung mechanics, three terms must first be defined: *compliance*, *elastic recoil*, and *resistance*. The interplay of these forces determines how well ventilation occurs in the neonatal lung, which differs in several respects from the adult lung. These forces, and their relevance to ventilation in the neonate, are discussed in this section.

COMPLIANCE

The term *compliance* refers to the ease with which a tissue may be stretched or distended. Mathematically, compliance (C_L) is expressed as

$$C_L = \Delta V / \Delta P$$

where ΔV is a change in lung volume and ΔP reflects the change in pressure required to effect that volume change.[94]

When compliance is measured during active breathing, the result is called *dynamic compliance*. This form of compliance is difficult to measure, given that it is rate dependent and is also influenced by lung volume. *Static compliance*, in contrast, is measured immediately before and after lung movements. Another term for static compliance is *elastance*, which is the inverse of elastic recoil.

A basic principle of compliance, whether dynamic or static, is that smaller lungs have less compliance and greater elastic recoil. In comparison with the adult's, the neonate's chest wall is very compliant. This design allows it to be compressed during passage through the birth canal without rib fractures; it then allows for further growth and development.[95–97] The infant's chest wall has been described as a loose-fitting glove surrounding the neonatal lung.[89] The clinical implications of this highly compliant chest wall are related to the ease with which lung collapse is possible in the neonate. The low elastic recoil pressure of the neonatal lung and the high compliance of the thorax result in the majority of tidal breathing being done at near the closing capacity (the volume at which lung regions are closed to the main bronchi). This contributes to the possibility of collapse and affects gas distribution.

The mechanical liabilities of a highly compliant chest wall after delivery include a compromised ability to produce large tidal volumes, because large tidal volumes require the generation of larger pressures. Consequently, the newborn must do more work than an older infant to move the same amount of tidal volume.[97] This is especially true in preterm infants with lung diseases associated with decreased lung compliance. Lung disease increases the respiratory drive in an attempt to generate stronger diaphragmatic contractions with high inspiratory pressures that will expand stiff, noncompliant lungs.

The diaphragmatic force and the pliable chest wall lead to chest distortion. Therefore, a portion of the energy and force of the contraction is wasted. Retractions are the clinical sign of these distortions, indicating the degree of rib-cage inward collapse during forceful diaphragmatic contraction.[97] This increase in the work of breathing can lead to fatigue and eventually apnea.

In contrast to the chest wall, the parenchyma of the term neonatal lung is less compliant than that of the adult—and it is even less compliant in preterm infants. Lung compliance depends on the elastic characteristics of the parenchyma, connective tissue, and blood vessels, as well as on the surface tension found in the alveoli and the initial lung volume before inflation. The net result is that, in cases where disease further decreases parenchymal compliance, the neonatal chest configuration can resemble that of pectus excavatum, with marked sternal retractions. Chest wall compliance combined with lung compliance affects closing volume, closing capacity, expiratory reserve volume, and functional residual capacity. For the neonate, this means a high closing volume and closing capacity combined with a low expiratory reserve volume and low FRC—and a propensity toward lung collapse.[89]

Lung compliance in the healthy preterm infant is slightly less than in the term infant. Changes in lung compliance are sensed by stretch receptors of the lung. Coupled with signals from the spindle fibers of the respiratory muscles, information is transmitted to the respiratory center to modify the drive necessary to maintain ventilation. Lung disease usually leads to a decrease in lung compliance, which translates to a reduced volume change for a given pressure change.

Alterations in lung compliance occur with age; however, it takes just as much pressure to produce a normal tidal volume in the newborn as in the adult. The smaller the individual, the smaller the volume change for a given pressure change (4–6 mL/cmH$_2$O in infants and 100–150 mL/cmH$_2$O in adults).[70]

ELASTIC RECOIL

Elastic recoil forces are exerted by distensible tissue components, such as elastic connective tissue fibers, in the parenchyma of the lung and the chest wall itself. During inspiration, elastic components become stretched. As the muscles of inspiration relax, the elastic forces behave like springs, recoiling and returning the surrounding tissues to their original dimensions.

In addition to elastic tissue components, however, there is another contributor to elastic recoil: surface tension. When water molecules are aligned at the alveolar interface, they lack opposing molecules on one side (the air side). The intermolecular attractive forces are then unbalanced, and the molecules move away from the interface. This movement reduces the internal surface area of the lung and augments the elastic recoil of the lung.[70]

Surface tension generates an inward-directed force, which can be expressed as

$$P = 2T/r$$

where P is the pressure required to counterbalance the tendency of alveoli to collapse inward, T is the air-liquid surface tension, and r is the radius of the curvature of the airway (Figure 1-11). The preceding formula is known as Laplace's relationship, and it is implicit that smaller alveoli have a greater inward-directed pressure.

In the neonatal lung, surface tension is the single greatest contributor to elastic recoil. The most important determinant of surface tension, in turn, is surfactant.

FIGURE 1-11
Laplace's relationship for calculating the force generated by surface tension.

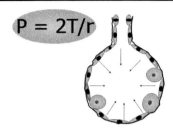

Key: P = pressure required to counterbalance tendency of alveoli to collapse inward; T = air-liquid surface tension; r = radius of curvature of airway.

Courtesy of William Diehl-Jones.

Pulmonary surfactant forms an insoluble surface film at the alveolar interface. This phospholipid-protein complex adsorbs to the interface to reduce surface tension and establish lung stability. Surfactant is stretched on inhalation and compressed on expiration; the compression allows for the pressure from surface tension to be lowered to physiologically near-zero values. The ability to achieve a low surface tension at low lung volumes (end-expiration) tends to stabilize the air spaces and prevent their closure. Without surfactant, the smaller alveoli would tend to empty into the larger ones.

Alveolar collapse occurs in a number of diseases, the most notable being RDS. In this condition, surfactant deficiency is directly related to the developmental immaturity of the lungs and to gestational age. Surfactant synthesis also depends on normal pH and pulmonary perfusion. Therefore, any pathology (such as asphyxia, hemorrhagic shock, or pulmonary edema) that interferes with these processes may lead to surfactant deficiency.[3,98,99]

RESISTANCE

Resistance is essentially the result of friction. It depends on (1) the size and geometric arrangement of the airways, (2) the viscous resistance of the lung tissue, and (3) the proportion of laminar to turbulent airflow. Resistance varies inversely with lung volume; therefore, the greater the lung volume, the less the resistance. The reason for this relationship is that airway diameter increases when the parenchyma expands.

Pulmonary resistance can be considered to have two components: viscous resistance and airway resistance.

1. **Viscous resistance** is generated by the movement of airway tissues past each other. Neonatal lungs have relatively fewer terminal air spaces and a higher

FIGURE 1-12
Pressure-volume loop showing relationship of tidal volume and tidal pressure to lung compliance.

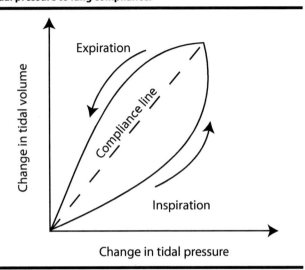

Courtesy of William Diehl-Jones.

amount of stromal tissue than adult lungs do. This gives the neonatal lung a greater level of viscous resistance during inflation and deflation. The contribution of viscous resistance to overall resistance is relatively low when compared to airway resistance (see below). The relative contribution of viscous resistance is higher in infants delivered by cesarean section, owing to higher levels of pulmonary interstitial fluid.[94] Coupled with the narrower lumen of the neonatal respiratory tree, there is a greater overall resistance in the neonatal respiratory system, offset only partially by the neonate's shorter airways. When viscous forces are altered in the neonate with lung pathology, increased pressure generation is needed to move air through the airways.

2. **Airway resistance,** the result of interactions between gas molecules and the walls of the respiratory system, plays the more significant role in impeding airflow, being responsible for as much as 80 percent of total pulmonary resistance. The smallness of the neonate's airways and nasopharynx increases airway resistance inherently. Pathology can exponentially alter resistance, contributing to ventilatory instability. Unfortunately, the use of endotracheal tubes and ventilatory circuits can also impede the flow of gas. For adequate support, delivery pressures may need to be adjusted in compensation.

In neonates and children younger than five years, the peripheral airways contribute most to airway resistance. This is secondary to the decreased diameter of the airways, especially in the periphery. The growth of the distal airways, in diameter and length, lags behind the growth of the proximal airways during the first five years of life. Therefore, a small decrement in airway caliber can lead to a very large increase in peripheral airway resistance.[100] This is seen in the early onset of clinical signs in the presence of disease in the neonate.

Resistance increases with decreasing gestational age and with specific lung diseases that are more prominent in low birth weight infants (such as RDS and bronchopulmonary dysplasia [BPD]). The respiratory muscles sense the increased resistance and increase ventilatory drive. In the infant with BPD, this may lead to an increase in pleural pressure to as much as 20–30 cmH$_2$O.

Changes in the caliber of the larynx or trachea because of edema and intubation also increase resistance. This effect may be quite pronounced because it generates resistance in the large airways, where resistance should be lowest.

Decreased airway and chest wall compliance can increase susceptibility to collapse and compression during expiration. In addition, the reduced FRC dramatically increases resistance in the preterm infant. Adequate ventilatory support can reduce resistance and stabilize the chest wall, making spontaneous respirations more effective.

Specific lung volumes and pressures are discussed later in this chapter. At this juncture, two terms bear defining: tidal volume and tidal pressure. *Tidal volume* refers to the volume of air that is displaced in the lungs during normal inspiration and expiration; *tidal pressure* refers to the change in pressure associated with tidal displacement. The relationship between tidal volume and tidal pressure can be depicted graphically in a pressure-volume loop (Figure 1-12), which also illustrates the relationship of these two parameters to lung compliance. In this graph, the slope of the dashed *compliance line* represents lung compliance. Clinically, the pressure-volume loop can be useful for monitoring the work associated with breathing, compliance, and resistance.[94] For example, the larger the volume inside the loop, the greater the work of breathing is for the neonate. If the compliance line is more horizontal than the baseline loop, this indicates that more pressure is needed to deliver a relatively low volume, and the lung is said to be less compliant. Conversely, a more vertical compliance line indicates a lung that is more compliant and more easily distended. Resistance can also be monitored; higher pressures within the same or diminished tidal

FIGURE 1-13
Lung volumes and capacities.

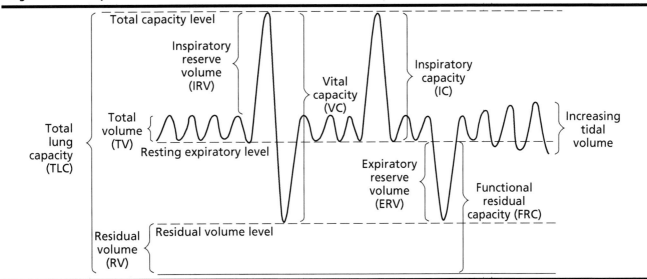

From: Fraser RG, and Paré JA. 1979. *Diagnosis of Diseases of the Chest*, 2nd ed., vol. 4. Philadelphia: Saunders. Reprinted by permission.

volume are indicative of higher resistance. Clinical uses of the pressure-volume loop are discussed in Chapter 5.

TIME CONSTANT

The time constant represents the time needed for a given lung unit to fill to 63 percent of its final capacity. It is also a measure of the product of lung resistance and compliance. Alveoli with shorter time constants fill faster than those with longer time constants. Nichols and Rogers observed that if resistance and compliance are equal in two adjacent lung units, the time constant will be the same, and there will be no redistribution of gases between the alveoli.[97] If the time constant of one unit is longer but the compliances remain equal, the two alveoli will eventually reach the same volume. The longer the time constant, however, the slower the filling will be because of increased resistance.

The time constant can also be lengthened by increasing compliance while keeping resistance the same. In this circumstance, the less compliant alveoli will fill faster than their adjacent, more compliant neighbors. This is because the less compliant alveoli have smaller volumes. Redistribution of gas will occur if inflation is interrupted prematurely because the pressure in the less compliant alveolus is greater than that in the adjacent lung unit.[97] In the normal lung, in which the alveoli are relatively stable and do not change much in size as a result of the effect of surfactant on the lung, this redistribution of gases is not a major factor.[97]

ANATOMY OF RESPIRATION

NEONATAL CHEST WALL

In adults, the intercostal muscles serve to stabilize the chest wall, preventing it from being inwardly deformed when the diaphragm contracts.[94] The newborn infant is at a biomechanical disadvantage to the adult. The neonate's chest is cylindrical; this places the ribs in a more horizontal position, shortening the course

TABLE 1-3
Infant Static Lung Volumes (mL/kg)

Total lung capacity (TLC)	63
Inspiratory capacity (IC)	33
Thoracic gas volume (Vtg)	30–36
Functional residual capacity (FRC)	30
Vital capacity (VC)	40
Closing capacity (CC)	35
Tidal volume (V_T)	6
Expiratory reserve volume (ERV)	7
Closing volume (CV)	12
Residual volume (RV)	23
ERV/FRC	0.23
RV/TLC	0.37
FRC/TLC	0.48
V_T/FRC	0.20

From: Smith CA. 1959. *The Physiology of the Newborn Infant*, 4th ed. Springfield, Illinois: Charles C. Thomas, 327. Reprinted by permission.

of the intercostal muscles and providing less mechanical advantage for stabilizing and elevating the ribs. Furthermore, the insertion of the diaphragm in infants is such that it pulls the bottom ribs inward and upward during inspiration. This has the effect of reducing overall lung capacity, which is exacerbated by the extra compliance of the chest wall. Neonates also have in the diaphragm relatively fewer slow-twitch muscle fibers, which fatigue much less easily than fast-twitch fibers.[101]

LUNG VOLUMES

The neonate has a total lung capacity of approximately 63 mL/kg of body weight. As shown in Figure 1-13, this total capacity encompasses both the portion of lung volume used in the normal course of breathing and the reserve and dead-space volumes. As clinicians, we are primarily concerned with two components of total lung capacity: tidal volume and FRC. Table 1-3 outlines the distribution of total lung capacity in the neonatal lung.

Tidal Volume

Tidal volume (the volume of gas inspired with each breath) plays a major role in alveolar minute ventilation and, ultimately, in the effectiveness of gas exchange. Tidal volume normally ranges between 6 and 8 mL/kg, but may be altered by a variety of disease states.

Functional Residual Capacity

FRC (the gas remaining in the lungs at the end of expiration) is established during the initial breaths. FRC takes the form of the alveolar reservoir at end-expiration, allowing for continuous gas exchange between respiratory efforts and stabilizing PaO_2. FRC normally comprises 30–40 percent of the total capacity of the lung and may change in volume from breath to breath.

Immediately following birth and the initial breath, FRC is low; but in healthy term infants, it increases rapidly with successive breaths. In preterm infants, FRC stays low until lung disease resolves. The goal is to keep FRC above the passive resting volume of the lung (reached after a totally relaxed expiration). The neonate's pliable chest wall, which lends itself to a low FRC, makes this difficult.

The role of FRC in the energy expenditure of the respiratory musculature is crucial. It minimizes the work of breathing while optimizing system compliance and maintaining a gas reservoir during expiration.[78]

RESPIRATORY PUMP

The movement of gas in and out of the lungs is based on the functioning of the respiratory pump, which consists of the rib cage and the respiratory muscles. The pump must move sufficient oxygen and carbon dioxide into and out of the lungs to replace the oxygen consumed and to wash out the carbon dioxide that accumulates in the alveoli. Ventilatory efforts in the neonate depend on the strength and endurance of the diaphragm; when these are insufficient, the neonate requires ventilatory assistance.[78]

Rib Cage and Chest Wall Muscles

The muscles of the rib cage consist of the external intercostal muscles (used during inspiration), the internal intercostal muscles (used during expiration), and the accessory muscles, including the sternocleidomastoid, pectoral, and scalene. The major role of these muscles is stabilization of the chest wall by tonic contraction during diaphragmatic excursion. If the muscles are unable to accomplish this goal, the chest wall is likely to collapse or distort during inspiratory efforts.

If these muscles are able to provide the needed stability, the contraction of the rib cage inspiratory muscles can contribute to thoracic volume. During sighing, the increase in tidal volume results largely from greater chest wall excursion.[102]

Diaphragm

The diaphragm insets on the lower six ribs, the sternum, and the first three lumbar vertebrae. It is innervated bilaterally by the phrenic nerves and exercises its efforts on the lung, rib cage, and abdomen. For the diaphragm to work optimally, the intercostal muscles must stabilize the rib cage, and the abdominal muscles should stabilize the abdomen.[83,103] In infants, coordination of the efforts of these muscle groups is almost nonexistent. During REM (rapid eye movement) sleep (the predominant sleep state in the neonate), the intercostal and abdominal muscles are ineffective, contributing to respiratory instability.[104]

The composition of the muscle fibers in the neonate differs from that of the adult. The neonatal diaphragm and intercostal muscles have a lower proportion of fatigue-resistant (type I) fibers (20 percent, compared with 60 percent in adults).[78,101,104] Type I fibers increase in number from 24 weeks gestation, when they compose 10 percent of total fiber content, to reach the adult proportion at eight months postnatal age.[104] Because of this developmental pattern, the neonate is particularly vulnerable to diaphragmatic muscle fatigue—especially when the work of breathing is greater than normal.[78,104] Decreasing gestational age potentiates this vulnerability.

The infant's diaphragm is attached to a chest wall that is more pliable than that of the adult. This can lead to distortion of the lower portion of the chest wall during contraction, especially if the contraction is forceful. The decreased efficiency of the contraction and reduced tidal volume can make ventilation less effective and require adjustments in respiratory pattern.[78]

CONTROL OF RESPIRATION

The goal of respiration is to meet the organism's oxygen and carbon dioxide metabolic demands by extracting oxygen from the atmosphere and removing carbon dioxide produced by the organism. The respiratory center is responsible for matching the level of ventilation to the metabolic demand. Assessment of metabolic needs and alteration of ventilation are accomplished by chemoreceptors.

The peripheral chemoreceptors (carotid and aortic bodies) sense oxygen and carbon dioxide tension; the central chemoreceptors (medullary) are sensitive to carbon dioxide and to hydrogen ion concentrations in the extracellular fluid of the brain. When the PaO_2 falls below the homeostatic set point, chemoreceptors increase the efferent neural activity to the brain's respiratory center, increasing ventilation. At birth, the neonate has a PaO_2 of 25 mmHg (sufficient for intrauterine growth), which increases to 50 mmHg during the first few breaths and then to 70 mmHg during the first hours.[76] This increase in oxygen tension exceeds the neonatal demand for oxygen, resulting in a relative "hyperoxia" at birth.

This change in oxygen tension causes the chemoreceptors to become inactive and to remain so for the first few days of life.[105] Thus, fluctuations in oxygen tension levels may not lead to a chemoreceptor response during these early days of life.[78] After this lag time, however, the chemoreceptors reset, becoming oxygen sensitive and playing a major role in the control of respiration.[106,107]

The neonate cannot maintain sustained hyperventilation efforts during hypoxia. Studies in infants and animals demonstrate that an initial hyperventilatory response is usually followed by a subsequent fall in ventilation and oxygen tensions.[77,108] The reasons for this lack of sustained response are unknown. Davis and Bureau speculate that it may be caused by feeble chemoreceptor

FIGURE 1-14
Effect of changes in pleural pressure (Ppl) in the lung.

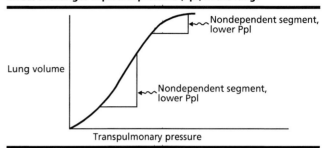

From: Nichols DG, and Rogers MC. 1987. Developmental physiology of the respiratory system. In *Textbook of Pediatric Intensive Care*, vol. 1, Rogers MC, ed. Philadelphia: Lippincott Williams & Wilkins, 88. Reprinted by permission.

output, the central inhibitory effect of hypoxia on ventilation, or changes in pulmonary mechanics.[78]

The neonate's response to carbon dioxide, though more mature than his response to hypoxia, is also limited during the early neonatal period. Neonates can increase ventilation by only three to four times their baseline ventilation, compared with the 10- to 20-fold increase adults can achieve.[78,109] The neonate's threshold of carbon dioxide tolerance is also higher initially, progressively declining over the first month of life.[78] This, too, may result from the increased $PaCO_2$ levels (45–50 mmHg) found in the fetal state and the need to reset chemoreceptors.

Modification of ventilatory patterns is dependent on inspiratory muscle strength, rib cage rigidity, airway resistance, and lung compliance. The status of these factors and the performance of the respiratory pump are controlled through specific reflex arcs.[78] Chemoreceptors provide information about the metabolic needs of the infant, mechanoreceptors provide information about the status of the respiratory pump, and the respiratory center integrates this information and establishes the ventilatory pattern that most efficiently meets the infant's needs.

Hypoxia is also known to alter ventilatory patterns. Premature infants manifest a biphasic response to a low inspired oxygen concentration: For the first minute of exposure, they show a rapid increase in ventilatory rate, followed by a decline in rate to baseline or below by three minutes.[110] It is believed that overactive peripheral chemoreceptors may be involved in this pattern and may contribute to apnea of prematurity (AOP).[87,111] Typically, AOP resolves with maturation of the infant, likely due to increased myelination of the brainstem.[112]

FIGURE 1-15
Gravity dependence of perfusion.

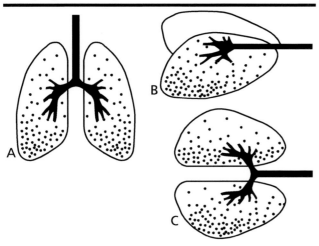

Blood is distributed to the most gravity-dependent areas of the lung.
A = upright; B = supine; C = side-lying

Adapted from: Malley WJ. 2005. *Clinical Blood Gases: Assessment and Intervention,* 2nd ed. Philadelphia: Saunders, 139. Reprinted by permission.

During a stable state (such as quiet sleep), each respiratory cycle is uniform in amplitude, duration, and waveform. Behavioral influences as well as sleep state (REM sleep) alter the regularity of breathing. The information received via chemoreceptors determines the inspiratory time, the expiratory time, the lung volume at which the breath should occur (FRC), the rate of inspiration, and the braking of the expiration.[113] The recruitment and adjustment of the various respiratory muscle groups result in the predetermined lung volume being achieved.[78]

DISTRIBUTION OF VENTILATION

DEAD-SPACE VENTILATION

A variable portion of each breath is not involved in gas exchange and is therefore wasted. That portion is considered dead-space ventilation. There are two types of dead space: (1) *anatomic dead space,* that volume of gas within the conducting airways that cannot engage in gas exchange, and (2) *alveolar dead space,* the collective volume of inspired gas that reaches an alveolus but does not participate in gas exchange because of inadequate perfusion of that alveolus.

The total (anatomic plus alveolar) dead space is termed *physiologic dead space.* Physiologic dead space is usually expressed as a fraction of the tidal volume, approximately 0.3 in infants and adults.[114] Infants

experiencing respiratory failure have elevated ratios of dead space to tidal volume. This elevated ratio results in hypoxia and hypercarbia unless it is counteracted by an increase in the amount of air expired per minute.[97]

PLEURAL PRESSURE

The differences in pleural pressure within the lung play a significant role in determining the distribution of gases. During spontaneous breathing, a greater proportion of gas is distributed to the dependent regions of the lung.[115] It is assumed that the increased negative intrapleural pressure in the bases of the lungs is the reason for this distribution pattern. Nichols and Rogers note that the smaller alveoli in the dependent lung regions lie on the steeper slope of the transpulmonary pressure–to–lung volume curve (Figure 1-14), resulting in a greater portion of tidal volume being directed to the dependent alveoli during normal breathing.[97] A greater portion of the pulmonary perfusion goes to the dependent regions as well, thereby matching ventilation and perfusion more closely (Figure 1-15). In addition, this distribution pattern is related to the initial preferential distribution of gases on inspiration to nongravity-dependent areas of the lung until just after the FRC is reached. What this means is that, at normal FRC, the apical alveoli are larger than the basal alveoli and the largest volume of resting gas is in the upper lung zones. As gas continues to fill the nondependent lung regions, the alveoli in the upper regions become so full that further inflation is more difficult than expanding the alveoli in the lower lung regions. At this point, which is reached when the inspired gas volume is slightly above the normal FRC, additional gas preferentially ventilates the lung bases. Consequently, most of the gas inhaled during normal breathing actually ventilates the lung bases.

Pleural pressure increases from the apex to the base of the lung, so alveoli become smaller at the base. Smaller alveoli are on the steep portion of the pressure-volume (compliance) curve; thus, a given change in transpulmonary pressure produces a greater increase in volume in the smaller alveoli.

CLOSING CAPACITY

During quiet breathing in the neonate (especially the preterm neonate), lung volumes can be reduced below FRC, with dependent regions of the lung being closed to the main bronchi (closing capacity). When the closing capacity exceeds the FRC, the ventilation-perfusion ratio drops, and hypoxia and hypercarbia can be seen. If total atelectasis ("whiteout" on chest x-ray) exists, then closing capacity exceeds not only FRC but also tidal volume, and the alveoli in the affected portions of the lung are closed during expiration and inspiration.

The use of end-expiratory pressure in the form of positive end-expiratory pressure or continuous distending pressure is designed to raise FRC above closing capacity.[97] This approach is employed in the neonatal population when chest wall compliance leads to marked distortion and altered lung volumes, as well as with disease states associated with alveolar collapse (such as RDS).

The greater closing capacity seen in children under 6 years of age and adults over 40 is probably a result of decreased elastic recoil in the lung.[99,116] Elastic recoil is the property that allows the lung to retract away from the chest wall, creating a subatmospheric pressure in the intrapleural space. The decrease in elastic recoil seen in younger children and older adults leads to an increase in subatmospheric pressure in the intrapleural spaces and airway closure in dependent regions.[97]

Perfusion

Alveolar ventilation is dependent on the airways and the pulmonary vasculature. Pulmonary vascular muscle thickness is a function of gestational age: The preterm infant has smooth muscle that is less well developed. This incomplete development results in a drop in pulmonary vascular resistance much sooner after delivery than in term infants, predisposing the preterm infant to a faster onset of congestive heart failure and left-to-right shunting.[97] This relatively rapid reduction in pulmonary vascular resistance, combined with the potential for fluid overload, can result in opening of extrapulmonary shunts, leading to hypoxia and further respiratory deterioration.

Vascular Pressures and Resistance

There are three categories of intravascular pressure associated with the pulmonary circulation: pulmonary artery pressure, transmural pressure, and perfusion pressure. The interactions and relationships among these pressures affect the flow of blood in the lung and are implicated in the distribution of blood flow.

Pulmonary Artery Pressure

Pulmonary artery pressure is a measure of the systolic, diastolic, and mean arterial pressures in the pulmonary artery in reference to atmospheric pressure at the level of the heart. After birth, pulmonary artery pressure falls as the lungs inflate; adult pressures are not achieved until several months have passed.[117] Normal

FIGURE 1-16
Pulmonary perfusion zones.

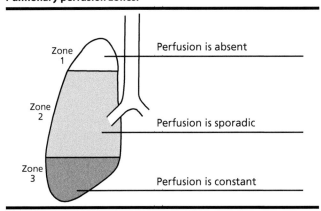

From: Malley WJ. 2005. *Clinical Blood Gases: Assessment and Intervention,* 2nd ed. Philadelphia: Saunders, 140. Reprinted by permission.

systolic, diastolic, and mean pressures in the adult are 22, 8, and 15 mmHg, respectively. Normal values for the neonate have not been established.[89,97]

Transmural Pressure

Transmural pressure is the difference between pressures inside and outside the lung. How transmural pressure is measured depends on the level of the measurement. At upper levels, transmural pressure is the gradient between pulmonary artery pressure and pleural pressure; at the pulmonary capillaries, it is the difference between pleural pressure and alveolar pressure.[118]

Capillary transmural pressure provides the hydrostatic pressure that tends to force fluid out of the capillaries and into the pulmonary interstitium. This is counterbalanced by oncotic pressure forces. The greater the capillary transmural pressure, the more distended the lung and the greater the flow.

Perfusion Pressure

Perfusion pressure is the pressure gradient between two points in the circulation (downward flow). This cascade is needed for blood to flow appropriately. In the pulmonary circulation, perfusion pressure is measured as the difference between pulmonary artery pressure and left atrial pressure.

Perfusion pressure divided by pulmonary blood flow provides a calculated value for pulmonary vascular resistance. An increase in flow, as occurs with activity, produces a drop in pulmonary vascular resistance secondary to the recruitment of additional pulmonary capillaries.[119,120]

FIGURE 1-17
Ventilation-perfusion ratios.

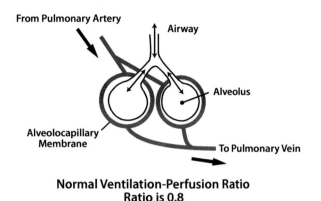

Normal Ventilation-Perfusion Ratio
Ratio is 0.8

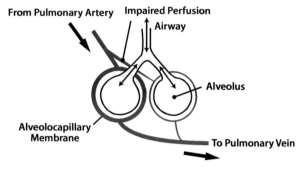

High Ventilation-Perfusion Ratio
Common cause is pulmonary embolus

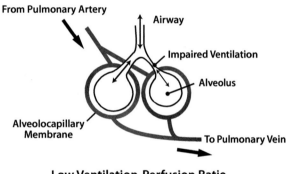

Low Ventilation-Perfusion Ratio
Result is hypoxemia with ↓ PaO_2

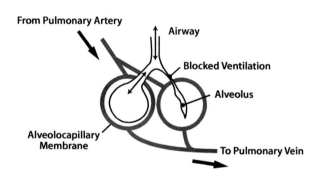

SHUNT (very low) Ventilation-Perfusion Ratio
Result is hypoxemia with ↓ PaO_2 and $PaCO_2$

Courtesy of William Diehl-Jones.

Pulmonary Blood Flow

In the adult, most pulmonary blood flow is distributed to the dependent regions of the lungs because of gravitational forces. Figure 1-16 illustrates the zonal distribution of perfusion. In zone 1 (apex of the lung), the alveolar pressure is greater than the pulmonary arterial and venous pressures. As a result, the pulmonary vessels collapse, and there is a concomitant loss of gas exchange and wasted ventilation.[121]

In zone 2 (middle of the lung), pulmonary artery pressure exceeds alveolar pressure, and blood flow resumes. The perfusion pressure increases as blood flows downward, resulting in a linear increase in blood flow. Slowing of blood flow occurs when the pulmonary venous and alveolar pressures are equal.[121]

In zone 3 (base of the lung), pulmonary venous and arterial pressures increase, exceeding alveolar pressure. In the more dependent regions of this zone, the transmural pressure increases (resulting in dilation of the vessels), and blood flow increases.[121]

Postural differences between the upright adult and the supine-lying infant probably explain pulmonary blood distribution in the infant, but this has not been explicated. The general principles likely still apply, however. Wasted ventilation in the apexes resulting from lack of perfusion is presumably much less likely in the supine position, helping to balance some of the limitations of the neonatal lung.

Numerous factors can influence the distribution of pulmonary blood flow in the lung. One of the most significant for the neonate is hypoxia. Alveolar hypoxia causes vasoconstriction. If generalized, hypoxia may increase intravascular pulmonary artery pressure, which is greater in infants than in adults.[99,122]

Ventilation-Perfusion Matching

Efficient gas exchange in the lungs requires matching pulmonary ventilation ($\dot{V}_A$) and perfusion ($\dot{Q}_C$). Ventilation-perfusion mismatching is the most common reason for hypoxia in the newborn and a frequent result of the liabilities of the neonatal respiratory system. The interaction between ventilation and perfusion is expressed as a ratio ($\dot{V}_A/\dot{Q}_C$) that reflects the relationship between alveolar ventilation and capillary perfusion for the lung as a whole.

Air space ventilation should be adequate to remove the carbon dioxide delivered there from the blood, and air space perfusion should be no greater than that which allows oxygenation and complete saturation of the blood in its brief passage through the alveolar capillaries. Ideal efficiency would occur if ventilation were perfectly matched to perfusion, yielding an ideal ratio of 1:1; in practice, this is approximately 0.8. Normal and abnormal ventilation-perfusion ratios are demonstrated in Figure 1-17.

In the healthy adult, capillary blood spends 0.75 seconds in the alveolus, and oxygen–carbon dioxide exchange occurs across the 0.5-micron alveolar-capillary membrane. As the blood leaves the alveolus, the blood gas tensions are identical to those of the alveolar gas. The gas tensions achieved at equilibrium depend on the following factors:[123–126]

1. Ventilation rate
2. Membrane thickness
3. Membrane area
4. Capillary blood flow
5. Venous gas tensions
6. Inspired gas tensions

The ability to achieve equilibrium rapidly depends on (1) the area of exchange being large enough to allow the blood to be spread thinly over the vessel wall and (2) the blood and gas being actively mixed together.[123]

Matching ventilation to perfusion depends largely on gravity. Both ventilation and perfusion increase with further distance down the lung, with perfusion increasing more than ventilation. The right ventricular pressure is inadequate to fully perfuse lung apexes. Lung weight leads to a relatively greater negative intrapleural pressure at the apex than at the base. This means, according to Krauss, that "apical alveoli are better expanded and receive a smaller portion of each tidal volume than those at the bases (p. 59)."[124] Along with this, there is reduced perfusion in the apexes, creating a high ratio of ventilation to perfusion.[126,127]

A ventilation-perfusion ratio of zero indicates a shunt. In this situation, no ventilation takes place during the passage of blood through the lungs. Blood from the pulmonary capillaries arrives in the left atrium with the same gas tensions it had when it entered the lungs. An example of an intrapulmonary shunt would be the perfusion of an atelectatic area of the lung.

High $\dot{V}_A/\dot{Q}_C$ ratios are the result of increased dead space. They occur if the blood is spread in an extremely thin film over a very large surface area or if the blood is vigorously mixed with large volumes of air. In these circumstances, equilibrium occurs, but a large amount of ventilation is required.[123] There is wasted ventilation in anatomic conducting airways and/or in poorly perfused alveoli (alveolar dead space). Thus, a large amount of ventilation is wasted on a relatively small amount of blood without significantly changing the oxygen content. This inefficient gas exchange eventually results in carbon dioxide retention.

Alveolar underventilation results in low $\dot{V}_A/\dot{Q}_C$ ratios. In these situations, ventilation is low in relation to perfusion, but not entirely absent. Low $\dot{V}_A/\dot{Q}_C$ ratios are also found in those with diseases (such as asthma or cystic fibrosis) in which airway obstruction reduces ventilation to alveolar units. The blood perfusing the underventilated alveoli is not completely oxygenated, and a smaller amount of carbon dioxide is removed. These partial venoarterial shunts contribute this blood to the arterial stream, creating a venous admixture, which is reflected in an elevated $PaCO_2$ and decreased partial pressure of oxygen in arterial blood (PaO_2).

Abnormalities of $\dot{V}_A/\dot{Q}_C$ may be secondary to (1) too much or too little ventilation to an area with normal blood flow, (2) too much or too little blood flow with normal ventilation, or (3) some combination of the two (see Figure 1-17). Whatever occurs, the lung's regulatory mechanisms work to achieve and maintain the ideal. In areas where $\dot{V}_A/\dot{Q}_C$ is high and carbon dioxide levels are low, local airway constriction reduces the amount of ventilation going to the area. When the opposite occurs, the airways dilate to increase ventilation to the area and improve carbon dioxide exchange. Where oxygenation is also affected and low alveolar oxygen concentrations are found, the lung reduces blood flow to the region. These mechanisms are finite, however.

In the newborn, most of the ventilated areas are well perfused, and there is little dead space. But significant amounts of perfusion are wasted on unexpanded air spaces (intrapulmonary shunts). The newborn's lower PaO_2 demonstrates the widened alveolar-to-arterial-oxygen-tension gradient, reflecting the increased venous admixture. Although perfusion of unexpanded air spaces may play a significant role in venous admixture, the continued right-to-left shunting through transitional circulatory circuits contributes to the situation. Because of developmental immaturity, the premature infant is at even greater risk of shunting and venous admixture than is the term newborn.[128]

Shunting and wasted ventilation are normal features of the newborn lung. Wasted ventilation results from the transition from fluid-filled to air-filled lungs, where alveoli are underventilated but normally perfused. These effects begin to dissipate after one or two hours of air breathing. During the first few days of life, the neonatal lung has a greater shunt component and a larger proportion of low $\dot{V}_A/\dot{Q}_C$ areas than the adult lung, although tidal volume, alveolar volume, and dead-space volume per breath (when expressed in mL/kg) are similar.

SUMMARY

The respiratory system undergoes rapid structural and functional changes from the moment when its precursors are recognizable (approximately five weeks postconception) until it must take over the task of gas exchange at birth. Even then, it is not fully formed, continuing to develop after birth under the influence of both genetics and the environment. Several hormonal axes are involved in modulating respiratory structures and function. In particular, much attention has been focused on the biochemistry and regulation of pulmonary surfactant, which for the neonate are critical factors in preventing atelectasis and modifying alveolar structure.

Transition from the intrauterine to the extrauterine environment is an event that takes several days to achieve, with initial responses being aligned with the fetal state. Knowledge of the differences between the two states and the progression toward extrauterine stability can guide clinical assessment and therapeutic interventions.

The respiratory muscles have exercised and trained to take over the function of the respiratory pump, although fatigue may develop quickly. Intercostal muscles can stabilize the chest wall so that effective ventilation can be achieved. Difficulties arise when disease or immaturity is encountered. These infants possess little reserve to increase ventilatory efforts, as well as only limited ability to sustain increased respiratory activity. The capacity to recruit accessory muscles, the use of laryngeal braking (grunting), and the mobilization of new alveoli

help improve gas exchange and increase the pulmonary surface area.[78]

For infants greater than 28 weeks gestational age, these mechanisms may be employable, although the degree to which they can be used and their efficiency may vary from infant to infant. Further research into the physiology and molecular biology of neonatal respiration will undoubtedly provide more clinical tools for supporting respiration in the neonate.

REFERENCES

1. Hsia CC. 2004. Signals and mechanisms of compensatory lung growth. *Journal of Applied Physiology* 97(5): 1992–1998.
2. Moore KL, and Persaud TVN. 2003. *The Developing Human: Clinically Oriented Embryology*, 7th ed. Philadelphia: Saunders, 608.
3. Bucher U, and Reid L. 1961. Development of the intrasegmental bronchial tree: The pattern of branching and development of cartilage at various stages of intra-uterine life. *Thorax* 16(3): 207–218.
4. Emery JL. 1970. The postnatal development of the human lung and its implications for lung pathology. *Respiration* 27(supplement): S41–S50.
5. Reid LM. 1984. Structural development of the lung and pulmonary circulation. In *Respiratory Distress Syndrome*, Ravio K, et al., eds. London: Academic Press, 1–18.
6. Inselman LS, and Mellins RB. 1981. Growth and development of the lung. *Journal of Pediatrics* 98(1): 1–15.
7. Guttentag S, and Ballard PL. 2005. Lung development: Embryology, growth, maturation, and developmental biology. In *Avery's Diseases of the Newborn*, 8th ed., Taeusch HW, Ballard RA, and Gleason CA, eds. Philadelphia: Saunders, 601–615.
8. Roth-Kleiner M, and Post M. 2003. Genetic control of lung development. *Biology of the Neonate* 84(1): 83–88.
9. Ang SL, and Rossant J. 1994. HNF-3 beta is essential for node and notochord formation in mouse development. *Cell* 78(4): 561–574.
10. Stahlman MT, Gray ME, and Whitsett JA. 1998. Temporal-spatial distribution of hepatocyte nuclear factor-3beta in developing human lung and other foregut derivatives. *Journal of Histochemistry and Cytochemistry* 46(8): 955–962.
11. Ioannides AS, et al. 2002. Dorsoventral patterning in oesophageal atresia with tracheo-oesophageal fistula: Evidence from a new mouse model. *Journal of Pediatric Surgery* 37(2): 185–191.
12. Litingtung Y, et al. 1998. Sonic hedgehog is essential to foregut development. *Nature Genetics* 20(1): 58–61.
13. Keijzer R, et al. 2001 The transcription factor GATA6 is essential for branching morphogenesis and epithelial cell differentiation during fetal pulmonary development. *Development* 128(4): 503–511.
14. Moens CB, et al. 1992. A targeted mutation reveals a role for N-myc in branching morphogenesis in the embryonic mouse lung. *Genes and Development* 6(5): 691–704.
15. Moessinger AC, et al. 1990. Role of lung fluid volume in growth and maturation of the fetal sheep lung. *Journal of Clinical Investigation* 86(4): 1270–1277.
16. Braems G. 2003. Fetal hypoxemia on a molecular level: Adaptive changes in the hypothalamic-pituitary-adrenal (HPA) axis and the lungs. *European Journal of Obstetrics, Gynecology, and Reproductive Biology* 110(supplement 1): S63–S69.
17. Acarregui MJ, Snyder JM, and Mendelson CR. 1993. Oxygen modulates the differentiation of human fetal lung in vitro and its responsiveness to cAMP. *American Journal of Physiology* 264(5 part 1): L465–L474.
18. American Thoracic Society ad hoc Statement Committee. 2004. Mechanisms and limits of induced postnatal lung growth. *American Journal of Respiratory and Critical Care Medicine* 170(3): 319–343.
19. Haworth SG, McKenzie SA, and Fitzpatrick ML. 1981. Alveolar development after ligation of left pulmonary artery in newborn pig: Clinical relevance to unilateral pulmonary artery. *Thorax* 36(12): 938–943.
20. Preston IR. 2007. Clinical perspective of hypoxia-mediated pulmonary hypertension. *Antioxidants & Redox Signaling* 9(6): 711–721.
21. Townsley MI, et al. 1994. Altered pulmonary microvascular reactivity to norepinephrine in canine pacing-induced heart failure. *Circulation Research* 75(2): 347–356.

22. Hislop A. 2005. Developmental biology of the pulmonary circulation. *Paediatric Respiratory Reviews* 6(1): 35–43.

23. Harned HS. 1978. Respiration and the respiratory system. In *Perinatal Physiology*, Stave U, ed. New York: Plenum, 53–101.

24. Hislop A, and Reid LM. 1977. Formation of the pulmonary vasculature. In *Development of the Lung*, Hodson WA, ed. New York: Marcel Dekker, 37–86.

25. Mendelson CR, et al. 1981. Multihormonal regulation of surfactant synthesis by human fetal lung *in vitro*. *Journal of Clinical Endocrinology and Metabolism* 53(2): 307–317.

26. Thurlbeck WM. 1975. Postnatal growth and development of the lung. *American Review of Respiratory Disease* 111(6): 803–844.

27. Hallman M. 1984. Development of pulmonary surfactant. In *Respiratory Distress Syndrome*, Ravio K, et al., eds. London: Academic Press, 33–50.

28. Meyrick B, and Reid LM. 1977. Ultrastructure of alveolar lining and its development. In *Development of the Lung*, Hodson WA, ed. New York: Marcel Dekker, 135–214.

29. Bleasdale JE, and Johnston JM. 1985. Developmental biochemistry of lung surfactant. In *Pulmonary Development: Transition from Intrauterine to Extrauterine Life*, Nelson GH, ed. New York: Marcel Dekker, 47–73.

30. Milner AD, Saunders RA, and Hopkin IE. 1978. Effects of delivery by caesarean section on lung mechanics and lung volume in the human neonate. *Archives of Disease in Childhood* 53(7): 545–548.

31. Ikegami M, et al. 2005. Surfactant protein D influences surfactant ultrastructure and uptake by alveolar type II cells. *American Journal of Physiology. Lung Cellular and Molecular Physiology* 288(3): L552–L561.

32. Farrell PM, and Ulane RE. 1981. The regulation of lung phospholipid metabolism. In *Physiological and Biochemical Basis for Perinatal Medicine*, Monset-Couchard M, and Minkowski A, eds. New York: S. Karger, 11–31.

33. Wessels NK. 1977. *Tissue Interactions and Development*. Menlo Park, California: Benjamin Cummings.

34. Van Golde LM. 1976. Metabolism of phospholipids in the lung. *American Review of Respiratory Disease* 114(5): 977–1000.

35. Liggins GC. 1969. Premature delivery of fetal lambs infused with glucocorticoids. *Journal of Endocrinology* 45(4): 515–523.

36. Ballard PL. 1981. Hormonal regulation of the surfactant system. In *Physiological and Biochemical Basis for Perinatal Medicine*, Monset-Couchard M, and Minkowski A, eds. New York: S. Karger, 42–53.

37. Hitchcock KR. 1979. Hormones and the lung. Part I: Thyroid hormones and glucocorticoids in lung development. *Anatomical Record* 194(1): 15–39.

38. Pope TS, and Rooney SA. 1987. Effects of glucocorticoid and thyroid hormones on regulatory enzymes of fatty acid synthesis and glycogen metabolism in developing fetal rat lung. *Biochimica et Biophysica Acta* 918(2): 141–148.

39. Fiascone J, et al. 1986. Differential effect of betamethasone on alveolar surfactant and lung tissue of fetal rabbits. *Pediatric Research* 20: 428A.

40. Smith BT. 1979. Lung maturation in the fetal rat: Acceleration by injection of fibroblast-pneumocyte factor. *Science* 204(4397): 1094–1095.

41. Ramin SM, et al. 2004. The effects of dexamethasone and betamethasone on surfactant protein-B messenger RNA expression in human type II pneumocytes and human lung adenocarcinoma cells. *American Journal of Obstetrics and Gynecology* 190(4): 952–959.

42. Vidaeff AC, et al. 2004. In vitro quantification of dexamethasone-induced surfactant protein B expression in human lung cells. *Journal of Maternal-Fetal & Neonatal Medicine* 15(3): 155–159.

43. Beneke S, and Rooney SA. 2001. Glucocorticoids regulate expression of the fatty acid synthase gene in fetal rat type II cells. *Biochimica et Biophysica Acta* 1534(1): 56–63.

44. Yoshida I, Ban N, and Inagaki N. 2004. Expression of ABCA3, a causative gene for fatal surfactant deficiency, is up-regulated by glucocorticoids in lung alveolar type II cells. *Biochemical and Biophysical Research Communications* 323(2): 547–555.

45. Arai H, et al. 2005. Dexamethasone-induced prenatal alveolar wall thinning is associated with a decrease in EIIIA+ fibronectin isoform in the fetal rat lung. *Biology of the Neonate* 87(2): 113–120.

46. Landmann E, et al. 2004. Phospholipid profile in tracheal aspirates of very preterm neonates: Effect of prenatal betamethasone administration. European *Journal of Obstetrics, Gynecology, and Reproductive Biology* 115(1): 15–16.

47. Purdy IB, and Wiley DJ. 2004. Perinatal corticosteroids: A review of research. Part I: Antenatal administration. *Neonatal Network* 23(2): 15–30.

48. Bizzarro MJ, and Gross I. 2004. Effects of hormones on fetal lung development. *Obstetrics and Gynecology Clinics of North America* 31(4): 949–961, xii.

49. Ballard PL, et al. 1980. Transplacental stimulation of lung development in the fetal rabbit by 3,5-dimethyl-3'-isopropyl-L-thyronine. *Journal of Clinical Investigation* 65(6): 1407–1417.

50. Gonzales LW, et al. 1986. Glucocorticoids and thyroid hormones stimulate biochemical and morphological differentiation of human fetal lung in organ culture. *Journal of Clinical Endocrinology and Metabolism* 62(4): 678–691.

51. Gross I, and Wilson CM. 1982. Fetal lung in organ culture. Part IV: Supra-additive hormone interactions. *Journal of Applied Physiology* 52(6): 1420–1425.

52. Kresch MJ, and Gross I. 1987. The biochemistry of fetal lung development. *Clinics in Perinatology* 14(3): 481–507.

53. Ballard PL, et al. 1986. Human pulmonary surfactant apoprotein: Effects of development, culture and hormones on the protein and its mRNA. *Pediatric Research* 20: 422A.

54. Pope TS, and Rooney SA. 1987. Opposing effects of glucocorticoid and thyroid hormones on the fatty acid synthetase activity in cultured fetal rat lung. *Federation Proceedings* 46: 2005A.

55. Smith BT. 1979. Biochemistry and metabolism of pulmonary surface-active material. In *The Surfactant System and the Neonatal Lung*, Mead Johnson Symposium on Perinatal and Developmental Medicine, no. 14. Evansville, Indiana: Mead Johnson, 12–16.

56. Ballard PL, Hovey ML, and Gonzales LK. 1984. Thyroid hormone stimulation of phosphatidylcholine synthesis in cultured fetal rabbit lung. *Journal of Clinical Investigation* 74(3): 898–905.

57. Rooney SA, et al. 1979. Thyrotropin-releasing hormone increases the amount of surfactant in lung lavage from fetal rabbits. *Pediatric Research* 13(5 part 1): 623–625.

58. Crowther CA, Alfirevic Z, and Haslam RR. 2004. Thyrotropin-releasing hormone added to corticosteroids for women at risk of preterm birth for preventing neonatal respiratory disease. *Cochrane Database of Systematic Reviews* (2): CD000019.

59. Dobbs LG, and Mason RJ. 1979. Pulmonary alveolar type II cells isolated from rats. Release of phosphatidylcholine in response to beta-adrenergic stimulation. *Journal of Clinical Investigation* 63(3): 378–387.

60. Corbet AJ, et al. 1978. Effect of aminophylline and dexamethasone on secretion of pulmonary surfactant in fetal rabbits. *Pediatric Research* 12(7): 797–799.

61. Smith BT, et al. 1975. Insulin antagonism of cortisol action on lecithin synthesis by cultured fetal lung cells. *Journal of Pediatrics* 87(6 part 1): 953–955.

62. Gross I, et al. 1980. The influence of hormones on the biochemical development of fetal rat lung in organ culture. Part II: Insulin. *Pediatric Research* 14(6): 834–838.

63. Sosenko IR, Hartig-Beecken I, and Frantz ID. 1980. Cortisol reversal of functional delay of lung maturation in fetuses of diabetic rabbits. *Journal of Applied Physiology* 49(6): 971–974.

64. Miakotina OL, Dekowski SA, and Snyder JM. 1998. Insulin inhibits surfactant protein A and B gene expression in the H441 cell line. *Biochimica et Biophysica Acta* 1442(1): 60–70.

65. Abdel-Ratif ME, and Osborn DA. 2011. Pharyngeal instillation of surfactant before the first breath for prevention of morbidity and mortality in preterm infants at risk of respiratory distress syndrome. *Cochrane Database of Systematic Reviews* (3): CD008311.

66. Norlin A, and Folkesson HG. 2001. Alveolar fluid clearance in late-gestational guinea pigs after labor induction: Mechanisms and regulation. *American Journal of Physiology. Lung Cellular and Molecular Physiology* 280(4): L606–L616.

67. Kemp PJ, and Kim KJ. 2004. Spectrum of ion channels in alveolar epithelial cells: Implications for alveolar fluid balance. *American Journal of Physiology. Lung Cellular and Molecular Physiology* 287(3): L460–L464.

68. Milner AD, and Vyas H. 1982. Lung expansion at birth. *Journal of Pediatrics* 101(6): 879–886.

69. Mescher EJ, et al. 1975. Ontogeny of tracheal fluid, pulmonary surfactant, and plasma corticoids in the fetal lamb. *Journal of Applied Physiology* 39(6): 1017–1021.

70. Burgess WR, and Chernick V. 1982. *Respiratory Therapy in Newborn Infants and Children*. New York: Thieme-Stratton.

71. Alcorn D, et al. 1977. Morphological effects of chronic tracheal ligation and drainage in the fetal lamb lung. *Journal of Anatomy* 123(3): 649–660.

72. Perlman M, Williams J, and Hirsch M. 1976. Neonatal pulmonary hypoplasia after prolonged leakage of amniotic fluid. *Archives of Disease in Childhood* 51(5): 349–353.

73. Bryan AC, and Bryan MH. 1978. Control of respiration in the newborn. *Clinics in Perinatology* 5(2): 269–281.

74. Zapletal A, Paul T, and Samanek M. 1976. Pulmonary elasticity in children and adolescents. *Journal of Applied Physiology* 40(6): 953–961.

75. Liggins GC, and Kitterman JA. 1981. Development of the fetal lung. In *The Fetus and Independent Life*, Ciba Foundation Symposium. London: Pitman, 308–330.

76. Strang LB. 1989. Solute and water transport across the pulmonary epithelium: A new chapter in lung physiology inaugurated by Alfred Jost. *Biology of the Neonate* 55(6): 355–365.

77. Marchal F. 1987. Neonatal apnea. In *Neonatal Medicine*, Stern L, and Vert P, eds. New York: Masson, 409–427.

78. Davis GM, and Bureau MA. 1987. Pulmonary and chest wall mechanics in the control of respiration in the newborn. *Clinics in Perinatology* 14(3): 551–579.

79. Liu M, et al. 1992. Stimulation of fetal rat lung cell proliferation in vitro by mechanical stretch. *American Journal of Physiology. Lung Cellular and Molecular Physiology* 263(3 part 1): L376–L383.

80. Hanson TN, and Corbet A. 2005. Anomalies of the airways, mediastinum, and lung parenchyma. In *Avery's Diseases of the Newborn*, 8th ed., Taeusch HW, Ballard RA, and Gleason CA, eds. Philadelphia: Saunders, 737–757.

81. Hanson TN, Corbet A, and Ballard RA. 2005. Disorders of the chest wall, pleural cavity, and diaphragm. In *Avery's Diseases of the Newborn*, 8th ed., Taeusch HW, Ballard RA, and Gleason CA, eds. Philadelphia: Saunders, 759–777.

82. Clyman RI. 2005. Patent ductus arteriosus in the premature infant. In *Avery's Diseases of the Newborn*, 8th ed., Taeusch HW, Ballard RA, and Gleason CA, eds. Philadelphia: Saunders, 816–826.

83. Boddy K, Dawes GS, and Robinson J. 1975. Intrauterine fetal breathing movements. In *Modern Perinatal Medicine*, Gluck L, ed. Chicago: Year Book Medical, 381–389.

84. Patrick JE, et al. 1978. Human fetal breathing movements and gross fetal body movements at weeks 34 to 35 of gestation. *American Journal of Obstetrics and Gynecology* 130(6): 693–699.

85. Patrick J. 1977. Measurement of human fetal breathing movements. In *Mead Johnson Symposium on Perinatal and Developmental Medicine*, no. 12. Evansville, Indiana: Mead Johnson.

86. Kitterman JA, and Liggins GC. 1980. Fetal breathing movements and inhibitors of prostaglandin synthesis. *Seminars in Perinatology* 4(2): 97–100.

87. Al-Matary A, et al. 2004. Increased peripheral chemoreceptor activity may be critical in destabilizing breathing in neonates. *Seminars in Perinatology* 28(4): 264–272.

88. Strang LB. 1977. Pulmonary circulation at birth. In *Neonatal Respiration, Physiological and Clinical Studies*. Oxford: Blackwell Scientific, 111–137.

89. Nelson NM. 1976. Respiration and circulation after birth. In *Physiology of the Newborn Infant*, 4th ed., Smith CA, and Nelson NM, eds. Springfield, Illinois: Charles C. Thomas, 117–262.

90. Jaykka S. 1954. A new theory concerning the mechanism of the initiation of respiration in the newborn: A preliminary report. *Acta Paediatrica* 43(5): 399–410.

91. Gruenwald P. 1963. Normal and abnormal expansion of the lungs of newborn infants obtained at autopsy. Part III: Opening pressure, maximal volume, and stability of expansion. *Laboratory Investigation* 12: 563–576.

92. Karlberg P, et al. 1962. Respiratory studies in newborn infants. Part II: Pulmonary ventilation and mechanics of breathing in the first minutes of life, including the onset of respiration. *Acta Paediatrica Scandinavica* 51(2): 121–136.

93. Klaus M, et al. 1962. Alveolar epithelial cell mitochondria as a source of the surface-active lung lining. *Science* 137: 750–751.

94. Wood B. 2003. Physiologic principles. In *Assisted Ventilation of the Neonate*, 4th ed., Goldsmith JP, and Karotkin EH, eds. Philadelphia: Saunders, 15–40.

95. Agostoni E. 1959. Volume-pressure relationships of the thorax and lung in the newborn. *Journal of Applied Physiology* 14: 909–913.

96. Avery ME, and Cook CD. 1961. Volume-pressure relationships of lungs and thorax in fetal, newborn, and adult goats. *Journal of Applied Physiology* 16: 1034–1038.

97. Nichols DG, and Rogers MC. 1987. Developmental physiology of the respiratory system. In *Textbook of Pediatric Intensive Care*, vol. 1, Rogers MC, ed. Philadelphia: Lippincott Williams & Wilkins, 83–111.

98. Henry JN. 1968. The effect of shock on pulmonary alveolar surfactant. Its role in refractory respiratory insufficiency of the critically ill or severely injured patient. *Journal of Trauma* 8(5): 756–773.

99. Said SI, et al. 1965. Pulmonary surface activity in induced pulmonary edema. *Journal of Clinical Investigation* 44: 458–464.

100. Hogg JC, et al. 1970. Age as a factor in the distribution of lower-airway conductance and in the pathologic anatomy of obstructive lung disease. *New England Journal of Medicine* 282(23): 1283–1287.

101. Keens TG, and Ianuzzo CD. 1979. Development of fatigue-resistant muscle fibers in human ventilatory muscles. *American Review of Respiratory Disease* 119(2 part 2): 139–141.

102. Thach BT, and Taeusch HW. 1976. Sighing in newborn human infants: Role of inflation-augmenting reflex. *Journal of Applied Physiology* 41(4): 502–507.

103. Mantell CD. 1976. Breathing movements in the human fetus. *American Journal of Obstetrics and Gynecology* 125(4): 550–553.

104. Escobedo MB. 1982. Fetal and neonatal cardiopulmonary physiology. In *Practical Neonatal Respiratory Care*, Schreiner RL, and Kisling JA, eds. New York: Raven Press, 1–18.

105. Blanco CE, Hanson MA, and McCooke HB. 1985. Studies *in utero* of the mechanisms of chemoreceptor resetting. In *The Physiologic Development of the Fetus and the Newborn*, Jones CT, and Nathaniels PW, eds. London: Academic Press, 639–642.

106. Bureau MA, and Begin R. 1982. Postnatal maturation of the respiratory response to O_2 in awake newborn lambs. *Journal of Applied Physiology* 52(2): 428–433.

107. Girard F, Lacaisse A, and Dejours P. 1960. Le stimulus O_2 ventilatoire a la periode neonatale chez l'homme. *Journal de Physiologie* 52: 108–109.

108. Albersheim S, et al. 1976. Effects of CO_2 on immediate ventilatory response to O_2 in preterm infants. *Journal of Applied Physiology* 41(5 part 1): 609–611.

109. Guthrie RD, et al. 1981. Development of CO_2 sensitivity: Effects of gestational age, postnatal age, and sleep state. *Journal of Applied Physiology* 50(5): 956–961.

110. Martin RJ, et al. 1998. Persistence of the biphasic ventilatory response to hypoxia in preterm infants. *Journal of Pediatrics* 132(6): 960–964.

111. Nock ML, et al. 2004. Relationship of the ventilatory response to hypoxia with neonatal apnea in preterm infants. *Journal of Pediatrics* 144(3): 291–295.

112. Mathew OP. 2011. Apnea of prematurity: Pathogenesis and management strategies. *Journal of Perinatology* 31(5): 302–310.

113. Widdicombe JG. 1981. Nervous receptors in the respiratory tract. In *Regulation of Breathing*, part 1, Hornbein TF, ed. New York: Marcel Dekker, 429–472.

114. Polgar G, and Weng TR. 1979. The functional development of the respiratory system from the period of gestation to adulthood. *American Review of Respiratory Disease* 120(3): 625–695.

115. Rehder K, et al. 1979. Ventilation-perfusion relationship in young healthy awake and anesthetized-paralyzed man. *Journal of Applied Physiology* 47(4): 745–753.

116. Mansell A, Bryan C, and Levison H. 1972. Airway closure in children. *Journal of Applied Physiology* 33(6): 711–714.

117. Dawes GS, et al. 1953. Changes in the lungs of the new-born lamb. *Journal of Physiology* 121(1): 141–162.

118. Boyden EA. 1977. Development and growth of the airways. In *Development of the Lung*, Hodson WA, ed. New York: Marcel Dekker, 3–35.

119. Robotham JL, et al. 1980. A physiologic assessment of segmental bronchial atresia. *American Review of Respiratory Disease* 121(3): 533–540.

120. Macklem PT. 1971. Airway obstruction and collateral ventilation. *Physiological Reviews* 51(2): 368–436.

121. West JB, Dollery CT, and Naimark A. 1964. Distribution of blood flow in isolated lung: Relation to vascular and alveolar pressures. *Journal of Applied Physiology* 19: 713–724.

122. James LS, and Rowe RD. 1957. The pattern of response of pulmonary and systemic arterial pressures in newborn and older infants to short periods of hypoxia. *Journal of Pediatrics* 51(1): 5–11.

123. Marshall BE, and Marshall C. 1980. Continuity of response to hypoxic pulmonary vasoconstriction. *Journal of Applied Physiology* 49(2): 189–196.

124. Krauss RV. 1979. Ventilation-perfusion relationship in neonates. In *Neonatal Pulmonary Care*, Thibeault DW, and Gregory GA, eds. Menlo Park, California: Addison-Wesley, 54–69.

125. Farhi LE. 1966. Ventilation-perfusion relationship and its role in alveolar gas exchange. In *Recent Advances in Respiratory Physiology*, Caro CG, ed. Philadelphia: Lippincott Williams & Wilkins, 148–197.

126. West JB. 1966. Regional differences in blood flow and ventilation in the lung. In *Recent Advances in Respiratory Physiology*, Caro CG, ed. Philadelphia: Lippincott Williams & Wilkins, 198–254.

127. Bryan AC, Mansell AL, and Levinson H. 1977. Development of the mechanical properties of the respiratory system. In *Development of the Lung*, Hodson WA, ed. New York: Marcel Dekker, 445–468.

128. West JB. 1970. *Ventilation, Blood Flow, and Gas Exchange*, 2nd ed. Oxford: Blackwell Scientific.

2 Pathophysiology of Acute Respiratory Distress

Susan Orlando, DNS, APRN, NNP-BC

Considering the complex series of cardiorespiratory changes that occurs at birth, it is not surprising that the transition to extrauterine life does not always proceed smoothly. Neonatal respiratory disorders account for the majority of admissions to intensive care units and result in significant morbidity and mortality.

Once the infant shows signs of respiratory distress, prompt diagnosis is essential. Respiratory distress may be related to structural problems such as poor lung development or defects of the chest wall or diaphragm. Biochemical and physical immaturity may exist. Abnormalities in the central nervous system may cause alterations in the respiratory regulatory apparatus. Perfusion abnormalities may impair gas exchange. Aspiration and infection can also occur.

Not all infants with respiratory distress have a respiratory disease (Figure 2-1). In some cases, congenital heart disease may be difficult to distinguish from primary lung disease. Labored breathing may also result from a metabolic problem. The coexistence of other factors, such as cold stress and polycythemia, may compound respiratory distress. Most neonatal respiratory problems are treated medically, but a number of conditions that present with respiratory distress may require surgical intervention. Institution of appropriate therapy requires an accurate diagnosis. Knowledge of the pathophysiology of neonatal pulmonary diseases is essential to ensure comprehensive management. This chapter discusses the pathophysiology of the most common pulmonary disorders that present as acute respiratory distress in the newborn period.

RESPIRATORY DISTRESS SYNDROME

Respiratory distress syndrome (RDS), also known as hyaline membrane disease and surfactant deficiency syndrome, is the major pulmonary problem occurring in the neonate. This syndrome affects approximately 40,000 infants annually in the U.S. Nearly 65 percent of these infants are born at gestational ages of 30 weeks or less.[1] Infants of 37–40 weeks gestational age rarely develop RDS. The prematurity rate is the main reason RDS remains a major neonatal problem. The frequency of RDS, which primarily affects preterm infants less than 35 weeks gestational age, increases inversely with gestational age. However, susceptibility to RDS depends more on the neonate's stage of lung maturity than on precise gestational age. Table 2-1 lists risk factors known to predispose the neonate to developing RDS.

Despite significant advances in understanding the pathophysiology of the disease, RDS ranks eighth among the top ten causes of neonatal deaths. Extreme prematurity; congenital anomalies; chromosomal abnormalities; bacterial sepsis; maternal complications of pregnancy; and complications of the placenta, cord, and fetal membranes currently outrank RDS as causes of neonatal mortality.[2] A sizable reduction in infant mortality from RDS has been linked to the introduction of exogenous surfactant therapy. However, the largest reduction in mortality from RDS in the U.S. occurred during the 15-year period before surfactant replacement therapy was introduced.[3] Regionalized neonatal care, improvements in mechanical ventilation, antenatal corticosteroid therapy, and surfactant replacement therapy have had a cumulative effect on reducing mortality from RDS.

RDS is often the most acute problem of the very immature infant. Numerous complications associated with

FIGURE 2-1
Differential diagnosis of respiratory distress in the newborn period.

Presentation with ± cyanosis, ± grunting, ± retractions, ± tachypnea, ± apnea, ± shock, ± lethargy						
Respiratory				**Extrapulmonary**		
Common	*Less Common*	*Rare*	*Heart*	*Metabolic*	*Brain*	*Blood*
Respiratory distress syndrome (hyaline membrane disease)	Pulmonary hemorrhage	Airway obstruction (upper), e.g., choanal atresia	Congenital heart disease	Metabolic acidosis	Hemorrhage	Acute blood loss
Transient tachypnea	Pneumothorax	Space-occupying lesion, e.g., diaphragmatic hernia, lung cysts, etc.	Patent ductus arteriosus (acquired)	Hypoglycemia	Edema	Hypovolemia
Meconium aspiration	Immature lung syndrome			Hypothermia	Drugs	Twin–twin transfusion
Primary pulmonary hypertension (persistent fetal circulation)		Hypoplasia of the lung		Septicemia	Trauma	Hyperviscosity
Pneumonia, especially Group B Streptococcus						

Adapted from: Martin RJ, Sosenko I, and Bancalari E. 2001. Respiratory problems. In *Care of the High-Risk Neonate,* 5th ed., Klaus MH, and Fanaroff AA, eds. Philadelphia: Saunders, 251. Reprinted by permission.

shortened gestation and preterm birth can prolong hospitalization and add enormous costs. Most infants with RDS do not die from primary lung disease but from complications directly associated with RDS, such as air leak syndrome, intraventricular hemorrhage, pulmonary hemorrhage, or chronic lung disease, or from extreme prematurity itself. Chronic lung disease in infants with birth weights of less than 1,000 g has been identified as a significant predictor of later neurodevelopmental impairment.[4] Efforts aimed at preventing RDS can be expected to improve morbidity and mortality, leading to significant cost savings and improved health for low birth weight infants.

Maternal antenatal steroid therapy reduces neonatal mortality and the incidence of RDS in preterm infants. Additional short-term benefits of this type of therapy include a decreased incidence of intraventricular hemorrhage, lower oxygen and ventilatory support requirements, and improved circulatory stability.[5] A single course of antenatal steroids is currently recommended for women at risk of delivery between the 24th and 34th week of gestation. Initiation of maternal treatment at least 24 hours before delivery produces the greatest benefit for the infant. Treated infants born at 24–28 weeks gestation experience less severe RDS than untreated infants, and disease incidence and mortality are reduced in treated infants born at 29–34 weeks gestation. The benefits of antenatal corticosteroids are additive to those gained from surfactant therapy. Risk and benefit data are insufficient to support the use of higher or repeat doses of antenatal corticosteroids, however.[6,7]

Other factors thought to produce a "sparing effect"— that is, to lessen the severity of RDS in the at-risk population—include maternal toxemia, heroin addiction, prolonged rupture of membranes, and chronic intrauterine stress leading to fetal growth restriction. Chronic fetal stress increases production of endogenous corticosteroids and results in accelerated lung maturity because the effect on surfactant production is similar to that seen with antenatal steroid therapy.

ETIOLOGY AND PATHOPHYSIOLOGY

Normal postnatal pulmonary adaptation requires the presence of adequate amounts of surface-active material to line the air spaces. In the normal lung, surfactant is continually formed, oxidized during breathing, and replenished. Surfactant provides alveolar stability by decreasing the forces of surface tension and preventing alveolar collapse at expiration. This allows more complete gas exchange between the air space and the capillary blood. Additional advantages of surfactant include increased lung compliance, decreased work of breathing, decreased opening pressure, and enhanced alveolar fluid clearance. (More detailed discussions of surfactant can be found in Chapters 1 and 11.)

The development of RDS is thought to begin with surfactant deficiency (Figure 2-2). This deficiency results from insufficient surfactant quantity, abnormal surfactant composition and function, or disruption of surfactant production. A combination of these factors may be present. The phospholipid composition of surfactant changes with gestational age.

Inability to maintain a residual volume of air in the alveoli on expiration results in extensive atelectasis. The reduced volume at the end of expiration requires the generation of high pressures to re-expand the lung with each breath (Figure 2-3).

TABLE 2-1
Risk Factors for Development of RDS

Prematurity

Male sex

Maternal diabetes

Perinatal asphyxia

Second-born twin

Familial predisposition

Cesarean section without labor

Infants with RDS have abnormal ventilation-perfusion relationships. Hypoxia results from right-to-left shunting of blood through the foramen ovale, causing significant venous admixture of arterial blood. The ductus arteriosus relaxes in response to hypoxia, allowing left-to-right shunting of blood. In addition, intrapulmonary shunting occurs as blood is directed away from areas of the lung that are ventilated, resulting in hypercarbia. Acidemia, hypercapnia, and hypoxia increase pulmonary vasoconstriction.

The presence of large amounts of fetal lung fluid in preterm infants contributes to early alveolar flooding. The development of alveolar edema adds to the compromised lung function as protein-rich interstitial fluid fills the alveolar air spaces. When ventilation is initiated, distal lung units tend to remain fluid filled and undistended while more proximal airways dilate to accommodate the ventilatory volume. With expiration, the fluid moves to the proximal airways as the lung collapses. The cyclic movement of fluids erodes the bronchiolar epithelium. Within hours of birth, hyaline membranes are formed from serum proteins such as fibrinogen and albumin, and cell debris is created from bronchiolar and epithelial damage.[1]

CLINICAL PRESENTATION

Infants with RDS develop typical signs of respiratory distress immediately after birth or within the first six hours of life. The usual presentation includes a combination of grunting, intercostal retractions, cyanosis, nasal flaring, and tachypnea. In the very small infant, the disease usually manifests itself as respiratory failure at birth. The presence of apnea in the early stage of the disease is an ominous sign: It usually indicates hypoxemia and respiratory failure; it may also reflect thermal instability or sepsis.

The clinical course is variable in terms of severity. There is usually a pattern of increasing oxygen dependence and poor lung function in which surfactant

FIGURE 2-2
Pathophysiology of respiratory distress syndrome.

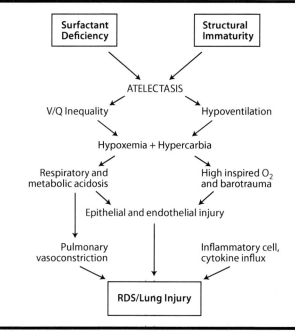

From: Martin RJ, Sosenko I, and Bancalari E. 2001. Respiratory problems. In *Care of the High-Risk Neonate,* 5th ed., Klaus MH, and Fanaroff AA, eds. Philadelphia: Saunders, 254. Reprinted by permission.

FIGURE 2-3
Pressure-volume curves of normal newborn lung and RDS lung.

Comparison of the pressure-volume curve of a normal infant *(solid line)* with that of a newborn with respiratory distress syndrome *(dotted line)*. Note that very little hysteresis (i.e., the difference between the inspiratory and expiratory limbs) is observed in the respiratory distress syndrome curve because of the lack of surfactant for stabilization of the alveoli after inflation. The wide hysteresis of the normal infant's lung curve reflects changes (reduction) in surface tension once the alveoli are opened and stabilized.

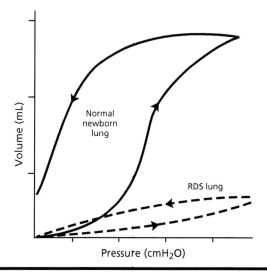

From: Keszler M, and Abukaker MK. 2011. Physiologic principles. In *Assisted Ventilation of the Neonate,* 5th ed., Goldsmith JP, and Karotkin EH, eds. Philadelphia: Saunders, 23. Reprinted by permission.

FIGURE 2-4
AP view of the chest of an infant with respiratory distress syndrome (hyaline membrane disease).

Note the reticulogranular appearance of the lung fields and the extension of air bronchograms.

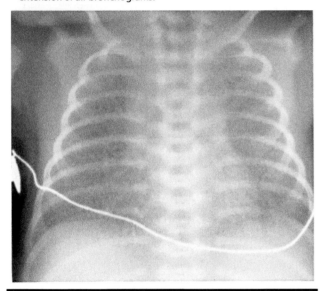

use exceeds the rate of surfactant production. After 48–72 hours of age, most infants begin to show signs of recovery. Oxygenation and ventilation improve, while retractions and respiratory rate decreases. The timing of clinical improvement coincides with a spontaneous diuresis.

A different clinical course may be seen in infants treated with surfactant therapy. These infants often have rapid improvements in oxygenation and a decreased need for ventilator support.[8] Despite surfactant therapy, some extremely low birth weight infants may experience a worsening in their respiratory distress after an initial period of improvement. A postsurfactant slump has been described after the first week of life in infants who require increased oxygen and ventilatory support. Repeat doses of surfactant resulted in improvement in oxygenation and ventilation.[9]

Infants with RDS are predisposed to developing a symptomatic patent ductus arteriosus (PDA)—left-to-right shunting through the ductus arteriosus causing compromised cardiovascular or pulmonary function relative to the magnitude of the shunt. The incidence of a symptomatic PDA in infants less than 30 weeks gestational age with RDS is 75–80 percent.[10] In infants with the most severe RDS, a large left-to-right shunt may be present on the first day of life without the characteristic ductal murmur.

A significant degree of shunting through the patent ductus results in diminished blood flow to the lower aorta and systemic hypoperfusion. Most of the left ventricular output is diverted back to the lungs. The brain, gut, kidneys, and myocardium may not receive adequate perfusion. Tissue mottling, diminished capillary filling, acidemia, and oliguria may result, mimicking the clinical picture of septicemia, intracranial hemorrhage, or a metabolic disorder. In very small infants, pharmacologic measures may fail to close the PDA, resulting in a prolonged recovery phase and ventilator dependence. Surgical intervention becomes necessary for these infants.

DIAGNOSIS: RADIOGRAPHIC FINDINGS

Characteristic features of RDS can be identified on x-ray (Figure 2-4). The lung fields show a fine reticulogranular pattern and marked underaeration, leading to a small lung volume. The most distinguishing finding is peripheral extension and persistence of air bronchograms. Prominent air bronchograms represent aerated bronchioles superimposed on a background of nonaerated alveoli. Granularity is attributed to the presence of distended terminal airways (alveolar ducts and terminal bronchioles) seen against a background of alveolar atelectasis.[11] These characteristic features of RDS progress as the disease worsens, but initiation of mechanical ventilation and surfactant replacement therapy alter the natural progression of radiologic changes.

Treatment with positive-pressure ventilation commonly results in lung fields that appear coarser than before treatment was instituted. A pattern of small bubbles replaces the granularity. This finding reflects overdistention of the terminal airways. On expiration, these bubbles can empty, producing a "whiteout" effect. This pattern occurs because the alveoli are underaerated and lack residual air (functional residual capacity), which results in empty lungs on expiration. When RDS is severe, the lung fields may appear completely opaque, and it may be impossible to distinguish the borders of the heart.

In the recovery phase of RDS, alveolar aeration occurs, and granularity disappears as surfactant production and function improve. The lung fields clear from the periphery inward and from the upper to the lower lobes. The lungs become large and radiolucent and frequently appear hyperaerated.[12] Surfactant therapy usually results in more rapid clearing and aeration of the lungs for infants at 32 weeks gestation and older. Uneven clearing and aeration of the lungs result from uneven distribution of the surfactant preparation.[11] Some infants with RDS develop chronic lung disease following treatment with supplemental oxygen, positive pressure ventilation, and surfactant replacement therapy. It may be difficult to distinguish the early x-ray findings in these infants from those of an infant in the recovery stages of RDS.

TREATMENT AND NURSING CARE

Therapy for infants with RDS begins with anticipation of the preterm birth and administration of antenatal corticosteroids. Once the infant is born, therapy is directed at providing support for respiratory and cardiovascular insufficiency. Surfactant replacement therapy is routinely used in many infants requiring intubation and mechanical ventilation. Immediate administration of appropriate therapy can be life saving. Preventing alveolar atelectasis, hypoxia, and hypercarbia are the main goals of therapy. General supportive measures must also be maximized. (See Chapter 4 for a detailed discussion of nursing care.) Maintenance of adequate oxygenation and ventilation are nursing care priorities. Meticulous attention must be paid to ensuring a thermoneutral environment. Fluid intake must be carefully balanced to avoid overload and complications related to a PDA. Acid-base disturbances, such as metabolic acidosis and respiratory acidosis, are frequently present in infants with RDS and require careful monitoring. Prophylactic antibiotic therapy may be used until the possibility of infection is ruled out.

Oxygen must be administered carefully to provide adequate amounts to tissues without risk of oxygen toxicity. (See Chapter 10 for a detailed discussion of complications of therapy.) An arterial oxygen tension (PaO_2) between 50 and 70 torr is satisfactory for most infants. A high inspired oxygen concentration may be required to maintain the arterial oxygen tension within an acceptable range. Frequent or continuous monitoring of arterial blood gases is essential during the acute phase of the disease. Pulse oximeters provide noninvasive means of obtaining immediate information on the infant's oxygenation status. Surfactant replacement is a major component of treatment for infants with RDS. Natural surfactant preparations are administered via an endotracheal tube using a side port or catheter to deliver the drug into the trachea. (See Chapter 11 for a discussion of surfactant preparations.) Prophylactic exogenous surfactant replacement may be initiated shortly after birth in infants at risk for RDS. This approach means that some infants receive therapy when their disease is

mild or never develops. Prophylactic administration of surfactant is associated with a decreased risk of pneumothorax, pulmonary interstitial emphysema, and death. However, the risk of the infant's developing a PDA and pulmonary hemorrhage increases.[13] Some clinicians administer surfactant therapy as a rescue treatment once the diagnosis of RDS is confirmed. Infants requiring mechanical ventilation for respiratory distress shortly after birth have demonstrated a decreased incidence of chronic lung disease when surfactant was administered within the first two hours of life.[14] Some infants with severe RDS may require multiple doses of surfactant. Others may be intubated only for administration of surfactant and then extubated to nasal continuous positive airway pressure (NCPAP). The combination of surfactant therapy followed immediately by institution of NCPAP has been shown to shorten the duration of respiratory support and eliminate the need for later mechanical ventilation in some infants.[15]

Timely transfer of infants with RDS to a special care unit should be considered when the infant is born in a facility where staff lack experience in caring for low birth weight infants with multisystem problems. Surfactant replacement therapy requires a person skilled in intubation and management of mechanical ventilation. Nursing and respiratory therapy personnel must be available to monitor the infant constantly. Institutional protocols for surfactant therapy should be available. Routine use of surfactant replacement therapy in facilities without a full range of services and expertise is not recommended.[16] Survival rates for very low birth weight infants are higher for those born in hospitals providing a high level of care to a high volume of sick infants.[17]

The decision to initiate ventilator therapy should be made on an individual basis. Variables that must be considered include birth weight, gestational age, postnatal age, results of the chest x-ray, progression of disease, and blood gas values. More immature and smaller infants, who will have a greater incidence of fatigue and apnea, are more likely to require mechanical ventilation even when their oxygen requirements are low. The goal of ventilator therapy is to provide the most effective gas exchange with the least risk of lung damage. Complications such as barotrauma, air leaks, oxygen toxicity, subglottic stenosis, pulmonary infections, cerebral hemorrhage, and retinopathy of prematurity are known to occur with intubation and ventilation. (See Chapter 10.)

Approximately one-third of preterm infants with RDS develop chronic lung disease.[18] However, rates

FIGURE 2-5
AP view of the chest in an infant with transient tachypnea of the newborn.

There is a typical pattern of streaky perihilar densities representing resorption of fluid through the pulmonary veins and lymphatics. The lungs are overaerated.

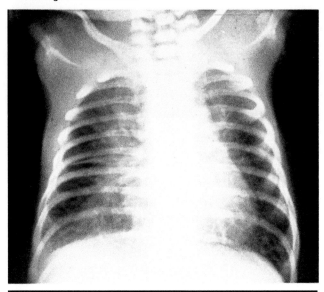

of chronic lung disease vary widely among neonatal intensive care units.[19] Use of conventional mechanical ventilation predisposes the infant with RDS to chronic lung disease as a result of lung injury from overdistention. Elective high-frequency oscillatory ventilation as initial ventilatory support has been studied, but no significant overall reduction in chronic lung disease has been identified. Adverse effects on short- and long-term neurologic outcomes remain a concern with this approach.[20] High-frequency oscillatory ventilation has been used to rescue preterm infants with severe RDS when conventional ventilation techniques have failed. However, there is concern that the benefit gained in terms of decreasing chronic lung disease is offset by the risk of an increase in the number and severity of intraventricular hemorrhages and the incidence of periventricular leukomalacia.[21]

A less severe form of chronic lung disease may be seen in low birth weight infants with only mild RDS. The cause of chronic lung disease in these infants is related to factors other than severity of the initial lung disease and need for mechanical ventilation with high inspired oxygen concentrations. Patent ductus arteriosus, nosocomial infection, and high fluid intake in the first days of life contribute to the development of chronic lung disease in infants with only mild RDS.[22,23] Although

treatment options have increased since the mid-1980s, RDS continues to be a major problem for preterm infants. Advances in assisted reproductive technology have resulted in more multiple gestations. Since 1990, the rate of twin births has increased by 25 percent.[24] The rising multiple-birth rate is contributing to an increase in the number of infants born preterm. Use of tocolytic agents coupled with antenatal steroid therapy is reducing mortality, morbidity, and RDS in premature infants. However, preterm birth remains a major contributing factor for RDS. More research is needed to determine the best combination approach to treating RDS at specific gestational ages and degrees of disease severity. Surfactant type, timing of surfactant administration, and ventilatory support options are key elements in developing better protocols for practice that will improve outcomes for infants with RDS.

TRANSIENT TACHYPNEA OF THE NEWBORN

Transient tachypnea of the newborn (TTN) represents one of the most common causes of respiratory distress in the immediate newborn period. Other names for TTN include wet lung disease and Type II respiratory distress syndrome.

ETIOLOGY AND PATHOPHYSIOLOGY

Delayed postnatal resorption of normal lung fluid is the most likely explanation for the clinical findings in infants with TTN. *In utero*, the fetus's potential airways and air spaces are filled with fluid formed by the fetal lung (active Cl^- [fluid] secretion). Resorption of fetal lung fluid begins with the onset of labor and its accompanying catecholamine surge. In the mature lung, this catecholamine surge also initiates Na^+ absorption, which is enhanced by the increase in oxygen tension.[25] Lung fluid is also cleared before the first breath by the "thoracic squeeze" that occurs during vaginal delivery and by the pulmonary veins and lymphatics. Factors that predispose infants to wet lung disease include prematurity, cesarean section delivery without labor, breech delivery, hypervolemia, hypoproteinemia, maternal asthma, and prolonged maternal hypotonic fluid administration. Premature infants undergo less thoracic compression than term infants because their thoraxes are smaller. The normal thoracic squeeze is absent in infants delivered by cesarean section, resulting in an increased volume of interstitial and alveolar fluid and a decreased thoracic gas volume during the first few hours after birth.[26] More lung fluid is present in infants born by cesarean section without labor because lung fluid absorption begins in early labor. Premature infants are more hypoproteinemic than term infants. A lower plasma oncotic pressure may result in delayed resorption of lung fluid. Hypervolemia may increase capillary and lymphatic hydrostatic pressures. Elevated central pressure may result from placental transfusion and delayed clearance of lung fluid through the thoracic duct. Maternal asthma is thought to affect the infant's response to circulating catecholamines and to alter sodium transport and fluid resorption in the lung epithelium.[27] Administration of hypotonic fluid to the mother results in a smaller osmotic gradient, reducing fluid resorption in the infant because less fluid is pulled from the lung.

An excess of interstitial fluid in the lung causes air trapping. The resulting hyperinflation is one mechanism that can raise pulmonary vascular resistance. When pulmonary vascular resistance is higher than systemic vascular resistance, the fetal pattern of circulation can occur, with shunting through the ductus arteriosus and foramen ovale. Severe hypoxemia results.[28]

CLINICAL PRESENTATION

Term and late preterm infants with TTN usually present with an increased respiratory rate and mild cyanosis. Many of these infants are born by cesarean section. There is often a history of maternal sedation resulting in mild depression at birth. Substernal retractions and expiratory grunting may be present in varying degrees of severity. The clinical signs and symptoms of TTN may mimic those seen in the early phase of RDS or Group B streptococcal pneumonia. The diagnosis of TTN is usually made by excluding other, less benign, causes of respiratory distress. (See Figure 2-1 and **DIAGNOSIS: RADIOGRAPHIC FINDINGS**.)

The most common presentation of TTN is one in which the respiratory rate is normal for the first hour of life and gradually increases during the next 4–6 hours. The rate usually peaks between 6 and 36 hours of life, then gradually returns to normal by 48–72 hours. The maximum rate may reach 120 breaths per minute. Mild hypercarbia, hypoxemia, and acidosis may be present at 2–6 hours.[29]

Blood gases most frequently show a mild respiratory acidosis, which resolves within 8–24 hours. Retained lung fluid interferes with alveolar ventilation, resulting in hypercarbia. Maldistribution of ventilation and ongoing perfusion of nonventilated areas of the lung cause mild to moderate hypoxemia. Some infants may show signs of mild pulmonary vascular lability; others may demonstrate more severe hypoxemia.[30] Two distinct clinical presentations of TTN may be seen based on oxygen requirements. Infants with mild, or classical, TTN typically require less than 40 percent oxygen. Infants with severe disease need more than 60 percent oxygen and will have echocardiographic findings of pulmonary hypertension and right-to-left shunting.[31]

Physical examination may reveal a barrel-shaped chest. Consequently, subcostal retractions may be less prominent. As the respiratory symptoms improve, the chest resumes a more normal size. Retained lung fluid may obstruct the lower airways, resulting in overdistention from a ball-valve effect. Grunting in infants with TTN may be associated with forced expiration as a result of partial airway obstruction from retained lung fluid rather than a means of increasing intra-alveolar pressure as lung compliance worsens.[26]

DIAGNOSIS: RADIOGRAPHIC FINDINGS

Because the presenting signs of TTN are commonly found in other neonatal respiratory diseases, the radiographic pattern becomes the key to diagnosis. The characteristic finding is prominent perihilar streaking and fluid in the interlobar fissures. The prominent perihilar streaking may represent engorgement of the periarterial lymphatics that function in the clearance of alveolar fluid. There may be small collections of liquid, particularly at the costophrenic angles. There is progressive clearing of lung fluid from the periphery to centrally and from upper to lower lung fields. Within 48–72 hours, the chest x-ray is normal.[12]

Hyperaeration of the lungs is evidenced by flattened hemidiaphragms and an increased anterior-posterior (AP) chest diameter. One factor differentiating infants with RDS from those with TTN is lung size. The lungs appear small and granular in infants with RDS; in those with TTN, the lungs are usually large and granular (Figure 2-5).

Clinicians rely on radiographic findings and the clinical presentation of the infant to diagnose TTN. A new approach to early diagnosis of TTN includes use of ultrasound. Differences in lung echogenicity between the upper and lower lung fields have been described in infants with TTN in the first hour after birth. In a study done by Copetti and Cattarossi, very compact comet-tail artifacts were seen in the inferior lung fields, but these were rare in the superior fields. This unique finding of "double lung point" was not observed in other common causes of neonatal respiratory distress such as RDS,

FIGURE 2-6
Cycle of hypoxemia in persistent pulmonary hypertension of the newborn.

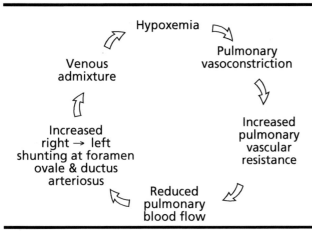

From: Keszler M, and Abukaker MK. 2011. Physiologic principles. In *Assisted Ventilation of the Neonate*, 5th ed., Goldsmith JP, and Karotkin EH, eds. Philadelphia: Saunders, 41. Reprinted by permission.

pneumothorax, atelectasis, pneumonia, or pulmonary hemorrhage.[32] Additional tools for diagnosis of TTN may include the early use of ultrasound as a means of ruling out other causes of neonatal respiratory distress.

Treatment and Nursing Care

TTN is usually a self-limited condition requiring supplemental oxygen and supportive care. Continuous positive airway pressure may be used in severe cases. (See Chapter 8.) Pulse oximetry allows noninvasive assessment of oxygenation. The infant should be carefully monitored and maintained in a thermoneutral environment.

Fluid and electrolyte requirements should be met with intravenous fluids during the acute phase of the disease. Oral feedings are contraindicated because of rapid respiratory rates. If pneumonia is suspected initially, antibiotics may be administered prophylactically. When hypoxemia is severe and tachypnea continues, persistent pulmonary hypertension may complicate the infant's clinical condition, and aggressive medical management may be required to break the cycle of hypoxemia (Figure 2-6).

Neonatal Pneumonia

Pneumonia must be considered in every newborn infant with asphyxia or respiratory distress at birth. Pneumonia is the most common neonatal infection, resulting in significant morbidity and mortality. Nearly 20 percent of all stillborn infants autopsied have a congenitally acquired pulmonary infection.[33] The mortality rate is approximately 20 percent for infants who have perinatally acquired pneumonia; the rate approaches 50 percent for those who acquire the infection in the postnatal period.[34] Recent declines in the incidence of Group B streptococcal disease have been linked to perinatal prevention strategies implemented in the 1990s. Although clinical guidelines for screening and treating colonized mothers have reduced the incidence of this disease, it remains a leading cause of morbidity and mortality.[35]

Etiology and Pathophysiology

Neonatal pneumonia can occur as part of a generalized septicemia or as a primary infection. It is often difficult to distinguish the two. Infectious agents include bacteria, viruses, protozoa, mycoplasmas, and fungi.

Pneumonia may be acquired *in utero*, during labor or delivery, or postnatally. Examination of the placenta and umbilical cord may provide the first evidence suggesting the presence of congenital pneumonia, which may result from the transplacental passage of organisms such as cytomegalovirus, herpes, varicella, and enterovirus. Listeria, *Mycobacterium tuberculosis*, and *Treponema pallidum* are less common agents.

Ascending infection from the maternal genital tract before or during labor is the more common route of contamination. The major predisposing factor is prolonged rupture of fetal membranes, although bacteria can enter the amniotic fluid through intact membranes. Rupture of the membranes for more than 24 hours, excessive obstetric manipulation, prolonged labor with intact membranes, maternal urinary tract infection, and maternal fever have all been linked to congenital pneumonia.[36] Fetal tachycardia and loss of beat-to-beat variability in the fetal heart rate pattern during labor may reflect the fetal response to infection.

Organisms that normally inhabit the maternal genital tract are responsible for infecting the neonate at risk. Bacterial contamination of the infant always occurs during vaginal delivery. Organisms enter the oropharynx and gastrointestinal tract *in utero* when the fetus swallows contaminated amniotic fluid. Aspiration of contaminated secretions present in the oropharynx may follow a complicated labor and delivery. Group B Streptococcus (GBS), *Escherichia coli*, *Klebsiella pneumoniae*, and Enterococcus commonly cause infection in the neonate. The likelihood of neonatal pneumonia caused by GBS increases when an untreated, colonized mother has other risk factors such as prolonged rupture of membranes, intrapartum fever, and signs of chorioamnionitis.[37]

Chlamydia, herpes simplex, and *Candida albicans* can infect the fetus during passage through the birth canal; however, manifestations of pneumonia may not appear until days after birth. Genital mycoplasmas are gaining increased recognition as a significant cause of perinatal infection.[38]

Ureaplasma urealyticum and *Mycoplasma hominis* may be transmitted vertically from the mother to the developing fetus *in utero* or at delivery. *U. urealyticum* has been the agent most commonly linked with histologic chorioamnionitis and is also linked to the development of chronic lung disease in the low birth weight infant.[39,40]

Pneumonia during the postnatal period can also result from a nosocomial infection. The neonate may acquire pathogenic organisms by droplets spread from hospital personnel, other infected infants, or parents. Unwashed hands, contaminated blood products, infected human milk, and open skin lesions are recognized modes of transmitting various pathogens to the susceptible neonate.

Viral pneumonia caused by respiratory syncytial virus or adenovirus may occur in epidemic proportions in the intensive care unit. The most common nosocomial fungal infection is caused by *C. albicans.* Widespread use of broad-spectrum antibiotics and central lines places the very low birth weight infant at high risk for pulmonary candidiasis.

Immaturity of the lungs and immune system causes the neonate to be more susceptible to pulmonary infection. An immature ciliary apparatus leads to suboptimal removal of inflammatory debris, mucus, and pathogens. In addition, the neonatal lung has an insufficient number of pulmonary macrophages for intrapulmonary bacterial clearance.[41] This is evidenced by a lack of significant pulmonary neutrophil accumulation, observed at postmortem examination, in neonates with pneumonia. The newborn infant has deficiencies in the neutrophil inflammatory system, as shown by the frequency of neutropenia during serious infection, a high bacterial attack rate, and a high mortality rate.[42]

Infants who require admission to intensive care units are at higher risk for colonization of the upper respiratory tract with pathogenic organisms than are those who are not admitted. Factors predisposing the NICU patient to pneumonia include liberal use of antibiotics, overcrowding and understaffing, invasive procedures such as endotracheal intubation and suctioning, contaminated respiratory support equipment, and frequent invasion of the protective skin barrier for blood sampling and parenteral fluid administration.[43] The specific organisms that colonize the respiratory tracts of NICU infants are influenced by the choice of antibiotics routinely used in that neonatal intensive care unit and the resident flora of the nursery. Airway colonization with organisms such as *Pseudomonas aeruginosa, Klebsiella pneumoniae, Enterobacter cloacae,* and *Escherichia coli* may be seen in very low birth weight infants requiring prolonged mechanical ventilation. Some infants become colonized with multiple Gram-negative and Gram-positive organisms. Asymptomatic infants may be colonized and not infected. However, ventilator-associated pneumonia (VAP) is more common in symptomatic, colonized infants with positive blood cultures.[44] VAP leads to increased length of stay in the NICU and high mortality rates. The frequency of infection and the risk of death from VAP increase with decreasing gestational age.[45]

CLINICAL PRESENTATION

Clinical signs characteristic of neonatal pneumonia are nonspecific. Some infants with pneumonia demonstrate no pulmonary symptoms. More often, the presentation includes subtle neurologic signs. The key to early diagnosis is a high index of suspicion. Temperature instability, lethargy, poor peripheral perfusion, apnea, tachycardia, and tachypnea are common early signs. The presence of tachypnea, cyanosis, grunting, retractions, and nasal flaring focuses attention on the pulmonary system. These clinical signs indicative of possible pneumonia are also present in other causes of respiratory distress. (See Figure 2-1)

More specific clinical signs, such as characteristic skin lesions, may be found in association with congenital pneumonia caused by Candida, herpes simplex, or *T. pallidum.* Hepatosplenomegaly and jaundice suggest a congenital viral infection. Symptoms of intrapartal infection may be delayed for hours following aspiration of infected amniotic fluid because of the incubation period necessary before the onset of infection. In preterm infants, it is often difficult initially to distinguish between pneumonia and RDS. Some at-risk infants may have pneumonia in combination with RDS or TTN.

DIAGNOSIS

The chest radiograph is important in detecting pneumonia; however, appropriate bacterial and viral cultures are needed to identify the specific organism. Rapid screening tests allow earlier initiation of appropriate therapy.

FIGURE 2-7
AP view of the chest in an infant with pneumonia.

Note the patchy, asymmetric pulmonary infiltrates.

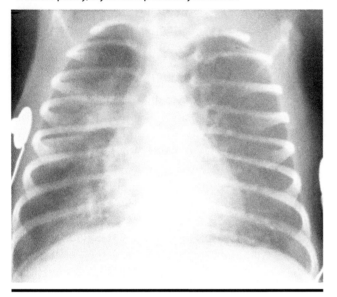

Laboratory Tests

Latex agglutination assay of body fluids detects specific antigens and aids in rapid diagnosis of early neonatal sepsis and pneumonia. It is recommended, however, that antigen test kits be used only as an adjunct to other diagnostic tests and not as a substitute for bacterial culture.[46] Blood cultures, which are usually positive in infants with congenital pneumonia, should be obtained on all infants with suspected pneumonia.[47]

The best indirect indication of congenital infection and pneumonia is the presence of bacteria on a Gram's stain of a tracheal aspirate obtained during the first 8 hours of life.[48] A culture of tracheal secretions obtained through a newly inserted endotracheal tube or by tracheal aspiration through a catheter under direct laryngoscopy during the first 12 hours of life has proved useful in diagnosing neonatal bacterial pneumonia.[47] Because of rapid colonization, results of tracheal cultures obtained later may be difficult to interpret. The most definitive method of diagnosis is culture and Gram's stain of pleural fluid, but the procedural risks may result in increased morbidity and outweigh any benefits.

The neutrophil count is valuable in identifying infants with congenital pneumonia or septicemia. Neutropenia in the presence of respiratory distress during the first 72 hours of life suggests bacterial disease. In addition, an increase in the ratio of immature to total neutrophils on the leukocyte differential is frequently observed during neonatal infection.[49]

Radiographic Findings

Chest x-ray examinations are required to support the diagnosis of pneumonia and to distinguish it from other causes of respiratory distress. In some cases, no abnormalities will be found if the studies are performed soon after the onset of symptoms, but radiologic diagnosis should be possible within 24–72 hours. Patchy opacifications become more impressive during subsequent days. In some infants, an area of radiopacification is present but may be attributed to atelectasis. Bilateral homogenous consolidation is a common finding when the pneumonia has been acquired *in utero.*

A wide spectrum of findings is commonly seen following aspiration of infected amniotic fluid: Mild cases may be evidenced by patchy, bilateral bronchopneumonic infiltrates; severe cases may show diffuse bilateral alveolar infiltrates in the lungs with moderate hyperaeration.[12] Although it is difficult to distinguish RDS from Group B streptococcal pneumonia radiologically, the presence of pleural effusions suggests pneumonia. *Pleural effusions are common with bacterial infections but rare with viral infections.*[11] Serial chest radiographs are useful in following the course of the disease and for assessing the effectiveness of treatment (Figure 2-7).

TREATMENT AND NURSING CARE

Antibiotic therapy should be instituted immediately following appropriate diagnostic studies and before identifying a pathogenic organism. The initial choice of therapy is broad-spectrum parenteral antibiotics. Therapeutic agents such as ampicillin and gentamicin or cefotaxime will provide coverage for the majority of neonatal infections caused by organisms found in the maternal genital flora. Azithromycin is a newer alternative treatment to erythromycin for neonatal respiratory infections caused by *U. urealyticum* as well as *Chlamydia trachomatis.*[50]

Many nosocomial infections are caused by organisms that have developed resistance to commonly used antibiotics. Once the pathogen has been identified and sensitivity patterns obtained, therapy can be altered to provide the most effective agent. A combination of antibiotics may be used for synergistic effect. The length of antibiotic therapy should be guided by the response of the infant and the identity of the pathogen. The average duration of therapy is 10 to 14 days, but may be longer in severe cases.

Antifungal therapy should be initiated in infants with pneumonia caused by Candida. Amphotericin B, flucytosine, and fluconazole have been used in neonates to treat fungal infections. Amphotericin B and flucytosine used in combination have a synergistic antifungal effect.[51] Careful monitoring of renal and hepatic function is required during therapy.

Viral pathogens respond to a limited number of drugs. When herpes simplex infection is suspected, acyclovir or vidarabine should be used. A small number of infants with cytomegalovirus infection (CMV) have been treated with ganciclovir. Infants with congenital CMV infection may have irreversible damage; those with acquired infection may show clinical improvements in respiratory status following treatment.[52,53] More research is needed to determine the best treatment strategy given available antiviral drugs.[54]

In addition to antimicrobial therapy, the neonate with pneumonia requires careful monitoring of oxygenation and acid-base status. Supplemental oxygen and ventilatory assistance are often necessary. Volume expanders, blood products, and buffers may be needed for the infant with cardiovascular collapse from septic shock. Exchange transfusion, granulocyte transfusion, and administration of intravenous gamma globulin have all been utilized in cases of overwhelming sepsis when conventional therapy has failed.[55] Extracorporeal membrane oxygenation (ECMO) has also been used in attempts to improve survival rates in neonates with little chance of survival.[56]

MECONIUM ASPIRATION SYNDROME

The passage of meconium by the fetus *in utero* is estimated to occur in 8–29 percent of all deliveries.[57] However, meconium passage is seen primarily in fetuses born at or beyond term and among those who are small for gestational age or have umbilical cord complications and compromised uteroplacental circulation. During breech deliveries, meconium passage is common and is often ignored.

When meconium-stained amniotic fluid is detected, careful and continuous monitoring of fetal well-being is required during labor. The passage of meconium into the amniotic fluid is considered a sign of fetal distress when accompanied by fetal heart rate abnormalities.[58] Increased stillbirth and neonatal mortality rates have been associated with meconium staining. In the U.S., approximately 520,000 infants are born meconium stained annually. Five percent of these (about 26,000) develop meconium aspiration syndrome, and more than 4 percent (about 1,000) die from the disease. Approximately 30 percent of infants with meconium

aspiration syndrome (about 7,800) require mechanical ventilation. Pneumothoraces occur in at least 2,900 of those infants requiring mechanical ventilation.[59] A decline in the number of postterm births has been identified as the most important factor in reducing the incidence of meconium aspiration syndrome by one-third.[60]

ETIOLOGY AND PATHOPHYSIOLOGY

Meconium is first produced during the fifth month of gestation. It is free of bacteria and contains residuals of gastrointestinal secretions. The pathophysiologic stimuli that trigger the fetal passage of meconium are not clearly understood.

The following theories have been proposed to explain the relationship between fetal hypoxia and the passage of meconium *in utero*.[57]

- Fetal gut ischemia resulting from decreased perfusion during the "diving reflex"
- Hyperperistalsis following an episode of intestinal ischemia
- Vagal stimulation elicited by umbilical cord compression, resulting in increased peristalsis and anal sphincter dilation

Meconium passage *in utero* is considered by some to be a normal physiologic function of term and postterm fetuses, indicating fetal maturity.[58] It is rarely observed in fetuses of less than 37 weeks gestation.

Fetal breathing movements occur in the healthy fetus at a rate of 30–70 times per minute. Normally, fluid from the airways moves out into the amniotic fluid with fetal respiratory movements. During an episode of fetal asphyxia, these movements cease, and apnea occurs. As the asphyxial episode continues, apnea is replaced by deep gasping. Amniotic fluid containing particulate material may be inhaled into the trachea and large bronchi, and the infant may demonstrate airway obstruction at birth. After the onset of air breathing, meconium migrates rapidly to the distal airways.

The amount of meconium passed into the amniotic fluid affects the appearance and viscosity of the fluid. Amniotic fluid containing meconium may have a light green tinge or the consistency and appearance of thick pea soup. Yellow, or "old," meconium-stained fluid indicates prolonged fetal hypoxia and is an ominous sign.[61]

Mechanical obstruction of the airways with meconium particles results in a ball-valve phenomenon. Complete obstruction of the smaller airways results in atelectasis of alveoli distal to the obstruction. Partial airway obstruction results in areas of overexpansion as air passes around the obstruction to inflate the

FIGURE 2-8
Pathophysiology of meconium aspiration syndrome.

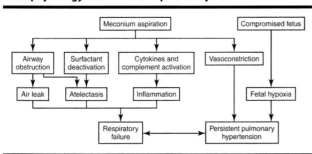

From: Abu-Shaweesh JM. 2011. Respiratory disorders in preterm and term infants. In *Fanaroff & Martin's Neonatal-Perinatal Medicine,* 9th ed, Martin RJ, Fanaroff AA, and Walsh MC, eds. St. Louis: Elsevier Mosby, 1158. Reprinted by permission.

alveoli. As the airway collapses around the obstruction during expiration, residual air becomes trapped distally. Pneumothorax occurs when the overdistended alveoli rupture and air leaks into the pleural space. Pneumomediastinum results when extra-alveolar air moves through interstitial tissue to the mediastinum.

The chemical composition of meconium causes local toxic effects. Bile salts, pancreatic enzymes, desquamated intestinal epithelium, and biliverdin in meconium initiate a chemical pneumonitis that further compromises pulmonary function (Figure 2-8).[62] Surfactant function is disrupted by serum and nonserum proteins and fatty acids, leading to atelectasis, decreased lung compliance, and hypoxia.[63]

CLINICAL PRESENTATION

Typically, an infant with meconium aspiration syndrome has a history of fetal distress and meconium-stained amniotic fluid. The classic postmature infant shows signs of weight loss with little subcutaneous fat remaining. The umbilical cord may be thin, with minimal Wharton's jelly. The nails, umbilical cord, and skin may be meconium stained. Respiratory distress at birth may be mild, moderate, or severe.

Tracheal occlusion by a meconium plug causes severe, gasping respirations; marked retractions; and poor air exchange. The severity of meconium aspiration syndrome is related to the amount of aspirated meconium. In mild cases, hypoxemia is present but easily corrected with minimal oxygen therapy; tachypnea is present but usually resolves within 72 hours. A low partial pressure of carbon dioxide in arterial blood ($PaCO_2$) and normal pH may be seen. Infants with moderate disease gradually worsen during the first 24 hours.

Severely affected infants have neurologic and respiratory depression at birth resulting from the hypoxic insult that precipitated the passage of meconium. They develop respiratory distress with cyanosis, nasal flaring, grunting, retracting, and tachypnea. The chest appears overinflated. Coarse crackles are common. Diminished breath sounds or heart tones may indicate a pulmonary air leak. Arterial blood gases typically show hypoxemia and acidosis. These infants have combined respiratory and metabolic acidosis secondary to respiratory failure and asphyxia. Because of large intrapulmonary shunts and persistence of fetal circulation patterns, hypoxemia is often profound despite administration of 100 percent oxygen.

DIAGNOSIS: RADIOGRAPHIC FINDINGS

Chest radiographs should be obtained to confirm the diagnosis of meconium aspiration and to rule out pulmonary air leaks. The classic radiographic picture of meconium aspiration syndrome includes coarse, patchy, irregular pulmonary infiltrates. Areas of irregular aeration are common, with some appearing atelectatic and others appearing emphysematous. Hyperaeration of the chest with flattening of the diaphragm is frequently seen. Pneumothorax and pneumomediastinum are common. Chemical pneumonitis may be apparent after 48 hours.[11,12] Massive aspiration is characterized by a "snowstorm" appearance. The extent of clinical and radiographic findings depends on the amount of meconium aspirated into the lungs (Figure 2-9).

TREATMENT AND NURSING CARE

Intrapartum and Immediate Postpartum Interventions

Prevention is the key to managing the infant at risk for meconium aspiration. Continuous electronic fetal monitoring is an essential tool for identifying the fetus in distress following passage of meconium *in utero.* Amnioinfusion (infusion of normal saline into the amniotic sac during labor) is used to correct oligohydramnios and decrease vagal stimulation caused by cord compression.[64] In prospective randomized studies, infants identified with thick meconium who received amnioinfusion had significantly fewer low one-minute Apgar scores, less meconium below the cords, and a significantly lower incidence of operative delivery.[65] However, other studies report continued occurrence of meconium aspiration syndrome and no improvement in neonatal outcome following prophylactic amnioinfusion for thick meconium.[66] Current evidence does not support routine use of amnioinfusion to dilute meconium stained amniotic fluid. Furthermore, the intervention requires systematic study in clinical trials.[67] Several studies have demonstrated decreased mortality and morbidity when meconium is removed from the mouth, pharynx, and trachea before the onset of breathing.[68–70] More recent evidence from a multicenter trial failed to show a positive effect from oropharyngeal and nasopharyngeal suctioning before the delivery of the shoulders in meconium-stained infants.[71] Current recommended practice does not include routine intrapartum suctioning of infants delivered through meconium-stained amniotic fluid.[72,73]

Some investigators have questioned the need for routine tracheal suctioning at the birth of meconium-stained infants who are delivered vaginally and have a one-minute Apgar score of more than 8. In a prospective study, meconium-stained but vigorous infants who made their first inspiratory effort before being handed to the pediatrician did not benefit from immediate tracheal suctioning.[74] Furthermore, case reports have demonstrated that aggressive airway management during and immediately after birth does not always prevent aspiration of meconium.[75] The Neonatal Resuscitation Program guidelines recommend no tracheal suctioning for infants with strong respiratory efforts, good muscle tone, and a heart rate greater than 100 beats per minute. Direct tracheal suctioning is recommended for the meconium-stained infant with depressed respiratory effort, poor muscle tone, and a heart rate less than 100 beats per minute. This procedure should be accomplished before the infant makes repeated inspiratory efforts.

Universal precautions should be taken. Suctioning should always precede positive-pressure ventilation. Meconium aspirator devices and regulated wall suction should be utilized to effectively clear meconium from the airway. The urgent need for oxygenation and ventilation in these infants should not be ignored.[76,77]

Nursery Management

Supportive respiratory therapy is required for infants who develop meconium aspiration syndrome. The infant should be monitored continuously for tachypnea. Frequent assessment of blood gases is essential. The need for oxygen and assisted ventilation is dictated by arterial blood gas values. Continuous monitoring of oxygenation by pulse oximetry will alert the nurse to early deterioration. Ventilatory assistance is indicated when adequate oxygenation cannot be achieved or maintained in a high concentration of oxygen. Respiratory failure commonly occurs in severe cases of meconium aspiration and may

FIGURE 2-9
AP view of the chest in an infant with meconium aspiration syndrome.

There are areas of patchy, asymmetric alveolar consolidation and volume loss in addition to areas of overexpansion resulting from obstruction (ball-valve effect). The lung fields are hyperexpanded.

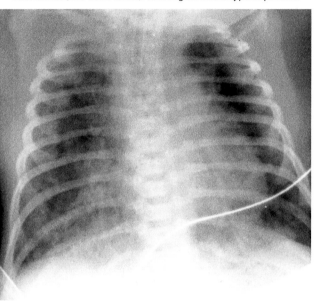

necessitate prolonged assisted ventilation. Once the infant requires assisted ventilation, morbidity and mortality increase. Sedatives and neuromuscular blocking agents may be added to the therapeutic regime when the infant's own ventilatory efforts interfere with the effectiveness of mechanical ventilation.

Gastric lavage is used to remove meconium-stained fluid from the stomach and reduce the chance of further aspiration with vomiting. There is no evidence from studies to support this practice.[78] As noted under **DIAGNOSIS: RADIOGRAPHIC FINDINGS,** chest radiographs should be obtained to confirm the diagnosis of meconium aspiration and rule out pulmonary air leaks.

Chest physiotherapy (CPT) is used in many neonatal units to assist in mobilization of secretions and prevent accumulation of debris in the airway of neonates with respiratory distress. Percussion, vibration, and tracheal instillation of saline followed by suctioning are commonly performed in the delivery room and nursery following aspiration of meconium-stained amniotic fluid. There are no randomized controlled trials demonstrating positive short- or long-term effects of this therapy in neonates. Some infants may show signs of acute clinical deterioration with further hypoxemia and the need for increased oxygen following chest physiotherapy. There is insufficient evidence to support the use of chest physiotherapy for meconium aspiration syndrome.[79]

Broad-spectrum antibiotic therapy is indicated when infection is suspected. Appropriate cultures should be obtained before starting therapy. Prophylactic use of antibiotics is a common practice in infants with meconium aspiration syndrome because it is difficult to distinguish on the chest radiograph from superimposed bacterial pneumonia. However, there is no evidence to suggest that prophylactic antibiotic therapy improves outcomes in nonventilated infants with meconium aspiration syndrome. No difference in duration of tachypnea, oxygen requirement, or need for NCPAP has been reported in a group of untreated, nonventilated infants with meconium aspiration syndrome. In the absence of perinatal risk factors for infection, these infants did not receive antibiotic therapy and had no evidence of bacteremia, pneumonia, or meningitis.[80]

There is no reported increase in bacteremia among meconium-stained infants when compared to non-stained infants. The decision to use antibiotic therapy for these infants is based on each infant's course.[81]

Surfactant replacement therapy early in the course of respiratory failure may reduce the severity of the disease in some infants. Surfactant therapy has been shown to reduce pulmonary air leaks, duration of mechanical ventilation and oxygen therapy, as well as length of hospital stay.[82] Further research is needed to determine the optimal timing, preparation, and method of surfactant administration for infants with meconium aspiration syndrome.

The infant should be carefully monitored for signs of seizure activity reflecting anoxic cerebral injury. Anticonvulsant therapy may be required. Metabolic derangements such as hypoglycemia and hypocalcemia require appropriate therapy and monitoring. Fluid balance is critical in these infants because cerebral edema and inappropriate secretion of antidiuretic hormone often occur following an asphyxial insult. Fluid restriction may be initiated early in the course of the disease. Careful monitoring of urine output is essential in the postasphyxial stage. Hematuria, oliguria, and anuria may indicate anoxic renal damage.

Recovery from meconium aspiration syndrome usually occurs within three to seven days in infants who do not require assisted ventilation. Those requiring assisted ventilation are usually ventilator dependent for three to seven days. Although the infant may be weaned successfully from assisted ventilation, tachypnea may persist for weeks. Pulmonary air leaks, persistent pulmonary

hypertension, and pulmonary barotrauma often complicate the course of the disease. Prolonged ventilator therapy predisposes these infants to bronchopulmonary dysplasia with resulting oxygen dependency. More long-term deficits may be seen as sequelae of asphyxia.

The major cause of death in infants with meconium aspiration syndrome is respiratory failure. As noted earlier, surfactant replacement therapy may improve oxygenation and reduce the incidence of pulmonary air leaks. In some cases, however, the infant cannot be adequately oxygenated and ventilated with conventional respiratory support. Timely transfer to a tertiary level neonatal intensive care unit is essential. High-frequency ventilation and inhaled nitric oxide have been used for infants with respiratory failure and severe hypoxemia unresponsive to conventional mechanical ventilation. The combined use of surfactant, inhaled nitric oxide, and high-frequency oscillatory ventilation has resulted in a significant decrease in the need for the most invasive therapies such as ECMO.[83,84]

Careful consideration should be given before initiating treatment with high-frequency oscillatory ventilation and inhaled nitric oxide in facilities where ECMO is not available. Collaborative agreements with an ECMO center and a mechanism for timely transport of the infant are recommended.[85] Once nitric oxide therapy is initiated, transfer should take place without interruption of the treatment. A transport incubator equipped with a nitric oxide delivery system is required for these infants. Abrupt discontinuation of therapy can cause acute deterioration, with severe hypoxemia and possible death.[86,87] When all other treatment options fail to reverse respiratory failure, ECMO has been used in many of these infants to improve survival.[88]

PERSISTENT PULMONARY HYPERTENSION OF THE NEWBORN

Persistent pulmonary hypertension of the newborn (PPHN) is a clinical syndrome characterized by cyanosis secondary to shunting of unoxygenated blood through the ductus arteriosus and foramen ovale. Gersony and colleagues originally described this condition in infants with no parenchymal lung disease or cardiac lesion who developed central cyanosis shortly after birth; they applied the term "persistence of the fetal circulation" to these infants.[89] Other terms have also been used to describe infants who, during the first few days of life, have cyanosis and respiratory disease, but no structural cardiac lesion. These monikers include progressive pulmonary hypertension, persistence of fetal cardiopulmonary circulation, and pulmonary vascular obstruction.

Because of the variable criteria used to define the syndrome, the true incidence of PPHN is unknown. It was reported in 1.9 infants per 1,000 live births in a multicenter study, although rates as high as 6.8 per 1,000 live births were documented in one of the centers. Half of the infants had high-risk factors, including abnormal fetal heart rate tracings, meconium-stained amniotic fluid, and low Apgar scores. These infants frequently required delivery room interventions.[90]

ETIOLOGY AND PATHOPHYSIOLOGY

Although elevated pulmonary vascular resistance is the key pathophysiologic element in the syndrome, there is a wide spectrum of etiologies. Classification according to etiology helps us understand the pathophysiology and manage the condition.

Pulmonary artery pressure is the product of pulmonary blood flow and pulmonary vascular resistance. Most of infants with PPHN have elevated pulmonary vascular resistance; few have increased pulmonary blood flow as an important component of their PPHN. Pulmonary artery pressure may be equal to or greater than systemic arterial pressure in infants with PPHN. Right ventricular and right atrial pressures rise.

When right atrial pressure exceeds left atrial pressure and pulmonary arterial pressure is greater than systemic pressure, blood flow changes to follow the path of least resistance. Desaturated blood returning to the right heart is shunted into the systemic circulation through the foramen ovale and ductus arteriosus. This right-to-left shunt causes hypoxemia secondary to venous admixture. Hypoxemia increases pulmonary vasoconstriction, and the cycle continues (see Figure 2-6).

Persistent pulmonary hypertension may occur in association with a wide spectrum of neonatal diseases (Table 2-2). Gersony classifies the causes of pulmonary hypertension in terms of cardiopulmonary pathophysiology as follows: (1) pulmonary venous hypertension, (2) functional obstruction of the pulmonary vascular bed, (3) pulmonary vascular constriction, (4) decreased pulmonary vascular bed, and (5) increased pulmonary blood flow.[91]

The time period during which pulmonary vasoconstriction occurs may clarify the pathophysiology of PPHN. Etiologies can be categorized into intra uterine, intrapartum, and postpartum periods. The terms *primary*, or *idiopathic*, and *secondary* have also been

TABLE 2-2
Clinical Conditions Associated with Persistent Pulmonary Hypertension of the Newborn

Pathophysiologic	Anatomic
Uteroplacental insufficiency	Diaphragmatic hernia
Perinatal asphyxia	Hypoplastic lungs
Hematologic	**Cardiac**
Polycythemia	Myocardial dysfunction
Hyperviscosity	Congenital heart defects
Metabolic	**Respiratory**
Hypocalcemia	Aspiration syndromes
Hypoglycemia	Infection Group B β Streptococcus
Hypothermia	Hyaline membrane disease
	Transient tachypnea of the newborn
Other	
Maternal drugs (aspirin, indomethacin, phenytoin, lithium)	

used to describe PPHN. Regardless of the classification used, it is essential to understand that a combination of etiologies may be responsible for PPHN. Many infants with PPHN also have a parenchymal lung disease causing intrapulmonary shunting. Meconium aspiration syndrome, bacterial pneumonia, or surfactant deficiency syndrome may be the primary disease leading to the development of PPHN.

CLINICAL PRESENTATION

Infants presenting with clinical evidence of PPHN are usually more than 32 weeks gestational age and born following complications of pregnancy, labor, or delivery. The syndrome occurs most commonly in term or post-term infants following an intrauterine or intrapartum asphyxial episode. Onset of symptoms is usually immediate in infants with congenital diaphragmatic hernia or severe asphyxia. Others may have a more subtle presentation, but most infants at risk have clinical manifestations before 24 hours of age. Clinical symptoms may initially be indistinguishable from those of cyanotic congenital heart disease.

There is marked variability in the clinical course of PPHN. Evidence of respiratory distress may be mild to severe. Signs of heart failure may be present in more adversely affected infants. Central cyanosis may be present despite a high inspired oxygen concentration. Arterial blood gases reveal severe hypoxemia and metabolic acidosis. Arterial PaO_2 values or oxygen saturation values may fluctuate widely when the infant is handled or stressed. The $PaCO_2$ is usually normal but may be mildly elevated. Physical examination reveals varying degrees of respiratory distress and cyanosis.

FIGURE 2-10
A. Preductal and postductal sampling sites. B. Right-to-left shunt across the patent ductus arteriosus. C. Right-to-left shunt across the foramen ovale.

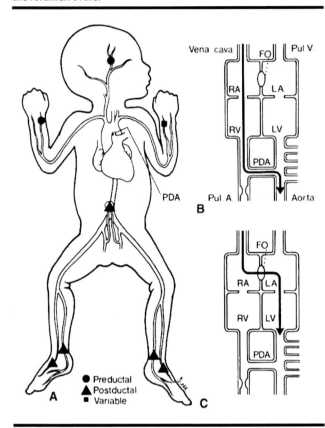

From: Durand DJ, and Mickas NA. 2011. Blood gases: Technical aspects and interpretation. In *Assisted Ventilation of the Neonate*, 5th ed., Goldsmith JP, and Karotkin EH, eds. Philadelphia: Saunders, 301. Reprinted by permission.

A single, loud, second heart sound or a narrowly split second heart sound with a loud pulmonic component is heard. A long, harsh systolic murmur may be heard at the lower left sternal border. This murmur is the result of tricuspid insufficiency. Inspection of the chest reveals a hyperactive precordium with a prominent right ventricular impulse that is visible or easily palpable at the lower left sternal border.

The chest may be barrel-shaped following aspiration of meconium or the use of high positive inflating pressures with mechanical ventilation. Retractions are present when pulmonary compliance is decreased. Peripheral perfusion is often poor, and pulses are diminished.

DIAGNOSIS

Radiographic Findings

There is no classic x-ray finding in PPHN because the etiologies are varied. The chest radiograph may show normal or decreased pulmonary vascular markings. When the syndrome is complicated by pulmonary disease, such as meconium aspiration, pneumonia, or hyaline membrane disease, the x-ray findings will reflect the primary pulmonary disorder. Cardiomegaly is a frequent finding on the initial chest x-ray and may be present without clinically detectable cardiac dysfunction.[92] The more severely affected infants with PPHN may show signs of heart failure. Pleural effusions, pulmonary venous congestion, and marked cardiomegaly may be seen when there is myocardial dysfunction.

Diagnostic Workup

PPHN should be suspected in any infant who has hypoxemia that is out of proportion to the severity of lung disease present. Parenchymal lung disease is the most common etiology of hypoxemia. However, persistent pulmonary hypertension often complicates the clinical course of infants with primary lung disease.

Differential diagnosis includes, most importantly, cyanotic heart disease. A series of noninvasive bedside tests can be performed using arterial blood gas determinations to differentiate between cyanotic heart disease and pulmonary parenchymal disease. These include the hyperoxia test, preductal and postductal arterial blood sampling, and echocardiography.[93] Pulse oximetry monitors can also be used to follow trends in oxygen saturation levels.

The hyperoxia test is used in term infants to differentiate between the fixed right-to-left shunt in congenital heart disease or PPHN and a ventilation-perfusion mismatch as seen in parenchymal lung disease. The infant is placed in a 100 percent oxygen concentration for five to ten minutes before an arterial oxygen pressure is determined. If a ventilation-perfusion problem is the cause of the hypoxemia, oxygen will diffuse into the poorly ventilated areas of the lung, and the PaO_2 will usually rise above 100 mmHg. A right-to-left shunt is demonstrated when the PaO_2 remains low in 100 percent oxygen. However, this shunt may be secondary to congenital heart disease or PPHN. Further evaluation is needed to determine if the right-to-left shunt is occurring at the ductal level.

Preductal and postductal arterial sampling are used to demonstrate the presence of a right-to-left shunt through the ductus arteriosus. Preductal samples can be obtained from the right radial or either temporal artery; postductal sites most frequently sampled include the umbilical, femoral, and posterior tibial arteries (Figure 2-10). The left radial artery may represent a mixture of preductal and postductal blood because of the proximity of the left subclavian artery to the ductus arteriosus.

Preductal and postductal arterial blood samples must be obtained simultaneously from the quiet infant if they are to be considered reliable. Strategic placement of two pulse oximeters can aid in determining the presence of a shunt. Preductal pulse oximeter readings can be obtained by placing the probe on the right hand; either foot can be used to obtain postductal oxygen saturation readings. In the hypoxemic infant, a PaO_2 difference greater than 15–20 mmHg indicates significant right-to-left shunting at the ductal level. If the test reveals no difference in PaO_2 between preductal and postductal sites, pulmonary hypertension cannot yet be ruled out because shunting may be primarily at the atrial level (see Figure 2-10). Additional testing is needed to differentiate between PPHN and cyanotic heart disease.

Echocardiography is used to confirm the presence of a structurally normal heart in infants with PPHN. It can also be used to measure the ratio of the systolic time intervals of the right ventricle: The ratio of the right ventricular pre-ejection period to the right ventricular ejection time is elevated in infants with pulmonary hypertension.[94] Two-dimensional echocardiography with color Doppler flow can be used to define the direction and location of shunting through the foramen ovale or the ductus arteriosus. The degree of pulmonary hypertension can also be estimated. When myocardial ischemia is present, an electrocardiogram shows ST segment depression. Invasive diagnostic tests such as cardiac catheterization and pulmonary artery pressure monitoring are rarely needed to make the diagnosis of PPHN.

TREATMENT AND NURSING CARE

When the fetus has been identified to be at risk for persistent pulmonary hypertension, the first step in prevention is skilled resuscitation and stabilization. Preventing hypoxemia, acidosis, and hypothermia during the immediate newborn period is essential. The time, site, and delivery route of the fetus with a known risk factor for PPHN, such as congenital diaphragmatic hernia, may be scheduled to minimize intrapartum and postnatal stress.

The aim of therapy for infants with PPHN is to correct hypoxemia by reversing right-to-left shunting. This is accomplished by decreasing pulmonary artery pressure or elevating the systemic arterial blood pressure. Treatment is often complex and includes mechanical ventilation, drug therapy, and supportive care.

Mechanical Ventilation

Treatment with mechanical ventilation should be individualized based on the underlying cause of pulmonary hypertension. The main goal is to improve oxygenation. Initially, the fraction of inspired oxygen (FiO_2) should be increased until the PaO_2 is greater than 50 mmHg postductally. In most cases, the infant will require an FiO_2 of 0.70 or more to maintain a PaO_2 of 50 mmHg or greater. Mechanical ventilation is most effective when it is begun early in the course of the disease. Ventilator management strategies may include use of conventional mechanical ventilation, high-frequency jet ventilation, or high-frequency oscillatory ventilation. Ventilation strategies are modified when parenchymal lung disease is identified as the etiology of the infant's pulmonary hypertension. If the infant fails to respond to initial ventilator therapy, adjunct therapies may include surfactant administration or inhaled nitric oxide. Surfactant deficiency as well as surfactant inactivation can lead to pulmonary hypertension. A combination of surfactant therapy and high-frequency ventilation may be required for some infants with pulmonary hypertension caused by respiratory distress syndrome or meconium aspiration syndrome. A different ventilator strategy may be required for those with pulmonary hypertension due to lung hypoplasia.

Mechanical hyperventilation using high rates and high inspiratory pressure to induce hypocarbia has been widely used in infants to improve oxygen transfer into the blood, when there is evidence of pulmonary hypertension. Each infant has a critical level of $PaCO_2$ at which optimum oxygenation occurs because of a decrease in pulmonary vascular resistance and in right-to-left shunting.[93] However, significant reductions in carbon dioxide levels in the blood can have adverse effects on the neonate, and there are many unanswered questions regarding the risk to benefit ratio of this therapy. Induced hypocarbia and alkalosis shift the oxygen-hemoglobin dissociation curve farther to the left, which reduces oxygen release at the tissue level. Venous blood return to the heart is impeded, and cardiac output is reduced when extremely high inspiratory pressure and ventilatory rates are used. Hypotension and reduced cardiac output cause a further reduction in oxygenation. Induced hypocarbia can diminish cerebral blood flow and increase cerebrospinal fluid lactate levels.[95] The degree and duration of hypocarbia have been linked to poor neurologic outcomes in preterm and term infants managed by hyperventilation. The worst outcomes were seen in infants who were hyperventilated twice as long as infants without abnormalities. Affected infants spent a significantly greater time in an alkalotic state with their $PaCO_2$ less than 25 mmHg.[96] Periventricular leukomalacia, cerebral palsy, abnormal cognitive development, hearing loss, and chronic lung disease have been identified as detrimental effects of hyperventilation in neonates.[97] Many clinicians have abandoned this treatment strategy because of ventilator-induced lung injury and adverse cerebral effects.[98,99]

The use of hyperventilation in management of the infant with PPHN has also decreased since the introduction of nitric oxide therapy. However, when nitric oxide therapy is not available, a variety of ventilation techniques may be used in attempts to stabilize the infant until transport can occur.

Some clinicians prefer a gentle ventilation approach over hyperventilation. The goal of this approach is to minimize barotrauma while maintaining a PaO_2 between 50 and 70 mmHg. $PaCO_2$ is maintained in the 40–60 mmHg range. The appropriate peak inspiratory pressure is determined by clinical assessment of chest excursion. This conservative approach has been used successfully to manage a group of infants with PPHN and severe respiratory failure.[100] Others have successfully treated infants with a combined approach using gentle ventilation and inhaled nitric oxide.[101]

The risk of barotrauma and pulmonary air leaks during conventional ventilator therapy may lead some clinicians to choose high-frequency ventilators as an alternative method to achieve adequate lung inflation. (See Chapter 12.) The goal is to optimally inflate the lungs and lower carbon dioxide levels while using lower proximal airway pressures. However, the risk of extreme hyperventilation is present. Once adequate lung volume is achieved with high-frequency ventilation, improved response to supplemental therapies such as surfactant and inhaled nitric oxide may be seen.[102]

Infants with PPHN often demonstrate extreme lability. Regardless of the ventilation strategy used, weaning should be done cautiously while the pulmonary vasculature is reactive because aggressive decreases in FiO_2 may result in pulmonary vasospasm and sudden hypoxemia. Oxygen concentration is decreased cautiously, 1 percent

at a time. If the PaO_2 remains greater than 120 mmHg, weaning should continue. High peak inflating pressure should also be decreased cautiously, provided that carbon dioxide levels remain within the desired range and adequate oxygenation is maintained. Many infants receiving inhaled nitric oxide therapy show a significant decrease in the amount of ventilator support required to maintain adequate oxygenation.[103]

The transitional phase of PPHN is the point in the disease process when the hypoxemia no longer results from pulmonary artery hypertension but from chronic parenchymal lung disease.[104] This change usually occurs at 3 to 5 days of age. During the transition phase, $PaCO_2$ can be allowed to rise by decreasing ventilator settings. Caution must be taken to ensure that no sudden decline in PaO_2 occurs. Failure to wean from high pressures and rates during the transition phase can result in severe barotrauma. Each infant must be carefully evaluated to determine the best ventilatory approach to reverse the severe hypoxemia while causing the least amount of harm.

Drug Therapy

A variety of pharmacologic agents has been used in managing PPHN. Most infants receive some combination of analgesia and sedation during the course of mechanical ventilation; however, there is no accepted standard to guide clinical practice. Sedation may be utilized early in the course of treatment if the infant's spontaneous respiratory efforts are not synchronous with the ventilator. Intravenous midazolam infusions for sedation of infants requiring mechanical ventilation are commonly used in the NICU. Data from a review of randomized, controlled trials indicate infants treated with midazolam had a statistically higher incidence of hypotension, adverse neurologic events, and a longer length of stay in the NICU.[105] There are no studies comparing outcomes of preterm and term infants with a specific diagnosis of PPHN who were sedated with midazolam. Further research is needed to determine whether identified risks outweigh the benefits infants may receive from this therapy.

Opioids are effective in reducing behavioral and physiologic indicators of pain and stress in mechanically ventilated infants.[106] Morphine or fentanyl is commonly administered in bolus doses followed by a continuous infusion. Morphine sulfate is administered to decrease the infant's spontaneous activity and resistance to controlled ventilation. Careful blood pressure monitoring is essential because systemic hypotension is a known adverse effect and can worsen PPHN. Fentanyl is useful in infants with PPHN because it prevents pain-induced increases in pulmonary vascular resistance. Hemodynamic stability is maintained in infants receiving fentanyl because the drug causes less histamine release than morphine.[107]

Skeletal muscle paralysis may be pharmacologically induced with agents such as pancuronium bromide when sedation fails to produce a desired improvement in oxygenation and ventilation. Meticulous nursing care and continuous assessment of all bodily functions are required when neuromuscular blocking agents are used.

Volume expanders and pressor agents may be required to maintain normal blood pressure. When vascular volume has been restored and hypotension still exists, dopamine may be utilized to increase myocardial contractility, cardiac output, and blood pressure. Improvement in oxygenation may be seen when systemic blood pressure is greater than pulmonary blood pressure. Dobutamine is sometimes used in combination therapy with dopamine.

Surfactant replacement therapy is used when the PPHN is complicated by the coexistence of parenchymal lung disease. Early administration of surfactant may reduce the need for more invasive interventions.

Before inhaled nitric oxide was available, success with pharmacologic therapy for infants with PPHN was varied and unpredictable. No available drug had selective pulmonary vasodilator effects. Side effects such as systemic hypotension caused further deterioration. Critically ill infants with severe hypoxemia and evidence of pulmonary hypertension respond to inhaled nitric oxide with significant improvement in oxygenation. (See Chapter 13.) The need for further treatment with ECMO is reduced when inhaled nitric oxide is used to interrupt the cycle of hypoxemia.[84] Other novel therapies have been studied in centers where nitric oxide therapy was not available. A pilot study of sildenafil use in infants with PPHN demonstrated steady improvements in oxygenation with no detrimental effect on blood pressure.[108] However, there have been no large clinical trials to determine the safety, efficacy, and long-term effects of sildenafil use in the neonatal population.[109] More research is needed before sildenafil can be considered as standard therapy in treatment of PPHN in countries where nitric oxide is available.

Supportive Care

Protocols for minimal stimulation are utilized for infants with PPHN in many neonatal centers. The infant may be secluded in a quiet, darkened room with restrictions on caregivers and visitors. The infant's sensitivity to noise and handling during the acute stage of the disease is manifested by sudden and prolonged periods of hypoxia. Nursing care should be organized and coordinated to prevent unnecessary disturbances.

Pulse oximetry may be utilized simultaneously at preductal and postductal sites. Continuous arterial blood pressure monitoring is imperative. In term infants, the mean systemic arterial pressure should be maintained above 50 mmHg. Maintaining systolic pressures between 60 and 80 mmHg reduces the systemic to pulmonary pressure gradient, resulting in a decreased right-to-left shunt.[72] Vasopressor therapy is usually required to attain this.

Fluid balance must be maintained to ensure adequate intravascular volume and blood pressure. Central venous pressure monitoring may aid in determining adequacy of fluid replacement. General nursing care measures to ensure maintenance of skin integrity are essential because these infants may not tolerate frequent position changes.

Despite ventilatory, pharmacologic, and supportive therapies, some infants do not survive. Others have been saved with ECMO therapy.[110] Long-term follow-up care is necessary for all survivors because they are at increased risk for abnormal neurodevelopmental outcomes, including cognitive delays and hearing loss.[111] Whatever the treatment, the outcome for infants with PPHN varies according to the etiology and severity of the disease. The optimal approach to treating the infant with PPHN remains to be determined through clinical trials.

SUMMARY

Most infants admitted to neonatal intensive care units have respiratory disorders. Understanding the pathophysiology associated with each disease process is essential to ensure timely and comprehensive management. Knowledge of clinical presentation and etiology in relation to gestational age assists in differential diagnosis. The goal of therapy for neonatal respiratory disorders is the maintenance of adequate oxygenation and ventilation. Advances in antenatal care affect the prematurity rate and lessen the incidence of respiratory disorders related to immaturity. Technologic advances including exogenous surfactant, new modes of ventilation, ECMO, and inhaled nitric oxide therapy have improved outcomes for many infants with severe respiratory disease.

REFERENCES

1. Raja JU. 1988. Hyaline membrane disease. In *Neonatal Cardiopulmonary Distress*, Emmanouilides GC, and Baylen G, eds. Chicago: Year Book Medical Publishers, 54–55.

2. Heron M. 2011. Deaths: Leading causes for 2007. *National Vital Statistics Reports* 59(8): 1–95.

3. Lee K, et al. 1999. Trend in mortality from respiratory distress syndrome in the United States, 1970–1995. *Journal of Pediatrics* 134(4): 434–440.

4. Hack M, et al. 2000. Neurodevelopment and predictors of outcomes of children with birth weights of less than 1000 g: 1992–1995. *Archives in Pediatric and Adolescent Medicine* 154(7): 725–731.

5. National Institutes of Health. 1994. Effect of corticosteroids for fetal maturation on perinatal outcomes. *NIH Consensus Statement* 12(2): 1–24.

6. National Institutes of Health. 2000. Antenatal corticosteroids revisited: Repeat courses. *NIH Consensus Statement* 17(2): 1–18.

7. Crowther CA, and Harding JE. 2003. Repeat doses of prenatal corticosteroids for women at risk of preterm birth for preventing neonatal respiratory disease. *Cochrane Database of Systematic Reviews* (2): CD003935.

8. Suresh GK, and Soll RF. 2005. Overview of surfactant replacement trials. *Journal of Perinatology* 25(supplement 2): S40–S44.

9. Katz LA, and Klein JM. 2006. Repeat surfactant therapy for postsurfactant slump. *Journal of Perinatology* 26(7): 414–422.

10. Cotton RB. 1987. The relationship of symptomatic patent ductus arteriosus to respiratory distress in preterm newborn infants. *Clinics in Perinatology* 14(3): 621–633.

11. Swischuk LE. 2004. *Imaging of the Newborn Infant and Young Child, 5th ed.* Philadelphia: Lippincott Williams & Wilkins, 31, 41, 45.

12. Wesenberg RL. 1973. *The Newborn Chest.* Hagerstown, Maryland: Harper & Row, 45–46, 62, 74–83, 119–124.

13. Soll RF. 1998. Prophylactic synthetic surfactant for preventing morbidity and mortality in preterm infants. *Cochrane Database of Systematic Reviews* (3): CD001079.

14. Yost CC, and Soll RF. 1999. Early versus delayed selective surfactant treatment for neonatal respiratory distress syndrome. *Cochrane Database of Systematic Reviews* (3): CD001456.

15. Dani C, et al. 2004. Early extubation and nasal continuous positive airway pressure after surfactant treatment for respiratory distress syndrome among preterm infants <30 weeks' gestation. *Pediatrics* 113(6): e560–e563.

16. American Academy of Pediatrics, Committee of Fetus and Newborn. 1999. Surfactant replacement therapy for respiratory distress syndrome. *Pediatrics* 103(3): 684–685.

17. Phibbs CS, et al. 2007. Level and volume of neonatal intensive care and mortality in very-low-birth-weight infants. *New England Journal of Medicine* 356 (21): 2165–2175.

18. Northway WH Jr. 1992. An introduction to bronchopulmonary dysplasia. *Clinics in Perinatology* 19(3): 489–495.

19. Payne NR, et al. Reduction of bronchopulmonary dysplasia after participation in the Breathsavers Group of the Vermont Oxford Network Neonatal Intensive Care Quality Improvement Collaborative. *Pediatrics* 118(supplement 2): S73–S77.

20. Henderson-Smart DJ, et al. 2003. Elective high frequency oscillatory ventilation versus conventional ventilation for acute pulmonary dysfunction in preterm infants. *Cochrane Database of Systematic Reviews* (4): CD000104.

21. Bhuta T, and Henderson-Smart DJ. 1998. Rescue high frequency oscillatory ventilation versus conventional ventilation for pulmonary dysfunction in preterm infants. *Cochrane Database of Systematic Reviews* (3): CD000438.

22. Rojas MA, et al. 1995. Changing trends in the epidemiology and pathogenesis of neonatal chronic lung disease. *Journal of Pediatrics* 126(4): 605–610.

23. Marshall DD, et al. 1999. Risk factors for chronic lung disease in the surfactant era: A North Carolina population-based study of very low birth weight infants. *Pediatrics* 104(6): 1345–1350.

24. Martin JA, and Park MM. 1999. Trends in twin and triplet births: 1980–1997. *National Vital Statistics Reports* 47(24): 1–16.

25. Bland RD. 2005. Lung fluid balance during development. *NeoReviews* 6(6): e255–e267.

26. Milner AD, Saunders RA, and Hopkin IE. 1978. Effects of delivery by caesarean section on lung mechanics and lung volume in the human neonate. *Archives of Disease in Childhood* 53(7): 545–548.

27. Demissie K, et al. 1998. Maternal asthma and transient tachypnea of the newborn. *Pediatrics* 102(1 part 1): 84–90.

28. Bucciarelli RL, et al. 1976. Persistence of fetal cardiopulmonary circulation: One manifestation of transient tachypnea of the newborn. *Pediatrics* 58(2): 192–197.

29. Sundell H, et al. 1971. Studies on infants with Type II respiratory distress syndrome. *Journal of Pediatrics* 78(5): 754–764.

30. Bonta BW. 1988. Transient pulmonary vascular lability: A form of mild pulmonary hypertension of the newborn not requiring mechanical ventilation. *Journal of Perinatology* 8(1): 19–23.

31. Halliday HL, McClure G, and Reid MM. 1981. Transient tachypnoea of the newborn: Two distinct clinical entities? *Archives of Disease in Childhood* 56(5): 322–325.

32. Copetti R, and Cattarossi L. 2007. The "double lung point": An ultrasound sign diagnostic of transient tachypnea of the newborn. *Neonatology* 91(3): 203–209.

33. Merritt TA. 1984. Respiratory distress. In *Assessment of the Newborn: A Guide for the Practitioner*, Ziai M, Clark T, and Merritt TA, eds. Boston: Little, Brown, 168.

34. Dennehy PH. 1987. Respiratory infections in the newborn. *Clinics in Perinatology* 14(3): 667–682.

35. Puopolo KM, Madoff LC, and Eichenwald EC. 2005. Early-onset group B streptococcal disease in the era of maternal screening. *Pediatrics* 115(5): 1240–1246.

36. Schrag S, and Schuchat A. 2005. Prevention of neonatal sepsis. *Clinics in Perinatology* 32(3): 601–615.

37. Benitz WE, Gould JB, and Druzin ML. 1999. Risk factors for early-onset Group B streptococcal sepsis: Estimation of odds ratios by critical literature review. *Pediatrics* 103(6): e77.

38. Waites KB, Katz B, and Schelonka, RL. 2005. Mycoplasmas and ureaplasmas as neonatal pathogens. *Clinical Microbiology Reviews* 18(4): 757–789.

39. Cassell GH, et al. 1988. Association of *Ureaplasma urealyticum* infection of the lower respiratory tract with chronic lung disease and death in very-low-birth-weight infants. *Lancet* 2(8605): 240–245.

40. Sanchez PJ, and Regan JA. 1988. *Ureaplasma urealyticum* colonization and chronic lung disease in low birth weight infants. *Pediatric Infectious Disease Journal* 7(8): 542–546.

41. Reid L. 1977. Influence of the pattern of structural growth of lung on susceptibility to specific infectious diseases in infants and children. *Pediatric Research* 11(3 part 2): 210–215.

42. Christensen RD, Thibeault DW, and Hall RT. 1986. Neonatal bacterial and fungal pneumonia. In *Neonatal Pulmonary Care*, 2nd ed., Thibeault DW, and Gregory GA, eds. Norwalk, Connecticut: Appleton & Lange, 580.

43. Hudome SM, and Fisher MC. 2001. Nosocomial infections in the neonatal intensive care unit. *Current Opinion in Infectious Diseases* 14(3): 303–307.

44. Cordero L, et al. 2000. Ventilator-associated pneumonia in very-low-birth-weight infants at the time of nosocomial bloodstream infection and during airway colonization with *Pseudomonas aeruginosa. American Journal of Infection Control* 28(5): 333–339.

45. Apisarnthanarak A, et al. 2003. Ventilator-associated pneumonia in extremely preterm neonates in a neonatal intensive care unit: Characteristics, risk factors, and outcomes. *Pediatrics* 112(6 part 1): 1283–1289.

46. U.S. Food and Drug Administration. 1997. FDA safety alert: Risks of devices for direct detection of Group B streptococcal antigen. Rockville, Maryland: Department of Health and Human Services.

47. Sherman MP, Chance KH, and Goetzman BW. 1984. Gram's stains of tracheal secretions predict neonatal bacteremia. *American Journal of Diseases of Children* 138(9): 848–850.

48. Sherman MP, et al. 1980. Tracheal aspiration and its clinical correlates in the diagnosis of congenital pneumonia. *Pediatrics* 65(2): 258–263.

49. Manroe BL, et al. 1979. The neonatal blood count in health and disease. Part I: Reference values for neutrophilic cells. *Journal of Pediatrics* 95(1): 89–98.

50. Asmar BI, and Abdel-Haq NM. 2005. Macrolides, chloramphenicol, and tetracyclines. In *Neonatal and Pediatric Pharmacology: Therapeutic Principles in Practice*, 3rd ed., Yaffe SJ, and Aranda JV, eds. Philadelphia: Lippincott Williams & Wilkins, 403–408.

51. Steinbach WJ, and Perfect JR. 2005. Antifungal agents. In *Neonatal and Pediatric Pharmacology: Therapeutic Principles in Practice*, 3rd ed., Yaffe SJ, and Aranda JV, eds, Philadelphia: Lippincott Williams & Wilkins, 459–474.

52. Schleiss MR. 2005. Antiviral therapy of congenital cytomegalovirus infection. *Seminars in Pediatric Infectious Disease* 16(1): 50–59.

53. Brayer C, et al. 2004. Bronchopulmonary dysplasia and cytomegalovirus pneumonia. *Archives de Pédiatrie* 11(3): 223–225.

54. Smets K, et al. 2006. Selecting neonates with congenital cytomegalovirus infection for ganciclovir therapy. *European Journal of Pediatrics* 165(12): 885–890.

55. Wasserman RL. 1983. Unconventional therapies for neonatal sepsis. *Pediatric Infectious Disease Journal* 2(6): 421–423.

56. Short BL, Miller MK, and Anderson KD. 1987. Extracorporeal membrane oxygenation in the management of respiratory failure in the newborn. *Clinics in Perinatology* 14(3): 737–748.

57. Bacsik RD. 1977. Meconium aspiration syndrome. *Pediatric Clinics of North America* 24(3): 463–479.

58. Fenton AN, and Steer CM. 1962. Fetal distress. *American Journal of Obstetrics and Gynecology* 83(1): 354–362.

59. Wiswell TE, and Bent RC. 1993. Meconium staining and the meconium aspiration syndrome. *Pediatric Clinics of North America* 40(5): 955–981.

60. Yoder BA, et al. 2002. Changing obstetric practices associated with decreasing incidence of meconium aspiration syndrome. *Obstetrics and Gynecology* 99(5 part 1): 731–739.

61. Brown CA, et al. 1957. Meconium staining of the amniotic fluid: A marker of fetal hypoxia. *Obstetrics and Gynecology* 9(1): 91–103.

62. Tyler DC, Murphy J, and Cheney FW. 1978. Mechanical and chemical damage to lung tissue caused by meconium aspiration. *Pediatrics* 62(4): 454–459.

63. Whitsell J, et al. 2005. Acute respiratory disorders. In *Neonatology: Pathophysiology and Management of the Newborn*, 6th ed., MacDonald MG, Seshia MM, and Mullett MD, eds. Philadelphia: Lippincott Williams & Wilkins, 553–577.

64. Miyazaki FS, and Nevarez F. 1985. Saline amnioinfusion for relief of repetitive variable decelerations: A prospective randomized study. *American Journal of Obstetrics and Gynecology* 153(3): 301–306.

65. Pierce J, Gaudier FL, and Sanchez-Ramos L. 2000. Intrapartum amnioinfusion for meconium-stained fluid: Meta-analysis of prospective clinical trials. *Obstetrics and Gynecology* 95(6 part 2): 1051–1056.

66. Xu H, Hofmeyr J, Roy C, and Fraser W. Intrapartum amnioinfusion for meconium stained amniotic fluid: A systematic review of randomized controlled trials. *British Journal of Obstetrics and Gynaecology* 114(4): 383–390.

67. ACOG Committee on Obstetric Practice. 2006. ACOG Committee Opinion Number 346. Amnioinfusion does not prevent meconium aspiration syndrome. *Obstetrics and Gynecology* 108(4): 1053–1055.

68. Carson BS, et al. 1976. Combined obstetric and pediatric approach to prevent meconium aspiration syndrome. *American Journal of Obstetrics and Gynecology* 126(6): 712–715.

69. Ting P, and Brady JP. 1975. Tracheal suction in meconium aspiration. *American Journal of Obstetrics and Gynecology* 122(6): 767–771.

70. Gregory GA, et al. 1974. Meconium aspiration in infants—A prospective study. *Journal of Pediatrics* 85(6): 848–852.

71. Vain NE, et al. 2004. Oropharyngeal and nasopharyngeal suctioning of meconium-stained neonates before delivery of their shoulders: Multicentre, randomized controlled trial. *Lancet* 364(9434): 597–602.

72. Aguilar AM, and Nestor NE. 2011. The suctioning in the delivery room debate. *Early Human Development* 87(supplement 1): S13–S15.

73. Perlman JM, et al. 2010. Part 11: Neonatal resuscitation: 2010 international consensus on cardiopulmonary resuscitation and emergency cardiovascular care science with treatment recommendations. *Circulation* 122(16 supplement 2): S516–S538.

74. Linder N, et al. 1988. Need for endotracheal intubation and suction in meconium-stained neonates. *Journal of Pediatrics* 112(4): 613–615.

75. Davis RO, et al. 1985. Fatal meconium aspiration syndrome occurring despite airway management considered appropriate. *American Journal of Obstetrics and Gynecology* 151(6): 731–736.

76. Wiswell TE, et al. 2000. Delivery room management of the apparently vigorous meconium-stained neonate: Results of the multicenter, international collaborative trial. *Pediatrics* 105(1 part 1): 1–7.

77. Kattwinkel J, ed. 2011. *Textbook of Neonatal Resuscitation*, 6th ed. Elk Grove Village, Illinois: American Academy of Pediatrics and American Heart Association, 37–70.

78. Narchi H, and Kulaylat N. 1999. Is gastric lavage needed in neonates with meconium-stained amniotic fluid? *European Journal of Pediatrics* 158(4): 315–317.

79. Hough JL, Flenady, V, Johnson L, Woodgate PG. 2008. Chest physiotherapy for reducing respiratory morbidity in infants requiring ventilatory support. *Cochrane Database of Systematic Reviews* (3): CD006445.

80. Lin HC, et al. 2005. Role of antibiotics in management of non-ventilated cases of meconium aspiration syndrome without risk factors for infection. *Biology of the Neonate* 87(1): 51–55.

81. Wiswell TE, and Henley MA. 1992. Intratracheal suctioning, systemic infection, and the meconium aspiration syndrome. *Pediatrics* 89(2): 203–206.

82. Soll RF, and Dargaville P. 2000. Surfactant for meconium aspiration syndrome in full term infants. *Cochrane Database of Systematic Reviews* (2): CD002054.

83. Finer NN, and Barrington KJ. 2006. Nitric oxide for respiratory failure in infants born at or near term. *Cochrane Database of Systematic Reviews* (4): CD000399.

84. Hintz SR, et al. 2000. Decreased use of neonatal extracorporeal membrane oxygenation (ECMO): How new treatment modalities have affected ECMO utilization. *Pediatrics* 106(6): 1339–1343.

85. American Academy of Pediatrics, Committee on Fetus and Newborn. 2000. Use of inhaled nitric oxide. *Pediatrics* 106(2 part 1): 344–345.

86. Kinsella JP, et al. 2002. Use of inhaled nitric oxide during interhospital transport of newborns with hypoxemic respiratory failure. *Pediatrics* 109(1): 158–161.

87. Davidson D, et al. 1999. Safety of withdrawing inhaled nitric oxide therapy in persistent pulmonary hypertension of the newborn. *Pediatrics* 104(2 part 1): 231–235.

88. Heiss KF, and Bartlett RH. 1989. Extracorporeal membrane oxygenation: An experimental protocol becomes a clinical service. *Advances in Pediatrics* 36: 117–136.

89. Gersony WM, Duc GV, and Sinclair JC. 1969. "PFC" syndrome (persistence of the fetal circulation). *Circulation* 40(supplement 3): S87.

90. Walsh M, and Stork E. 2001. Persistent pulmonary hypertension of the newborn: Rational therapy based on pathophysiology. *Clinics in Perinatology* 28(3): 609–627.

91. Gersony WM. 1984. Neonatal pulmonary hypertension: Pathophysiology, classification, and etiology. *Clinics in Perinatology* 11(3): 517–524.

92. Henry GW. 1984. Noninvasive assessment of cardiac function and pulmonary hypertension in persistent pulmonary hypertension of the newborn. *Clinics in Perinatology* 11(3): 627–640.

93. Fox WW, and Duara S. 1983. Persistent pulmonary hypertension of the neonate: Diagnosis and management. *Journal of Pediatrics* 103(4): 505–514.

94. Riggs T, et al. 1977. Neonatal circulatory changes: An echocardiographic study. *Pediatrics* 59(3): 338–344.

95. Plum F, and Posner JB. 1967. Blood and cerebrospinal fluid lactate during hyperventilation. *American Journal of Physiology* 212(4): 864–870.

96. Bifano EM, and Pfannenstiel A. 1988. Duration of hyperventilation and outcome in infants with persistent pulmonary hypertension. *Pediatrics* 81(5): 657–661.

97. Ambalavanan N, and Carlo WA. 2001. Hypocapnia and hypercapnia in respiratory management of newborn infants. *Clinics in Perinatology* 28(3): 517–531.

98. Gannon CM, Wiswell TE, and Spitzer A. 1998. Volutrauma, $PaCO_2$ levels, and neurodevelopmental sequelae following assisted ventilation. *Clinics in Perinatology* 25(1): 159–174.

99. Walsh MC, and Stork EK. 2001. Persistent pulmonary hypertension of the newborn: Rational therapy based on pathophysiology. *Clinics in Perinatology* 28(3): 609–627.

100. Wung JT, et al. 1985. Management of infants with severe respiratory failure and persistence of the fetal circulation, without hyperventilation. *Pediatrics* 76(4): 488–494.

101. Gupta A, et al. 2002. Inhaled nitric oxide and gentle ventilation in the treatment of pulmonary hypertension of the newborn—A single-center, 5-year experience. *Journal of Perinatology* 22(6): 435–441.

102. Kinsella JP, and Abman SH. 1998. Inhaled nitric oxide and high frequency oscillatory ventilation in persistent pulmonary hypertension of the newborn. *European Journal of Pediatrics* 157(supplement 1): S28–S30.

103. Sadiq HF, et al. 2003. Inhaled nitric oxide in the treatment of moderate persistent pulmonary hypertension of the newborn: A randomized controlled, multicenter trial. *Journal of Perinatology* 23(2): 98–103.

104. Sosulski R, and Fox WW. 1982. Hyperventilation therapy for persistent pulmonary hypertension of the neonate and occurrence of a transition phase. *Pediatric Research* 16: 309A.

105. Ng E, Taddio A, and Ohlsson A. 2003. Intravenous midazolam infusion for sedation of infants in the neonatal intensive care unit. *Cochrane Database of Systematic Reviews* (1): CD002052.

106. Aranda JV, et al. 2005. Analgesia and sedation during mechanical ventilation in neonates. *Clinical Therapeutics* 27(6): 877–899.

107. Zenk KE, Sills JH, and Koeppel RM. 2003. *Neonatal Medications and Nutrition: A Comprehensive Guide*, 3rd ed. Petaluma, California: NICU Ink, 240–241, 411–414.

108. Baquero H, et al. 2006. Oral sildenafil in infants with persistent pulmonary hypertension of the newborn: A pilot randomized blinded study. *Pediatrics* 117(4): 1077–1083.

109. Shan PS, and Ohlsson A. 2011. Sidenafil for pulmonary hypertension in neonates. *Cochrane Database of Systematic Reviews* (8): CD005494.

110. O'Rourke PP, et al. 1989. Extracorporeal membrane oxygenation and conventional medical therapy in neonates with persistent pulmonary hypertension of the newborn: A prospective randomized study. *Pediatrics* 84(6): 957–963.

111. Lipkin PH, et al. 2002. Neurodevelopmental and medical outcomes of persistent pulmonary hypertension in term newborns treated with nitric oxide. *Journal of Pediatrics* 140(3): 306–310. (Comment in *Journal of Pediatrics*, 2002, 140(3): 284–287.)

NOTES

3 Neonatal Apnea

Ruben E. Alvaro, MD, FAAP

Apnea is a very common and troublesome disorder in newborns, especially in small premature infants. With the conquest of respiratory distress syndrome following the development of surfactant, the survival rate of very low birth weight (VLBW) infants has increased significantly. Not only are these tiny infants now surviving, but they are extubated and "forced" to breathe spontaneously sooner than in the past. As a result, apnea has now become one of the major clinical problems in our neonatal intensive care units. The prevalence of apnea increases exponentially with decrease in gestational age; it is seen in nearly 100 percent of infants born at <28 weeks gestational age.[1] Apneas are seen not only in spontaneously breathing infants (such as those recovering from lung diseases, feeding and growing preterm infants, and infants approaching discharge), but also in mechanically ventilated and critically ill infants.

This chapter reviews some important aspects of neonatal apnea, with emphasis on apnea of prematurity. Its objective is to identify the physiologic alterations in control of breathing that predispose infants to apnea, as well as to examine relevant treatment approaches for this condition.

DEFINITION

Apnea means cessation of respiratory airflow. Apnea is considered pathologic if it is prolonged (≥20 seconds) or associated with cyanosis; abrupt, marked pallor; hypotonia; or bradycardia.[2] However, what best defines *pathologic apnea* is not the duration of the respiratory pause, but the physiologic events resulting from the pause (i.e., the degree of bradycardia and desaturation the infant experiences). For example, VLBW infants (<1,500 g) do not tolerate apnea very well; they can develop significant bradycardia or desaturation with respiratory pauses lasting only 8 to 10 seconds. The term *apnea of infancy* generally refers to infants who are >37 weeks gestational age at onset of pathologic apnea. The term *apnea of prematurity* is reserved for pathologic apnea occurring in a premature infant that usually ceases by 37 weeks gestational age.[2]

Pathologic apnea should be differentiated from *periodic breathing*, which is characterized by recurring cycles of short respiratory pauses >3 seconds duration with <20 seconds of respiration between pauses (Figure 3-1). Although periodic breathing is considered by many to be a benign disorder, it may have the same physiopathologic root as apnea of prematurity. That would make apnea of prematurity just a further step in the basic disturbance that induces periodic breathing. Thus, the cyclic changes in respiratory frequency and tidal volume observed during periodic breathing may result, at least in part, from the instability of the respiratory center, an instability that in more severe form could manifest as apnea.[3] In support of this view, Al-Saedi and colleagues and Waggener and coworkers have found that long apneas (>20 seconds) are not random events, but are part of the underlying instability of the breathing pattern. These apneas are preceded by frequent apneas of shorter duration and by a decrease in respiratory frequency and minute ventilation (Figure 3-2).[4,5] That both disorders tend to decline in frequency with advancing postconceptional age, administration of methylxanthines, and a small increase in inspired oxygen further supports this view.

CLASSIFICATION

Apnea has traditionally been classified as central, obstructive, and mixed (Figure 3-3). This classification

FIGURE 3-1

Two respiratory flow patterns characteristic of periodic breathing (alternation between breathing periods and apnea) in two small preterm infants.

A. Ventilation/apnea ratio is approximately 2, and the infant hyperventilates in relation to episodes of regular breathing.
B. Ratio is 0.4, and the infant hypoventilates.

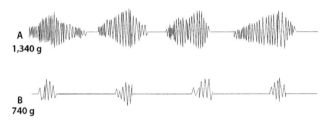

FIGURE 3-2

Likelihood of a prolonged apneic episode during the 11th minute of monitoring based on the number of apneic episodes in the preceding 10 minutes.

The risk of a prolonged apnea in the 11th minute increases significantly when the 11th minute is preceded by a period containing a large number of apneic episodes (more than ten) rather than by an apnea-free period.

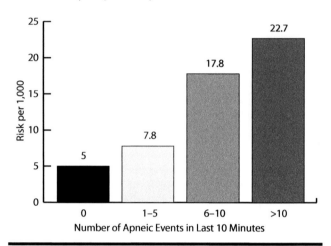

From: Al-Saedi SA, et al. 1997. Prolonged apnea in the preterm infant is not a random event. *American Journal of Perinatology* 14(4): 198. Reprinted by permission.

is based on the presence or absence of inspiratory muscle activity. In central apnea, airflow (usually measured at the nasal level) and inspiratory muscle activity (measured by diaphragmatic activity or by abdominal or thoracic movements) are absent. Obstructive apnea presents with absent airflow, but with inspiratory muscle activity throughout the apnea. This type of apnea is rare, tends to be of short duration (<10 seconds), and usually occurs before or after generalized body movements. Obstructive apnea that lasts longer (>20 seconds) is usually seen in infants born with Robin sequence (hypoplastic mandible); those who develop bronchopulmonary dysplasia; and those with severe neurologic problems such as intracranial hemorrhage, hydrocephalus, and severe asphyxia.[6,7] Mixed apnea has both central and obstructive components; this type of apnea is most commonly observed in small preterm infants. It can go undetected by transthoracic impedance and present with bradycardia or desaturations. Because most mixed apneas start with a central pause followed by obstruction, they comprise a progressively greater proportion of all apneas as apnea duration increases. The lack of central output during the initial central pause produces a loss of or decrease in airway smooth muscle tone, with concomitant airway collapse.[8] Consistent with this mechanism is the observation that short apneas are more likely central and that longer apneas (>15 seconds) are more likely mixed (Figure 3-4).[9]

PATHOPHYSIOLOGY

Although a significant amount of new knowledge regarding neonatal apnea has been acquired in the past 20 years, the exact mechanism that triggers apnea remains controversial. Immaturity of the respiratory center has been accepted as the key element for the pathogenesis of apnea of prematurity. However, *immaturity* is a vague term. Is this immaturity related to an immaturity of the synaptic connections between the respiratory neurons in the brainstem? Is it, instead, related to the neurotransmitters and neuromodulators that cause either inhibition (such as γ-aminobutyric acid [GABA], adenosine, endorphins, and prostaglandins) or stimulation (such as glutamate and aspartate) of respiration? The exact manner in which all of these factors are altered during neonatal apnea remains unknown.

There are two factors that, together with other aspects of the immature respiratory feedback loop, play a major role in the high prevalence of periodic breathing and apnea in infants compared to adults. The first is increased peripheral chemoreceptor activity.

The most important peripheral chemoreceptors are located in the carotid bodies at the bifurcation of the common carotid arteries. These chemoreceptors respond to decreases in arterial PO_2 and pH and increases in arterial PCO_2. The relationship between firing rate and arterial PO_2 is very nonlinear, with very little response until the arterial PO_2 is reduced below 100 mmHg. At this point, the rate rapidly increases. The peripheral chemoreceptors are responsible for all the increase in

FIGURE 3-3
Examples of different type of apneas.

Central apneas occur when respiratory efforts are absent; obstructive apneas, when efforts are continuously present; and mixed apneas, when elements of both central and obstructive apneas are present.

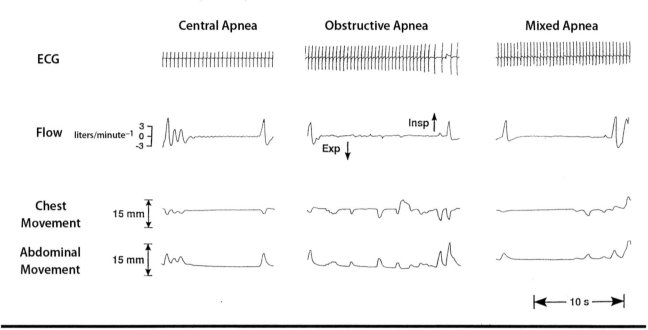

From: Al-Saedi SA, et al. 1997. Prolonged apnea in the preterm infant is not a random event. *American Journal of Perinatology* 14(4): 198. Reprinted by permission.

ventilation that occurs in response to hypoxemia. In the absence of these receptors, severe hypoxemia depresses respiration, presumably through a direct effect on the respiratory centers.

Research has shown that peripheral chemoreceptor activity is significantly increased in early life versus adulthood and in infants breathing periodically versus those breathing continuously.[10] This increased peripheral chemoreceptor activity corresponded to a lower arterial PO_2 in one of the groups of infants being studied. Thus, low arterial PO_2 leads to increased peripheral chemoreceptor activity and more instability of breathing because minor changes in PO_2 can greatly alter baseline ventilation. These findings support the hypothesis that the drive to breathe early in life depends on increased peripheral chemoreceptor activity and that this heightened peripheral chemoreceptor activity may play a role in disturbing the respiratory control system, leading to periodic breathing and apnea. That even a small amount of supplemental oxygen greatly reduces periodic breathing and apnea supports the notion that hypoxemia is a vital factor in the mechanism responsible for apnea in preterm infants (Figure 3-5).[11]

FIGURE 3-4
Incidence of apnea types at various apnea durations.

The graph shows a significant decrease in the proportion of central apneas with increasing apnea duration ($p<.001$). Conversely, there is a significant increase in the proportion of mixed apneas with increasing apnea duration ($p<.001$).

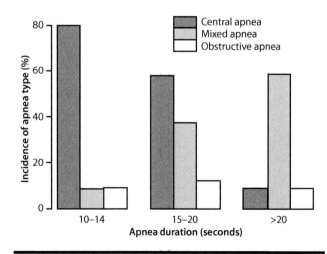

From: Butcher-Puech MC, et al. 1985. Relation between apnoea duration and type and neurological status of preterm infants. *Archives of Disease in Childhood* 60(10): 956. Reprinted by permission.

FIGURE 3-5
Change in respiratory pattern with gradual increase in inspired O$_2$.

Respiratory flow recorded in one preterm infant, age 16 days, 1,600 g. Note regularization of breathing pattern with increased inspired O$_2$.

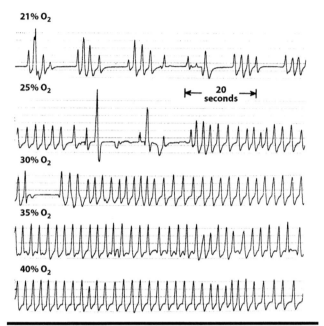

21% O$_2$

25% O$_2$

30% O$_2$

35% O$_2$

40% O$_2$

From: Weintraub Z, et al. 1992. Effects of inhaled oxygen (up to 40%) on periodic breathing and apnea in preterm infants. *Journal of Applied Physiology* 72(1): 117. Copyright by American Physiology Society. Reprinted by permission.

FIGURE 3-6
Relationship between CO$_2$ apneic threshold and baseline or actual PCO$_2$ levels in neonates and adults.

Because of the proximity of these two levels in neonates, PCO$_2$ is much more likely to dive below the apneic threshold in newborns than in adults.

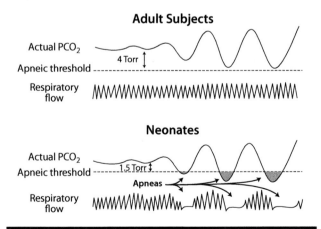

Adult Subjects

Actual PCO$_2$

Apneic threshold — 4 Torr

Respiratory flow

Neonates

Actual PCO$_2$
Apneic threshold — 1.5 Torr

Apneas

Respiratory flow

FIGURE 3-7
Increases in ventilatory sensitivity to inhaled CO$_2$ with increasing gestational age.

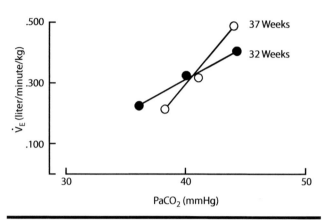

37 Weeks

32 Weeks

From: Rigatto H, Brady JP, and de la Torre Verduzco R. 1975. Chemoreceptor reflexes in preterm infants. Part II: The effects of gestational and postnatal age on the ventilatory response to inhaled carbon dioxide. *Pediatrics* 55(5): 617. Reprinted by permission.

The second factor is the PCO$_2$ apneic threshold, which is the minimal PCO$_2$ level that sustains respiration. When the CO$_2$ level decreases below this minimal level, breathing stops. This notion of a CO$_2$ apneic threshold is crucial to our understanding of periodic breathing and apnea in humans. Research has suggested that the closer the eupneic PCO$_2$ is to the threshold PCO$_2$, the more prone the infant is to instability of breathing.[12] Khan and associates have shown that the average CO$_2$ apneic threshold in preterm infants is only 1.5 torr lower than the actual or baseline PCO$_2$, whereas, in adults, it is approximately 5 torr lower.[13] This narrow difference between eupneic and apneic PCO$_2$ in neonates is likely related to a low baseline PCO$_2$ caused by a decrease in metabolism triggered by hypoxemia. Thus, the great variability in tidal volume with major oscillations in PCO$_2$ under normal circumstances together with the closeness of the CO$_2$ apneic threshold to the baseline CO$_2$ likely contribute to the high prevalence of periodic breathing in infants compared to adults (Figure 3-6).[3]

Studies have shown that inhalation of low concentrations of CO$_2$ regularizes breathing and decreases apnea time in preterm infants. Although the exact mechanism by which CO$_2$ inhalation reduces apnea is not completely understood, it is likely related to decreased

FIGURE 3-8
Steady-state CO$_2$ response curves at different inspired O$_2$ concentrations in preterm infants.

The lower the inspired O$_2$, the flatter the response to CO$_2$.

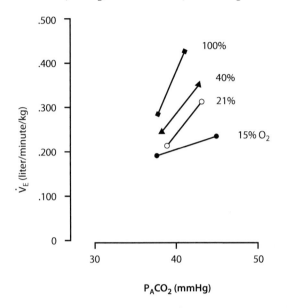

From: Rigatto H, de la Torre Verduzco R, and Gates DB. 1975. Effects of O$_2$ on the ventilatory response to CO$_2$ in preterm infants. *Journal of Applied Physiology* 39(6): 898. Reprinted by permission.

FIGURE 3-9
Comparison of CO$_2$ sensitivity obtained from ventilatory responses to changing alveolar PCO$_2$ in preterm infants with and without apnea.

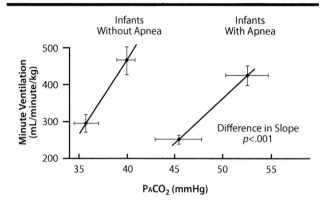

Adapted from: Gerhardt T, and Bancalari E. 1984. Apnea of prematurity: Part I: Lung function and regulation of breathing. *Pediatrics* 74(1): 60. Reprinted by permission.

FIGURE 3-10
Percent change in ventilation when 15 percent O$_2$ was substituted for 21 percent O$_2$ in preterm infants (solid circles) and 12 percent O$_2$ was substituted for 15 percent O$_2$ in adult subjects (open circles).

Preterm infants on 15 percent O$_2$ do not sustain hyperventilation, and ventilation decreases toward the end of five minutes.

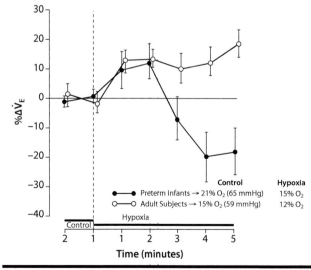

From: Sankaran K, et al. 1979. Immediate and late ventilatory response to 100% and 15% O$_2$ in preterm infants and adult subjects. *Pediatric Research* 13(8): 876. Reprinted by permission.

breath-to-breath fluctuations of arterial PCO$_2$, raising and stabilizing it above the apneic threshold.[14]

An aspect of the immature respiratory feedback loop that plays a role is the ventilatory response to CO$_2$. This primarily measures the activity of the central chemoreceptors located in the brain stem. The response is normally measured by having the subject inhale CO$_2$ mixtures or rebreathe from a bag so that the inspired PCO$_2$ gradually rises. The ventilatory response to CO$_2$ is expressed as the change in minute ventilation with changes in alveolar or arterial PCO$_2$. This response has been shown to increase from 32 to 37 weeks gestational age and from 2 to 27 days postnatal age. This increase likely relates to the growing maturity of the central nervous system (Figure 3-7).[15,16]

One of the most intriguing findings in preterm infants, compared with adult subjects, is their opposite response to CO$_2$ when various concentrations of O$_2$ are administered. In adults, the lower the inspired O$_2$ concentration, the steeper the response to CO$_2$. In the preterm infant, a progressive decrease in inspired O$_2$ concentration causes a significant flattening of CO$_2$ responsiveness (Figure 3-8).[17] This paradoxical response is likely related to the central depressive effect of hypoxia.

FIGURE 3-11
Changes in ventilatory variables in response to 15 percent O₂ in preterm infants ≤1,500 g.

Left: A sustained decrease in ventilation occurred in both sleep states, mainly because of a decrease in breathing frequency. **Right:** Percentage changes in ventilation show that during REM sleep, ventilation decreased significantly more than in quiet sleep as a result of a lack of increase in tidal volume. Values are mean ± SEM.[‡]

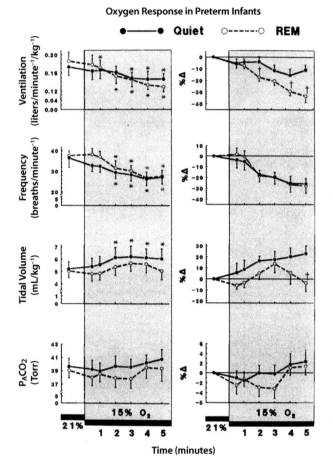

Oxygen Response in Preterm Infants

●——● Quiet   ○-----○ REM

15% O₂   21%   1 2 3 4 5

Time (minutes)

* $p \le .05$ compared with control
† $p \le .05$ between sleep states
‡ SEM = standard error of the mean

From: Alvaro R, et al. 1992. Small preterm infants (less than or equal to 1,500 g) have only a sustained decrease in ventilation in response to hypoxia. *Pediatric Research* 32(4): 405. Reprinted by permission.

Although Gerhardt and Bancalari reported in 1984 that preterm infants with apnea have a decreased ventilatory response to CO_2 compared with infants without apnea, a clear cause-effect relationship between the decreased response to CO_2 and apnea of prematurity has not yet been firmly established.[18] Both might simply represent aspects of a decreased respiratory drive (Figure 3-9).

Another aspect is the ventilatory response to hypoxia, which measures primarily the activity of the peripheral chemoreceptors located in the carotid bodies. This response is measured by having the subject inhale a concentration of O_2 less than that of room air (usually 12–15 percent) so that the arterial PO_2 gradually decreases. The ventilatory response to hypoxia is expressed as the percent change in ventilation in response to a change in alveolar or arterial PO_2. This response is also unique in preterm infants and is characterized by the classical biphasic response consisting of an initial increase in ventilation that lasts one to two minutes, followed by a decline in breathing toward the end of five minutes, often below baseline ventilation (Figure 3-10).[19,20] The initial hyperventilation is similar to that seen in adult subjects and results from stimulation of the peripheral chemoreceptors. The late decline in ventilation is poorly understood, but it is likely related to the central depressant effect of hypoxia mediated by GABA,[21] adenosine,[22] endothelin,[23] and endorphins,[24] which overrule the peripheral stimulant effect. In very small infants (<1,500 g), the initial hyperventilatory phase is entirely absent, and only a decrease in ventilation is observed (Figure 3-11).[16] Although the exact relationship between this hypoxic ventilatory depression and neonatal apnea is not completely clear, it is likely a significant factor in the appearance of periodic breathing and the delay in recovery after episodes of apnea. This is discussed further in the following section.

A third factor is pulmonary and airway reflexes. Lung distention is associated with a decrease in inspiratory time and prolongation of expiratory time, mediated by stimulation of slowly adapting receptors innervated by myelinated vagal fibers (the well-known Hering-Breuer inflation reflex).[25-27] This reflex is much more active in the newborn period than in adult life and may cause significant apnea when stimulated. The role that this reflex plays in apnea of prematurity is controversial. However, as in the adult, the reflex is likely not significant during normal breathing.

Rapid compression of the lower ribs produces instant diaphragmatic inhibition through an intercostal phrenic inhibitory reflex.[28] This reflex may be stimulated during the chest distortion that frequently occurs in preterm infants during rapid eye movement (REM) sleep and may be an important contributor to periodic breathing and apnea.

The immaturity of other pulmonary reflexes may also play a role in some apneas. This may apply especially to those reflexes associated with decreased lung volume (Hering-Breuer deflation reflex),[25] airway obstruction (gamma system), endotracheal suctioning of intubated infants (irritant reflexes), and in the pulmonary congestion observed in preterm infants with significant left-to-right shunting through the patent ductus arteriosus (J receptors).

Reflexes originating in the upper airway play an important role, not only in triggering apnea episodes, but also in terminating them. The same stimulation of chemoreceptors and mechanoreceptors of the upper airway that produces cough and increases breathing in adults could trigger a fatal apnea in preterm infants.[29,30] This reflex-induced apnea is mediated through the superior laryngeal nerve.[29–31] It is observed with severe gastroesophageal reflux (GER) and with mechanical stimulation of the back of the pharynx with suctioning or when introducing a nasogastric tube.[32] This reflex-induced apnea is also present in preterm infants inhaling high concentrations of CO_2 (approximately 8 percent). This apnea is not present in term neonates or adults under the same circumstances, suggesting that maturation plays an important role in triggering this reflex.[33,34]

Sleep state is also a factor. It is accepted today that sleep modulates breathing and may predispose infants to periodic breathing and apnea. It is also known that periodic breathing and apnea occur more commonly during REM sleep.[35–38] Because infants sleep most of the time and spend approximately 33 percent of their sleep time in REM sleep (whereas adult subjects sleep only 20 percent of the time and spend approximately 20 percent of their sleep time in REM sleep), sleep is likely to have a greater effect on breathing patterns in infants than in adults.

Several physiologic factors favor the appearance of periodic breathing and apnea during REM sleep. First, during REM sleep, the intercostal muscles are inactivated, exaggerating the tendency of the upper rib cage to collapse during normal inspiration.[39] As mentioned previously, this would enhance chest distortion and asynchronous breathing (abdominal expansion during inspiration accompanied by inward movement of the rib cage), which through the intercostal-phrenic-inhibitory reflex may cause apnea.[28] Second, REM sleep also inhibits the expiratory activity of the adductor muscles of the larynx, preventing closure of the airway during expiration.[40] This, together with the loss of intercostal tone, would decrease lung volume, leading to hypoxemia, respiratory instability, and apnea. Third, sighs are very common in neonates and are more frequent in REM than in quiet sleep.[41] The increased presence of sighs likely relates to the increased tendency of lung volume to decrease; sighs restore lung volume.

However, it has been shown that sighs may trigger a run of periodic breathing and apneas by decreasing PCO_2 below the threshold level for apnea.[42]

CLINICAL PROBLEMS ASSOCIATED WITH APNEA

Although most apneas in newborns represent a disorder of the central control of breathing secondary to immaturity, apnea may also result from a variety of clinical conditions that frequently affect newborn infants.

Apnea occurring immediately after birth in term infants is usually associated with maternal oversedation and/or a result of excessive oropharyngeal secretions in the neonate. Infection (sepsis, meningitis, necrotizing enterocolitis) is a very frequent cause of neonatal apnea. Term or preterm infants displaying apnea should be promptly evaluated and treated for infection, especially when the frequency and/or the severity of the apnea suddenly worsens. Although the precise mechanism by which infection presents with apnea is not clear, toxic central depression appears to be involved. In older infants, respiratory syncytial virus (RSV) infection may initially present with severe apnea.

Disturbances of the central nervous system may also be associated with apnea. Intracranial hemorrhage (very common in small preterm infants), asphyxia, and malformations of the brain (Arnold-Chiari malformation) may cause apnea.[43] Central hypoventilation (Ondine's curse) is a rare but devastating disorder that can present as apnea in an otherwise normal infant. Metabolic disorders such as hypoglycemia, hypocalcemia, and electrolyte imbalance, although rare now because of stricter clinical controls, can precipitate apnea. Clinical conditions that cause decreased oxygen delivery (such as severe anemia, hypoxemia, shock, and a patent ductus arteriosus) may also predispose infants to apnea. Hyperthermia, whether iatrogenic or secondary to an infection, is another well-known precipitating factor for apnea, especially in small preterm infants. Medications given to the mother before delivery (narcotics, magnesium sulfate) or directly to the infant (prostaglandin E_1 to maintain ductal patency, narcotics, benzodiazepines, and barbiturates for sedation) can produce apnea in neonates. Pulmonary conditions that cause mechanical restrictions or hypoxemia (such as severe respiratory distress syndrome, airway obstruction, and thoracic dystrophies) can cause apnea likely secondary to increased work of breathing causing respiratory muscle fatigue.

FIGURE 3-12
Cerebral blood flow velocity (CBFV) and coefficient of variation (CV) of CBFV in four respiratory patterns.

Note that mean CBFV was similar in the four respiratory patterns (p= NS). However, the CV of CBFV was significantly higher (p<.05) in periodic and apneic breathing than during regular and irregular respiratory patterns. Values are mean ± SEM.[†]

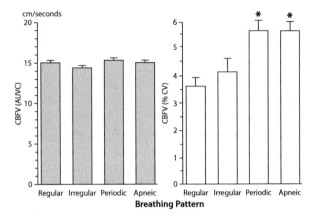

* p<.05
† SEM = standard error of the mean
Key: AUVC = area under velocity curve

From: Rehan VK, et al. 1996. Influence of sleep state and respiratory pattern on cyclical fluctuations of cerebral blood flow velocity in healthy preterm infants. *Biology of the Neonate* 69(6): 362. Reprinted by permission.

GER has been implicated as a cause of neonatal apnea. This has contributed to the widespread use of antireflux medications to treat apnea of prematurity.[44,45] Although GER is a near-universal phenomenon in preterm infants, its overall role in the pathogenesis of apnea of prematurity remains unclear. We can conclude from recent studies using continuous pH monitoring and esophageal impedance that GER does not contribute significantly to the overall frequency of apnea in preterm infants and that the use of antireflux medications for the treatment of apnea of prematurity can no longer be supported.[46–49]

CONSEQUENCES OF APNEA

HYPOXEMIA

Most infants experience a decrease in oxygenation following an apneic episode; the severity of the hypoxemia is directly related to the duration of the respiratory pause. Also, apnea with an obstructive component decreases oxygenation more than does purely central apnea.[13] However, in a number of apneas, the decrease in oxygenation cannot be explained solely by a lack of ventilation because the hypoxemia develops so rapidly and with such severity. In these cases, the primary event causing or contributing to the hypoxemia may

be right-to-left intrapulmonary shunting that in turn may cause respiratory depression and further aggravate hypoxemia. This intrapulmonary shunting may occur secondary to distal airway closure triggered by intermittent falls in lung volume below normal functional residual capacity during repeated apneic pauses.[50] Closure of the small airways may even occur during continuous breathing as a result of the infant's very compliant chest wall and the immaturity of the bronchiolar wall supporting tissues.[51,52] This small-airway closure may also occur as a result of activation of C-fiber nerve endings by secretions or inflammation (lower respiratory tract infections).[53,54] Other potential triggers for small-airway closure may include autonomic activity (GER), airway hypoxia (bronchopulmonary dysplasia), and a fall in cardiac output (cyanotic breath-holding spells).[55–60]

BRADYCARDIA

A decrease in heart rate may begin within 1.5 to 4 seconds of the onset of an apnea.[61,62] Because bradycardia usually follows the onset of hypoxemia, it has been postulated that, in the majority of episodes, apnea or hypoventilation, with a concomitant fall in lung volume, is the initiating event. The decrease in oxygen saturation that follows would cause bradycardia as a result of hypoxic stimulation of the peripheral chemoreceptors.[63] The rapid fall in heart rate observed during some apneic episodes may also be related to a complex reflex similar to the diving reflex of the seal. This reflex is characterized by the occurrence of apnea with superior laryngeal and trigeminal nerve stimulation producing a greatly enhanced bradycardia.[64] This inhibitory reflex may be triggered by activation of laryngeal receptors during swallowing, causing simultaneous apnea and bradycardia.[34]

CHANGES IN BLOOD PRESSURE

Short apnea associated with mild bradycardia is accompanied by an increase in systolic blood pressure. This systolic blood pressure rise is caused by an increase in stroke volume resulting from a greater filling volume of the heart during bradycardia (Starling's law).[34,65] A decrease in systemic blood pressure may occur with more severe apnea and bradycardia.

CHANGES IN CEREBRAL BLOOD FLOW

The lack of cerebrovascular autoregulation in infants means that cerebral blood flow mirrors changes in arterial blood pressure. In our laboratory, we studied the relationship between apnea and cerebral blood flow. In the first study, in term infants, we found that cerebral blood flow remained stable during central apneas as a result of an increase in flow velocity with each heartbeat to compensate for the decrease in heart rate that accompanied those apneas. In the second study, this one in preterm infants, we studied the influence of sleep state and different respiratory patterns on cerebral blood flow. We found that although flow velocity was similar during the different sleep states and respiratory patterns, variability or fluctuations in cerebral blood flow were greater during REM sleep and during periodic breathing and apnea than during regular respiratory patterns (Figure 3-12).[66,67]

DIAGNOSIS

The high incidence of apnea in preterm infants makes respiratory and cardiovascular monitoring mandatory in infants <35 weeks gestational age, as well as in high-risk infants >35 weeks gestational age. Most neonatal intensive care units rely on a combination of heart rate and impedance alarm systems, supplemented by oxygen saturation monitors. Although impedance electrodes fail to detect obstructive or mixed apneas, the heart rate and the oxygen saturation monitors should detect the bradycardia and oxygen desaturation that are usually associated with these events. For precise diagnosis of airway obstruction, more specific techniques are required; these include pneumotachography, nasal thermistors, plethysmography, and end-tidal carbon dioxide monitoring. Such techniques are rarely used in routine clinical practice, however. In our neonatal unit, respiratory alarms are set at 20 seconds, heart rate monitors set at 80 beats per minute, and the oxygen saturation monitors set at 80 percent to monitor for apnea.

If apnea presents in a term infant or in a preterm infant who is unwell or who experiences a sudden increase in the number or severity of apneic episodes, the infant should be investigated for other associated clinical problems, as previously discussed.

GENERAL SUPPORTIVE TREATMENT

Maintenance of optimal metabolic and biochemical balance is important in preventing many apneic episodes. The first consideration to be made is whether the apnea is severe enough to warrant further investigation and then treatment. The factors to be considered are the frequency and duration of the apneic episodes as well as their severity as measured by the degree of bradycardia, oxygen desaturation, and the type of stimulation needed

to terminate the event. In general, the smaller the infant, the more aggressive one should be in preventing apnea.

In VLBW infants, the temperature should be kept at the lower end of the thermoneutral range.[68,69] These infants should also be kept in the prone position with the head elevated because this position improves oxygenation and decreases the number of apneas, bradycardias, and desaturations.[70,71] Although there are no controlled trials to evaluate the benefits or possible harm of increases in inspired oxygen concentration, it is important to maintain these infants relatively well oxygenated, avoiding hyperoxemia (PaO_2 >70–80 mmHg). An oscillating water mattress used for kinesthetic stimulation has been found to be ineffective and is presently not recommended.[72]

MEDICAL TREATMENT

METHYLXANTHINES

Methylxanthines have become the treatment of choice for apnea of prematurity in the past 30 years. Since the initial report by Kuzemko and Paala in 1973, several studies have confirmed the efficacy of methylxanthines in reducing both the number of apneic episodes and the use of mechanical ventilation in preterm infants.[73,74] A major mechanism of action of methylxanthines is competitive antagonism of adenosine, a well-known respiratory inhibitor. Thus, xanthines have been shown to increase minute ventilation, improve CO_2 sensitivity, decrease the hypoxic depression of breathing, and enhance diaphragmatic activity.[75]

The most commonly used xanthines are theophylline and caffeine. Although they are similarly effective, caffeine has several advantages over theophylline and has become the preferred methylxanthine in the treatment of apnea. Its toxicity is lower and half-life longer, and there is less need for therapeutic drug monitoring.[76] Side effects of xanthines include tachycardia, cardiac dysrhythmias, feeding intolerance, increased metabolic rate and oxygen consumption, irritability, and, much less frequently, seizures. Adenosine is neuroprotective during ischemic episodes. By blocking it, methylxanthines have the potential to exacerbate ischemic brain damage during neonatal hypoxemia. Evidence from the late 1990s identifies the importance of the adenosine receptor system on neurodevelopment and behavior and of the potential for methylxanthines to permanently disrupt this ontogeny.[77–79] However, a recent multicenter trial comparing caffeine with a placebo in VLBW infants (CAP trial) showed a reduction of bronchopulmonary

FIGURE 3-13
Effect of CPAP on number of apneic episodes ≥10 seconds in ten infants.

Mixed and obstructive apnea decrease significantly during both periods of CPAP, with no effect on central apnea.

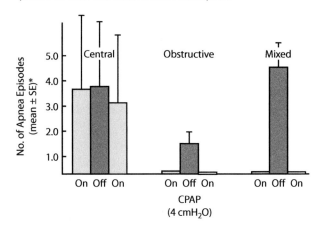

* SE = standard error

From: Miller MJ, Carlo WA, and Martin RJ. 1985. Continuous positive airway pressure selectively reduces obstructive apnea in preterm infants. *Journal of Pediatrics* 106(1): 92. Reprinted by permission.

dysplasia and improved rate fo survival without neuro-developmental disability at 18–21 months in the caffeine group.[80,81] In view of these results and its lower toxicity, caffeine would be the preferred drug for the treatment of apnea.[82]

CONTINUOUS POSITIVE AIRWAY PRESSURE (CPAP)

Nasal CPAP has been shown to be very effective in the treatment of apnea of prematurity.[83] Several mechanisms could be involved. The most important effects could be secondary to an improvement in lung volume and functional residual capacity, thereby improving oxygenation. Nasal CPAP decreases mainly mixed and obstructive apneas by splinting the upper airway (Figure 3-13).[84] Low levels of positive end-expiratory pressure (PEEP) (between 3 and 6 cmH$_2$O) are usually effective in treating apnea.[85] Higher pressures are more effective only in cases of laryngotracheomalacia. In small preterm infants, high levels of PEEP may increase the work of breathing and lead to muscle fatigue.

Improvements in nasal CPAP delivery using nasal intermittent positive pressure ventilation (NIPPV) in a synchronized or nonsynchronized mode and variable-flow nasal CPAP may increase the effectiveness of nasal CPAP for the treatment of apnea of prematurity.[86–88] NIPPV may improve patency of the upper airway by creating intermittently elevated pharyngeal pressures,

FIGURE 3-14
Apnea rate (top) and apnea time (bottom) decrease significantly in preterm infants with inhalation of low concentrations of CO$_2$.

Values are mean ± SEM.[†]

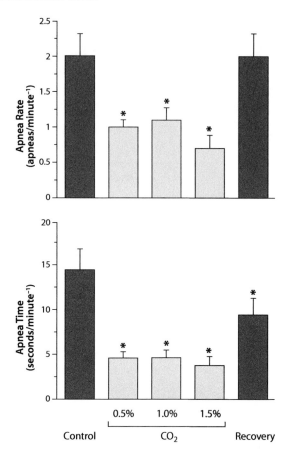

* $p<.05$
† SEM = standard error of the mean

From: Al-Saif S, et al. 2001. Inhalation of low (0.5%–1.5%) CO$_2$ as a potential treatment for apnea of prematurity. *Seminars in Perinatology* 25(2): 103. Reprinted by permission.

thus activating respiratory drive. Variable-flow nasal CPAP uses a more sophisticated prong that entrains gas on inspiration and shunts gas away from the infant on exhalation, minimizing device-dependent imposed work of breathing. This new form of nasal CPAP seems to recruit lung volume more effectively and to reduce the work of breathing compared with constant-flow nasal CPAP.[89] Several randomized trials are currently under way to test the effectiveness and safety of these new devices. Although a high-flow nasal cannula (1–2.5 liters/minute) can also generate positive distending pressure and has recently been suggested as an alternative modality for the treatment of apnea of prematurity, its safety has not been properly evaluated.[90]

FIGURE 3-15
Although inhalation of low concentrations of CO_2 (~1 percent) seems to be effective in reducing the number and severity of apneas in most infants, it was less effective than theophylline.

Values are mean ± SEM.[‡]

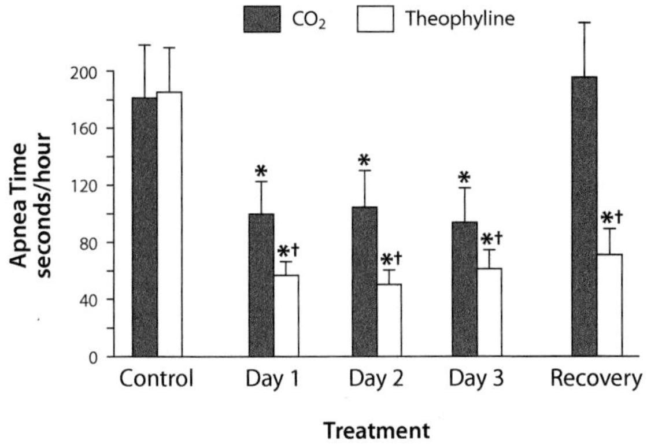

* $p<.05$ compared with control
† $p<0.05$ compared with CO_2
‡ SEM = standard error of the mean

Adapted from: Alvaro R, et al. 2012. CO_2 inhalation as a treatment for apnea of prematurity: A randomized double-blind controlled trial. The *Journal of Pediatrics* 160(2): 252–257, by American Academy of Pediatrics. Reproduced with permission of Mosby, Inc., in the format Journal via Copyright Clearance Center.

CO_2 INHALATION

Because CO_2 is the physiologic stimulus for breathing and it is known that most of the apnea in preterm infants occurs when the baseline CO_2 level decreases below the threshold for apnea, inhalation of low concentrations of CO_2 could be more physiologic and effective and produce fewer side effects than pharmacologic stimulants in the treatment of apnea. Earlier studies have shown that inhalation of low concentrations of CO_2 (0.5–1.5 per cent) through nasal prongs is effective in reducing the number of apneas in preterm infants (Figure 3-14). This was accompanied by an increase in minute ventilation and oxygenation. Breathing became more regular with each higher concentration of CO_2, during both REM and quiet sleep.[14] In a recent randomized, controlled, double-blind study comparing the use of theophylline and CO_2 inhalation for apnea of prematurity, we have shown that although inhalation of low concentrations of CO_2 seems to be effective in reducing the number and severity of apneas in most infants, it was less effective than theophylline (Figure 3-15). The less effectiveness of CO_2 treatment compared with theophylline was likely related to the variability of the delivery of CO_2 in the clinical situation. While no significant adverse side effects were found in the CO_2 group, infants in the theophylline group showed significantly more episodes of emesis, tachycardia, and jitteriness.[91] These findings suggest that inhalation of low concentrations of CO_2, as used in that study, cannot be considered an alternative to theophylline in the treatment of apnea of prematurity. Further studies should investigate the effect of different concentratons of CO_2 in preterm infants with significant apneas despite treatment with methylaxanthines.

MECHANICAL VENTILATION

When severe apnea persists in spite of previous therapeutic attempts, endotracheal intubation and artificial ventilation may be needed. Minimal ventilatory settings should be used to allow for spontaneous ventilatory efforts and to minimize the risk of barotrauma. We prefer the use of a volume guarantee ventilatory mode using tidal volumes of approximately 4 mL/kg and short inspiratory times. The PEEP used is generally determined by lung pathology. The length of ventilatory support depends on the cause of the apnea, but is usually short.

RESOLUTION OF APNEA, RELATIONSHIP TO SUDDEN INFANT DEATH SYNDROME (SIDS), AND THE USE OF HOME MONITORING

The incidence of periodic breathing and apnea decreases as gestational and postnatal age increase. Most infants stop having significant episodes of apnea by the time they are able to control temperature and be fed entirely by breast or bottle—usually between 35 and 36 weeks postconceptional age. However, in extremely small preterm infants (those born <28 weeks gestation), apnea can persist beyond 40 weeks postconceptional age. Beyond 43 to 44 weeks postconceptional age, the incidence of cardiorespiratory events in preterm infants is similar to that in term infants.[92]

The hypothesis that apnea is the pathophysiologic precursor of SIDS was first proposed in 1972.[93] Despite extensive independent research since that time, the apnea theory has never been proved. A multicenter consortium, the Collaborative Home Infant Monitoring Evaluation (CHIME) Study Group, analyzed 29,000 days of monitoring data on 1,079 infants. They found that events previously described as "pathologic" were actually quite common, as determined by the presence of apnea/bradycardia events that exceeded the conventional alarm threshold in 43 percent of healthy term infants; 2.3 percent of those events were extreme. The risks for conventional or extreme events were not increased in the group with a history of one or more severe apparent life-threatening events or in the siblings of two or more SIDS victims. The group of preterm infants in the study had an increased incidence of both types of events, but the events disappeared once the infants reached 43 weeks postconceptional age.[92] However, the peak incidence of SIDS in preterm infants is well beyond that age.

Most cases of SIDS can be prevented by proper sleep position, use of proper infant bedding, elimination of pre- and postnatal exposure to tobacco smoke, and breastfeeding.[94] The remaining cases are likely associated with high environmental temperature, severe GER, congenital anomalies, viral infections, fatty acid metabolic disorders, abnormal mast cell function, interleukin 10 genotype, prolonged QT interval, and infanticide cases.[95–99] These residual causes of SIDS are unlikely to be prevented by home monitoring. Furthermore, the CHIME study found a high frequency of obstructive events that would have been missed by the transthoracic impedance monitors used for most home monitoring.

The American Academy of Pediatrics recommends that home cardiorespiratory monitoring *not* be prescribed to prevent SIDS. Home cardiorespiratory monitoring may be warranted for premature infants at high risk of recurrent episodes of apnea, bradycardia, and hypoxemia after hospital discharge, but it should be discontinued at approximately 43 weeks postmenstrual age.[100]

DEVELOPMENTAL OUTCOME

The clinical significance and long-term consequences of persistent apnea, bradycardia, and desaturation remain subjects of considerable debate. Separating the consequences of preterm birth from the effects of apnea of prematurity has proved difficult. Most preterm infants with significant apnea have other adverse perinatal and postnatal factors that are associated with poor neurodevelopmental outcomes. Those factors include perinatal asphyxia, intraventricular hemorrhage, periventricular leukomalacia, sepsis, bronchopulmonary dysplasia, and necrotizing enterocolitis, to mention a few. Moreover, many of these conditions by themselves can cause apnea.

Reports of long-term follow-up of high-risk infants have shown controversial results. Taylor and colleagues found that apnea of prematurity was among the factors that predicted poor neurodevelopmental outcome in a cohort of preterm infants followed to early school age.[101] Other studies, however, have failed to demonstrate a significant correlation between apnea of prematurity and poor neurologic outcome.[102–104] Clinical

trials now under way or proposed will help to identify whether these cardiorespiratory events are associated with long-term consequences, are markers for neurodevelopmental disturbances, and/or are associated with sleep-disordered breathing later on in life.

SUMMARY

Apnea is one of the most common clinical problems that we face in our neonatal units, especially now that smaller and more immature infants are surviving. Most apneas are of unknown etiology. They represent a disturbance of the respiratory control system, a system that is both poorly understood and improves with advancing gestational and postnatal age. Decreased response to CO_2, hypoxemia, immaturity of the pulmonary and upper airway reflexes, as well as the influence of sleep, predispose preterm infants to one or multiple incidents of apnea. More knowledge of the physiologic factors that control the respiratory center and its maturation will help us to better understand the mechanisms that trigger these apneas. Administration of respiratory stimulants and the use of nasal CPAP are, in general, very effective treatments for apnea of prematurity. Caffeine, being one of the safest and most cost-effective therapies, should now be considered the preferred drug for the treatment of apnea of prematurity. Further studies should investigate the effect of different concentrations of CO_2 in preterm infants with significant apneas despite treatment with methylxanthines. Peer-reviewed evidence indicates that newborn apnea and apnea of prematurity are neither predictive of nor precursors of SIDS. Home cardiorespiratory monitoring should not be prescribed to prevent SIDS. The clinical significance and long-term consequences of persistent apnea, bradycardia, and desaturation remain subjects of considerable debate.[105]

REFERENCES

1. Barrington K, and Finer N. 1991. The natural history of the appearance of apnea of prematurity. *Pediatric Research* 29(4 part 1): 372–375.

2. National Institutes of Health Consensus Development Conference on Infantile Apnea and Home Monitoring, Sept. 29 to Oct. 1, 1986. *Pediatrics* 79(2): 292–299.

3. Rigatto H. 2000. Periodic breathing. In *Sleep and Breathing in Children. A Developmental Approach*, Loughlin GM, Carroll JL, and Marcus CL, eds. New York: Marcel Dekker, 237–272.

4. Al-Saedi SA, et al. 1997. Prolonged apnea in the preterm infant is not a random event. *American Journal of Perinatology* 14(4): 195–200.

5. Waggener TB, et al. 1984. Apnea duration is related to ventilatory oscillation characteristics in newborn infants. *Journal of Applied Physiology* 57(2): 536–544.

6. Butcher-Puech MC, et al. 1985. Relation between apnoea duration and type and neurological status of preterm infants. *Archives of Disease in Childhood* 60(10): 953–958.

7. Fajardo C, et al. 1993. The incidence of obstructive apneas in preterm infants with and without bronchopulmonary dysplasia. *Early Human Development* 32(2-3): 197–206.

8. Mitchell RA, Herbert DA, and Baker DG. 1985. Inspiratory rhythm in airway smooth muscle tone. *Journal of Applied Physiology* 58(3): 811–920.

9. Lee D, et al. 1987. A developmental study on types and frequency distribution of short apneas (3 to 15 seconds) in term and preterm infants. *Pediatric Research* 22(3): 344–349.

10. Al-Matary A, et al. 2004. Increased peripheral chemoreceptor activity may be critical in destabilizing breathing in neonates. *Seminars in Perinatology* 28(4): 264–272.

11. Weintraub Z, et al. 1992. The effects of inhaled oxygen (up to 40%) on periodic-breathing and apnea in preterm infants. *Journal of Applied Physiology* 72(1): 116–120.

12. Xie A, et al. 2002. Apnea-hypopnea threshold for CO_2 in patients with congestive heart failure. *American Journal of Respiratory and Critical Care Medicine* 165(9): 1245–1250.

13. Khan A, et al. 2005. Measurement of the CO_2 apneic threshold in newborn infants: possible relevance for periodic breathing and apnea. *Journal of Applied Physiology* 98: 1171–1176.

14. Al-Saif S, et al. 2001. Inhalation of low (0.5%–1.5%) CO_2 as a potential treatment for apnea of prematurity. *Seminars in Perinatology* 25(2): 100–106.

15. Frantz ID III, et al. 1976. Maturational effects on respiratory responses to carbon dioxide in premature infants. *Journal of Applied Physiology* 41(1): 41–45.

16. Rigatto H, Brady JP, and De la Torre Verduzco R. 1975. Chemoreceptor reflexes in preterm infants. Part II: The effects of gestational and postnatal age on the ventilatory response to inhaled carbon dioxide. *Pediatrics* 55(5): 614–620.

17. Rigatto H, De la Torre Verduzco R, and Gates DB. 1975. Effects of O_2 on the ventilatory response to CO_2 in preterm infants. *Journal of Applied Physiology* 39(6): 896–899.

18. Gerhardt T, and Bancalari E. 1984. Apnea of prematurity. Part I: Lung function and regulation of breathing. *Pediatrics* 74(1): 58–62.

19. Cross KW, and Oppe TE. 1952. The effect of inhalation of high and low concentrations of oxygen on the respiration of the premature infant. *Journal of Physiology* 117(1): 38–55.

20. Rigatto H, Brady JP, and De la Torre Verduzco R. 1975. Chemoreceptor reflexes in preterm infants. Part I: The effect of gestational and postnatal age on the ventilatory response to inhalation of 100% and 15% oxygen. *Pediatrics* 55(5): 604–613.

21. Young RSK, et al. 1993. Effect of anoxia on excitatory amino acids in brain slices of rats and turtles: *In vitro* microdialysis. *American Journal of Physiology* 264(4 part 2): 716–719.

22. Lopes JM, et al. 1994. The role of adenosine on the hypoxic ventilatory response of the newborn piglet. *Pediatric Pulmonology* 17(1): 50–55.

23. Dreshraj IA, et al. 1993. Endothelin-1 (ET1) acting on central chemosensitive areas causes respiratory depression in piglets. *Pediatric Research* 33: 1923A.

24. DeBoeck C, et al. 1984. Naloxone reduces decrease in ventilation induced by hypoxia in newborn infants. *Journal of Applied Physiology* 56(6): 1507–1511.

25. Hering E, and Breuer J. 1868. Die Selbststeurung der Athmung durch den nervus vagus. *Sitzber Deut Akad Wiss Wein* 57: 672–677.

26. Cross KW, et al. 1960. The response of the newborn baby to inflation of the lungs. *Journal of Physiology* 151: 551–565.

27. Martin RJ, et al. 1978. The effect of lung volume on expiratory time in the newborn infant. *Journal of Applied Physiology* 45(1): 18–23.

28. Knill R, and Bryan AC. 1976. An intercostal-phrenic inhibitory reflex in human newborn infants. *Journal of Applied Physiology* 40(3): 352–356.

29. Goding GS, Richardson MA, and Trachy RE. 1987. Laryngeal chemoreflex: Anatomic and physiologic study by use of the superior laryngeal nerve in piglet. *Otolaryngology—Head and Neck Surgery* 97(1): 28–38.

30. Lee JC, Stoll BG, and Downing SE. 1977. Properties of the laryngeal chemoreflex in neonatal piglets. *American Journal of Physiology* 233(1): R30–R36.

31. Harding R. 1984. Function of the larynx in the fetus and newborn. *Annual Review of Physiology* 46: 645–659.

32. Pickens DL, Schefft D, and Thach BT. 1988. Prolonged apnea associated with upper airway protective reflexes in apnea of prematurity. *American Review of Respiratory Disease* 137(1): 113–118.

33. Alvaro RE, et al. 1993. A developmental study of the dose response of the upper airway reflex to CO_2. *American Review of Respiratory Disease* 148(4 part 1): 1013–1017.

34. Miller AJ. 1976. Characterization of the postnatal development of superior laryngeal nerve fibers in the postnatal kitten. *Journal of Neurobiology* 7(6): 483–493.

35. Mosso A. 1898. *Life of Man on the High Alps*. London: T. Fisher Unwin, 45.

36. Prechtl H. 1974. The behavioural states of the newborn infant. *Brain Research* 76(2): 185–212.

37. Rigatto H, and Brady JP. 1972. Periodic breathing and apnea in preterm infants. Part I: Evidence for hypoventilation possibly due to central respiratory depression. *Pediatrics* 50(2): 202–218.

38. Rigatto H, and Brady JP. 1972. Periodic breathing and apnea in preterm infants. Part II: Hypoxia as a primary event. *Pediatrics* 50(2): 219–228.

39. Henderson-Smart DJ, and Read DJC. 1979. Reduced lung volume during behavioral active sleep in the newborn. *Journal of Applied Physiology* 46(6): 1081–1085.

40. Harding R, Johnson P, and McClelland ME. 1980. Respiratory function of the larynx in developing sheep and the influence of sleep state. *Respiration Physiology* 40(2): 165–169.

41. Alvarez JE, et al. 1993. Sighs and their relationship to apnea in the newborn infant. *Biology of the Neonate* 63(3): 139–146.

42. Fleming PJ, et al. 1984. The development of stability of respiration in human infants: Changes in ventilatory responses to spontaneous sighs. *Journal of Physiology* 347: 1–16.

43. Henderson DJ, and Cohen GL. 1987. Interaction of central and peripheral factors in the irregular breathing and apnea of newborn infants. In *Neurobiology of the Control of Breathing*. Von Euler C, and Lagercrantz H, eds. New York: Raven Press, 67–73.

44. Spitzer AR, et al. 1984. Awake apnea associated with gastroesophageal reflux: A specific clinical syndrome. *Journal of Pediatrics* 104(2): 200–205.

45. Menon AP, Schefft GL, and Thack BT. 1985. Apnea associated with regurgitation in infants. *Journal of Pediatrics* 106(4): 625–629.

46. De Ajuriaguerra M, et al. 1991. Gastroesophageal reflux and apnea in prematurely born infants during wakefulness and sleep. *American Journal of Diseases of Children* 145(10): 1132–1136.

47. Kimball AL, and Carlton DP. 2001. Gastroesophageal reflux medications in the treatment of apnea in premature infants. *Journal of Pediatrics* 138(3): 355–360.

48. Peter CS, et al. 2002. Gastroesophageal reflux and apnea of prematurity: No temporal relationship. *Pediatrics* 109(1): 8–11.

49. Di Fiore JM, et al. 2005. Apnea is not prolonged by acid gastroesophageal reflux in preterm infants. *Pediatrics* 116(5): 1059–1063.

50. Poets CF, and Southall DP. 1991. Patterns of oxygenation during periodic breathing in preterm infants. *Early Human Development* 26(1): 1–12.

51. Mortola JP, et al. 1982. Dynamics of breathing in infants. *Journal of Applied Physiology: Respiratory, Environmental and Exercise Physiology* 52(5): 1209–1215.

52. Burri PH. 1984. Fetal and postnatal development of the lung. *Annual Review of Physiology* 46: 617–628.

53. Smith JJ, Lemen RJ, and Taussig LM. 1987. Mechanisms of viral-induced lower airway obstruction. *Pediatric Infectious Disease Journal* 6(9): 837–842.

54. Martinez FD, Taussig LM, and Morgan WJ. 1990. Infants with upper respiratory illnesses have significant reduction in maximal expiratory flow. *Pediatric Pulmonology* 9(2): 91–95.

55. Barnes PJ. 1986. Neural control of human airways in health and disease. *American Review of Respiratory Disease* 134(6): 1289–1314.

56. See CC, et al. 1989. Gastroesophageal reflux–induced hypoxemia in infants with apparent life-threatening event(s). *American Journal of Diseases of Children* 143(8): 951–954.

57. Tay-Uyboco JS, et al. 1989. Hypoxic airway constriction in infants of very low birth weight recovering from moderate to severe bronchopulmonary dysplasia. *Journal of Pediatrics* 115(3): 456–459.

58. Green M, and Widdicombe JG. 1966. The effects of ventilation of dogs with different gas mixtures on airway calibre and lung mechanics. *Journal of Physiology* 186(2): 363–381.

59. Ohlsson J, Middaugh M, and Hlastala MP. 1989. Reduction of lung perfusion increases VA/Q heterogeneity. *Journal of Applied Physiology* 66(5): 2423–2430.

60. Southall DP, Samuels MP, and Talbert DG. 1990. Recurrent cyanotic episodes with severe arterial hypoxaemia and intrapulmonary shunting: A mechanism for sudden death. *Archives of Disease in Childhood* 65(9): 953–961.

61. Vyas H, Milner AD, and Hopkin IE. 1981. Relationship between apnoea and bradycardia in preterm infants. *Acta Paediatrica Scandinavica* 70(6): 785–790.

62. Poets CF, et al. 1993. The relationship between bradycardia, apnea, and hypoxemia in preterm infants. *Pediatric Research* 34(2): 144–147.

63. Henderson-Smart DJ, et al. 1986. Incidence and mechanism of bradycardia during apnoea in preterm infants. *Archives of Disease in Childhood* 61(3): 227–232.

64. Angel-James JE, et al. 1981. Lung inflation: Effects on heart rate, respiration, and vagal afferent activity in seals. *American Journal of Physiology* 240(2): H190–H198.

65. Girling DJ. 1972. Changes in heart rate, blood pressure, and pulse pressure during apnoeic attacks in newborn babies. *Archives of Disease in Childhood* 47(253): 405–410.

66. Rehan V, et al. 1995. The effects of central apneas on cerebral blood flow velocity (CBFV) in healthy term infants. *Journal of Pediatrics* 126(6): 979–982.

67. Rehan V, et al. 1996. The influence of sleep state and respiratory pattern on cyclical fluctuations of cerebral blood flow velocity (CBFV) in healthy preterm infants. *Biology of the Neonate* 69(6): 357–367.

68. Samuels MP, and Southall DP. 1992. Recurrent apnea. In *Effective Care of the Newborn Infant*, Sinclair JC, and Bracken MB, eds. New York: Oxford University Press, 385–397.

69. Lagercrantz H. 1992. What does the preterm infant breathe for? Controversies on apnea of prematurity. *Acta Paediatrica* 81(10): 733–736.

70. Kurlak LO, Ruggins NR, and Stephenson TJ. 1994. Effect of nursing position on incidence, type, and duration of clinically significant apnoea in preterm infants. *Archives of Disease in Childhood. Fetal and Neonatal Edition* 71(1): F16–F19.

71. Jenni OG, et al. 1997. Effect of nursing in the head elevated tilt position (15 degrees) on the incidence of bradycardia and hypoxemic episodes in preterm infants. *Pediatrics* 100(4): 622–625.

72. Osborn DA, and Henderson-Smart DJ. 2004. Kinesthetic stimulation for preventing apnea in preterm infants. *Cochrane Database of Systematic Reviews* (3): CD000499.

73. Kuzemko JA, and Paala J. 1973. Apnoeic attacks in the newborn treated with aminophylline. *Archives of Disease in Childhood* 48(5): 404–406.

74. Henderson-Smart DJ, and Steer P. 2004. Methylxanthine treatment for apnea in preterm infants. *Cochrane Database of Systematic Reviews* (3): CD000140.

75. Aubier M, et al. 1981. Aminophylline improves diaphragmatic contractility. *New England Journal of Medicine* 305(5): 249–252.

76. Natarajan G, Lulic-Botica M, and Aranda JV. 2007. Pharmacology review: Clinical pharmacology of caffeine in the newborn. *Neoreviews* 8(5): e214–e221.

77. Etzel BA, and Guillet R. 1994. Effect of neonatal exposure to caffeine on adenosine A_1 receptor ontogeny using autoradiography. *Brain Research. Developmental Brain Research* 82(1-2): 223–230.

78. Weaver DR. 1996. A_1-adenosine receptor gene expression in fetal rat brain. *Brain Research. Developmental Brain Research* 94(2): 205–223.

79. Ledent C, et al. 1997. Aggressiveness, hypoalgesia and high blood pressure in mice lacking the adenosine A_2-receptor. *Nature* 388(6643): 674–678.

80. Schmidt B, et al. 2006. Caffeine therapy for apnea of prematurity. *New England Journal of Medicine* 354(20): 2112–2121.

81. Schmidt B, et al. 2007. Long-term effects of caffeine therapy for apnea of prematurity. *New England Journal of Medicine* 357(19): 1893–1902.

82. Henderson-Smart DJ, and De Paoli. 2010. Methylxanthine treatment for apnoea in preterm infants. *Cochrane Database of Systematic Reviews* (12): CD000140.

83. Davis PG, and Henderson-Smart DJ. 2004. Nasal continuous positive airways pressure immediately after extubation for preventing morbidity in preterm infants. *Cochrane Database of Systematic Reviews* (3): CD000143.

84. Miller MJ, Carlo WA, and Martin RJ. 1985. Continuous positive airway pressure selectively reduces obstructive apnea in preterm infants. *Journal of Pediatrics* 106(1): 91–94.

85. Al-Alaiyan S, et al. 1993. Effects of different levels of nasal CPAP (NCPAP) on ventilation and short apneas in preterm infants. *Pediatric Research* 33: 199A.

86. De Paoli AG, Davis PG, and Lemyre B. 2003. Nasal continuous positive airway pressure versus nasal intermittent positive pressure ventilation for preterm neonates: A systematic review and meta-analysis. *Acta Paediatrica* 92(1): 70–75.

87. Lemyre B, Davis PG, and De Paoli AG. 2004. Nasal intermittent positive pressure ventilation (NIPPV) versus nasal continuous positive airway pressure (NCPAP) for apnea of prematurity. *Cochrane Database of Systematic Reviews* (3): CD00272.

88. Moretti C, et al. 1999. Comparing the effects of nasal synchronized intermittent positive pressure ventilation (nSIPPV) and nasal continuous positive airway pressure (NCPAP) after extubation in very low birth weight infants. *Early Human Development* 56(2-3): 167–177.

89. Pandit PB, et al. 2001. Work of breathing during constant- and variable-flow nasal continuous positive airway pressure in preterm neonates. *Pediatrics* 108(3): 682–685.

90. Sreenan C, et al. 2001. High flow nasal cannulae in the management of apnea of prematurity: A comparison with conventional nasal continuous positive airway pressure. *Pediatrics* 107(5): 1081–1083.

91. Alvaro R, et al. 2012. CO_2 inhalation as a treatment for apnea of prematurity: A randomized double-blind controlled trial. *Journal of Pediatrics* 160(2): 252–257.

92. Ramanathan R, et al. 2001. Cardiorespiratory events recorded on home monitors: Comparison of healthy infants with those at increased risk for SIDS. *JAMA* 285(17): 2199–2207.

93. Steinschneider A. 1972. Prolonged apnea and the sudden infant death syndrome: Clinical and laboratory observations. *Pediatrics* 50(4): 646–654.

94. Jobe AH. 2001. What do home monitors contribute to the SIDS problem? *JAMA* 285(17): 2244–2245.

95. Boles RG, et al. 1998. Retrospective biochemical screening of fatty acid oxidation disorders in postmortem livers of 418 cases of sudden death in the first year of life. *Journal of Pediatrics* 132(6): 924–933.

96. Gold Y, Goldberg A, and Sivan Y. 2000. Hyper-releasability of mast cells in family members of infants with sudden infant death syndrome and apparent life-threatening events. *Journal of Pediatrics* 136(4): 460–465.

97. Summers AM, et al. 2000. Association of IL-10 genotype with sudden infant death syndrome. *Human Immunology* 61(12): 1270–1273.

98. Zupancic JA, et al. 2000. Cost-effectiveness and implications of newborn screening for prolongation of QT interval for the prevention of sudden infant death syndrome. *Journal of Pediatrics* 136(4): 481–489.

99. American Academy of Pediatrics. 2001. Distinguishing sudden infant death syndrome from child abuse fatalities. *Pediatrics* 107(2): 437–441.

100. American Academy of Pediatrics. 2003. Apnea, sudden infant death syndrome, and home monitoring. *Pediatrics* 111(4): 914–916.

101. Taylor HG, et al. 1998. Predictors of early school age outcomes in very low birth weight infants. *Journal of Developmental and Behavioral Pediatrics* 19(4): 235–243.

102. Tudehope DI, et al. 1986. Apnoea in very low birth weight infants: Outcome at 2 years. *Australian Paediatric Journal* 22(2): 131–134.

103. Koons AH, et al. 1993. Neurodevelopmental outcome of infants with apnea of infancy. *American Journal of Perinatology* 10(3): 208–211.

104. Levitt GA, et al. 1988. Outcome of preterm infants who suffered neonatal apnoeic attacks. *Early Human Development* 16(2-3): 235–243.

105. Martin RJ, and Fanaroff AA. 1998. Neonatal apnea, bradycardia, or desaturation: Does it matter? *Journal of Pediatrics* 132(5): 758–759.

Notes

4 Nursing Assessment and Care of the Neonate in Acute Respiratory Distress

Kathleen Koszarek, NNP-BC, MSN
Dawn Ricouard, RNC-NIC, BSN

Nursing care is a vital contributor to a positive outcome for the critically ill neonate experiencing acute respiratory distress. The caregiver at the bedside integrates knowledge of and skills in many aspects of care, including developmental physiology, pathophysiology, and the psychosocial needs of the patient and family. No other health care professional spends as many hours at the patient's bedside. This intense, lengthy contact allows the nurse to become totally familiar with the infant's status and promotes an awareness of the subtle cues that warn of a change in his clinical condition. In addition, nurses are an essential communication link in the implementation of family-centered care. One study identified nurses as the health care provider who spent the most time explaining the infant's condition to the parents and were viewed by them as the best source of information about their baby.[1] The impact of nursing care on neonatal morbidity and mortality should never be underestimated, and each unit's nurses must be aware of its standards of care and outcome statistics.

This chapter discusses components of respiratory care for the neonate, from delivery through NICU admission, routine care procedures, and planning for discharge. Special attention is given to clinical assessment, basic nursing care measures, and parent support issues.

RESUSCITATION

Responsibility for the neonate precedes the infant's admission to the NICU. Preparations for resuscitation and an orderly admission must begin before the birth. Essential to this preparation is an awareness of the maternal-fetal factors that place the neonate at risk. Absolute prediction of infant status at delivery is not possible, but a thorough knowledge of the perinatal history allows the clinician to identify risk factors for the neonate and to begin anticipatory measures. Pulmonary immaturity must be anticipated with preterm delivery; asphyxia is seen more often in term infants with congenital anomalies or those experiencing fetal distress. Table 4-1 lists high-risk antepartum and intrapartum conditions that are associated with respiratory depression or distress in the neonate at delivery.

Any institution that provides perinatal health services must have an adequately staffed and equipped resuscitation room. This means having trained personnel available from the moment of delivery to receive the infant for whom acute respiratory distress is anticipated. Any perinatal center delivering intrapartum care must have an individual capable of providing emergency care for the infant. The Neonatal Resuscitation Program is a formal education program, developed by the American Academy of Pediatrics and the American Heart Association.[2] It helps to ensure that personnel are adequately trained.[3,4] When resuscitative measures are required, an orderly approach optimizes results (Figure 4-1).

The need for resuscitation is based on the infant's clinical presentation and response as well as anticipation of likely problems. The infant's Apgar score does not determine whether resuscitation is needed, but this score has become a standard for quantifying and conveying the infant's initial clinical presentation in the first several minutes of life (Table 4-2). When the 5-minute score is less than 7, additional scores should be assigned every 5 minutes until the score is 7 or greater for up to 20 minutes.[2,4] Despite this instrument's simplicity,

TABLE 4-1
Risk Factors for Neonatal Respiratory Depression at Delivery

Antepartum Factors	Intrapartum Factors
Maternal diabetes	Emergency cesarean section
Gestational hypertension or preeclampsia	Forceps or vacuum-assisted delivery
Chronic hypertension	Breech or other abnormal presentation
Fetal anemia or isoimmunization	
Previous fetal or neonatal death	Premature labor
Bleeding in second or third trimester	Precipitous labor
	Chorioamnionitis
Maternal infection	Prolonged rupture of membranes (>18 hours before delivery)
Maternal cardiac, renal, pulmonary, thyroid, or neurologic disease	
	Prolonged labor (>24 hours)
Polyhydramnios	Macrosomia
Oligohydramnios	Category 2 or 3 fetal heart rate patterns
Premature rupture of membranes	
	Use of general anesthesia
Fetal hydrops	Uterine tachysystole with fetal heart rate changes
Postterm gestation	
Multiple gestation	Narcotics administered to mother within 4 hours of delivery
Size-dates discrepancy	
Drug therapy, such as magnesium	Meconium-stained amniotic fluid
	Prolapsed cord
Adrenergic agonists	Abruptio placentae
Maternal substance abuse	Placenta previa
Fetal malformation or anomalies	Significant intrapartum bleeding
Diminished fetal activity	
No prenatal care	
Mother older than 35 years	

From: Kattwinkel J, ed. 2011. *Textbook of Neonatal Resuscitation,* 6th ed. Elk Grove Village, Illinois: American Academy of Pediatrics and American Heart Association, 16. Reprinted by permission.

FIGURE 4-1
Steps of resuscitation.

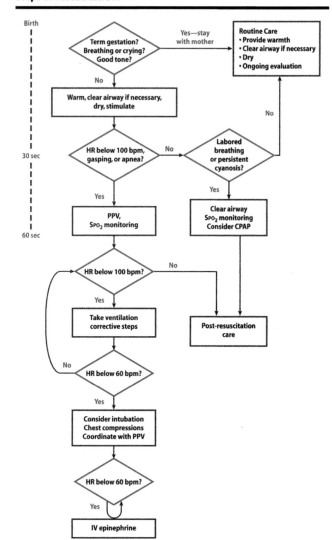

Key: HR = heart rate; SPO$_2$ = oxygen saturation; bpm = beats per minute; PPV = positive pressure ventilation; CPAP = continuous positive pressure ventilation.

From: Kattwinkel J, ed. 2011. *Textbook of Neonatal Resuscitation,* 6th ed. Elk Grove Village, Illinois: American Academy of Pediatrics and American Heart Association, 21. Reprinted by permission.

improper and biased scoring occurs, and the observer must make an effort to use the scale as objectively as possible.[5] A cord blood gas drawn from the umbilical artery can be used to determine the presence of acidemia in the fetus just before birth. The mean umbilical artery pH is 7.26 for the term infant, and an umbilical artery pH <7.10 is considered fetal acidemia.[6] Along with the appropriate resuscitation equipment, each delivery area must have resuscitation information available for quick reference. This information includes resuscitative drug doses, appropriate endotracheal tube sizes for various infant weights, depth of insertion for umbilical lines, and emergency phone numbers needed to mobilize a resuscitation team.

Nursing responsibilities during resuscitation include the following:

- Correctly position the infant's airway, suction the airway as needed, and deliver oxygen (O$_2$) and bag and mask manual ventilation as required.
  - Attach pulse oximeter probe. Adjust the fractional concentration of oxygen as appropriate using an oxygen blender to avoid both overly low and high oxygen saturations.
- Monitor heart rate. Recheck the heart rate every 30 seconds while aggressive resuscitation is under way, and place the infant on a cardiac monitor if available.

TABLE 4-2
Apgar Scoring Criteria

Sign	0	1	2
Color	Blue or pale	Acrocyanotic	Completely pink
Heart rate	Absent	<100 bpm	>100 bpm
Reflex irritability	No response	Grimace	Cry or active withdrawal
Muscle tone	Limp	Some flexion	Active motion
Respiration	Absent	Weak cry, hypoventilation	Good, crying

Adapted from: Kattwinkel J, ed. 2011. *Textbook of Neonatal Resuscitation*, 6th ed. Elk Grove Village, Illinois: American Academy of Pediatrics and American Heart Association, 35. Reprinted by permission.

TABLE 4-3
Delivery Room Inspection of Infant

General: Inspect for inappropriate growth for dates or asymmetry of growth. Assess for presence of major birth defects or birthmarks, checking trunk front and back as well as extremities and entire length of spine. Note head shape, fontanels, and suture lines. Check genitalia for normalcy.

Neurologic: Note posture, muscle tone, activity, and responsiveness.

Respiratory: Auscultate breath sounds, assessing air entry and equality. Inspect movement of the thorax and rate and regularity of respirations.

Cardiac: Note underlying skin color and assess perfusion. Auscultate cardiac sounds, noting rate, rhythm, and presence or absence of murmur. Note point of maximal impulse. Palpate brachial and femoral pulses.

Abdomen: Palpate for presence of kidneys and for abdominal masses.

- Monitor the infant's temperature, continue to dry the infant as needed, remove wet linen from the infant, use the servocontrol mechanism and calibrate the radiant warmer controls, and continually assess the newborn's temperature to prevent hyperthermia and hypothermia, both of which can be harmful to the infant.[7]
  - Immediately wrap extremely low birth weight (ELBW) infants, with limited or no drying, in an occlusive polyethylene wrap or polyethylene bag to decrease evaporative heat loss while still allowing warming by overhead heaters.[8]
  - Delivery room temperatures of at least 25°C (77°F) are recommended for the ELBW infant.[9]
- Assist with procedures such as endotracheal intubation, umbilical line placement, and chest tube placement.
- Draw up and administer resuscitation medications as ordered by the physician; verify that dose and route of administration are correct.
- Initiate and continue chest compressions as per protocol.
- Check whole blood glucose via a reagent strip, notify the health care provider, start a peripheral intravenous (IV) line, and administer IV fluids if required.
- Place identification bands on the infant before he leaves the delivery room, and verify the birth record, including maternal identification number, infant sex, and date and time of birth.
- To establish the infant's risk factors, complete a history and a physical assessment no later than two hours after birth.

The nurse must be aware of the overall care needs of the infant in acute distress and the hospital protocol specific for resuscitation of the neonate.

Each institution should have a specific protocol to prevent hypothermia in the very low birth weight (VLBW) and ELBW infant because this weight group is at high risk. One successful strategy is to use polyethylene film wrap or polyethylene bags to keep the VLBW or ELBW infant warm.[10–12] Although the focus is usually on preventing hypothermia, the neonate is also at risk for complications of hyperthermia, which is believed to worsen the impact of asphyxia.[13] Research supports the neuroprotective effects of induced hypothermia in infants who have suffered hypoxic-ischemic brain injury, demonstrating improvement in developmental outcomes and decrease in mortality.[14–17]

Each unit should have a protocol in place to rapidly identify those infants at risk for asphyxial hypoxic-ischemic encephalopathy and who qualify for therapeutic hypothermia. The infants need continuous monitoring to prevent excessive hypothermia prior to transport to a cooling center or prior to initiation of the cooling protocol. Adequate ventilation should be maintained, avoiding hyper- and hypoxemia; hypotension and hypoglycemia must be identified and treated to limit the negative effects of asphyxia.[18] Unless the infant is a candidate for therapeutic hypothermia, nursing efforts should continue to be directed at maintaining a thermoneutral environment.

Further examination of the infant should be done in the delivery room or resuscitation area to identify any abnormalities that require immediate treatment. A brief examination routine can provide valuable information regarding the infant's status (Table 4-3).

Anticipation of problems extends to the nursery as well. A well-prepared nursery environment includes a heat source for temperature stabilization, cardiorespiratory and oxygen saturation monitoring equipment, blood pressure monitoring equipment, blended oxygen and regulated suction availability, a manual resuscitator with appropriately sized face masks, supplies for immediate vascular access, emergency drugs, and intubation supplies. Constant attention to the patient's respiratory status is maintained during the admission procedure. Medical and nursing procedures carried out on any infant in acute respiratory distress should be coordinated and modified to minimize stress that could lead to further compromise.

ADMISSION AND TRANSITION

Immediate assessment procedures include auscultation of cardiac and breath sounds as well as recording vital signs, including heart rate, respiratory rate, blood pressure, temperature, and oxygen saturation. Blood glucose and hematocrit should be measured by the time the infant is one hour of age. Weight may be estimated if the infant is too compromised to tolerate the stressful weighing procedure. If the infant is weighed, the utmost care must be taken to ensure adequate ventilation and oxygenation during the process. Monitoring equipment (cardiorespiratory, temperature, and oxygen saturation) needs to be applied as quickly as is feasible.

Common sense can be used to determine which procedures can be delayed. Although measurements and gestational age assessment are vital pieces of information, they should not be obtained to the detriment of the infant. Table 4-4 lists admission procedures to be done within a reasonable time frame, patient status permitting.

The first six hours of life are a period of transition for the newborn. Some infants exhibit acute distress at delivery; others develop signs and symptoms of ineffective adaptation to extrauterine life over the first hours. Not every infant who exhibits difficulty during transition will require extraordinary supportive measures, but careful assessment and monitoring will ensure that supportive measures are in place when needed to prevent infant compromise. An awareness of "expected" behavior and clinical presentation can assist the nurse in identifying those infants who are not successfully adapting to extrauterine life.

Normal recovery from the birth process has been outlined by Desmond and coworkers, who describe a characteristic series of changes in vital signs and physical behavior during the first hours of life (Figure 4-2). A

TABLE 4-4
NICU Admission Procedures

- Check identification bands and compare to accompanying paperwork.
- Weigh infant.
- Place in prewarmed radiant warmer or incubator, and connect temperature probe.
- Attach cardiorespiratory monitoring and pulse oximetry probe.
- Provide supplemental oxygen and assisted ventilation as ordered.
- Obtain and record vital signs (heart rate, temperature, respiratory rate, and blood pressure); measure point-of-care hematocrit and capillary blood glucose.
- Auscultate chest and abdomen to assess quality of heart tones, breath sounds, and bowel sounds.
- Establish peripheral IV access/assist with umbilical line placement.
- Implement priority orders, including medications, IV fluids, and diagnostic studies as ordered.
- Obtain and record perinatal history.
- Complete physical and gestational age assessment of infant.
- Orient family to equipment, environment, and unit guidelines.
- Initiate nursing care plan.

normal transition period can be divided into two major periods of reactivity:[19]

1. The first 60 minutes of life have been identified as a period of reactivity characterized by an alert infant, with open eyes, intense activity, and increased muscle tone. This initial period is followed by an unresponsive interval occurring between one and four hours of age and lasting two to four hours.
2. The infant then moves into a second period of reactivity and exhibits variable levels of responsiveness and a tendency toward increased muscle tone.

The immature infant exhibits a prolonged period of unresponsiveness following the first period of reactivity, with the second period of reactivity beginning later than in a healthy term infant. Medications given to the mother before delivery can also alter the time sequence, and infants requiring resuscitation exhibit a general neurologic decline, evidenced by hypotonia and decreased response to stimuli, following the first reactivity period.[19,20]

THERMOREGULATION

Excessive cooling or heating is detrimental to the neonate. Heat balance in the newborn is the result of internal heat production and heat supplied by external sources measured against heat loss.

FIGURE 4-2
Newborn adaptations following birth.

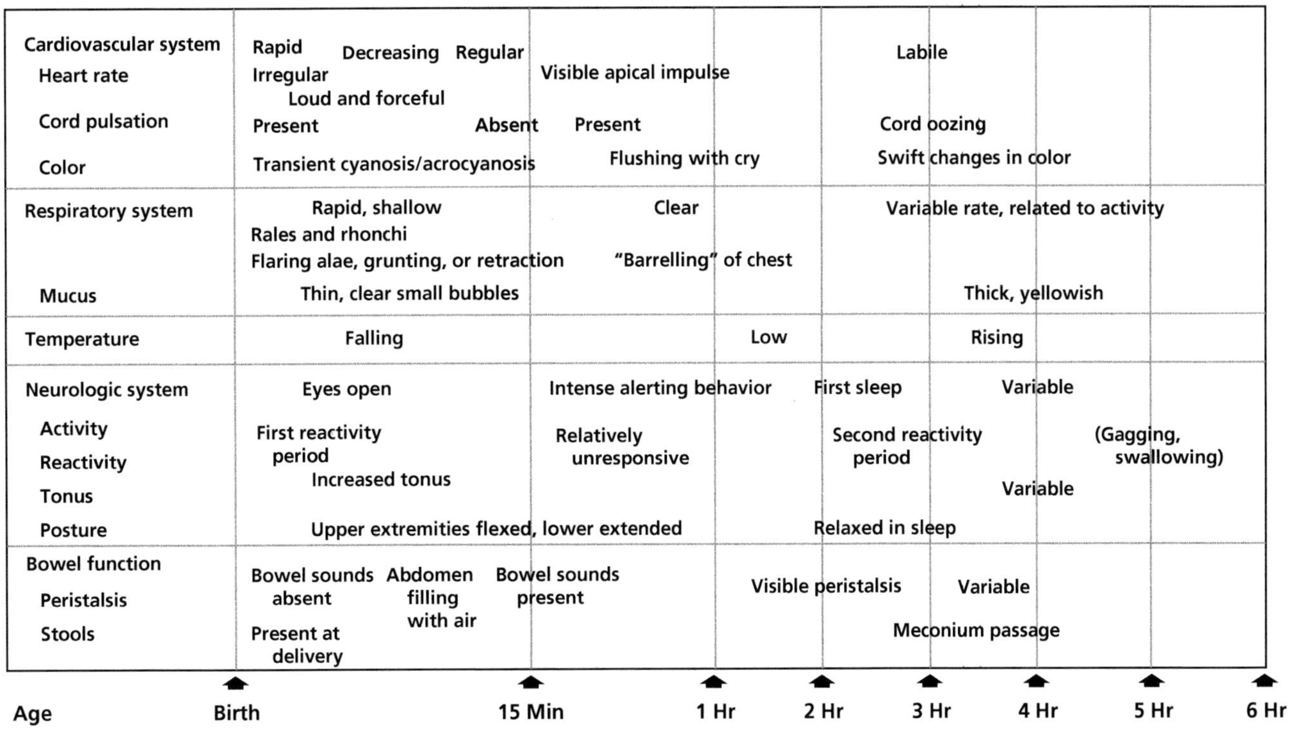

Cardiovascular system	Rapid Decreasing Regular				Labile			
Heart rate	Irregular	Visible apical impulse						
	Loud and forceful							
Cord pulsation	Present Absent	Present			Cord oozing			
Color	Transient cyanosis/acrocyanosis	Flushing with cry			Swift changes in color			
Respiratory system	Rapid, shallow	Clear			Variable rate, related to activity			
	Rales and rhonchi							
	Flaring alae, grunting, or retraction	"Barrelling" of chest						
Mucus	Thin, clear small bubbles				Thick, yellowish			
Temperature	Falling		Low		Rising			
Neurologic system	Eyes open	Intense alerting behavior	First sleep		Variable			
Activity	First reactivity	Relatively		Second reactivity			(Gagging,	
Reactivity	period	unresponsive		period			swallowing)	
Tonus	Increased tonus				Variable			
Posture	Upper extremities flexed, lower extended		Relaxed in sleep					
Bowel function	Bowel sounds Abdomen Bowel sounds			Visible peristalsis	Variable			
Peristalsis	absent filling present							
Stools	with air				Meconium passage			
	Present at delivery							
Age	**Birth**	**15 Min**	**1 Hr**	**2 Hr**	**3 Hr**	**4 Hr**	**5 Hr**	**6 Hr**

From: Desmond MM, et al. 1963. The clinical behavior of the newly born. Part 1: The term baby. *Journal of Pediatrics* 62(3): 311. Reprinted by permission.

HEAT PRODUCTION

A neonate has three basic methods of heat production, although they are not all fully developed or totally efficient immediately after birth:

1. **Shivering.** Shivering produces heat through muscle activity; however, an immature nervous system limits this reaction in the term infant, and it is not available to the preterm infant. The term infant may shiver only in response to a profound drop in core body temperature.[21,22]

2. **Voluntary muscle activity.** The infant may generate heat by crying or moving and attempt to reduce heat loss by seeking changes in position that limit exposed skin surface. This response is attenuated in preterm infants as well as in compromised infants, especially those who are sedated, physically restrained, or have experienced brain injury.[6,21]

3. **Metabolic heat production.** The main method of heat production in the newborn is chemical (nonshivering) thermogenesis. This process requires an increase in metabolic rate (and a resultant increased oxygen consumption). The central regulating mechanism for temperature control is situated in the hypothalamus. Thermal receptors are located in the skin. In the infant, the most sensitive thermal receptors are located in the trigeminal region of the face. Stimulation of these receptors leads to heat-conserving responses such as vasoconstriction and results in an increase in metabolic rate and brown adipose tissue (BAT) metabolism.[6] Warming of the facial skin, as with an excessively heated oxyhood, when the infant's body is cold suppresses the needed increase in metabolic rate.[6,21]

BAT, which is stored prenatally in the mediastinum, interscapular, paraspinal, and perirenal areas, is the primary fuel source used by the neonate for metabolic heat production. The sympathetic nervous system and hormonal mediators control BAT metabolism.[23] Oxygen, glucose, and adenosine triphosphate are required for the combustion of fatty acids to produce heat. In response to cold stress, brown fat is rapidly metabolized for heat production. Metabolism of this tissue results in the breakdown of triglycerides into glycerol and fatty acids. However, hypoxia, acidosis, and hypoglycemia can all adversely affect this process.[6,23] Under conditions of stress, epinephrine is also released, activating the

TABLE 4-5
Nursing Measures to Decrease Heat Loss[6,21,132,133]

Conduction	Prewarm line and equipment that will be in contact with infant.
	Utilize portable chemical warming mattress or heating mattress.
Convection	Use radiant overhead warmer for procedures.
	Use sleeves over portholes on incubator.
	Stretch plastic film wrap over plastic frame or side guards of radiant warmer.
	Use polyethylene wrap as a blanket only if infant airway is protected and skin is mature enough to resist sticking to wrap and then tearing.
	Transport infant in enclosed, warmed incubator.
	Keep infant away from air drafts.
	Warm delivered gases.
Evaporation	Keep infant dry; change wet linen promptly.
	Bathe under radiant warmer and in a draft-free environment.
	Cover infant with heat shield.
	If in radiant warmer and intubated, cover infant with plastic-film-wrap blanket.
	Increase humidity in incubator.
	Warm and humidify delivered gases.
	Use of semiocclusive polyurethane dressings and topical emollients remains controversial.
Radiation	Keep infant away from outside windows (or cold walls).
	Place infant in double-walled incubator.
	Use incubator covers.
	Keep nursery environmental temperature at 24°C (≥75°F).
	Dress medically stable infants who are in incubators or open cribs with hats, gowns, and booties.

utilization of glycogen stores. Glycolysis may be inhibited, however, in the presence of lipolysis, which occurs during the utilization of brown fat.

Heat production abilities can be quickly exhausted in the term infant, and brown fat, once metabolized, is not replaced. Central nervous system damage, shock, hypoxia, and drugs, such as anesthetics, muscle relaxants, and sedatives, reduce the infant's metabolic response to cold.[6,21,22] Premature infants have limited ability to increase their metabolic rate, have minimal BAT and glycogen stores, and may have impaired oxygenation secondary to lung disease—all of which puts them at increased risk for hypothermia.

Heat Loss

Thermoregulation is further complicated by the neonate's susceptibility to heat loss, or thermolysis. The newborn's body surface is large compared with total body mass, thereby accelerating heat loss. Heat reaches the body surfaces by direct conduction through body tissue or via the circulation. Constriction of peripheral vessels keeps internal heat, generated by normal metabolic processes, from being lost to the external environment. However, this mechanism is compromised during periods of vasodilation associated with phases of shock or when drugs that produce vasodilation are given. Newly born premature infants have limited subcutaneous tissue to serve as an insulation layer and have an extremely thin epidermal skin layer, both of which increase caloric losses.[21,24,25] Vasoconstriction and vasodilation in response to thermal stimulation are attenuated as well in the preterm newborn, but this response does mature by two to three weeks postnatal age.[26]

Thermolysis occurs as heat moves from the body core to the surface and then from the body surface to the environment. Heat transfer occurs through four mechanisms:

1. *Conduction* refers to heat transfer through solids, liquids, or gases. It is dependent on physical contact between surfaces of different temperatures. In the infant, heat is transferred from the body surface to cooler objects in contact with the infant's skin.

2. *Convection* refers to heat transfer via mass flow of moving air. Air molecules adjacent to the infant's skin are heated by the skin, and these heated molecules expand and diffuse away from the skin. Air currents accelerate heat loss.

3. *Evaporation* refers to loss of heat from a surface when a given amount of liquid is converted to a gas. Evaporative heat loss is similar to heat loss from convection, but in evaporation gas, molecules transport water rather than kinetic energy. Evaporative heat loss is accelerated by low environmental humidity.

4. *Radiation* refers to transmission of heat by electromagnetic waves from the surface of one mass to another; it does not require direct contact. Heat is transferred to cooler objects, with the rate of transfer dependent on temperature gradient, distance, and surface area.

Practical application of these principles can be made to many aspects of nursing care and incorporated into nursing care procedures (Table 4-5). Ideally, infants are cared for in environmental temperatures and conditions that permit maintenance of normal core temperature when oxygen consumption and metabolic rate at rest are minimal. This has been called the infant's thermoneutral environment. Thermal environment components are environmental air temperature, radiant surfaces, ambient airflow, and relative humidity. Although environmental air temperature is usually easily monitored and maintained, factors such as the temperature of radiant surfaces, airflow, and humidity are more difficult to assess and control.

Because thermal needs vary with weight and gestational age, the proper thermoneutral environment for each infant should be estimated from available graphs and then adjusted accordingly, with the goal of maintaining infant temperature between 36.5°C and 37.3°C (97.7°F and 99.1°F) axillary.[6]

THERMAL INSTABILITY

Thermal instability—whether it results in hypothermia or hyperthermia—places the infant at risk for further complications. Diligent bedside care can markedly decrease the incidence of these complications. Cold-stressed infants, if capable, will increase their metabolic rate to produce heat, thereby increasing calorie consumption. Poor weight gain and hypoglycemia are consequences of this higher calorie consumption. The increased metabolic rate requires oxygen as fuel, and increased oxygen consumption may produce tissue hypoxia and a resultant metabolic acidosis. An increase in indirect (unconjugated) bilirubin can occur in the presence of acidosis. Secondary effects of cold stress will also cause metabolic acidosis as a consequence of vasoconstriction and fat metabolism. Pulmonary vasoconstriction can occur, leading to further hypoxia, acidosis, and increasing severity of respiratory distress and pulmonary vascular resistance (Figure 4-3).[6] No evidence-based practice for rewarming the infant is currently available.

Although hypothermia is the more common neonatal condition, hyperthermia may also occur very readily in the neonate. Hyperthermia is usually iatrogenic, resulting from inappropriate heat from radiant warmers or incubators, servocontrol malfunction or misplaced probe, phototherapy lights, excessive clothing and blankets, or excessive exposure to direct sunlight. Hyperthermia may also be an indication of sepsis, dehydration, or neurologic compromise. The overheated neonate's system attempts to release heat by increasing blood flow to the skin. This can result in hypotension and greater insensible water loss leading to dehydration. Hyperthermia increases metabolic demands and results in more oxygen consumption, especially in preterm infants. Hyperthermia is also associated with tachycardia, tachypnea, poor weight gain, hypoxia, and metabolic acidosis.[6]

FIGURE 4-3
Physiologic consequences of cold stress.

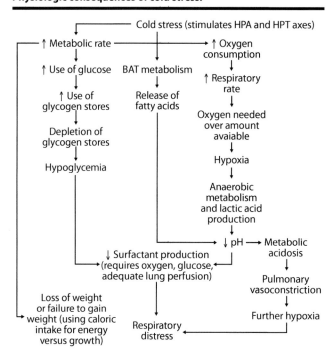

Key: BAT = brown adipose tissue; HPA = hypothalamic-pituitary-adrenal; HPT = hypothalamic-pituitary-thyroid.

From: Blackburn ST. 2007. *Maternal, Fetal, and Neonatal Physiology: A Clinical Perspective,* 3rd ed. Philadelphia: Saunders, 718. Reprinted by permission.

Although newborns have mature sweat glands by 36 weeks gestational age, heat-induced sweating requires a greater thermal stimulus than in adults. Heat-induced sweating is even less developed in preterm infants than in term newborns. The functional ability of the sweat glands does improve rapidly with chronologic age and matures rapidly during the first weeks after birth, but sweating still remains an inefficient means of thermal homeostasis.[26,27]

ASSESSMENT OF GESTATIONAL AGE

Newborns should be classified by birth weight, gestational age, and intrauterine growth to identify existing or potential problems (Figure 4-4). Unique problems or risk factors can be associated with an infant's gestational age, birth weight, and appropriateness of growth.

Weight alone is an inadequate predictor of gestational age (Figure 4-5). The neonate's gestational age can be estimated from the mother's menstrual history or prenatal ultrasound examination. Ultrasound dating, especially when it is done before 20 weeks gestation, is a very accurate predictor. Admitting nursing or medical staff

FIGURE 4-4
Neonatal morbidity by birth weight and age.

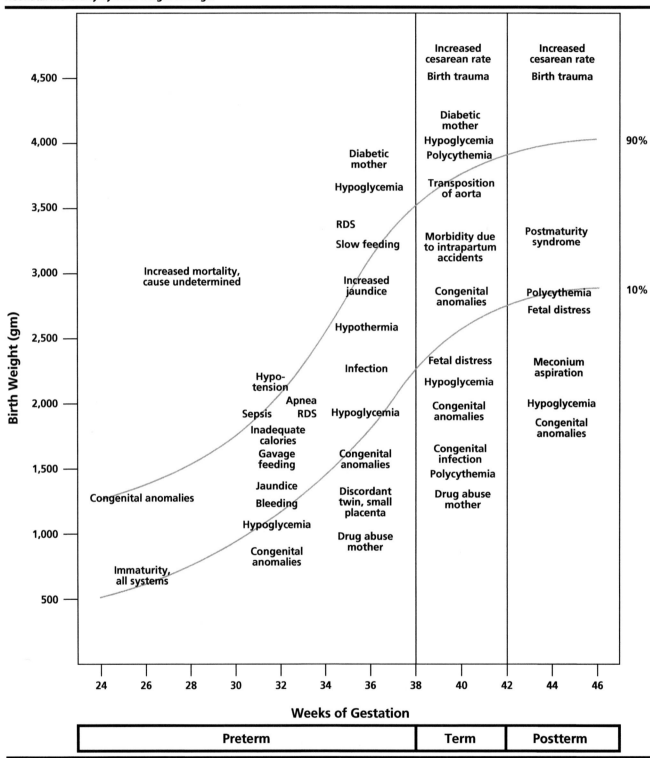

From: Lubchenco LO. 1976. *The High Risk Infant.* Philadelphia: Saunders, 122. Reprinted by permission.

usually perform a physical assessment using a clinical assessment tool to assist in estimating gestational age. The most widely used assessment tools incorporate both neurologic and physical criteria. Neurologic criteria are usually less biased than physical criteria by intrauterine growth restriction (IUGR) and birth weight, although they may be affected by central nervous system insult or trauma. Use of physical criteria alone may result in an overestimation of maturity in the presence of IUGR.[28] The Ballard maturational score may be used on newborns as young as 20 weeks gestation (Figure 4-6).[29]

Gestational age assessment is most accurate when done early; accurate identification of infants at risk is essential. The results of even a properly done gestational age examination can vary approximately two weeks (plus or minus) from actual gestation. Despite this limitation, gestational age assessment remains a valuable tool.

OVERALL CLINICAL ASSESSMENT

Particular attention should be paid to the infant's clinical presentation. Presenting clinical signs may indicate the etiology of the respiratory distress, and sequential monitoring traces the progression of the respiratory disease. An orderly approach to physical examination provides a consistent, complete assessment.

Initial assessment procedures in the nursery are essential to establish a baseline of information. Because this is often the patient's first complete physical examination, each nursing unit needs an established format for this procedure (Table 4-6). A comprehensive approach to the examination of the newly born infant, including gestational age assessment, is presented in *Physical Assessment of the Newborn*.[30] The nursing admission note must be exact, including the infant's name, age, sex, admitting diagnosis, mode of admission, pertinent findings from the examinations, and any significant perinatal history. All of the data will be used to prepare a nursing plan of care for the neonate.

Assessment interventions must be tempered by an appreciation of the infant's tolerance for such stressful procedures. Any critically ill infant should be monitored with pulse oximetry to assist in assessing tolerance. Some clinicians prefer to group their caregiving tasks; others space them, believing that doing so decreases stress. The superiority of either method is unclear, but it is certain that the infant should be allowed to recover from any procedure, as evidenced by normalization of transcutaneous oxygen value or pulse oximetry saturation, heart rate and color, before further stressful

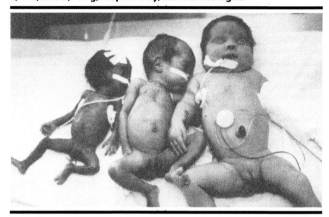

FIGURE 4-5
Three infants, same gestational age (32 weeks) weighing 600, 1,400, and 2,750 g, respectively, from left to right.

From: Korones S. 1986. *High-Risk Newborn Infants,* 4th ed. Philadelphia: Mosby, 118. Reprinted by permission.

procedures are implemented. Evaluation of the infant's tolerance following care measures should guide the caregiver's subsequent approach to interventions with that particular infant.

CLINICAL ASSESSMENT OF RESPIRATORY STATUS

Clinical assessment of the infant's respiratory status entails inspection, auscultation, palpation, and occasionally percussion and transillumination.

INSPECTION

The assessment begins with basic observation. Color is judged, looking at generalized color as well as that of the oral mucous membranes. Cyanosis is a blue discoloration of the skin, nail beds, and mucous membranes resulting from hemoglobin that is desaturated, or not carrying a maximum amount of oxygen. Fetal hemoglobin, which makes up the majority of the newborn's hemoglobin, is easily saturated with oxygen but does not release oxygen to the tissue as readily as adult hemoglobin does. High saturations are thus associated with lower levels of partial pressure of oxygen in arterial blood (PaO_2) (see **PULSE OXIMETRY** later in this chapter). In the newborn infant, clinical cyanosis does not occur until severe hypoxia is present. Because cyanosis reflects desaturated hemoglobin, a baby with a higher hemoglobin (polycythemia) will appear cyanotic at a higher PaO_2 than an anemic baby whose PaO_2 may be quite low before cyanosis becomes visible.

The presence of oral or nasal secretions is noted. Chest movement is evaluated, including depth of respirations,

FIGURE 4-6
Ballard maturational score.

Neuromuscular Maturity

Neuromuscular Maturity Sign	Score							Record Score Here
	-1	0	1	2	3	4	5	
Posture								
Square Window (Wrist)	>90∞	90∞	60∞	45∞	30∞	0∞		
Arm Recoil		180∞	140∞–180∞	110∞–140∞	90∞–110∞	<90∞		
Popliteal Angle	180∞	160∞	140∞	120∞	100∞	90∞	<90∞	
Scarf Sign								
Heel to Ear								

Total Neuromuscular Maturity Score

Maturity Rating

Score	Weeks
-10	20
-5	22
0	24
5	26
10	28
15	30
20	32
25	34
30	36
35	38
40	40
45	42
50	44

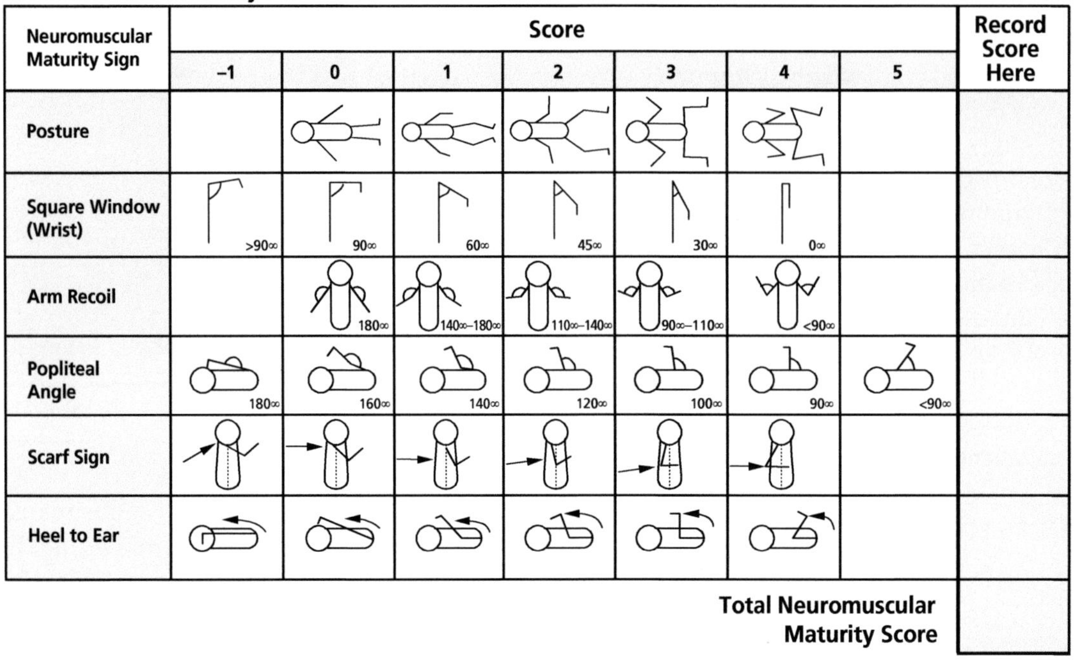

Physical Maturity

Physical Maturity Sign	Score							Record Score Here
	-1	0	1	2	3	4	5	
Skin	sticky friable transparent	gelatinous red translucent	smooth pink visible veins	superficial peeling and/or rash, few veins	cracking pale areas rare veins	parchment deep cracking no vessels	leathery cracked wrinkled	
Lanugo	none	sparse	abundant	thinning	bald areas	mostly bald		
Plantar Surface	heel-toe 40–50 mm:-1 <40 mm:-2	>50 mm no crease	faint red marks	anterior transverse crease only	creases anterior 2/3	creases over entire sole		
Breast	imperceptible	barely perceptible	flat areola no bud	stippled areola 1–2 mm bud	raised areola 3–4 mm bud	full areola 5–10 mm bud		
Eye/Ear	lids fused loosely: -1 tightly: -2	lids open pinna flat stays folded	slightly curved pinna; soft; slow recoil	well-curved pinna; soft but ready recoil	formed and firm; instant recoil	thick cartilage ear stiff		
Genitals (Male)	scrotum flat, smooth	scrotum empty faint rugae	testes in upper canal rare rugae	testes descending few rugae	testes down good rugae	testes pendulous deep rugae		
Genitals (Female)	clitoris prominent and labia flat	prominent clitoris and small labia minora	prominent clitoris and enlarging minora	majora and minora equally prominent	majora large minora small	majora cover clitoris and minora		

Total Physical Maturity Score

From: Ballard JL, et al. 1991. New Ballard score, expanded to include extremely premature infants. *Journal of Pediatrics* 119(3): 418. Reprinted by permission.

TABLE 4-6
History and Physical Examination

History	
Maternal:	Age, gravida, para (term and preterm delivery), abortions, living children
	Blood type, hepatitis B status, serology (date and results), other available lab results
	Medical problems and complications of pregnancy
	Use of alcohol, tobacco, or recreational drugs
Labor and delivery:	Labor spontaneous or induced; complications of labor; fetal monitoring
	Rupture of membranes: hours prior to delivery, character of fluid
	Medications given
	Fetal presentation; delivery (vaginal or cesarean section; indication); use of forceps
	Apgar at 1 and 5 minutes (also 10, 15, 20 minutes if indicated); specify lost points
	Resuscitation measures required
Family:	Mother/father: married, single, cohabitating, apart, father in contact, occupations, identified social problems
	Environment: living arrangements, telephone

Physical Examination	
Vital signs:	Temperature (axillary)
	Pulse
	Respirations
	Blood pressure (central or peripheral, four limbs)
	Oxygen saturation
	Blood glucose
	Hematocrit
General:	Resting posture, activity, gross abnormality or overt distress, color
Skin:	Condition, texture, lanugo, vernix; note meconium staining, pallor, plethora, jaundice, hemangioma, nevi, rash, excoriation, petechiae, bruises, subcutaneous fat
Head:	General shape; note molding, caput, cephalhematoma, craniotabes, sutures, fontanels (anterior and posterior); hair texture
Eyes:	Size and shape, clarity of lenses, reactivity of pupils, blink; note hemorrhage, edema, discharge
Nose:	Shape, including nasal bridge; patency; note drainage, nasal flaring
Ears:	Cartilaginous development, position of earlobe, shape of auricle, external auditory canal
Mouth:	Palate, natal teeth, tongue (size), lips and mucous membranes (color), symmetry and movement
Neck:	Trachea position, movement; note masses or webbing
Chest:	Clavicles, symmetry; diameter of breast buds; note retractions, abnormal rate or respiratory pattern
Lungs:	Breath sounds, equality, character; note grunt, crackles, rhonchi, wheezes, rubs, stridor, bowel sounds
Cardiovascular system:	Point of maximal impulse, heart rhythm and rate; murmur (quality, radiation, location of intensity); peripheral pulses—femoral, brachial, radial (equality); peripheral perfusion
Abdomen:	Shape, muscle tone, size of liver; note any masses palpated; umbilicus abnormalities; number of vessels, drainage, inflammation
Genitourinary system:	Female: Labia and clitoris development; note discharges, abnormalities in voiding
	Male: Length of penis, urethral orifice position; testicular descent and scrotal development (rugae); note hernia or hydrocele, abnormalities in voiding
Anus:	Position, patency, stools
Extremities:	Symmetry, range of motion, positioning of feet and hands; number, shape, length of digits; appearance of nails; palmar creases; hip click
Spine:	Alignment; note sacral dimple, scoliosis, midline defects
Neurologic system:	Tone, responsiveness, cry (character, intensity, frequency); behavior (alertness, irritability); reflexes (suck, grasp, Moro); note tremors, paralysis (facial, brachial, lower extremities)

FIGURE 4-7
Retraction sites.

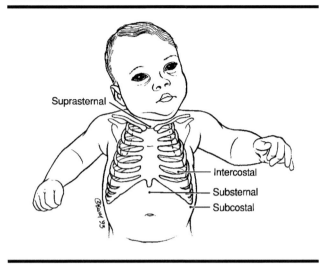

Suprasternal

Intercostal

Substernal

Subcostal

Illustration by Elizabeth Weadon Massari.

TABLE 4-7
Silverman-Andersen Retraction Score

Stage 0	Stage 1	Stage 2
Upper chest and abdomen rise synchronously	Lag or minimal sinking of upper chest as abdomen rises	"Seesaw" sinking of upper chest with rising abdomen
No intercostal sinking on inspiration	Just visible sinking of intercostal spaces on inspiration	Marked sinking of intercostal spaces on inspiration
No xiphoid retraction	Just visible xiphoid retraction	Marked xiphoid retractions
No nasal flaring	Nasal flaring minimal	Marked nasal flaring
No expiratory grunt	Expiratory grunt heard with stethoscope onl	Expiratory grunt heard with naked ear

Adapted from: Silverman WA, and Andersen DH. 1956. A controlled clinical trial of effects of water mist on obstructive respiratory signs, death rate, and necropsy findings among premature infants. *Pediatrics* 17(1): 1–10. Reprinted by permission.

symmetry, and synchrony. The rate of respiration is counted for a full minute. Tachypnea is the most frequent indicator of respiratory disease, although an infant in severe respiratory failure may exhibit slow, gasping respirations or experience episodes of apnea.

Because the cartilage in the infant's chest wall is soft, airway resistance or lung disease may cause visible retractions as the infant generates high negative intrathoracic pressures to inflate the lung. Retractions can be intercostal (between the ribs) or subcostal (immediately below the rib cage). Sternal as well as suprasternal and substernal retractions may be present (Figure 4-7). Severe lung disease with decreased lung compliance can also produce paradoxical breathing or "see-saw" respirations, a sign of significant work of breathing. "Seesaw" respirations are characterized by retraction of the chest wall and a rising abdomen on inspiration. Nasal flaring may also be identified during inspiration. Flaring is the result of widening of the nasal alae in an attempt to decrease upper airway resistance.

The Silverman-Andersen scale was developed to provide an objective means of assessing the progression or improvement of respiratory distress (Table 4-7). This scale is especially useful in assisting the novice during a complete evaluation. As experience is gained in caring for the critically ill neonate, the nurse will be able to recognize patterns of clinical signs and symptoms associated with specific disease states. For example, a round barrel chest is seen with volume-trapping (obstructive) disorders such as transient tachypnea of the newborn and meconium

aspiration syndrome; retractions and hypoexpansion are present with restrictive (atelectatic) disease such as respiratory distress syndrome (RDS, hyaline membrane disease). (Chapter 2 discusses the pathophysiology and clinical presentation of RDS more specifically.)

AUSCULTATION

Auscultation is performed to determine air movement and quality of breath sounds. Grunting, a sound produced when air is exhaled against a partially closed glottis, may be audible without the aid of a stethoscope. Grunting reflects the infant's attempt to delay expiration and increases gas exchange by increasing end-expiratory pressure and lung volume.

Auscultation of the chest should progress in an orderly manner, with the examiner comparing and contrasting each side of the chest for equality of breath sounds (Figure 4-8). Breath sounds in neonates are higher pitched than in adults, and there is less difference in sound intensity between inspiration and expiration, especially in smaller infants. Normal breath sounds would be classified as bronchovesicular, defined as a medium volume and pitch, heard equally during inspiration and expiration.[31] Because sound is easily transmitted through the small chest of the newborn, the clinician has to be able to identify subtle differences, assessing and documenting the presence of crackles, wheezes, grunting, or other extraneous sounds (Table 4-8). While listening to the infant's chest, the examiner should also listen for heart tones, as well as the presence of any murmurs. It is important to note the

FIGURE 4-8
Sequence for breath sound auscultation: Anterior and posterior chest.

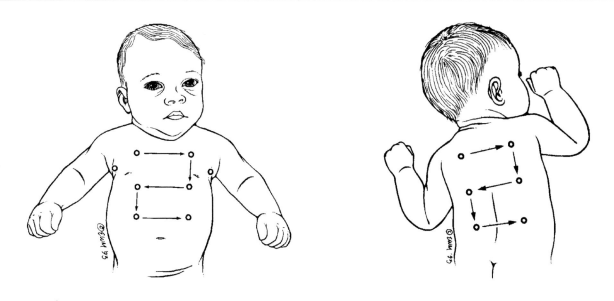

Illustration by Elizabeth Weadon Massari.

cardiac point of maximal intensity (PMI). A shift in PMI can indicate such problems as a pneumothorax.

PALPATION

Palpation of the chest is important to the assessment of the newborn with respiratory distress. The clinician should be alert to any masses, chest wall edema, or subcutaneous emphysema. Table 4-9 gives an overview of the examination of the newborn chest.

PERCUSSION AND TRANSILLUMINATION

Percussion can sometimes be a useful tool for the experienced practitioner to determine a change in consistency of underlying tissue. The examiner places one finger against the infant's chest and uses the index finger of the other hand to tap that finger. As the examiner moves the finger over the chest and continues to tap it, a difference in resonance can indicate a change

TABLE 4-8
Adventitious Lung Sounds

Term	Description
Crackles	Discontinuous: Early crackles occur in first half of inspiration, late crackles, in second half. Early crackles suggest atelectatic alveoli; late crackles suggest alveolar air trapping.
• Fine crackles	High pitch, low amplitude, short duration: Early fine crackles originate in collapsed small distal airways that snap open on inspiration.
• Coarse crackles	Low pitch, high amplitude, long duration: Early coarse crackles are associated with pneumonia and surfactant-deficiency respiratory distress; late coarse crackles sound like hook and loop separating and are found in pulmonary interstitial emphysema.
Wheezes	Continuous, high pitch, musical: Duration is long, but may not be heard through entire respiratory cycle. Sound is generated by air passing at high velocity through narrowed airway. Higher flow rates produce higher pitch. Heard with diseases such as bronchopulmonary dysplasia, gastroesophageal reflux, tracheomalacia/bronchomalacia, and tracheal webs.
Rhonchi	Continuous, low pitch: Occur on inspiration and expiration. Associated with secretions or stricture in larger airways. Improve or clear with cough or suctioning.
Stridor	Rough, harsh sound associated with narrowing of upper airways; worse during inspiration, but may be present in both phases of respiratory cycle. Multiple associated conditions including vocal cord paralysis, subglottic stenosis, and postextubation edema.

Adapted from: Fletcher MA. 1998. *Physical Diagnosis in Neonatology*. Philadelphia: Lippincott Williams & Wilkins, 303–401.

TABLE 4-9
Examination of the Newborn Chest

	Normal Findings	Abnormal Findings
Inspect	Oval chest shape, narrow at top and flares at bottom with narrow anteroposterior diameter	Bulging of chest
		Concavity of chest
	Prominent xiphoid process	Increased anteroposterior diameter (barrel chest)
	Flexible chest wall, mild retractions with crying	Depressed sternum (pectus excavatum/funnel chest)
	Symmetric chest movement in synchrony with abdomen during respirations	Protuberant sternum (pectus carinatum/pigeon breast)
		Asymmetric chest wall movement, flail chest
	Breath rates 30–40/minute in term infants and 40–60/minute in preterm infants	Asynchronous respirations/paradoxical breathing ("seesaw")
		Retractions
	Nipples well formed and prominent, symmetrically positioned; may have milk secretion	Tachypnea
		Supernumerary nipples
	Pink color; harlequin color change	Erythema and tenderness of breasts
		Widely spaced nipples
		Central cyanosis, jaundice, pallor, mottling
		Precordial impulse visible beyond first hours of life in term infant
Palpate	Clavicles and ribs intact	Lump over clavicle
	Breast nodule 3–10 mm	Crepitus
	PMI left of lower sternum	Lack of breast tissue
		Shift in PMI
		Fremitus
Auscultate	Equal bronchovesicular breath sounds	Crackles, rhonchi, wheeze, stridor, rubs, bowel sounds in chest
	Lusty cry	Grunting
	No murmur or soft murmur	Cough
		Weak, whining, or high-pitched cry
		Hoarseness, stridor
		Harsh murmur (grade 2–3) in first hours of life

in underlying tissue mass. Percussion is normally not performed on small infants, but it may be used over the chest to identify the upper edge of the liver.

When a pneumothorax is suspected, transillumination of the chest can be used prior to chest x-ray to identify air pockets and allow for quick action and treatment. A chest x-ray should follow transillumination whenever a pneumothorax is suspected.

PULSE OXIMETRY

Pulse oximetry is a standard of care in the NICU. This noninvasive technique allows close oxygen monitoring in the neonate. To fully evaluate the infant's status, it is essential that the nurse at the bedside understand the information that is available via pulse oximetry. This understanding begins with knowledge of the physiology of O_2 transport in the blood.

BASICS OF OXYGEN TRANSPORT

Oxygen is transported in the blood in two physical forms. The majority is bound reversibly to hemoglobin

(Hb) within the red cell. This portion makes up 98 percent of the total blood O_2 content and is measured as oxygen saturation (SaO_2). The smaller portion of O_2, which makes up 2 percent of the total blood oxygen content, is dissolved in the plasma. It is this smaller, dissolved portion that is measured with arterial blood gas sampling as PaO_2. Gases such as oxygen, nitrogen, and carbon dioxide are dissolved in the blood. The force each gas exerts in the blood is termed the **partial pressure** of the respective gas. Through simple diffusion, gases move from an area of higher partial pressure to an area of lower partial pressure.

The partial pressure of the oxygen dissolved in the plasma is measured in mmHg (torr). The amount of oxygen bound to hemoglobin (SaO_2) is directly related to the PaO_2. Under this pressure, oxygen diffuses into the red blood cells, where it reacts and combines with hemoglobin to form oxyhemoglobin. The PaO_2, although a small percentage of total oxygen content, is significant because it determines the pressure gradient for oxygen diffusion and thus the amount of oxygen bound to hemoglobin.[32]

FIGURE 4-9
Comparison of hemoglobin saturation and PO$_2$.

Comparison between the dissociation curve of hemoglobin (curve A) and the amount of oxygen dissolved in plasma (curve B). Note that the hemoglobin is almost 100 percent saturated at PO$_2$ 80 mmHg. When fully saturated, 15 g Hb will bind 20.1 mL O$_2$.

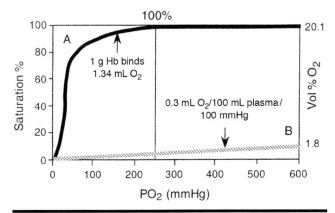

From: Duc G. 1971. Assessment of hypoxia in the newborn: Suggestions for a practical approach. *Pediatrics* 48(3): 469. Reprinted by permission.

Each Hb molecule can combine with four molecules of O$_2$. When fully saturated (combined) with oxygen, 1 g Hb carries 1.34 mL of O$_2$.

TISSUE OXYGENATION

Oxygen diffuses from the alveolus into the pulmonary capillary blood because the oxygen pressure (PO$_2$) in the alveolus is greater than the PO$_2$ in the pulmonary blood. At the tissue level, O$_2$ dissociates from hemoglobin into the plasma and diffuses into the cells. The diffusion of any gas is a direct function of its partial pressure, not its concentration, and the most important factor for tissue oxygenation is the partial pressure of oxygen in arterial blood as it equilibrates with the partial pressure of oxygen in the tissues.[33] The O$_2$ supply to the tissues depends on the oxygenation of Hb, the delivery of O$_2$, and the uptake and utilization of oxygen in the tissues.

The relationship between blood PaO$_2$ and the amount of O$_2$ bound to Hb is commonly expressed as hemoglobin-oxygen (Hb-O$_2$), hemoglobin's affinity for oxygen, and is curve shaped when graphed. It is known as the oxygen, or oxyhemoglobin, dissociation curve (Figure 4-9). On the steep portion of the curve, a large change in saturation is accompanied by only a small change in oxygen tension. This steep lower portion ensures an adequate O$_2$ supply to tissues by releasing large amounts of oxygen for relatively small decreases in partial pressure. The steep lower part of the dissociation curve means that the peripheral tissues can withdraw large amounts of O$_2$

TABLE 4-10
Factors Affecting Hemoglobin-Oxygen Affinity

Increased Hb-O$_2$ Affinity (shift to the left)	Decreased Hb-O$_2$ Affinity (shift to the right)
Alkalosis ↓ PCO$_2$	Acidosis ↑ PCO$_2$
Hypothermia ↓ 2,3-DPG (HbF)	Hyperthermia ↑ 2,3-DPG (HbA)

for only a small drop in capillary PO$_2$. This maintenance of blood PO$_2$ assists the diffusion of O$_2$ into the tissue cells.[34]

On the other end of the curve, as oxygenation increases, Hb saturation becomes a less sensitive index of oxygen tension, and a larger change in PaO$_2$ is reflected in only minor changes in hemoglobin saturation. The flat, upper section of the curve, which is principally concerned with O$_2$ uptake, ensures that arterial blood leaves the lung well saturated even when the partial pressure is reduced by lung disease or by high altitude. The flat upper portion means that even if the PO$_2$ in alveolar gas falls somewhat, loading of oxygen will be little affected. In addition, as the red cell takes up O$_2$ along the pulmonary capillary, a large partial pressure difference between alveolar gas and blood continues to exist, even when most of the oxygen has been transferred. This hastens the diffusion process.[33,34]

The affinity of hemoglobin for oxygen is modified by four factors: (1) hydrogen ion (H$^+$) concentration; (2) partial pressure of carbon dioxide (PCO$_2$), with most of the effect of PCO$_2$ attributed to its action on pH; (3) temperature; and (4) 2,3-diphosphoglycerate (2,3-DPG) concentration (Table 4-10). The substrate 2,3-DPG is produced by the enzyme system as a by-product of glucose metabolism. It occurs in response to chronically reduced O$_2$ delivery to the tissues, and it enhances the dissociation of oxygen from hemoglobin by competing with O$_2$ for iron-binding sites.

Increased values of these factors act to decrease the affinity of Hb for O$_2$. Decreased oxygen affinity means diminished O$_2$ uptake but its increased release at the tissues. Increased values for H$^+$, PCO$_2$, and temperature occur in tissues at sites of active metabolism. This aids in releasing O$_2$ from Hb, raising the local PO$_2$ and making oxygen more available for tissue uptake. These conditions are reversed in the lungs, where Hb uptake is more important.[32]

A decreased affinity of hemoglobin for oxygen, occurring with acidosis, hypercapnia, hyperthermia,

FIGURE 4-10
Oxyhemoglobin dissociation curve with right and left shifts.

An oxyhemoglobin dissociation curve with the normal P_{50} illustrated and the effect of right and left shifts of the curve shown. As the curve shifts to the right, the oxygen affinity of hemoglobin decreases, more oxygen is released at a given oxygen tension, and the P_{50} value increases. When the curve shifts to the left, there is increased oxygen affinity, less oxygen is released at a given oxygen tension, and the P_{50} value decreases. The dashed lines correlate the landmarks of the 30-60-90 rule for estimating oxygen saturation.

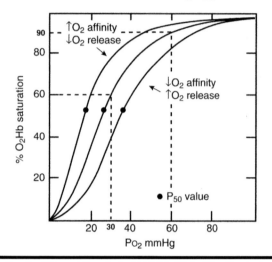

From: Barnhart SL, and Czervinske MP. 1995. *Clinical Handbook of Perinatal and Pediatric Respiratory Care*. Philadelphia: Saunders, 308. (Adapted from: Oski FA. 1972. Fetal hemoglobin, the neonatal red cell, and 2,3-diphosphoglycerate. *Pediatric Clinics of North America* 19[4]: 907–917.) Reprinted by permission.

or increased 2,3-DPG, is said to shift the oxygen dissociation curve to the right. This means that a specific point of oxygen saturation on the curve now correlates with a higher PO_2. Hb releases O_2 more readily when the affinity is decreased. A shift to the right improves oxygen unloading capacity to the tissues. But consider that a decreased affinity of hemoglobin for oxygen also affects hemoglobin's ability to saturate (or pick up oxygen) at the alveolar level. This decreased ability to saturate is usually not a factor because the lung normally is saturating at the upper, flat portion of the curve, where small changes in saturation can produce large changes in PO_2. However, an extreme shift to the right in the presence of major respiratory or cardiac disease almost always results in decreased oxygen content with poor oxygen pickup. This limits the amount of O_2 that can be given to the tissues regardless of how easily it can dissociate from the Hb. Tissue PO_2 is determined by a balance between (1) the rate of O_2 transport to the tissues in the blood and (2) the rate at which the oxygen is utilized by the tissues. Sudden and severe acidemia and/or hypercarbia cause decreased O_2 content and lowered oxygen availability to the tissues.

A shift to the left in the oxygen dissociation curve results when decreased values for (H^+), PCO_2, and temperature and lower levels of 2,3-DPG occur (Figure 4-10). Alkalosis, low CO_2 levels, and low temperatures increase hemoglobin's affinity for oxygen, allowing for greater uptake of oxygen. This increased affinity also results in diminished release of oxygen at the tissue level. Banked donor blood has decreased levels of 2,3-DPG, causing a shift to the left in the curve, and fetal hemoglobin (HbF) also exhibits an increased oxygen affinity.[6]

OXYGEN TRANSPORTATION IN THE FETUS AND NEWBORN

The hemoglobin structure is altered in the fetus such that Hb's affinity for O_2 is increased, resulting in higher O_2 saturation and blood oxygen content at relatively lower PaO_2 values. In the fetus, the higher hemoglobin affinity for oxygen is produced by a decreased response of HbF to 2,3-DPG. This increased affinity to saturate is important to the fetus because umbilical venous PO_2, the oxygenated blood supply to the fetus, is limited by the uterine venous PO_2. The fetal PaO_2 in the umbilical vein is about 28–32 mmHg.[6]

At term, 50–80 percent of cord blood is HbF, and preterm infants have higher levels of HbF than do term infants. Because HbF has an increased ability to saturate, the newborn's saturations may be high yet correlate with a low or marginal PaO_2. Newborns may look pink but have a low PaO_2, which is why skin color is not a totally reliable means of assessing oxygenation in a newly born infant. As fetal hemoglobin is replaced with adult-type hemoglobin over the first months of life, O_2 affinity decreases, but the oxygen-diffusing capacity to tissues improves. By four months of age, 90–95 percent of hemoglobin is the adult type.[6] This time frame is changed dramatically when neonates are transfused with adult packed red blood cells.

MEASURING BLOOD OXYGEN SATURATIONS

Pulse oximetry measures arterial oxygen saturation transcutaneously. Blood changes color with changing hemoglobin saturation. An oximeter is a spectrophotometric device that measures the differential absorption of light by oxygenated hemoglobin (oxyhemoglobin) and reduced, or deoxygenated, hemoglobin (deoxyhemoglobin) and reports the oxyhemoglobin saturations. Because oxyhemoglobin and deoxyhemoglobin absorb light at known fractions of wavelengths, the technology

TABLE 4-11
Advantages and Disadvantages of Pulse Oximetry[36,134,135]

Advantages	Disadvantages
Easy to apply; instrument calibration not required	Motion artifact, with frequent artifactual alarms
Rapid response to changes in blood oxygen	Does not allow precise estimation of PaO_2 at higher saturations
Probes noninvasive and can be left in place for extended periods of time, usually moved at least every 8 hours	SpO_2 may be clinically acceptable even though PaO_2 is low
	Accuracy of readings declines as saturations fall out of normal ranges
Does not heat skin or require strong adherence; not associated with significant cutaneous injury	Phototherapy or procedure lights can interfere with SpO_2 accuracy, giving falsely reassuring readings
May be used on infants of any size	Reduced arterial pulsations associated with hypothermia, vasoconstriction, shock, vasoactive drug infusion, severe edema, indwelling peripheral arterial catheter, blood pressure cuff; ineffective with asystole
High correlation of SpO_2 and PaO_2 in normal range of saturations	
	May pick up venous pulsations in severe right-sided heart failure
Reliability of sensor can be checked by comparison with electrocardiogram pattern	May be affected by darkly pigmented skin or high bilirubin level if light intensity is low
	Readings falsely elevated in the presence of dyshemoglobins, such as methemoglobin

requires a two-wavelength source and a photodetector. The oxygen saturation calculation is made by comparing the ratio of light absorption by the blood in the red color spectrum. Deoxyhemoglobin absorbs more red, and oxyhemoglobin absorbs more infrared light. As it expands and relaxes, the pulsating vascular bed changes the light path, allowing the oximeter to identify arterial blood. Most pulse oximeter monitors display either pulse waveforms or light-emitting diode (LED) lights that identify the tracking of the arterial blood flow pulse. The abbreviation used with pulse oximetry is SpO_2, referring to arterial oxygen saturation as measured by a pulse oximeter.[35]

CLINICAL USE OF PULSE OXIMETRY

Most oximeters measure functional saturation, which is the ratio of oxyhemoglobin to all hemoglobin measures. Because the amount of deoxygenated hemoglobin is important, visible cyanosis is often marked, and low SpO_2 readings are obtained when polycythemia is present despite a normal PaO_2. In anemia, the hemoglobin may be 100 percent saturated, but total oxygen content is low because of reduced carrying capacity. Thus, the reliability of pulse oximeters to measure O_2 content in infants with polycythemia or severe anemia is limited.

In clinical application, an oxygen saturation of less than 80 percent may provide insufficient O_2 to the tissues, particularly at the associated PaO_2 levels; but the presence of acceptable SpO_2 readings does not guarantee adequate tissue oxygenation or oxygen delivery to vital organs.[32] The patient's blood gas levels should be correlated with the SpO_2 periodically to help evaluate tissue oxygenation. Safe upper and lower saturation limits for the neonatal patient are usually defined for the individual patient, based on gestational age, postnatal age,

and clinical pathology. Generally, however, the lowest acceptable SpO_2 is 85 percent, and high acceptable limits are less than 95 percent when the infant is receiving supplemental oxygen.

The technology of pulse oximetry is dependent on pulsatile blood flow. Elements of the sensor, which consists of LEDs and a photodetector, must be placed directly opposite each other. The sensor is usually applied to a translucent pulsed extremity, such as a finger, hand, toe, or foot. For infants weighing less than 3 kg, the sensor should be wrapped across the palm of the hand or the ball of the foot. In larger infants, the bridge of the nose, the palm, the thumb, the great toe, or the index finger can be used. In infants weighing less than 1 kg, the lower calf or wrist has also been used. Because the photodetector is light sensitive, the probe must be shielded from external light with an opaque wrap. Direct sunlight, procedure or surgical lights, phototherapy lights, and infrared radiant heaters can interfere with sensor function. Table 4-11 lists advantages and disadvantages of pulse oximetry.

When the pulse oximeter is functioning properly, the pulse rate it displays should be within five beats/minute of the rate displayed on the cardiac monitor. The accuracy of the equipment varies by brand, but is generally ± 2–4 percent. Accuracy decreases and error in measurement increases progressively when blood saturation levels fall below 70 percent.[36]

"False" alarms resulting from motion artifact and low peripheral perfusion states continue to be an issue.[36] Newer pulse oximeters are designed to overcome these problems.[37–39] But the sizeable number of false alarms associated with pulse oximetry can be an issue for health care staff in the nursery. Excessive oximetry alarms may

FIGURE 4-11
Bedside reminder for infants under oxygen saturation targeting protocol.

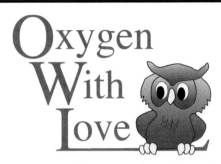

From: Ochsner Clinic Foundation with permission.

TABLE 4-12
Targeted Pre-ductal SpO$_2$ After Birth

Ranges of pre-ductal oximetry values during the first 10 minutes following birth of uncomplicated infants born at term. Data from original study adjusted to provide easily remembered targets.	
1 minute	60%–65%
2 minutes	65%–70%
3 minutes	70%–75%
4 minutes	75%–80%
5 minutes	80%–85%
10 minutes	85%–95%

Adapted from: Kattwinkel J, ed. 2011. *Textbook of Neonatal Resuscitation*, 6th ed. Elk Grove Village, Illinois: American Academy of Pediatrics and American Heart Association, 54. Reprinted by permission.

slow staff response time and may increase parental anxiety, not to mention the obvious risk to the patient of reduced staff responsiveness.

Using pulse oximetry in the clinical setting can begin in the delivery room, but even healthy infants can show decreased saturations in the first minutes of life (Table 4-12). Continuous monitoring should be done on any infant with acute respiratory distress and on those weaning from supplemental oxygen or ventilatory support. Infants with healthy lungs will exceed saturations of 95 percent when breathing room air, but in these circumstances, excessive PaO$_2$ does not occur. It is in the presence of supplemental oxygen that markedly increased PaO$_2$ levels occur.

Alarm parameters for the pulse oximeter vary with the clinical status of the infant and should be specified for each infant.[40] For example, an infant experiencing persistent pulmonary hypertension of the newborn may require saturations >95 percent until the pulmonary hypertension begins to resolve. In contrast, acceptable parameters for an infant with a cyanotic congenital heart lesion may be 75–85 percent in the absence of metabolic acidosis.

Clinicians need to be aware of the harmful effects of oxygen, especially in the preterm infant at risk for retinopathy of prematurity. Noninvasive monitoring of oxygen saturation is a very important tool in identifying estimated oxygen levels. NICUs should have specific protocols for oxygen saturation targeting for at-risk patients. Caregivers should consider identifying infants under such protocols by flagging their beds. The Seymour the owl "Oxygen with Love" identifier (Figure 4-11) is one creative way to communicate to all caregivers (physician, nurse, and respiratory, occupational, and physical therapists) that the patient is under an oxygen

saturation targeting protocol. Chapter 10 provides more information on the complications of oxygen therapy and the need to follow saturation levels closely. The pulse oximeter can alert the health care staff caring for the NICU patient to an acute or steady deterioration in status. Continuous monitoring also allows the nurse at the bedside to evaluate the infant's tolerance of nursing care measures and to adjust interventions to allow the patient time to stabilize, as evidenced by normalizing oxygen saturation levels.

BLOOD GAS SAMPLING

An adjunct to clinical assessment of respiratory disease is chemical assessment via blood gases. The infant's medical plan of care includes the frequency of blood gas determinations, and it is the responsibility of every nurse to be cognizant of each blood gas sample drawn. The nurse also needs to be aware of the status of the patient before the sample is obtained so it can be considered when the blood gas results are interpreted.

Assessment of any abnormalities identified and institution of treatment are often the responsibility of the staff nurse or respiratory therapist, working within the parameters established by the physician or neonatal nurse practitioner. Although the etiology of abnormalities can be complex and multifactorial, the nurse must have a basic knowledge of acid-base disorders to interpret blood gases. Chapter 6 discusses blood gas interpretation in detail.

The sample used for blood gas analysis can be drawn from either an arterial or a capillary source. Arterial blood is the more accurate of the two sources because it produces a reliable PaO$_2$ value. When arterial blood is not available, capillary blood can be used in the NICU

FIGURE 4-12
Location of radial artery.

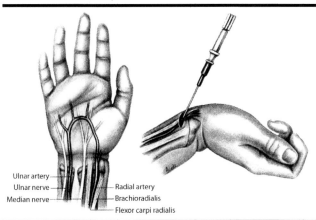

Ulnar artery
Ulnar nerve — Radial artery
Median nerve — Brachioradialis
— Flexor carpi radialis

Adapted from: Durand DJ, and Mickas NA. 2011. Blood gases: Technical aspects and interpretation. In *Assisted Ventilation of the Neonate,* 5th ed., Goldsmith JP, and Karotkin EH, eds. Philadelphia: Saunders, 295. Reprinted by permission.

patient population. Either method of sampling comes with risk factors, and the nurse or respiratory therapist drawing the sample needs to be aware of these factors during blood draws.

A common site for accessing arterial samples is the umbilical artery catheter (UAC). During sampling, it is important that the catheter be kept sterile to minimize the risk of infection associated with use of this line. The stopcock at the end of the UAC is used for the blood draw. To prevent clot formation, the blood withdrawn during the process to clear the line of fluids should be returned to the patient as soon as the sample has been collected. Before any fluid is flushed into the line, gently aspirate the line to remove any air at the connection site between the stopcock and the newly attached syringe. Closed tubing systems that limit entry points with the intent of lower infection risk are currently available for arterial lines. Aspiration and flushing of umbilical lines should be done slowly to avoid the negative cerebral hemodynamic effects that can be associated with rapid withdrawal of fluid from the line. Drawing blood should be coordinated to limit the number of entries into the line. It is vital to maintain the integrity of all connections to avoid iatrogenic hemorrhage. The nurse caring for the patient with umbilical lines must be alert to and meticulous in keeping air out of the catheter; massive air embolism is a fatal complication. If clots form in the line, they must be removed, if possible, or the UAC discontinued. Never flush a clot forward; doing so could cause thrombus embolization or infarction.[41] When a UAC is in place, the quality of the waveform and the perfusion

TABLE 4-13
Peripheral Arterial Puncture Procedure

Palpate the chosen artery.

If performing radial artery puncture, do a modified Allen's test: Gently squeeze hand to partially empty it of blood while applying pressure to both ulnar and radial arteries. Remove pressure from hand and ulnar artery. If entire hand flushes and fills with blood in <10 seconds, ulnar artery can supply the hand with blood, and radial artery can be punctured safely.

Apply antiseptic to infant's skin over the site of the artery. If artery is palpated after antiseptic has been applied, sterile gloves must be used.

Stabilize infant's extremity as necessary.

Check needle and syringe for proper function; use smallest possible needle to minimize trauma to artery; use 23-, 25-, or 27-gauge needle. Butterfly needle with long tubing may be helpful to coordinate puncture and aspiration by a second person.

Insert needle at a 15- to 25-degree angle with bevel down for a superficial artery and at a 30- to 45-degree angle with bevel up for a deep artery.

Position needle against direction of arterial blood flow. Insert needle into skin, and then puncture artery.

Pull needle back slowly until blood flows freely into needle.

Connect syringe to butterfly tubing, and gently aspirate amount of blood needed.

Withdraw needle quickly. Apply continuous pressure over and just above puncture site using a sterile 2 x 2-inch gauze for 5 minutes or longer until hemostasis is complete.

Before leaving bedside, make certain puncture site has stopped bleeding. Check distal circulation after puncture for pulse, capillary refill, color, and temperature.

Adapted from: Walton DM, and Short BL. 2007. Arterial puncture. In *Atlas of Procedures in Neonatology,* 4th ed., MacDonald MG, and Ramasethu J, eds. Philadelphia: Lippincott Williams & Wilkins, 89–92.

to the lower extremities and buttocks must be monitored closely; charting should reflect this assessment. Low doses of heparin (0.25–1 unit/mL) should be added to the fluid infused through the UAC. To decrease the risk of infection, arterial line tubing is changed every 72–96 hours; daily changes are needed if blood or lipids have been infused. Optimally, the UAC should not be left in place for more than five days, to decrease infection risk as well.[42]

When umbilical catheter placement is not possible, a peripheral arterial line (PAL) may be placed instead. As with the UAC, it is important to maintain sterility and to keep air out of the line when accessing blood from a PAL. The PAL should be stabilized and taped to allow an unobstructed view of the distal digits, and the extremity must be observed closely for signs of hypoperfusion or thrombosis; charting should reflect this assessment. Normally, the radial or posterior tibial artery is used, but the dorsalis pedis artery and the ulnar artery are alternatives.[43] These small distal arteries often exhibit a brief

FIGURE 4-13
Heel capillary sample technique. Use the shaded area when performing a heelstick in an infant.

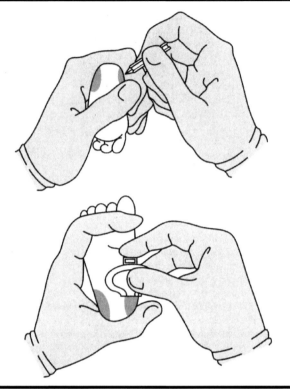

From: Gomella LG, and Haist SA, eds. 2007. *Clinician's Pocket Reference*, 11th ed. New York: McGraw-Hill, 280. Reprinted by permission.

TABLE 4-14
Complications of Capillary Blood Draw via Heelstick

Infection
Scarring
Calcaneus osteomyelitis
Calcified nodules
Nerve damage
Arterial laceration
Bruising
Cellulitis
Bleeding
Burns

From: Barnhart SL, and Czervinske MP. 1995. *Clinical Handbook of Perinatal and Pediatric Respiratory Care*. Philadelphia: Saunders, 312–313. Reprinted by permission.

spasm when flushed. Care must be taken to withdraw fluids slowly from and flush fluids slowly into the PAL.

When a UAC or a PAL is not available, intermittent arterial puncture to obtain arterial samples may be performed by the trained practitioner. This procedure inevitably disturbs the patient, leading to alteration in PaO_2 levels. This makes intermittent sticks a less desirable means of collecting arterial blood. Intermittent puncture can be performed on the radial, ulnar, posterior tibial, or dorsalis pedis artery (Figure 4-12). The femoral arteries are consider inappropriate for sampling, and brachial arteries should be used only for emergency access; the temporal arteries are not recommended because of the risk of neurologic damage.[44-46] Table 4-13 outlines the procedure for peripheral arterial puncture.

Many nurseries use capillary blood samples instead of intermittent arterial punctures when line placement is not feasible. Capillary samples can be obtained from punctures made with small lancets on the posterolateral aspects of the heel (Figure 4-13), taking care to avoid the curvature of the heel (calcaneus). Heel puncture in the calcaneus places the infant at risk for calcaneal

osteomyelitis. Neonatal lancets should be 2 mm or less in length, and there are lancets currently available for use with the premature infant set at depths 0.65–0.85 mm to avoid hitting bone.[47,48]

Arterialized capillary blood samples are obtained by heating the extremity for five minutes prior to the stick. This procedure increases vascularity to facilitate a better flow of blood and reduces the need for squeezing the extremity to obtain a blood sample.[48] The temperature of the warming chemical packets should not exceed 40°C (104°F).[45] Capillary samples from a well-perfused extremity can closely estimate arterial blood gas values with usually slightly lower pH and PCO_2 values, but with a significantly lower PaO_2 value.[49] Blood flow can also be facilitated by holding the puncture site lower than the rest of the extremity. The heel is encircled by the hand and index finger (see Figure 4-13). The puncture site should be prepped with alcohol or a topical iodophor solution before the stick. If an iodophor preparation is used, follow with a saline or alcohol wipe.[48] The alcohol should be completely dry before collecting blood to prevent hemolysis of the specimen. Using a neonatal lancet, puncture the skin, and wipe the first drop of blood away with a dry, sterile gauze pad. Avoid squeezing the heel because this will lower blood yield and increase cell lysis. Using moderate, firm pressure, collect the expressed blood in a capillary tube held downward from the collection site. Avoid repeated scooping along the skin surface because microclots that form in the blood on the skin can alter lab results.[48] A gentle rhythmic pumping, increasing and decreasing pressure, allows for capillary refill so as to keep a steady blood flow. When collecting the blood into a capillary tube, it is important not to allow air to contaminate the sample. Even small air bubbles mixed into the blood can lead to erroneously low PCO_2 and high PaO_2 levels. Falsely elevated serum glucose, serum potassium, and hematocrit and inaccurate blood gas values are known problems associated with heelstick sampling.[45] Capillary blood sampling is a painful procedure, and the nurse should offer the infant comfort measures, such as swaddling and nonnutritive sucking on a pacifier, during and after the procedure.[50] Once blood collection is completed, apply gentle pressure over the puncture site using a sterile gauze pad until the bleeding stops. Table 4-14 lists complications of capillary blood draw via heelstick.

RADIOLOGY OF THE NEWBORN CHEST

Radiographic examination is a medical standard of care for the neonate with respiratory distress. The frequency of such examinations is at the discretion of the physician or neonatal nurse practitioner, but in an emergency, the nurse is often the first health care provider available to view the film. On transport, it is usually the responsibility of the primary transport nurse to interpret available films.

The nurse's responsibility begins with the x-ray examination itself and includes knowledge of appropriate technique. Proper technique includes using the collimator light to identify the x-ray field and then tightly coning down the field size to provide a better quality film as well as to reduce radiation scatter. A properly positioned cassette with appropriate coning exposes only those structures that are to be evaluated. Nursing responsibility includes placing a small lead shield over the infant's reproductive organs to further limit radiation exposure and seeing that such objects as shields, which touch the infant, are cleaned properly if used for other patients. The bedside nurse needs to be aware, as well, of the impact of patient positioning on film interpretation. Head position, flexed or extended, changes endotracheal tube position in relation to the carina, and limb position affects catheter tip position of a peripherally inserted central catheter.[51] A rotated film skews the appearance of the lung fields and prevents the evaluation of a mediastinal shift. One side may falsely appear atelectatic, and the heart may obscure the left lung field.

The NICU staff nurse should have the basic knowledge necessary to recognize acute or dramatic changes in the infant's x-ray film and to convey this information to the physician if he or she is not immediately available to view the films. The best way for nurses to develop this skill is through consistent observation of the diagnostic interpretation of such films. Attending radiographic rounds, if the unit has them, is an excellent way to gain this experience.

REVIEWING IMAGE QUALITY

Interpretation of the x-ray film requires a systematic approach, beginning with evaluation of the quality of the film. Exposure, seen as density and contrast, is noted. Overpenetration results in a dark film, with the infant's lungs appearing hyperlucent or overaerated. Underpenetration produces a "white" film, giving the false impression of atelectasis or hypoexpansion.

Density and contrast can be evaluated by looking at the appearance of the stomach, which is usually partially filled with air, providing a baseline for comparison. The density of the spine and soft tissues can be assessed; they seem to disappear with overpenetration.[52] The technician documents on each film the settings used to obtain it. Use of consistent settings, with appropriate modification of the technique, is the best means of obtaining quality films.

Film interpretation continues with a survey of the infant's positioning. Rotation, if any, should be identified. On a nonrotated film, the ribs appear of equal length on either side of the vertebral column, and the clavicles appear symmetric. If the area to be exposed is not perpendicular to the beam from the x-ray tube, an oblique view will be obtained. Such a film slants all structures and misrepresents the positioning of indwelling tubes and lines. With proper angulation the clavicles will be at a 90-degree angle to the vertebral column. Errors can be avoided by proper positioning of the infant, who should be held flat and prevented from rolling to one side or the other. If the infant is to be held during the procedure, the staff member must wear a lead apron, and the staff member's hand must be coned out of the field.

Motion during the film can make assessment of the lung fields inaccurate. Evidence of motion is best detected by the blurring of normally distinct structures such as electrocardiograph lead wires.

Next the film should be evaluated for extraneous objects that may prevent interpretation or lead to a false conclusion. Radiopaque objects appear clearly on film and are thus easily identified. If possible, these objects should be removed from the field before the x-ray study to prevent obstruction of body structures. Electrocardiograph leads or temperature probes, for example, block viewing of structures and should be moved, if feasible. For an anterior-posterior chest film,

FIGURE 4-14
Method for determining the cardiothoracic ratio.

The sum of the horizontal projections from the vertical line (lines marked A and B) is the transverse diameter of the heart. The dotted line is the greatest internal diameter of the chest. The ratio between the transverse cardiac diameter and the internal diameter of the chest is the cardiac-to-thoracic ratio.

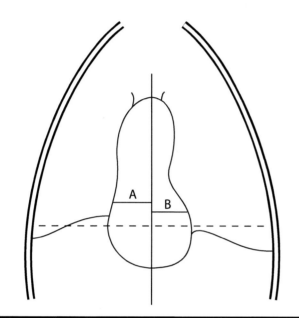

it is best to place electrocardiograph leads in the axillary line and to place skin sensors on the shoulder or abdomen.

Nonradiopaque objects do not appear clearly on the film, but leave shadows that may be difficult to differentiate from pathologic findings in the chest. Warming mattresses produce a waffle-like appearance that prevents any realistic interpretation of the film. Bunched linen or plastic tubings lying under or over the infant produce extraneous lines. Incubator tops often have a small hole used to insert tubings into the incubator. If an x-ray film is shot through this transparent plastic top, a small, circular bleb may appear on the film. Skin folds may be falsely interpreted as a pneumothorax. These are best identified on the film by following the skin fold line outside the thoracic cavity.

RECOGNIZING CLINICAL INDICATORS

After the film has been assessed for technical difficulties, a clinical examination can be started. Air or gas is radiolucent and leaves a dark gray or black image. Tissue and water are more dense than air or gas and are therefore more radiopaque, with a lighter image. Bone and metal, with the highest densities, produce a light gray or white image.

Examine the film systematically:

1. **Evaluate heart size, position, and shape.** Cardiac borders should be clear and distinct. The cardiac silhouette of the newborn is large, especially in the first 24 hours of life. Cardiac size is estimated by determining the cardiothoracic ratio. The longest horizontal diameter of the heart is divided by the greatest internal diameter of the chest (Figure 4-14). The heart normally measures half the width of the thorax, with a cardiothoracic ratio of 0.5, although the ratio in term and preterm newborns may be slightly larger, up to 0.65.[51–53] This measurement, used to determine cardiomegaly, is further limited in the neonate because a large thymic shadow or areas of atelectasis create a generous cardiac silhouette that may exceed this ratio. An expiratory film will do likewise.[53]

    Cardiomegaly is seen in infants with volume overload (Table 4-15). An extremely small silhouette is seen in infants who are hypovolemic or dehydrated or who have high intrathoracic pressure that is causing decreased venous return. Hypoinflation, lordosis, and rotation distort the cardiac silhouette.[48] Initially, the apex of the heart is elevated secondary to right ventricular hypertrophy associated with fetal circulation. Because the left ventricle predominates in extrauterine life, the cardiac apex descends caudally. The configuration is affected by the size of the thymus, but abnormal shapes can be seen with various congenital heart diseases. A globular shape is seen with hypoplastic left heart or coarctation of the aorta, an egg shape is seen with transposition of the great vessels, and a boot shape is seen with tetralogy of Fallot.

2. **Evaluate the mediastinum.** The space between the lungs contains the esophagus, trachea, thymus, heart, and major vessels. Displacement of the mediastinum is associated with free air in the pleural space.

3. **Survey the lung fields.** Pulmonary expansion can be determined by locating the level of the diaphragm. The right diaphragm is normally slightly higher than the left because of the liver. During inspiration, the dome of the right hemidiaphragm usually moves to the level of the eighth rib or below. The diaphragm will be higher if the lungs are severely hypoventilated or if the film was taken during the expiratory phase of respiration. Overinflated lungs appear hyperlucent, with their normally domed diaphragms flattened.

4. **Determine the aeration of the lungs.** Are the lungs clear (dark) or opaque (white)? Is there evidence of granularity, seen as coarseness or a "ground glass" appearance? Are there areas of streaking, haziness, or consolidation? Lung tissue should extend fully to the pleura.

Hyperlucent (extremely clear) areas over the entire lung or at its margins can indicate a pneumothorax (free air in the thoracic cavity surrounding the lung). A decubitus film (obtained by placing the unaffected side down and taking the film as an anteroposterior penetration) more clearly defines a pneumothorax because the free air rises to the uppermost area. Free air in the mediastinal area, called a pneumomediastinum, outlines the thymus, producing a sail or butterfly appearance. A pneumopericardium (free air around the heart) is seen as a complete halo encircling the heart.

5. **Assess pulmonary vascularity.** Vascular markings branch in a treelike fashion from the hilum, decreasing in size as they extend through the lung fields. The vascular and organ margins should be sharp. Hazy, indistinct margins suggest early pulmonary interstitial edema. Decreased pulmonary vascularity suggests persistent pulmonary hypertension of the newborn with a right-to-left shunt or congenital heart disease with obstructed pulmonary blood flow.

Table 4-16 lists the classic radiographic findings associated with the major neonatal respiratory pathologies. Because many of the abnormalities have similar radiographic findings, knowledge of the patient's history and clinical presentation is essential. A basic competence in x-ray film interpretation and familiarity with associated respiratory pathophysiology are invaluable to the nurse in providing appropriate patient care—including the ability to knowledgeably communicate patient status to the physician.

ROUTINE CARE

After the infant's admission to the NICU, a routine should be established regarding the frequency of assessment. This will be based upon the guidelines for care of an infant experiencing respiratory distress established by the NICU. Table 4-17 provides an example of such a guideline. Table 4-18 provides an example of routine nursing orders for the critically ill patient. Premature infants often tolerate handling poorly, so the

TABLE 4-15
Causes of Cardiomegaly Other Than Congenital Heart Anomalies

Hypervolemia and pulmonary edema and/or congenital heart disease	Mediastinal masses simulating cardiomegaly
• Cardiac ischemia secondary to brain asphyxia	• Teratomas
• Hypertrophic subaortic stenosis	• Liver herniation through an anterior defect of the diaphragm
• Cardiomyopathy	
• Intracardiac myxoma	
• Infant of diabetic mother	
• Patent ductus arteriosus	
• Hydrops fetalis	
• Arteriovenous malformation: brain or liver	
• Polycythemia	
• Erythrocythemia	
• Blood transfusions	

From: Dominguez R. 1992. *Diagnostic Imaging of the Premature Infant.* Philadelphia: Churchill Livingstone, 104. Reprinted by permission.

TABLE 4-16
Disorders Indicated by Abnormal Roentgenographic Patterns

Granular: Hyaline membrane disease, transient respiratory distress of the newborn, neonatal pneumonitis (especially Group B Streptococcus)

Bubbly: Hyaline membrane disease with overdistended terminal airways (associated with mechanical ventilation), pulmonary interstitial emphysema, bronchopulmonary dysplasia, Wilson-Mikity syndrome

Opaque: Absent or greatly reduced functional residual volume, pulmonary hemorrhage, bilateral chylothorax or hydrothorax

Vascular Congestion: Transient respiratory distress of the newborn, congenital heart disease >12 hours of age, myocardial dysfunction with congestive heart failure

Infiltrate: Pulmonary infections (viral and bacterial), meconium aspiration, amniotic fluid aspiration, segmental atelectasis, pulmonary hemorrhage, vascular congestion secondary to cardiac disease, transient respiratory distress of the newborn, early Wilson-Mikity syndrome

Hazy: Underaeration, pulmonary edema, healing phase of hyaline membrane disease, bilateral diaphragmatic paralysis

Overaerated, Clear: Hyperventilation, congenital heart disease with decreased pulmonary vascularity, central obstructing lesions (vascular ring or mediastinal mass)

Unequal Aeration: Secondary to mucus plugging or improper placement of endotracheal tube, unilateral pulmonary hypoplasia, congenital lobar emphysema

Hyperlucent: Pulmonary air leak

Adapted from: Swischuk LE. 1986. Radiology of pulmonary insufficiency. In *Neonatal Pulmonary Care,* 2nd ed., Thibeault DW, and Gregory GA, eds. Norwalk, Connecticut: Appleton-Century-Crofts, 235–279.

TABLE 4-17
Sample Guideline for Care of an Infant with Respiratory Distress[136–138]

Nursing Diagnosis: Impaired gas exchange/Ineffective breathing pattern

Expected Outcome: Infant will maintain adequate gas exchange, as shown by a lack of cyanosis, minimal retractions and flaring, vital signs within normal limits, adequate breath sounds, blood gases within parameters, oxygen saturations >85 percent, and ability to tolerate activities without signs of respiratory distress.

Nursing Interventions/Rationales:

- Monitor blood gases serially to assess acid-base balance and to detect deterioration.
- Minimize handling to prevent hypoxia; use pulse oximeter readings to modify care.
- Insert vented orogastric tube to prevent accumulation of air in gastrointestinal tract.
- Explain treatment rationale to infant's family to assist with family coping skills.
- Assess and document:

  Respiratory effort every 2 hours to detect changes.

  Breath sounds every 6 hours and as needed to detect deterioration.

  Vital signs every 2–6 hours and as needed to determine patient is stable.

  Oxygen saturations every hour to detect need for changes in oxygen being delivered.

  Ventilatory/oxygen parameters and alarm limits every 2 hours to detect changes.

  Response to analgesics or sedatives.

  Response to muscle relaxants, noting duration of effect, change in cardiovascular status, and need for continuation of paralysis.
- Monitor security of ETT to prevent accidental extubation.

Nursing Diagnosis: Ineffective airway clearance

Expected Outcome: Infant will maintain a clear airway, as evidenced by clear and equal breath sounds, lack of respiratory difficulty, and normal blood gases.

Nursing Interventions/Rationales:

- Suction nares and mouth as needed to prevent accumulation of secretions in upper airway.
- Place small roll under neck to promote optimal airway.
- Ensure chest physiotherapy and aerosolized respiratory treatments are done as ordered to promote clearance of secretions and bronchodilation.
- Suction ETT, using two-person technique or closed suction system, as indicated by clinical assessment, to prevent occlusion of airway.
- Reposition infant every 3–4 hours as tolerated to prevent accumulation of secretions in one area of the airway.
- Report absent or unequal breath sounds, tenacious secretions, significant increase in FiO_2 requirement (10% or greater), or clinical deterioration to facilitate quick and appropriate management of the patient.

TABLE 4-18
Nursing Care Guideline for Critically Ill Infants

Vital Signs

1. Temperature (axillary), pulse, and respirations:
   - Every hour or more frequently on critically unstable infants
   - Every 3–4 hours on all mechanically ventilated, continuous positive airway pressure (CPAP), or oxyhood patients
   - Every 4–6 hours on stable infants not in supplemental oxygen
2. Record blood pressure every hour on all unstable infants and all infants with arterial lines (Lines must be recalibrated every 12 hours and should be correlated with an indirect, peripheral blood pressure [BP] measurement.)
3. Take peripheral BP (documenting extremity used):
   - Every 3–4 hours on all stable, acute care infants without arterial lines
   - Every 24 hours on all infants
4. Record oxygen saturation:
   - Every hour or document more frequently on critically unstable infants
   - Every 3–4 hours on stable infants off CPAP and mechanical ventilation

Laboratory Tests

1. Hematocrit (label as central or peripheral):
   - On admission and every 8–12 hours on all unstable infants
   - Daily on stable, acute care infants; extended to weekly when out of supplemental oxygen or if infant is in a chronic, long-term phase of recovery
   - 4–24 hours after a blood transfusion
2. Blood glucose:
   - On admission and every 30 minutes to 1–2 hours until stable (60–150 mg/dL)
   - 2 hours after infant is placed on IV fluids or following a major change in dextrose concentration
   - Every 12 hours while infant is on IV fluids

Intake and Output

1. Compute every 8–12 hours
2. Calculate urine output (mL/kg/day) every 4–8 hours if urine output is low or excessively high
3. Record all fluid intake, including medications, flush solution used, and blood products
4. Record all output, including urine, blood, stool, gastric output, and drainage

Hand Washing

First and foremost, caregivers must wash their hands! Hand washing is the single most effective measure for the prevention of infection and cross-contamination.[54,55] According to the recommendation of the Centers for Disease Control and Prevention guidelines for hand washing for health care workers, initial hand washing before entering the NICU area should be aseptic. Rings, watches, and bracelets should be removed before hand washing and entering nursery areas. Artificial fingernails are not to be permitted.[4] Personnel should scrub

relative importance of all interventions must be weighed against their potential disturbance of the patient. The individual infant's care plan will adapt unit care guidelines to each patient.

their hands and arms to a point above the elbow thoroughly with an antiseptic soap. After vigorous washing, the hands should be rinsed completely and dried with a paper towel. Decontaminate the hands with an alcohol-based rub, or wash with antibacterial soap and water for at least ten seconds before and after each patient procedure. Decontaminate the hands before donning gloves and after removing them and after contact with inanimate objects in the immediate vicinity of the patient.[4,56–58] Alcohol-based products, foams or gels, can be used according to the manufacturer's recommendations, but are not appropriate for cleaning physically soiled hands.[4,57,59]

Vital Signs and Laboratory Values

Infants do not necessarily need to be disturbed to monitor their vital signs. Heart rate, blood pressure, and skin temperature values can usually be obtained from monitoring equipment. At least once every 12 hours, the nurse should correlate direct blood pressure readings with an indirect (cuff pressure) reading method. "Hands on" assessment should be done at the beginning of the nurse's shift to obtain baseline information and then every 4 to 8 hours, depending on patient status and unit protocol.

The nurse is responsible for verifying the proper functioning of all monitoring equipment, setting appropriate alarm limits for the patient, and analyzing the information gathered for significant changes. The nurse reviews and interprets changes in vital signs, evaluates temperature fluctuations and the thermal environment, carefully monitors urine output (mL/kg/hour), and compares fluid intake with output. Normal parameters for infant vital signs are as follows:

- Temperature (axillary): 36.5–37.3°C (97.7–99.1°F)
- Heart rate:
  Term infant: 80–160 beats per minute
  Preterm infant: 120–160 beats per minute
- Respiratory rate: 30–60 breaths per minute
- Blood pressure (term infant) (Figure 4-15):
  Systolic: 50–70 mmHg, increasing by four days of age to 60–90 mmHg
  Diastolic: 25–45 mmHg, with a slight rise by four days of age

The nurse also reviews hematocrit and serum glucose values, urine checks (specific gravity, glucose, protein, pH), stool checks (occult blood), acid-base status, recent laboratory studies, and outstanding laboratory test results. Each NICU should have available to the nursing staff a listing of normal laboratory values specific for its hospital laboratory. Laboratory values, properly interpreted, are instrumental in providing an accurate picture of the neonate's clinical condition.

Pain Assessment and Management

Many of the procedures and treatments for infants with respiratory distress are inherently painful.[60] Many tools are currently available for assessing neonatal pain.[61] Each nursing unit should have a pain assessment tool that has documented reliability and validity, is appropriate for the patient care population, and is practical in the clinical setting. Pain assessment should be done with every vital sign assessment and before and after every procedure.[62] Interventions range from comfort measures (e.g., pacifier, swaddling, and kangaroo care) to sucrose nipples, topical anesthetics, pharmacologic sedatives, and analgesics (Table 4-19). Chapter 11 covers pharmacotherapy in depth. The infant's response to the intervention should be assessed and documented. Further action should be taken until the infant is comfortable based on clinical assessment, including reevaluation with the pain scale.

One iatrogenic problem when aggressive and long-term pain management with opiates is necessary is neonatal withdrawal symptoms when medication is no longer necessary. This complication must be recognized and the infant provided with a supported transition off the medication. A neonatal abstinence scoring system is another infant care requirement, coupled with intervention strategies ranging from comfort measures to pharmacologic treatment. Again, the infant's response to the intervention should be assessed and documented, and further appropriate action should be taken until the infant's withdrawal signs and symptoms are reasonably controlled.[63] The parents may need additional reassurance because drug withdrawal changes the infant's behavior, and they may feel there is a social stigma attached to the need to wean opiates.

Endotracheal Tube Care

Endotracheal intubation with mechanical ventilation is a common management strategy for the clinically ill neonate with respiratory distress. Airway management is crucial to the well-being of the intubated infant and requires considerable time and attention by the bedside health care provider(s). Accidental extubation or endotracheal tube (ETT) occlusion can result in bradycardia, hypoxia, and the urgent need for reintubation. Repeated intubation can cause serious damage to the trachea, including subglottic stenosis, vocal cord

FIGURE 4-15
Systolic, diastolic, mean, and pulse pressures for newborns (based on birth weight) during the first 12 hours of life.

Linear regressions (broken lines) and 95% confidence limits (solid lines) of systolic (top left) and diastolic (bottom left) aortic blood pressures and mean pressure (top right) and pulse pressure (bottom right) on birth weight in healthy newborn infants during the first 12 hours after birth.

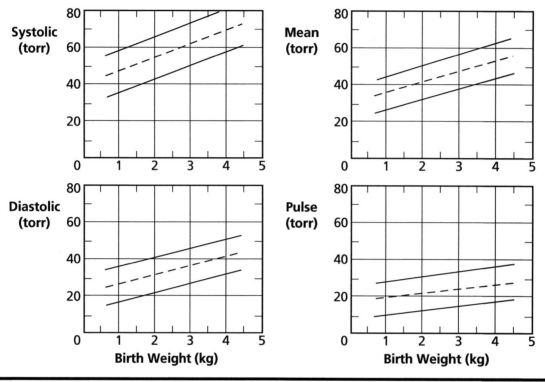

Adapted from: Versmold HT, et al. 1981. Aortic blood pressure during the first 12 hours of life in infants 610 to 4,220 grams. *Pediatrics* 67(5): 611. Reprinted by permission.

injury, and tracheal perforation.[64,65] On taking over the patient's care, the bedside nurse must know the optimal position of the ETT and the insertion depth for the suction catheter. With each assessment, the nurse should visually inspect the tube for movement and security of placement.

To maintain the patency of the artificial airway (the ETT), the nurse must also be able to identify when the patient is in need of suctioning. Indicators include visible secretions in the ETT, audible coarse rhonchi, or an acute change in vital signs or oxygen saturation level. Monitored ventilator parameters, such as reduced tidal volumes, can also indicate the need for suctioning.

Suctioning of the ETT can be done using one of two general approaches:

1. The suction catheter can be passed through a closed in-line suction system or via a modified ETT adapter that allows entry of the catheter without disconnecting the infant from mechanical ventilation.

2. The patient can be disconnected from mechanical ventilation and manually ventilated during suctioning. This should be done as a two-person procedure to ensure adequate ventilation of the infant during suctioning.

Closed suctioning is associated with fewer disturbances in heart rate and oxygenation during the suctioning process, but a Cochrane review was unable to find sufficient evidence to support one suctioning method over the other.[66–68] No matter which technique is used, key points, as outlined in Table 4-20, must be observed to minimize the side effects potentially associated with ETT suctioning.

Complications of suctioning can include cardiac arrhythmias and bradycardia, hypoxemia, changes in blood pressure and cerebral blood flow, intraventricular hemorrhage, barotrauma, tracheobronchial trauma (including perforation and hemorrhage), atelectasis, infection, and pneumothorax.[66,69,70] Figure 4-16 shows the type of card that should be placed at the bedside of an intubated infant or one with a tracheostomy to help prevent errors during suctioning.

TABLE 4-19
Potential Pain Interventions for the Infant[139–143]

Behavioral Interventions
Nonnutritive sucking (pacifier)
Sucrose pacifier
Positioning: flexed with limb containment and hands to midline
Rocking and holding
Environmental Interventions
Prewarm heel stick before procedure
Dim lighting and decrease noise to reduce stress response
Cluster care procedures
Local Anesthetics
Subcutaneous lidocaine
Penile nerve block for circumcision
Pharmacologic Interventions
Oral analgesics
Opioids
Sedatives in conjunction with opioids

TABLE 4-20
Key Points for Safe ETT Suctioning in Neonates[65,66,68,69,140,144,145]

Use suction catheter of appropriate size for ETT size; catheter should be half to two-thirds the diameter of the ETT.
Keep suction catheter sterile.
Do not insert catheter beyond tip of ETT; catheters should have markings at measured intervals; bedside card should indicate depth of suctioning (see Figure 4-16).
Mechanically regulated suction pressure should be set just high enough to move secretions into the catheter; generally, pressure should not exceed 100 mmHg, although clinical trials have not established a clear recommendation.
Monitor vital signs, including blood pressure and pulse oximetry readings, during the procedure. Evaluate for signs of increased respiratory distress or pain.
Pass catheter gently; if resistance is met, withdraw catheter slightly before suction is applied to avoid mucosa trauma.
Apply suction only as the suction catheter is withdrawn from the ETT.
Limit suction duration to 10 seconds.
Limit number of suction passes to number needed to clear secretions.
The routine use of saline is not recommended. Instill saline to lubricate suction catheter or to loosen tenacious secretions based on your hospital's protocol; limit volume of saline instilled to 0.1–0.2 mL/kg/body weight up to a maximum of 0.5 mL total dose.

Other considerations to minimize the risk of ventilator acquired pneumonia in the intubated patient include:

1. Appropriate and frequent oral care
2. Placement of an orogastric tube for decompression
3. Elevation of the head of the bed by 15 to 30 degrees
4. Limiting disconnection from the ventilator during patient repositioning
5. Correct hygiene when handling the ventilator circuit, including draining water from the circuit whenever it is moved, to prevent aspiration

These recommendations are derived from adult studies, but have been applied to the NICU patient to improve clinical practice.[71]

CHEST PHYSIOTHERAPY

Chest physiotherapy (CPT) is an effective means of facilitating removal of secretions and is sometimes used as part of the treatment regimen for a neonate experiencing respiratory distress. Airways may be obstructed by secretions and debris; examples of diseases with hypersecretion include cystic fibrosis and pneumonia. A patient with neuromuscular compromise, an ETT, or a tracheostomy is at risk as a result of damaged mucociliary clearance mechanisms and a limited ability to cough and clear secretions.

CPT is usually administered by either a respiratory therapist or nurse. Two techniques are used, augmented by appropriate positioning. Percussion is performed using a cupped hand or a well-padded cuplike appliance like a circular face mask. In term infants, percussion can be performed using a cupped hand, in preterm infants, by holding the three middle fingers in a tented position. If a face mask is used, the adapter should be plugged to maintain the air pocket that generates the movement (or hertz) that mobilizes debris.

The second method is manual application of vibration during expiration, using the fingertips.[66] Manual application of vibrations involves placing the fingers on the chest and moving them in a quivering or rapidly vibrating manner during the expiratory phase. Because of the difficulty of this procedure, vibrations are often done

FIGURE 4-16
Example of a bedside card to aid caregivers during suctioning of intubated infants.

Patient Label
ETT Placement and Suctioning Guide
Date Tube Inserted: _9/30/2012_
ETT Size: _3.0_ mm   ETT cut at _12_ cm
Secured with _green_ NEOBAR _7.5_ cm @ Lip
Suction Catheter Size: _6_ Fr.   Suction Depth: _17_ cm

FIGURE 4-17
Postural drainage.

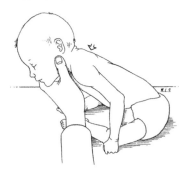

Drainage of the posterior segments of the upper lobe. The infant is leaned over at a 30° angle from the sitting position. The clinician claps and vibrates over the upper back on both sides.

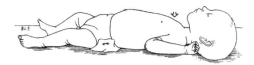

Drainage of the anterior segments of the upper lobe. While the infant is lying flat on the back, the clinician claps and vibrates between the nipples and the clavicle on both sides.

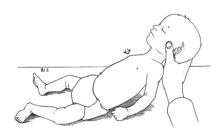

Drainage of the apical segment of the upper lobe. The infant is leaned backward about 30° from the sitting position, and the clinician claps or vibrates the clavicle on both sides.

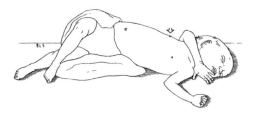

For drainage of the right middle lobe, the caregiver elevates the hips to about 5 inches above the head, rolls the infant backward one-quarter turn, and then claps and vibrates over the right nipple. For drainage of the lingular segments of the left upper lobe, the caregiver places the infant in the same position, but with the left side lifted upward, then claps and vibrates over the left nipple.

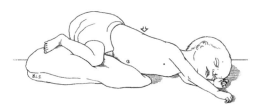

Drainage of the lateral basal segments of the lower lobes. The caregiver places the infant on the left side with the hips elevated to a level about 8 inches above that of the head. The caregiver rolls the infant forward one-quarter turn and then claps or vibrates over the lower ribs. Note that the position shown is for draining the right side. For draining the left side, the same procedure is followed, except that the infant is placed on the right side.

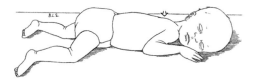

Drainage of the superior segments of the lower lobe. The clinician places the infant flat on the stomach and then claps or vibrates at top of the scapula on the back side of the spine.

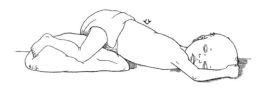

Drainage of the posterior basal segments of the lower lobe. The clinician places the infant on the stomach with the hips at a level 8 inches above that of the head, then claps and vibrates over the lower ribs close to the spine on both sides.

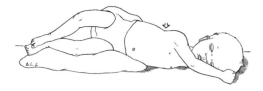

Drainage of the anterior basal segment of the lower lobes. The caregiver places the infant on the left side with the hips at a level about 8 inches above that of the head, then claps and vibrates just beneath the axilla. Note that for drainage of the opposite anterior basal segment, the infant is turned on the right side.

From: MacKendrick W, et al. 2011. Pulmonary care. In *Assisted Ventilation of the Neonate*, 5th ed., Goldsmith JP, and Karotkin EH, eds. Philadelphia: Saunders, 119. Reprinted by permission.

TABLE 4-21
Complications of Chest Physiotherapy

Hypoxemia	Aspiration
Tachypnea	Increased intracranial pressure
Increasing dyspnea	Increased intraventricular hemorrhage
Rib fractures	
Positional hypotension or hypertension	Bruising
	Cyanosis
Ventilation-perfusion alterations from postural changes	Hemorrhage (high risk in patients with recent tracheostomy or prosthetic cardiac patch)
Atelectasis	
Bronchospasm	
Increased oxygen consumption	Inadvertent extubation or mainstem intubation
Increased gastroesophageal reflux episodes	Displaced tube (chest tube or gastrostomy tube)
Vomiting	Cardiac arrhythmias

Adapted from: Barnhart SL, and Czervinske MP. 1995. *Clinical Handbook of Perinatal and Pediatric Respiratory Care.* Philadelphia: Saunders, 259. Reprinted by permission.

TABLE 4-22
Contraindications to Chest Physiotherapy

Absolute Contraindications	Relative Contraindications	Modified Positioning Required
Pulmonary hemorrhage	Unstable cardiac status	Increased intracranial pressure
Foreign body aspiration	Cardiac arrhythmias	Hypertension
Untreated tension pneumothorax	Immediate postoperative period following tracheostomy or tracheobronchial reconstruction	Abdominal distention
Displaced fracture of the ribs		Compromised diaphragm movement
		Continuous feedings
	Low platelet count (<50,000 cells/ mm^2)	Chest tube or gastrostomy tube in place
		Severe gastroesophageal reflux
		Premature infant at risk for intracranial hemorrhage

Adapted from: Barnhart SL, and Czervinske MP. 1995. *Clinical Handbook of Perinatal and Pediatric Respiratory Care.* Philadelphia: Saunders, 258. Reprinted by permission.

instead with a pulmonary vibrator or a padded electric toothbrush.[69,72]

Postural drainage (PD) utilizes gravity to facilitate the movement of secretions from the peripheral airways to the large airway and is part of CPT (Figure 4-17). There are often limitations on the positioning of critically ill infants; it can be difficult or even impossible to place them in the ideal position. Utilization of PD, including the upright and the head-down positions, should not be implemented without approval of the attending neonatologist.

The nurse must be aware of the potential for producing severe hypoxemia while performing CPT. Care must be taken with all infants not to cause soft tissue damage or to fracture ribs. This is especially true for premature infants and those at risk for rickets. Table 4-21 lists complications associated with the CPT procedure. The infant should have continuous cardiorespiratory monitoring and pulse oximetry monitoring in place during the procedure. The practitioner needs to constantly evaluate infant tolerance by being aware of heart rate, breathing pattern, skin color, and body temperature, as well as placement of all tubes and wires. Percussion and PD should not be done on infants who are at high risk for intraventricular hemorrhage. Table 4-22 lists contraindications to CPT and PD.

Although CPT is effective for assisting in the removal of tracheobronchial secretions in infants, the literature does not support its routine use.[66,73] CPT should be ordered only when control of secretions or atelectasis is a known problem. The frequency of percussion is every

two to eight hours, varying with patient diagnosis and tolerance. Therapy is given over three to five minutes, focusing on any areas of known atelectasis and avoiding the xiphoid process and the lower rib area over the liver and spleen.[72] PT after extubation was not found to reduce alveolar atelectasis, but did decrease the need for reintubation when given every one to two hours.[74]

ADMINISTRATION OF MEDICATIONS

A major nursing responsibility is the prompt and accurate administration of medications. Dosages of drugs given to the neonate are based on body weight, and every nurse must be capable of calculating such doses. Because doses and volumes are relatively small, extreme care is needed in the preparation and administration of medications. Complicating medication preparation and administration are the infant's possible fluid restriction and dependence on a continuous infusion of glucose. Drugs infused over several minutes or hours should be mixed with glucose solutions when compatible to provide optimal calories.

The literature is rich with information on drug doses, routes, and intervals, but often lacks the necessary information on minimum dilution volumes, administration rates, and drug compatibilities. Table 4-23 is a protocol sheet listing the information that should be available to the nurse for every drug administered in the NICU.

TABLE 4-23
Protocol of Essential Drug Information

Name: Generic name with trade names (indexed by both names)

Indication/Action: Class, indication/action of drug

Dose/Route/Interval: Dose (listed as a single dose, not as total daily dose), route, and interval of administration

Preparation: Type of fluid for reconstitution and dilution; preferred fluids listed first (see drug label for reconstitution instructions)

Administration Rate: Desired rate of administration

Other Pertinent Information: Drug levels, side effects, antidotes, incompatibilities

TABLE 4-24
Estimated Fluid Requirement for Term Infants

To Replace Loss from:	mL/kg
Insensible water loss	15–20
Urine	60–90
Stool*	10
Growth*	10–15
Water of oxidation	–15
Total	80–120

* On day 1 of life, these values should be 0 rising to the stated numbers by day 3.

From: Wassner SJ. 1990. Fluid therapy. In *Current Therapy in Neonatal-Perinatal Medicine,* part II, Nelson N, ed. Toronto: Decker, 153. Reprinted by permission.

FLUID REQUIREMENTS

Infants in respiratory distress are usually managed initially with intravenous fluids. Umbilical catheters and percutaneously inserted IV catheters are used. Central venous lines may be utilized if prolonged parenteral fluids are required. Nursing personnel are responsible for ongoing assessment to ensure both accuracy of the infusion rate and patency of the line. IV or catheter accidents can result in major iatrogenic complications.

Fluid requirements vary with gestational and chronologic age. Table 4-24 illustrates how fluid requirements are calculated for term infants. Fluid is required to replace water retained for growth. It is also required to replace water lost via urine, stool, or drainage (such as gastrointestinal or wound drainage), as well as fluid lost from the respiratory tract and via the skin (insensible water loss [IWL]). About 30 percent of IWL normally occurs through the respiratory tract as moisture in expired gas; the remaining 70 percent is lost through the skin.[75] IWL is especially significant in the neonate. It increases proportionally as birth weight and gestational age decrease.[76] Basal levels of IWL are 20 mL fluid/kg. This level is markedly increased in VLBW infants with larger surface area for size, immature skin with increased permeability, greater percentage of body water, increased skin blood flow in relation to metabolic rate, and higher respiratory rate.[6,75] Table 4-25 lists factors that can increase or decrease IWL in the neonate.

During the first week of life, physiologic diuresis causes a 5–10 percent weight loss in the neonate. Smaller preterm infants experience a higher fraction of weight loss, 10–15 percent, because of their proportionately larger percentage of extracellular water present at birth and their immature renal function, which produces more dilute urine.[6,75] Fluid requirements increase with postnatal age and the introduction of enteral feedings. When feedings begin, fecal water losses increase, and urine output increases in response to the enlarged renal solute.

NUTRITIONAL REQUIREMENTS

The healthy neonate has high nutrition requirements to support growth, but the ill neonate's nutritional needs are even greater. Enteral feedings are the ideal method of meeting caloric needs with a balanced diet. Unfortunately, the critically ill neonate may not be

TABLE 4-25
Factors Affecting Insensible Water Loss (IWL) in Neonates

Increases IWL

Immaturity (50%–300%)

Radiant warmer (50%–200%)

Forced convection incubator (30%–50%)

Phototherapy (40%–100%)

Respiratory distress

Elevated body or ambient temperature (A 1° increase in body temperature produces a 30% increase in IWL.)

Skin breakdown or injury

Congenital defects (omphalocele, gastroschisis, neural tube defect)

Motor activity, crying (up to 70%)

Other factors that increase metabolic rate

Decreases IWL

Plastic heat shields (30%–50%)

Double-wall incubator or heat shield (30%–50%)

Plastic blanket under radiant warmer (30%–50%)

High humidity (50%–100%)

Transport thermal blanket (70%)

Assisted ventilation with warmed and humidified air (20%–30%)

Increasing postnatal age

Semipermeable dressing or topical agents (50%)

From: Blackburn ST. 2007. *Maternal, Fetal, and Neonatal Physiology: A Clinical Perspective,* 2nd ed. Philadelphia: Saunders, 405. Reprinted by permission.

a candidate for enteral feedings in the first days of life or longer.

Parenteral Nutrition

Parenteral nutrition is begun with glucose infusions, usually 5 or 10 percent dextrose in water, depending on the infant's tolerance of the glucose load. Most infants can tolerate initial glucose loads of 4 to 8 mg/kg/minute.[6,77,78] If the VLBW infant cannot tolerate the glucose load, the intake should be decreased until serum glucose levels stabilize. If the glucose load is too low for the caloric needs of the infant or if he is unable to tolerate even minimal glucose intake, insulin therapy may be indicated to satisfy the required energy intake.[79] The glucose intake is increased gradually with a usual goal of 11–12 mg/kg/minute of glucose as long as hyperglycemia (blood glucose >150 mg/dL) does not develop.[77,78] A minimum of 50–60 kcal/kg/day, given as lipids and glucose, with 1.5 g/kg/day of amino acid solution, is needed to achieve positive nitrogen balance.[4] Glucose intolerance, as evidenced by a blood glucose level greater than 150 mg/dL and/or glucosuria greater than +1, can be precipitated by stress, thermal instability, sepsis, acidosis, or respiratory failure.

Protein can be provided by administration of a parenteral amino acid solution. The infant should be given a minimum of 1.5–2 g/kg/day of protein as soon after birth as possible. This can be increased within the first few days of life to 3 g/kg/day as long as renal and liver functions are adequate.[80] Preterm infants may require an even higher intake of up to 3.5–4 g/kg/day, but these levels may be difficult to achieve.[6,81] With a nonprotein intake of 80–85 kcal/kg/day and an amino acid intake of 3 g/kg/day, nitrogen retention may occur at a rate similar to that of the fetus.[4] Electrolytes, vitamins, minerals, and trace elements must also be provided as part of the parenteral solution.

Fat, given as an IV fat emulsion, can also be started by one to two days of age. Intravenous fat emulsions provide essential fatty acids and are an excellent source of calories in minimal fluid volumes because they are calorie dense compared with carbohydrates and protein. The infant is given 0.5–1 g/kg/day of fat, which is usually increased by 0.5 g/kg/day to 3 g/kg/day.[82] Preterm infants may not be able to tolerate the higher amounts. Serum turbidity is a poor predictor of hyperlipidemia; therefore, blood levels must be monitored. Serum triglyceride levels >150–200 mg/dL usually require a decrease in fat administration.[78]

Complications of parenteral nutrition include electrolyte imbalance, hypoglycemia, hyperglycemia, hypocalcemia, hypercalcemia, and hypophosphatemia. These problems can usually be corrected by manipulation of the solution. Primary complications, seen more frequently with prolonged administration, are hepatic dysfunction (cholestasis) and complications associated with central venous catheters (e.g., sepsis, thrombosis, cardiac tamponade) and peripheral venous access (e.g., infiltrates).[77]

Enteral Feedings

Enteral feedings should be started as soon as is feasible. They remain the best source of nutrition for the neonate—especially for the low birth weight infant who is particularly vulnerable to malnutrition. Human milk is ideal for starting enteral feedings in the VLBW infant.[83] Mothers of VLBW infants should be strongly encouraged to express breast milk for their infants if at all possible, even if they choose to express and store milk for just a short period of time. Even infants requiring mechanical ventilation should be considered candidates for early enteral feedings (Table 4-26).

A preterm infant usually must be started on gavage feedings in small volumes that are gradually increased over several days. Feeding guidelines can be utilized to achieve a consistent approach to advancing enteral feedings and have been shown to improve nutritional outcomes.[84–86] Each nurse should be capable of properly placing a gavage tube and correctly administering the feeding to the neonate.[87] Infants who use pacifiers during gavage feedings have been found to nipple feed earlier.[88–90] They are also discharged home earlier.[91] The infant's clinical status is assessed with each feeding or every two to four hours if feedings are continuous. Abdominal distention, regurgitation, absence of bowel sounds, bile-stained gastric aspirates, and large feeding residuals are indications of feeding intolerance. Table 4-27 outlines nursing considerations when administering enteral feedings.

Determination of the formula, volume, and route of feeding is based on the infant's gestational age, weight, and clinical status. Formula for term infants contains 20 kcal/oz. This is considered the caloric content of breast milk as well, although the actual caloric content can vary greatly. Supplements for breast milk are available to provide the additional calories, vitamins, and minerals required by premature infants. Utilization of breast milk requires special care measures by the mother and the nursery staff to prevent excessive bacterial

TABLE 4-26
Neonatal Enteral Feedings[92,146–152]

Route	Advantages	Disadvantages
Gastric (intermittent bolus)	Utilizes stomach capacity; promotes intestinal growth Utilizes digestive capabilities; promotes cyclical gut hormone secretions and bile flow Potential for greater absorption Tube easier to place and less likely than an indwelling tube to perforate gastrointestinal tract	Potential compromise in neonates with severe respiratory distress, delayed gastric emptying, esophageal chalasia, or during the use of nasal continuous positive airway pressure (CPAP) Bradycardia with tube placement Bypasses salivary and lingual enzymes
Gastric (continuous)	Reduces energy required for absorption of nutrients; minimizes volume given at any one time May be better tolerated by VLBW infants or by infants with bowel disease or severe cardiopulmonary disease	Increased risk of bacterial contamination of formula or breast milk Decreases fat content of breast milk
Transpyloric (continuous)	Useful in infants with significant delayed gastric emptying or severe gastroesophageal reflux with risk of aspiration Used in infants with gastric distention on nasal CPAP	As per continuous gastric feedings Risk of bowel perforation and aspiration Increased radiation exposure because of more frequent x-ray exams for placement Possible decreased absorption of potassium and fat Possible increased mortality; not recommended for routine use in the preterm infant

contamination. Use of breast milk in continuous feedings has been associated with high bacterial growth and loss of fat content in early studies.[92,93] Caution should be used and unit protocols followed to ensure that milk does not become contaminated. Steady growth can normally be achieved when the infant is receiving 110–120 kcal/kg/day. If the infant cannot tolerate the high fluid volumes necessary to achieve this goal, a modified formula of increased caloric density (24 kcal/oz) can be utilized. Special formulas for low birth weight infants contain additional protein, easily absorbed carbohydrates, and easily digested and absorbed lipids, along with additional electrolytes, minerals, trace metals, and vitamins needed to meet their infants' increased needs.[4]

The time when suck, swallow, and respirations are coordinated varies.[6,94,95] Generally, infants can begin successful nipple feeding by 32–34 weeks gestational age if they are alert and vigorous without respiratory distress.[96] For breastfeeding infants, "practice" sessions can be initiated when the infant is medically stable.

SKIN CARE

Skin integrity relates directly to neonatal well-being, and skin care is recognized as a vital nursing function. Skin maturity and integrity greatly affect thermoregulation, insensible water loss, chemical absorption, and susceptibility to infection (Table 4-28).

The skin is composed of three layers: epidermis, dermis, and subcutaneous fat. The epidermis is mature by 34 weeks gestation.[27] The outer layer of the epidermis, known as the stratum corneum (horny layer), is composed of several layers of flattened and dehydrated cells. It is tough and fairly impermeable. It constitutes a functional barrier against a variety of substances, protects against invasion by microorganisms, and is vital in decreasing both transepidermal water loss and heat loss.[27] The dermal-epidermal junction is a specialized attachment between the epidermis and the papillary, or outer, layer of the dermis. The dermis lies beneath the epidermis and is formed primarily of connective tissue (including collagen and elastic tissue). Structures found in the dermis include lymphatics, nerves and nerve endings, blood vessels, and the cutaneous appendage (pilosebaceous units, eccrine and apocrine sweat glands). Underlying the dermis is subcutaneous fat, first appearing around 14 weeks gestation, but not significant in quantity until near term. Subcutaneous fat absorbs shocks, stores energy, and maintains body heat.

When an infant is born prematurely, the stratum corneum is underdeveloped, and the dermal-epidermal junction is weak, resulting in markedly increased skin permeability. This is especially true of infants less than 34 weeks gestational age and 2–3 weeks chronological age. In infants born at less than 25 weeks gestation, skin maturation may take even longer, until 4–8 weeks chronological age.[26,27,97] Preterm infants also display functional immaturity of the sweat glands, altered vasomotor tone, and a deficit in the shivering reflex. Consequently, they are at increased risk for temperature instability, high insensible water loss, and skin injury.[26,98,99]

TABLE 4-27
Nursing Considerations for Infants Receiving Enteral Feedings

Trophic feedings are minimal-volume feedings (12–24 mL/kg/day) used to stimulate growth and maturation of the gastrointestinal tract.[153]

Minimal requirements for beginning enteral feedings include presence of bowel sounds, passage of initial meconium stool, and baseline assessment of abdominal girth.

Whenever possible, orogastric (OG) tubes are preferred over nasogastric (NG) feeding tubes so as to keep the nares open.

Placement of indwelling feeding tubes should be assessed on insertion, with documentation of centimeter mark placement entered on nursing flow sheet. Tube placement should be reassessed with each hands-on assessment of the patient.

Formula used for continuous feedings should be changed every 12 hours. If human milk is being given, it should be changed every 4 hours. It is best to infuse human milk with a syringe pump and microbore tubing to minimize the priming volume needed.

Mothers should be encouraged to collect breast milk. Guidelines for breast milk feedings include the following:[4]

    Freshly expressed milk is best.

    Freshly expressed milk should be labeled with the mother's name, the baby's name, and the date and time of pumping. It can be refrigerated for up to 48 hours.

    Frozen breast milk can be stored for 2–3 weeks in a home freezer or for 6–12 months in deep freeze.

    Thaw only the amount of milk that can be used in a 24-hour period. Breast milk should be thawed/heated in a water bath, never in the microwave.

    Advise parents that breast milk must be kept frozen during transport to and from the hospital.

    Freshly pumped breast milk should not be layered onto previously pumped milk.

OG/NG tubes used for intermittent gavage feedings should be assessed for placement at the time of placement and before each feeding.

During gavage feedings, nonnutritive sucking should be offered.

Intermittent gavage feedings should be administered by gravity flow unless otherwise ordered by physician.

Infants can be started on nipple feedings if:

    Their respiratory rate is <60 breaths/minute.

    They are 32–34 weeks corrected gestational age.

    They show ability to coordinate suck, swallow, and breathing activity.

    Behavioral cues (such as rooting, sucking on pacifier or fingers) are present.

Assessment for signs of feeding intolerance should be ongoing during all types of enteral feedings. Signs should be reported to appropriate medical personnel as they occur. Signs of feeding intolerance include:

    Increased abdominal girth measurements.

    Gastric residuals greater than the hourly rate with continuous feedings or bile-stained or bloody aspirates.

    Absence of bowel sounds.

    Presence of dilated bowel loops or abdominal discoloration.

    Increased number and/or severity of apnea and bradycardia spells.

    Vomiting.

    Bloody stools.

Adapted from: Lockwood CJ, and Lemons JA. 2007. *Guidelines for Perinatal Care*, 6th ed. Elk Grove Village, Illinois: American Academy of Pediatrics and American College of Obstetricians and Gynecologists, 205–301; and Newell SJ. 2000. Enteral feeding of the micropremie. *Clinics in Perinatology* 27(1): 221–234.

TABLE 4-28
Multiple Physiologic Roles of the Skin at Birth

Barrier to water loss

Thermoregulation

Infection control

Immunosurveillance

Acid mantle formation

Antioxidant function

Ultraviolet light photoprotection

Barrier to chemicals

Tactile discrimination

Attraction to caregiver

From: Hoath SB. 2011. Physiologic development of the skin. In *Fetal and Neonatal Physiology*, 4th ed., Polin RA, Fox WW, and Abman SH, eds. Philadelphia: Saunders, 684. Reprinted by permission.

Normally the stratum corneum is a diffusion barrier, aided by skin surface lipids (sebum). The infant born prematurely has an underdeveloped stratum corneum and thin layer of keratinocytes; the skin, therefore, is highly susceptible to percutaneous absorption of substances. Factors influencing absorption are temperature, hydration, perfusion, surface lipids, gestational and chronological age, condition of the skin, and the chemical and vehicle used.

The skin surface at birth is pH neutral. Acidic skin pH develops during the first few weeks after delivery, providing an acid mantle that has a bactericidal quality. Acid mantle development is delayed in the VLBW infant, and bathing with alkaline soaps alters the status of the acid mantle.[97,100]

Much work is directed to protecting the integrity of the VLBW infant's friable skin. There is evidence to support the use of emollients in the NICU patient.[10,101] Prophylactic application of topical ointments in the first days of the VLBW infant's life is not recommended because of concern over an increased incidence of infection.[102] Keeping the VLBW infant in a high-humidity environment remains an important means of protecting the fragile skin.

The skin care needs of the sick infant include preventing physical injury (stripping of the epidermis, thermal burns, pressure necrosis), preventing chemical injury (chemical infiltrates, chemical burns), minimizing IWL, minimizing risk of infection, and avoiding excessive transdermal absorption of topical agents. Table 4-29 provides a standard of care, listing nursing interventions designed to protect the integrity of the neonate's skin.

TABLE 4-29
Standard of Care for Neonatal Skin[4,6,8,132,137,154–156]

Nursing Diagnosis: Risk for impaired skin integrity

Expected Outcome: Infant will maintain intact skin integrity, with minimal trauma, and skin will have a moist to slightly dry and flaky quality.

Nursing Interventions/Rationales:

- Assess skin and document integrity, color, perfusion, turgor, temperature, and edema each shift and as needed to look for altered integrity.
- Notify physician of significant findings to ensure appropriate medical intervention.
- Minimize use of adhesives such as benzoin preparations to avoid epidermal stripping.
- Use alcohol sparingly to avoid chemical burns.
- Utilize pectin barriers and hydrogel- or hydrocolloid-backed adhesive electrodes; change as indicated by infant's skin integrity to avoid epidermal stripping.
- Use patience and water-soaked cotton balls when removing adhesives from infant skin to avoid epidermal stripping.
- Allow transparent dressings to peel off naturally to avoid epidermal stripping.
- Utilize sterile gauze with mild pressure for stasis of bleeding to prevent infection to the area.
- Avoid hot packs or heat-retaining plastic to avoid thermal burns.
- Avoid use of emollient and agents with preservatives and dyes to avoid chemical burns.
- Using sterile water, remove topical antiseptic on skin after procedures and before dressing applications to avoid chemical burns and systemic absorption.
- Rotate temperature probe sites a minimum of every 24 hours to avoid skin irritation.
- Turn infant every 4–6 hours and as needed, and utilize gel-filled positioning aid, egg-crate, or foam mattress to prevent pressure points.
- Avoid causing pressure points or constriction of blood flow with dressings, tubing, probes, or clothes to avoid altered tissue perfusion.
- Bathe acutely ill infants only in diaper area or where skin is soiled; bathe convalescent infants with soap only once or twice a week to avoid drying of the skin.
- Utilize less alkaline soaps (such as Lowila, Aveeno, Basis, Neutrogena, Purpose, or Oilatum) to avoid drying of the skin.
- Use a nonperfumed emollient (such as Eucerin or Aquaphor) to treat excessively dry skin.
- Treat IV infiltrates with hyaluronidase or with phentolamine if vasoconstrive agent infiltrates) to minimize chemical burns.
- Elevate and immobilize the area of IV infiltrates to reduce edema to the area.
- Do not use moist heat on IV infiltrates to avoid thermal burns.
- Use hydrogel dressings for extravasation injuries.
- Use semipermeable occlusive dressings over superficial wounds to promote more rapid epidermal barrier repair.

DEVELOPMENTAL CARE

Survival rates in the NICU have improved, but infants continue to be at risk for poor neurodevelopmental outcomes. Researchers have been assessing the caregiving environment and its impact on the growth and development of the fragile infant with the goal of improving both short-term and long-term developmental outcomes. Much research is still required to demonstrate consistent effects of developmental care interventions on clinical outcomes.[103] However, a strong base of information exists.

Studies have documented that the NICU environment can be overstimulating and that its complexity exceeds the ability of infants, especially those born preterm, to cope or adapt.[104–108] *Adaptation* is defined as a process in which bodily functions and behavioral responses are modified to promote an equilibrium between self and environment. According to Als and associates, adaptation in the infant is a function of neurophysiologic development and requires integrated functioning between his physiologic and behavioral systems.[109] Lack of adaptability can be attributed to a disruption in the infant's attempts to cope with environmental events such as light, noise, pain, and touch. This disruption may cause imbalances in autonomic, motor, and state subsystem functioning. Preterm infants are especially vulnerable because they have not attained integrated functioning between their physiologic and behavioral systems. If developmentally able, preterm infants will attempt to use self-regulatory mechanisms, such as sucking and hand-to-mouth maneuvers, to maintain balance and cope with disruptions, but these self-regulatory mechanisms are limited or absent in most preterm infants.

Concern exists that these imbalances in autonomic, motor, and state subsystem functioning, if not corrected, may result in late neurobehavioral sequelae and subsequent developmental delays.[104] Because there is a potential association between infant organization and developmental outcomes, all nursing care and the caregiving environment should support optimal infant development.[106,110]

Parents can contribute to optimal infant development by providing kangaroo care. Skin-to-skin contact, or kangaroo care, has been shown to correlate with infants who are more socially alert at six months with higher Bayley developmental scores in the mental and motor domains. In addition, mothers who provided kangaroo care were less depressed, perceived their infants as less abnormal, and showed more positive affect, touch, and adaptation to infant cues during the hospitalization period.[111]

Nurses can support the infant's developmental agenda by allowing and supporting stabilization of physiologic and behavioral functioning, which may ultimately improve developmental outcome. Table 4-30 provides an example of a generic developmental care plan. The physical environment of the NICU is part of the developmental care plan, with focus on how the unit supports or controls development issues such as light, sound, sleep patterns, pain, and promotion of family-centered care.[112] The reader is referred to *Developmental Care of Newborns and Infants: A Guide for Health Professionals,* which contains extensive information on this topic.[113]

CARE OF THE FAMILY

An essential component of care for the neonate is care for the neonate's parents and family. Parent care begins with a respect for these individuals' rights as parents and an understanding that they are individuals in a crisis situation. When someone's coping skills cannot deal with a problem or threat, the situation becomes a crisis. It is important to remember that it is the parents, not the health care team members, who define the magnitude or significance of the crisis. Reaction to a crisis causes a temporary disruption of one's normal psychological equilibrium, resulting in tension and discomfort. Feelings of guilt, anxiety, fear, shame, and helplessness may occur. As a result of this affective upset, the individual's cognitive process may be impaired, leading to confusion and disorganized behavior.[114,115]

Because parents usually anticipate a normal birth and a healthy infant, a crisis situation develops when these outcomes do not occur. Parents may perceive the premature infant as defective, even if otherwise healthy. The birth of a premature or critically ill infant may also be viewed as the mother's failure to produce a normal or complete child. The guilt feelings arising from such perceptions often discourage or prohibit closeness between parent and child, as well as between the parents themselves. Guilt, coupled with a life-threatening situation, interferes with the parents' ability to understand and deal with the problem.[116]

The initial phase of crisis is usually marked by a period of physical, functional, and emotional disorganization. Parents feel they cannot take on their parenting role because they do not have a child to care for. The hospital staff assumes the care of their infant, and the parents' feelings of inadequacy and disorganization intensify. They may mimic the physician or nurses in an attempt to define their role as parent. When they cannot perform at the same level as these professionals, further feelings of inadequacy develop.

Parents may use denial as a coping mechanism to control the disorganization the crisis precipitates. Withdrawal may be a form of denial, as well as part of the anticipatory grief for the potential loss of their child. Anger and resentment are also seen during this phase. Parents may direct their anger at themselves or displace it onto others, including family, friends, or health care workers.[117] Both physical and mental barriers hamper parents in their attempts to become acquainted with and form emotional ties to their child. Going home without their baby also reinforces their feelings of disappointment and failure.[118]

Family-centered care is a concept meant to support the family through this difficult process. Family-centered care is defined as the professional support of the child and family through a

TABLE 4-30
Example of a Developmental Care Plan[112,137,158–161]

Nursing Diagnosis: Risk for disorganized infant behavior

Expected Outcome: Infant will maintain equilibrium of physiologic status; will rest in flexed position, free from hyperextension; will tolerate handling and stimulation with minimal stress responses; and will demonstrate organized sleep states and calm, quiet alerting.

Nursing Interventions/Rationales:

- Recognize stress responses (signs of overstimulation) as:

    Mild stress response: Gaze aversion, yawning, hiccups, grimacing, tongue thrusting, slack jaw, bowel movements, sneezing, coughing

    Moderate stress response: Flushing, mottling, sighing, regurgitation, finger splaying, extension of arms and legs, jitteriness, jerky movement, limpness

    Severe stress response: Hypoxia, pallor, cyanosis, tachypnea, apnea, tachycardia, bradycardia, arrhythmia.

- Take steps to reduce causes of overstimulation to minimize stress.

- Support with blanket rolls or swaddle with blanket to promote flexed position.

- Place in prone position with arms and knees flexed or on side with hands in midline as often as possible to promote flexed position.

- Avoid sudden position changes; contain limbs during and after position changes to promote flexed position.

- Avoid large neck rolls to avoid hyperextended positioning.

- Do not lift feet when in prone position; rather, lift hips for diaper change to avoid hyperextended positioning.

- Avoid supine, "spread-eagle" position to avoid hyperextended positioning.

- Shade eyes and cover ears with soft gauze or blanket when in open warmer to decrease/minimize overstimulation and stress response.

- Coordinate care to minimize unnecessary handling to decrease/minimize overstimulation and stress response.

- Talk in a soft voice; then lightly touch before handling to decrease/minimize overstimulation and stress response.

- Provide a calm, quiet environment in unit to decrease/ minimize overstimulation and stress response.

- Provide pacifier, stroking, and/or touch to comfort at least twice a day and as needed during painful procedures to decrease/minimize overstimulation and stress response.

- Shade incubator and close portholes gently to decrease/minimize overstimulation and stress response.

- Do not awaken for routine vital signs to decrease/ minimize overstimulation and stress response.

- Keep dressed if condition warrants to decrease/ minimize overstimulation and stress response.

- Schedule periods during which nursery lights are dimmed to support circadian rhythms.

- Arrange for consistent caregivers to provide continuity of care.

- Teach/demonstrate to parents how to recognize early signs of stress and to provide social interaction based on infant's readiness and response to enable parents to contribute to their baby's development.

TABLE 4-31
Helpful Techniques for Communicating With Families of Infants In the NICU*

1. Maintain eye contact. Use touch and space appropriately.
2. Use the client's name. Address the individual formally as Mr., Mrs., or Ms.
3. Begin with a tone-setting statement that indicates the infant's status.
4. Briefly describe the infant's problem(s) in lay terms.
5. Follow with the correct medical term(s), verbal and written.
6. End with a continuity statement. Explain what will happen next, but avoid making any predictions about the infant's condition.

* These are general tips. Knowledge of the family's cultural background should be the basis for respectful communication.

process of involvement, participation, and partnership underpinned by empowerment and negotiation.[119] It may begin before the infant is born by providing the parents with educational material and information about the NICU. A tour of the NICU may also by appropriate. The health care team meets with the parents to discuss expected outcomes, potential problems, and risks (Table 4-31). Parents are given freer access to the NICU, greater depth of information, and more control in decision making for their child. Key to this concept is communication.

During hospitalization, families can be empowered by ongoing communication regarding the infant's clinical status and plan of care. This may include parental participation in daily rounds, being present during medical procedures, and frequent multidisciplinary care conferences.[120] Information should be factual, and health care providers should always be aware that conflicting opinions given by various team members contribute to parental stress. Nurses are an essential communication link between the infant, family, and medical staff.[1] But the parents should always have easy, readily available access to the physician.

Throughout the infant's hospitalization, parents' needs should be identified along with those of their infant. The perceptive nurse will identify the family's strengths and capitalize on them to assist them through a difficult time. The family's weaknesses, which are sometimes easy to see and in other instances hidden, will eventually affect the parents' ability to deal with their infant's problems. Once the parents move through the grief phase and work through their sense of failure, they can begin a phase of emotional adaptation and enter into a more positive relationship with their child. They begin to focus on their infant as an individual and

resume the task of interacting with him that began during the pregnancy.

In the case of well term infants, the parents get acquainted with their child during their early days together. They gather information about their infant and assess his attitude toward them. The well term infant can communicate in various ways, focusing on the human face and listening attentively to the human voice. The child will latch onto the mother by grasping, sucking, or rooting, and she interprets these behaviors as methods of seeking contact. Parents identify signals such as crying, smiling, babbling, and arm gestures as personal communications from the infant.[121]

Infant cues play a major part in the acquaintance process. Research has shown that, for many mothers, the first positive maternal feelings toward their infant are associated with the baby's responses to them.[122] Parents use the infant's behavior to judge or assess his attitude toward them. Unfortunately, the premature or critically ill newborn does not respond to the parents in the manner typical for a well term newborn. Preterm infants have less facial expression and fewer looking behaviors.[123] As they recover, the infants may be irritable, inconsolable, or easily exhausted. Such behaviors, as well as those exhibited by a neurologically abnormal infant, can hinder parent-infant interaction. Parents need to find ways to come to terms with their infant's abilities and inabilities.

To enable communication, mothers need to be able to recognize an infant cue (conveying a need or a bid for attention) and respond appropriately to it. Factors that contribute to ineffective maternal responsiveness may include prematurity, disorganized sleep-wake cycles, and irritability. Maternal factors include a labile emotional state, lack of social support, low self-esteem, fatigue, pain, depression, and socioeconomic stressors.[124] With a greater understanding of developmental care, nurses can help parents identify the subtle behavior cues and needs of the preterm infant, thus promoting the acquaintance process and positive maternal-infant interactions.[125]

Kangaroo care has been implemented in many nurseries to support positive parent-child interaction. The diaper-clad infant is placed directly on the mother's or father's chest, under the parent's clothing. The parent may hold the infant for several hours, and medically stable infants are allowed to nurse at the breast as desired.[126–128] Mothers reported an increased sense of mastery and enhanced self-esteem following several weeks of holding their babies in the skin-to-skin kangaroo position.[129] Kangaroo care was shown to be associated with lower levels of maternal depression, more sensitive parental care of the infant, and better home care of the infant after discharge.[111] However, parents may need periods of respite. Nurses must be sensitive to their emotional status, allowing them to decline kangaroo care without guilt. Table 4-32 provides a care plan dealing with general principles that health care team members can utilize to assist the NICU parent.

As parents of critically ill and premature infants adapt emotionally and attach to their infant, they should be encouraged to assume caregiving responsibilities that take into consideration the individuality of each parent, infant, and situation. Mastering caregiving skills reinforces the parenting role and diminishes feelings of inadequacy. Reluctance to assume this caregiving role may indicate that the parents are still grieving the anticipated loss of their child. Forcing them to assume responsibilities prematurely may reinforce their feelings of disorganization.

As parents move through this getting-acquainted phase, they start to recognize the special needs of their child. How is this infant like "normal" infants? How does he differ from "normal" infants? As parents recognize their infant's uniqueness and develop an understanding his needs, they begin to accept and integrate him into their family. These tasks may be only partially completed at the time of the infant's discharge, but they eventually must be accomplished to foster a positive parent-child relationship.

DISCHARGE PLANNING

Throughout hospitalization, the goal remains the infant's successful discharge. Discharge itself can be a crisis event for parents. Depending on each family member's stage of adjustment, he or she may be at a different level of readiness to learn, and readiness is a prerequisite for successful learning. As the parents work through the emotional upheaval of their infant's hospitalization, the nurse must continually assess their status and introduce health information and caregiving skills that they are capable of handling.

Effective discharge planning ensures continuity of care and appropriate discharge timing. Timely discharge decreases the risk of nosocomial infection to the infant, reduces costs for both the family and the hospital, allows the infant to assimilate to the family unit earlier, and should provide an atmosphere more conducive to infant stimulation and development.[130,131]

Ineffective discharge planning or advocacy of excessively early discharge for financial or other reasons increases the infant's risk for illness and rehospitalization. If discharge teaching is incomplete, if community resources are inadequate, or if the family or home situation is unacceptable, then discharge is inappropriate.

Successful discharge planning and discharge teaching develop a high degree of parental confidence and competence while maintaining the health of the infant. Both decrease the stress of transition to the home and encourage formation of a healthy family unit.

To achieve these goals, the entire process of discharge planning needs to be approached systematically. This begins with the initial assessment of the infant and the family at the time of the newborn's admission to the NICU and continues as additional information becomes available. Effective discharge planning requires ongoing patient and family assessment throughout the hospitalization.

The planning process should be organized through a single individual with input from the entire health care team. A discharge coordinator provides the expertise necessary to link the family and infant to available community services. The multidisciplinary team usually includes the parents, neonatal nurses (including the primary nurse), neonatologist, nurse practitioner or resident, primary care physician, social worker, and discharge planner. Other health care providers, such as the respiratory therapist, occupational therapist, physical therapist, or nutritionist, along with representatives of the necessary community services, participate as required.

To be ready for discharge, the high-risk infant should meet the following criteria:[4]

- A sustained pattern of weight gain of sufficient duration
- Ability to maintain normal body temperature while fully clothed in an open bed with normal ambient temperature (24–25°C or 75–77°F)
- Competent oral feeding, breast or bottle, without cardiorespiratory compromise (or parents capable of administering orogastric or gastrostomy feedings)
- Physiologically mature and stable cardiorespiratory function of sufficient duration
- Successful car seat trial, if indicated
- Receipt of appropriate immunizations
- Receipt of appropriate metabolic screening
- Assessment of hematologic status and institution of indicated therapy
- Assessment of nutritional risks and institution of indicated therapy and dietary modifications

TABLE 4-32
Care Plan for Optimizing Parental Coping[137,159,162–165]

Nursing Diagnosis: Risk for compromised family coping

Expected Outcome: Parent(s) will get appropriate meals and rest; will verbalize their feelings about their infant's illness and hospitalization; after initial shock and/or denial, will verbalize an understanding of their infant's condition, treatment, and progress; and will collaborate with health care team members regarding decisions about their infant.

Nursing Interventions/Rationales:

- Assist parent(s) in recognizing own health needs to meet own basic needs.
- Collaborate with social services in finding alternate housing, such as boarding home or hotel, to help individual meet own basic need for rest.
- Assist parents(s) with meals when appropriate to help individual meet own basic need for nutrition.
- Encourage parent(s) to draw on extended family support system to help meet own basic need for rest and emotional support.
- Assess individual and collective responses of family members to infant's condition and appearance.
- Provide a supportive climate to encourage parent(s) to feel comfortable sharing their concerns.
- Allow full expression of parents' feelings without minimizing or repudiating those feelings to encourage parents to express their concerns.
- Interpret hospital environment and events for parent(s) to help them understand the rationale for prescribed treatment regimens.
- Offer a brief explanation of infant's condition and treatment to facilitate parents' understanding.
- Refer pertinent questions to physician to facilitate parents' understanding.
- Reinforce or clarify explanations to ensure parents' understanding of treatment regimens.
- Recognize parents' ethnic/cultural background(s), and identify customs or attitudes that may affect interaction with health care personnel to help avoid miscommunication.
- Utilize primary nursing to provide a consistent caretaker who can develop a trusting relationship with parent(s).
- Allow parent(s) to ventilate anger and respond nondefensively to prevent buildup of pent-up anger.
- Offer other support avenues, such as social workers, pastoral care, and parent support groups, to prevent inappropriate anger toward staff.
- Arrange multidisciplinary family conferences for difficult or complex patients or family to facilitate the family's learning needs and give them the opportunity to express their concerns to the entire team.

Nursing Diagnosis: Risk for impaired parent/infant attachment

Expected Outcome: Parents will demonstrate positive attachment behaviors toward their infant and will participate in his care.

Nursing Interventions/Rationales:

- Provide an open visiting policy to encourage parental participation in infant care.
- Involve parent(s) in decisions about their infant's care, offering choices whenever possible to facilitate parents' feeling that they are participating in their baby's care.
- Encourage parent participation in basic care to help parents engage with their infant by meeting his needs. Be aware that parents can easily be intimidated by the expertise of the hospital staff.
- Identify and avoid attachment behavior by hospital staff that supersedes the parent's role to encourage parental attachment.
- Provide privacy at the infant's bedside to encourage parental participation in infant care.
- When medically appropriate, provide periods of skin-to-skin contact between parents(s) and infant (kangaroo care) to encourage parental attachment.
- Identify the infant's special characteristics to assist parent(s) in seeing him as a unique individual, encouraging parental attachment.
- Encourage parent(s) to bring clothes, hard plastic toys (must be able to be cleaned), or small articles of significant meaning (e.g., family photographs, sibling's artwork, religious articles) to encourage parental attachment.
- Encourage picture taking; provide parent(s) with photographs on special occasions, if unit has camera/photo printer, to encourage parental attachment.
- If parent(s) cannot visit, arrange set times to call with updates to maintain contact. Send weekly information letters to keep family involved in decisions about their child.
- Develop discharge plan early in hospitalization, encouraging parental input to encourage parent participation in infant care.

(continued on next page)

- Completion of indicated sensorineural assessments, hearing and funduscopy
- Completion of hospital course review if indicated, identification of unresolved medical problems, institution of indicated treatment plans and post-discharge referrals

The family and the home must also be evaluated for readiness. Ideally, at least two family members should be capable of and competent in infant care. Their knowledge base should include feeding (including formula preparation), basic infant care measures, safety precautions, administration of medications (dosage, timing, storage, signs of toxicity), understanding of early

TABLE 4-32
Care Plan for Optimizing Parental Coping[137,159,162–165] *(continued)*

Nursing Diagnosis: Knowledge deficit (learning need) regarding condition, prognosis, and treatment needs

Expected Outcome: Parent(s) will be able to verbalize their understanding of infant's present condition, planned treatment, and likely progress.

Nursing Interventions/Rationales:

- Prepare parent(s) for first contact with infant when possible to prevent fear of unknown.
- Provide tours of the NICU to parent(s) identified by the obstetrician as at high risk for delivering a preterm or ill infant to prepare them for environmental challenges.
- Explain to parent(s) what equipment is being used and why to help them understand treatment modalities being used.
- Encourage parent(s) to ask questions frequently to foster their understanding of the care being delivered.
- Coordinate information and explanations within the health care team, and document information in clinical notes to provide consistent information.
- Avoid information overload by carefully planning timing and content of information given to parent(s) to facilitate accurate recall of the information presented.
- Periodically review information with parent(s) to facilitate understanding of infant's status.
- Provide significant information to both parents to avoid confusion.
- Provide written literature or videotapes when appropriate to foster parent understanding of the care being delivered.
- Provide reference books on the unit, such as *Newborn Intensive Care: What Every Parent Needs to Know,* for the parents to read to facilitate understanding of ongoing physical, neurodevelopmental, and psychosocial needs of the infant and the family.[165]

---

indications of illness, and basic neonatal cardiopulmonary resuscitation.

Many infants are being discharged with complex multiple-system problems and are technology dependent. Caregivers must understand equipment operation, including maintenance and problem solving. They must be able to demonstrate the appropriate technique for each required special care procedure, such as artificial airway, gastrostomy, or ostomy care. Onsite evaluation of the home may be required to assess the availability of telephone access, electricity, in-house water supply, heating, and air conditioning (if appropriate). Financial resources must be available to the family as well, and home health visits are usually essential. Emergency intervention and transportation plans should also be in place.[4]

Discharge teaching is part of the implementation of discharge planning. The effective nurse uses every teaching opportunity to its fullest. To help the family move forward, the nurse must recognize and deal professionally with obstacles to learning, such as insecurity, anger, frustration, or guilt. Other common obstacles to learning may involve parents' intellectual capabilities or willingness to commit time. Table 4-33 provides guidelines for effective parent teaching.

Parents generally find inconsistent information extremely stressful. Standardized discharge teaching protocols promote continuity of care among those providing direct patient care. Giving videotaped and/or written teaching materials to the family before their rooming-in experience is helpful if the parents have the educational background to read and understand the

information. Rooming-in with their infant provides a less intense environment than the NICU for parents and allows extensive caregiving opportunities.

Evaluation of the discharge process is ongoing. A discharge checklist documents progress and ensures completion of the planning and teaching requirements. Follow-up visits and phone calls complete the evaluation process.

Key points for discharge planning include the following:[131]

1. Begin when the infant is admitted to the NICU.
2. Utilize a multidisciplinary team approach.
3. Confirm patient and family readiness for discharge.

TABLE 4-33
Guidelines for Effective Parent Teaching

1. Use "everyday" terms.
2. Utilize 2 or more modes of communication.
3. Recognize parent's limitations.
4. Make comparisons.
5. Repeat information.
6. Progress from simple to difficult.
7. Summarize information.
8. Check for understanding.
9. Encourage questions.
10. Allow expression of feelings.

From: Sumrall BC. 1990. Personal communication.

4. Clarify family involvement. Develop an informal but written contract for the technology-dependent neonate with complex care requirements.
5. Coordinate discharge planning through one individual, such as a primary nurse, social worker, or discharge planner.
6. Use a written, individualized discharge teaching plan.
7. Encourage rooming-in, if available.
8. Arrange appropriate follow-up: pediatric care, specialty services (such as cardiology, surgery, neurology, ophthalmology), early intervention programs, newborn follow-up, medical equipment supply, community support agencies, home health nursing, and respite care services.
9. Follow up with a telephone call two to three days after discharge.

SUMMARY

Nursing care of the infant in acute respiratory distress is all encompassing. Responsibilities begin with direct patient care and extend to the family of the infant. Although the focus of patient care activities is directed by the infant's diagnosis, the nurse provides total assessment and care. Each intervention with the neonate has a purpose and affects the infant's status. The effective nurse looks at each aspect of the neonate's care with the awareness that nursing activities sculpt the environment in which the infant lives. The neonate's well-being is truly in the hands of the nurse.

REFERENCES

1. Kowalski WJ, et al. 2006. Communicating with parents of premature infants: Who is the informant? *Journal of Perinatology* 26(1): 44–48.
2. Kattwinkel J, ed. 2011. *Textbook of Neonatal Resuscitation*, 6th ed. Elk Grove Village, Illinois: American Academy of Pediatrics and American Heart Association.
3. Committee on Perinatal Health. 1993. *Toward Improving the Outcome of Pregnancy: The 90s and Beyond.* White Plains, New York: March of Dimes Birth Defects Foundation.
4. Lockwood CJ, and Lemons JA. 2007. *Guidelines for Perinatal Care*, 6th ed. Elk Grove Village, Illinois: American Academy of Pediatrics and American College of Obstetricians and Gynecologists, 205–301.
5. Clark DA, and Hakanson DO. 1988. The inaccuracy of Apgar scoring. *Clinics in Perinatology* 8(3): 203–205.
6. Blackburn ST. 2007. *Maternal, Fetal, and Neonatal Physiology: A Clinical Perspective*, 3rd ed. Philadelphia: Saunders, 261, 318, 319, 339–368, 395–410, 443–467, 700–723.
7. Gunn A, and Bennet L. 2001. Is temperature important in delivery room resuscitation? *Seminars in Neonatology* 6(3): 241–249.
8. Watkinson M. 2006. Temperature control of premature infants in the delivery room. *Clinics in Perinatology* 33(1): 43–53.
9. Soll RF. 2008. Heat loss prevention in neonates. *Journal of Perinatology* 28(supplement 1): S57–S59.
10. Baumgart S, Harrsch SC, and Touch SM. 1999. Thermal regulation. In *Neonatology: Pathophysiology and Management of the Newborn*, 5th ed., Avery GB, Fletcher MA, and MacDonald MG, eds. Philadelphia: Lippincott Williams & Wilkins, 395–408.
11. Vohra S, et al. 1999. Effect of polyethylene occlusive skin wrapping on heat loss in very low birth weight infants at delivery: A randomized trial. *Journal of Pediatrics* 134(5): 547–551.
12. Vohra S, et al. 2004. Heat loss prevention (HELP) in the delivery room: A randomized controlled trial of polyethylene occlusive skin wrappings in very preterm infants. *Journal of Pediatrics* 145(6): 750–753.
13. Shankaran S. 2002. The postnatal management of the asphyxiated term infant. *Clinics in Perinatology* 29(4): 675–692.
14. Higgins RD, et al. 2006. Hypothermia and perinatal asphyxia: Executive summary of the National Institute of Child Health and Human Development workshop. *Journal of Pediatrics* 148(2): 170–175.
15. Laptook AR, and Cobertt RJ. 2002. The effects of temperature on hypoxic-ischemic brain injury. *Clinics in Perinatology* 29(4): 623–649.
16. Wyatt JS, et al. 2007. Determinants of outcomes after head cooling for neonatal encephalopathy. *Pediatrics* 119(5): 912–921.
17. Shah PS, Ohlsson A, and Perlman M. 2007. Hypothermia to treat hypoxic-ischemic encephalopathy. *Archives of Pediatric and Adolescent Medicine* 161(10): 951–958.
18. Volpe JJ. 2008. Hypoxic-ischemic encephalopathy: Clinical aspects. In *Neurology of the Newborn*, 5th ed., Volpe JJ, ed. Philadelphia: Saunders Elsevier, 400–488.
19. Desmond MM, Rudolph AJ, and Phitaksphraiwan P. 1966. The transitional care nursery: A mechanism for preventative medicine in the newborn. *Pediatric Clinics of North America* 13(3): 651–667.
20. Brazelton TB. 1961. Psychophysiologic reactions in the neonate. *Journal of Pediatrics* 58(4): 513–518.
21. Sedin G. 2006. Physical environment. In *Fanaroff and Martin's Neonatal-Perinatal Medicine: Diseases of the Fetus and Infant*, 8th ed., Martin RJ, Fanaroff AA, and Walsh MC, eds. Philadelphia: Mosby, 585–608.
22. Sahni R, and Schulze K. 2004. Temperature control in newborn infants. In *Fetal and Neonatal Physiology*, 3rd ed., Polin RA, Fox WW, and Abman SH, eds. Philadelphia: Saunders, 548–569.
23. Power GG, Blood AB, and Hunter CJ. 2004. Perinatal thermal physiology. In *Fetal and Neonatal Physiology*, 3rd ed., Polin RA, Fox WW, and Abman SH, eds. Philadelphia: Saunders, 541–547.
24. Sedin G. 2004. Physics and physiology of human neonatal incubation. In *Fetal and Neonatal Physiology*, 3rd ed., Polin RA, Fox WW, and Abman SH, eds. Philadelphia: Saunders, 570–581.
25. Topper WH, and Stewart TP. 1984. Thermal support for the very-low-birth-weight infant: Role of supplemental conductive heat. *Journal of Pediatrics* 105(5): 810–814.
26. Williams M. 2001. Skin of the premature infant. In *Textbook of Neonatal Dermatology*, Eichenfield LF, Frieden IJ, and Esterly NB, eds. Philadelphia: Saunders, 46–61.
27. Mancini AJ. 2001. Structure and function of newborn skin. In *Textbook of Neonatal Dermatology*, Eichenfield LF, Frieden IJ, and Esterly NB, eds. Philadelphia: Saunders, 18–32.
28. Dubowitz L, Dubowitz V, and Goldberg C. 1970. Clinical assessment of gestational age in the newborn infant. *Journal of Pediatrics* 77(1): 1–10.
29. Ballard JL, et al. 1991. New Ballard score, expanded to include extremely premature infants. *Journal of Pediatrics* 119(3): 417–423.
30. Tappero EP, and Honeyfield ME. 2009. *Physical Assessment of the Newborn*, 4th ed. Petaluma, California: NICU INK.
31. Fletcher MA. 1998. *Physical Diagnosis in Neonatology*. Philadelphia: Lippincott-Raven, 303–401.
32. Dear PR. 1987. Monitoring oxygen in the newborn: Saturation or partial pressure? *Archives of Disease in Childhood* 62(9): 879–881.
33. West J. 1985. *Respiratory Physiology—The Essentials*, 3rd ed. Philadelphia: Lippincott Williams & Wilkins, 67–83.
34. Hay W. 1987. The uses, benefits, and limitations of pulse oximetry in neonatal medicine: Consensus on key issues. *Journal of Perinatology* 4(7): 347–349.
35. Tin W, and Gupta S. 2006. Clinical issues regarding pulse oximetry. In *Manual of Neonatal Respiratory Care*, 2nd ed., Donn DM, and Sinha SK, eds. Philadelphia: Mosby, 124–127.
36. Salyer JW. 2003. Neonatal and pediatric pulse oximetry. *Respiratory Care* 48(4): 386–396.
37. Hay WW, et al. 2002. Reliability of conventional and new pulse oximetry in neonatal patients. *Journal of Perinatology* 22(5): 360–366.
38. Kugelman A, et al. 2004. Reflectance pulse oximetry from core body in neonates and infants: A comparison to arterial blood oxygen saturation and to transmission pulse oximetry. *Journal of Perinatology* 24(6): 366–371.
39. Sahni R, et al. 2003. Motion resistant pulse oximetry in neonates. *Archives of Disease in Childhood. Fetal and Neonatal Edition* 88(6): F505–F508.

40. Anderson CG, Benitz WE, and Madan A. 2004. Retinopathy of prematurity and pulse oximetry: A national survey of recent practices. *Journal of Perinatology* 24(3): 164–168.

41. Wortham BM, Gaitatzes CG, and Rais-Bahrami K. 2007. Umbilical artery catheterization. In *Atlas of Procedures in Neonatology*, 4th ed., MacDonald MG, and Ramasethu J, eds. Philadelphia: Lippincott Williams & Wilkins, 157–176.

42. O'Grady NP, et al. 2011. Guidelines for the prevention of intravascular catheter-related infections. Centers for Disease Control and Prevention. Retrieved from www.cdc.gov/hicpac/pdf/guidelines/bsi-guidelines-2011.pdf.

43. Massaro AN, Rais-Bahrami K, and Eichelberger MR. 2007. Peripheral arterial cannulation. In *Atlas of Procedures in Neonatology*, 4th ed. Philadelphia: Lippincott Williams & Wilkins, 186–198.

44. Duran DJ, Phillips B, and Boloker J. 2003. Blood gases: Technical aspects and interpretation. In *Assisted Ventilation of the Neonate*, 4th ed., Goldsmith JP, and Karotkin EH, eds. Philadelphia: Saunders, 279–292.

45. Gomella TL, et al. 2004. *Neonatology: Management, Procedures, On-Call Problems, Diseases, and Drugs*, 5th ed. New York: Lange Medical Books, 157–160, 182–183.

46. Walton DM, and Short BL. 2007. Arterial puncture. In *Atlas of Procedures in Neonatology*, 4th ed., MacDonald MG, and Ramasethu J, eds. Philadelphia: Lippincott Williams & Wilkins, 89–92.

47. Fischbach FT. 2004. *Manual of Laboratory and Diagnostic Tests*, 7th ed. Philadelphia: Lippincott Williams & Wilkins, 40.

48. Folk LA. 2007. Capillary heelstick blood sampling. In *Atlas of Procedures in Neonatology*, 4th ed. Philadelphia: Lippincott Williams & Wilkins, 93–96.

49. Yldzdas D, et al. 2004. Correlation of simultaneously obtained capillary, venous, and arterial blood gases of patients in a paediatric intensive care unit. *Archives of Disease in Childhood* 89(2): 176–180.

50. Holsti L, et al. 2004. Specific newborn individualized development care and assessment program movements are associated with acute pain in preterm infants in the neonatal intensive care unit. *Pediatrics* 114(1): 65–72.

51. Dominguez R. 1992. *Diagnostic Imaging of the Premature Infant*. New York: Churchill Livingstone, 87–116.

52. Kirpalani H, et al. 1999. The chest. In *Imaging of the Newborn Baby*, Kirpalani H, Mernagh J, and Gill G, eds. Edinburgh: Churchill Livingstone, 5–50.

53. Park MK. 1988. *Pediatric Cardiology for Practitioners*, 2nd ed. Chicago: Year Book, 54.

54. Brady MT. 2005. Health care–associated infections in the neonatal intensive care unit. *American Journal of Infection Control* 33(5): 268–275.

55. Chudleigh J, Fletcher M, and Gould D. 2005. Infection control in neonatal intensive care units. *Journal of Hospital Infection* 61(2): 123–129.

56. Lam BCC, Lee J, and Lau YL. 2004. Hand hygiene practices in a neonatal intensive care unit: A multimodal intervention and impact on nosocomial infection. *Pediatrics* 114(5): e565–e571.

57. Centers for Disease Control and Prevention. 2002. Guideline for hand hygiene in health-care settings. *MMWR* 51(RR-16): 1–45.

58. Gaitztzes CG, and Rais-Bahrami K. 2007. Aseptic preparation. In *Atlas of Procedures in Neonatology*, 4th ed. Philadelphia: Lippincott Williams & Wilkins, 21–27.

59. Polak JD, Ringler N, and Daugherty B. 2004. Unit based procedures: Impact on the incidence of nosocomial infections in the newborn intensive care unit. *Newborn and Infant Nursing Reviews* 4(1): 38–45.

60. Puchalski M, and Hummel P. 2002. The reality of neonatal pain. *Advances in Neonatal Care* 2(5): 233–247.

61. Duhn LJ, and Medves JM. 2004. A systematic integrative review of infant pain assessment tools. *Advances in Neonatal Care* 4(3): 126–140.

62. American Academy of Pediatrics Committee on Fetus and Newborn, and Canadian Paediatric Society Fetus and Newborn Committee. 2007. Prevention and management of pain in the neonate: An update. *Advances in Neonatal Care* 7(3): 151–160.

63. Zahorodny W, et al. 1998. The Neonatal Withdrawal Inventory: A simplified score of newborn withdrawal. *Developmental and Behavioral Pediatrics* 19(2): 89–93.

64. Sherman JM, et al. 1986. Factors influencing acquired subglottic stenosis in infants. *Journal of Pediatrics* 109(2): 322-327.

65. Rais-Bahrami K. 2007. Endotracheal intubation. In *Atlas of Procedures in Neonatology*, 4th ed., MacDonald MG, and Ramasethu J, eds. Philadelphia: Lippincott Williams & Wilkins, 241–255.

66. Parker A, and Greenough A. 2003. Physiotherapy. In *Neonatal Respiratory Disorders*, 2nd ed., Parker A, and Milner AD, eds. London: Arnold, 236–244.

67. Woodgate PG, and Flenady V. 2001. Tracheal suctioning without disconnection in intubated ventilated neonates. *Cochrane Database of Systematic Reviews* (2): CD003065.

68. Morrow BM, and Argent AC. 2008. A comprehensive review of pediatric endotracheal suctioning: Effects, indications, and clinical practice. *Pediatric Critical Care Medicine* 9(5): 465–477.

69. Hageman JR, et al. 2003. Pulmonary care. In *Assisted Ventilation of the Neonate*, 4th ed., Goldsmith JP, and Karotkin EH, eds. Philadelphia: Saunders, 91–105.

70. Kaiser JR, Gauss CH, and Williams DK. 2008. Tracheal suctioning is associated with prolonged disturbances of cerebral hemodynamics in very low birth weight infants. *Journal of Perinatology* 28(1): 34–41.

71. Norris SC, Barnes AK, and Roberts TD. 2009. When ventilator-associated pneumonias haunt your NICU—One unit's story. *Neonatal Network* 28(1): 59–66.

72. Walsh BK, and Davidson K. 2003. Airway clearance techniques and lung volume expansion. In *Perinatal and Pediatric Respiratory Care*, 2nd ed., Czervinske MP, and Barnhart SL, eds. Philadelphia: Saunders, 183–206.

73. Wallis C, and Prasad A. 1999. Who needs chest physiotherapy? Moving from anecdote to evidence. *Archives of Disease in Childhood* 80(4): 393–397.

74. Halliday HL. 2004. What interventions facilitate weaning from the ventilator? A review of the evidence from systematic reviews. *Paediatric Respiratory Reviews* 5(supplement A): S347–S352.

75. Bell EF, and Oh W. 2005. Fluid and electrolyte management. In *Neonatology: Pathophysiology and Management of the Newborn*, 6th ed., MacDonald MG, Seshia MMK, and Mullett MD, eds. Philadelphia: Lippincott Williams & Wilkins, 362–379.

76. Kerr BA, Starbuck AL, and Block SM. 2006. Fluid and electrolyte management. In *Handbook of Neonatal Intensive Care*, 6th ed., Merenstein GB, and Gardner SL, eds. Philadelphia: Mosby, 360.

77. Poindexter BB, Leitch CA, and Deene SC. 2006. Parenteral nutrition. In *Fanaroff and Martin's Neonatal-Perinatal Medicine: Diseases of the Fetus and Infant*, 8th ed., Martin RJ, Fanaroff AA, and Walsh MC, eds. Philadelphia: Mosby, 679–693.

78. Brine E, and Ernst JA. 2004. Total parenteral nutrition for premature infants. *Newborn and Infant Nursing Reviews* 4(3): 133–155.

79. Ziegler EE, Thureen PJ, and Carlson SJ. 2002. Aggressive nutrition of the very low birthweight infant. *Clinics in Perinatology* 29(2): 225–244.

80. Uhing MR, and Das UG. 2009. Optimizing growth in the preterm infant. *Clinics in Perinatology* 36(1): 165–176.

81. Deene SC. 2001. Protein and energy requirements in preterm infants. *Seminars in Neonatology* 6(5): 377–382.

82. Putet G. 2004. Lipids as an energy source for the premature and full-term infant. In *Fetal and Neonatal Physiology*, 3rd ed., Polin RA, Fox WW, and Abman SH, eds. Philadelphia: Saunders, 415–418.

83. Atkinson SA. 2000. Human milk feeding of the micropremie. *Clinics in Perinatology* 27(1): 235–247.

84. Kuzma-O'Reilly B, et al. 2003. Evaluation, development, and implementation of potentially better practices in neonatal intensive care nutrition. *Pediatrics* 111(4): e461–e470.

85. Patole SK, and de Klerk N. 2005. Impact of standardized feeding regimens on incidence of neonatal necrotising enterocolitis: A systematic review and meta-analysis of observational studies. *Archives of Disease in Childhood. Fetal and Neonatal Edition* 90(2): F147–F151.

86. Street JL, et al. 2006. Implementing feeding guidelines for NICU patients <2000 g results in less variability in nutrition outcomes. *Journal of Parenteral and Enteral Nutrition* 30(6): 515–518.

87. Weibley TT, et al. 1987. Gavage tube insertion in the premature infant. *American Journal of Maternal Child Nursing* 12(1): 24–27.

88. Fucile S, Gisel E, and Lau C. 2002. Oral stimulation accelerates the transition from tube to oral feeding in preterm infants. *Journal of Pediatrics* 141(2): 230–236.

89. Harding CM, Law J, and Pring T. 2006. The use of non-nutritive sucking to promote functional sucking skills in premature infants: An exploratory trial. *Infant* 2(6): 238–240, 242–243.

90. Sheppard JJ, and Fletcher KR. 2007. Evidenced-based interventions for breast and bottle feeding in the neonatal intensive care unit. *Seminars in Speech and Language* 28(3): 204–212.

91. Pinelli J, and Symington A. 2005. Non-nutritive sucking for promoting physiologic stability and nutrition in preterm infants. *Cochrane Database of Systematic Reviews* (4): CD001071.

92. Greer F, McCormick A, and Locker J. 1984. Changes in fat concentration of human milk during delivery by intermittent bolus and continuous mechanical pump infusion. *Journal of Pediatrics* 105(5): 745–749.

93. Lemons P, et al. 1983. Bacterial growth in human milk during continuous feeding. American *Journal of Perinatology* 1(1): 76–80.

94. Simpson C, Schanler RJ, and Lau C. 2002. Early introduction of oral feeding in preterm infants. *Pediatrics* 110(3): 517–522.

95. Thoyre SM, Shaker CS, and Pridham KF. 2005. The early feeding skills assessment for preterm infants. *Neonatal Network* 24(3): 7–16.

96. Hadley LB, and West D. 1999. *Developmental and Behavioral Characteristics of Preterm Infants.* Petaluma, California: NICU INK, 12–15.

97. Hoath S. 2004. Physiologic development of the skin. In *Fetal and Neonatal Physiology*, 3rd ed., Polin RA, Fox WW, and Abman SH, eds. Philadelphia: Saunders, 597–611.

98. Rutter N. 1988. The immature skin. *British Medical Bulletin* 44(4): 957–970.

99. Solomon LM, and Esterly NB. 1973. *Neonatal Dermatology.* Philadelphia: Saunders, 1–22.

100. Rutter N. 1987. Percutaneous drug absorption in the newborn: Hazards and uses. *Clinical Pediatrics* 14(4): 911–930.

101. Lund C, et al. 1986. Evaluation of a pectin-based barrier under tape to protect neonatal skin. *Journal of Obstetric, Gynecologic, and Neonatal Nursing* 15(1): 39–44.

102. Conner JM, Soll RF, and Edwards WH. 2003. Topical ointment for preventing infection in preterm infants. *Cochrane Database of Systematic Reviews* (4): CD001150.

103. Symington A, and Pinelli J. 2006. Developmental care for promoting development and preventing morbidity in preterm infants. *Cochrane Database of Systematic Reviews* (2): CD001814.

104. Graven S, et al. 1992. The high-risk infant environment. Part I: The role of the neonatal intensive care unit in the outcome of high-risk infants. *Journal of Pediatrics* 12(2): 164–172.

105. DePaul D, and Chambers SE. 1995. Environmental noise in the neonatal intensive care unit: Implications for nursing practice. *Journal of Perinatal and Neonatal Nursing* 8(4): 71–76.

106. Als H, et al. 1986. Individualized behavioral and environmental care for the very low birth weight preterm infant at high risk for bronchopulmonary dysplasia: Neonatal intensive care unit and developmental outcome. *Pediatrics* 78(6): 1123–1132.

107. Gottfried AW, Hodgman JE, and Brown KW. 1984. How intensive is newborn intensive care? An environmental analysis. *Pediatrics* 74(2): 292–294.

108. Wolke D. 1987. Environmental neonatology. *Archives of Disease in Childhood* 62(10): 987–988.

109. Als H, et al. 1982. Toward a research instrument for the Assessment of Preterm Infant's Behavior (APIB). In *Theory and Research in Behavioral Pediatrics*, Fitzgerald HE, Lester BM, and Yogman MW, eds. New York: Plenum, 35–63.

110. Als H, et al. 2004. Early experience alters brain function and structure. *Pediatrics* 113(4): 846–857.

111. Feldman R, et al. 2002. Comparison of skin-to-skin (kangaroo) and traditional care: Parenting outcomes and preterm infant development. *Pediatrics* 110(1): 16–26.

112. National Association of Neonatal Nurses. 1994. *Infant and Family-Centered Developmental Care Guidelines.* Glenview, Illinois: NANN.

113. Kenner C, and McGrath JM. 2010. *Developmental Care of Newborns and Infants: A Guide for Health Professionals*, 2nd ed. Chicago: National Association of Neonatal Nurses.

114. Aguilera DC, and Messick JM. 1978. *Crisis Intervention: Theory and Methodology.* Philadelphia: Mosby-Year Book, 62–79.

115. Lam C. 1982. Crisis intervention in respiratory distress. *Journal of the California Perinatal Association* 2(2): 104–107.

116. Klaus JH, and Kennell MH. 1982. *Parent-Infant Bonding*, 2nd ed. Philadelphia: Mosby-Year Book, 151–161.

117. Sammons W, and Lewis J. 1985. *Premature Babies—A Different Beginning.* Philadelphia: Mosby, 42–45.

118. Mercer R. 1990. *Parents at Risk.* New York: Springer, 154–166.

119. Cone S. 2007. The impact of communication and the neonatal intensive care environment on parent involvement. *Newborn and Infant Nursing Reviews* 7(1): 33–38.

120. American Academy of Pediatrics Committee on Hospital Care. 2003. Family-centered care and the pediatrician's role. *Pediatrics* 112(3): 691–697.

121. Brazelton TB, Koslowski B, and Main M. 1974. The origins of reciprocity: The early mother-infant interaction. In *The Effect of the Infant on Its Caregiver*, Lewis M, and Rosenblum L, eds. New York: Wiley, 49–76.

122. Robson K, and Moss H. 1970. Patterns and determinants of maternal attachment. *Journal of Pediatrics* 77(6): 976–985.

123. Bozzette M. 2007. A review of research on premature infant-mother interaction. *Newborn and Infant Nursing Reviews* 7(1): 49-55.

124. Amankwaa LC, Pickler RH, and Boonmee J. 2007. Maternal responsiveness in mothers of preterm infants. *Newborn and Infant Nursing Reviews* 7(1): 25–30.

125. Kleberg A, Westrup B, and Stjernqvist K. 2000. Developmental outcome, child behaviour and mother-child interaction at 3 years of age following Newborn Individualized Developmental Care and Intervention Program (NIDCAP) intervention. *Early Human Development* 60(2): 123–135.

126. Anderson GE. 1991. Current knowledge about skin-to-skin (kangaroo) care for preterm infants. *Journal of Perinatology* 11(3): 216–226.

127. Ludington-Hoe SM, et al. 1994. Kangaroo care: Research results, and practice implications and guidelines. *Neonatal Network* 13(1): 19–27.

128. Ludington-Hoe SM, et al. 2004. Randomized controlled trial of kangaroo care: Cardiorespiratory and thermal effects on healthy preterm infants. *Neonatal Network* 23(3): 39–48.

129. Affonso D, et al. 1993. Reconciliation and healing for mothers through skin-to-skin contact provided in an American tertiary level intensive care nursery. *Neonatal Network* 12(3): 25–32.

130. Brooten D, et al. 1986. A randomized clinical trial of early hospital discharge and home follow-up of very-low-birth-weight infants. *New England Journal of Medicine* 315(15): 934–939.

131. Zotkiewicz TT. 2010. Home at last. In *Newborn Intensive Care: What Every Parent Needs to Know*, 3rd ed., Zaichkin J, ed. Elk Grove Village, Illinois: American Academy of Pediatrics, 467–523.

132. Friedman M, and Baumgart S. 2005. Thermal regulation. In *Neonatology: Pathophysiology and Management of the Newborn*, 6th ed., MacDonald MG, Seshia MM, and Mullett MD, eds. Philadelphia: Lippincott Williams & Wilkins, 445–457.

133. L'Herault J, Petroff L, and Jeffery J. 2001. The effectiveness of a thermal mattress in stabilizing and maintaining body temperature during transport of very-low-birth weight newborns. *Applied Nursing Research* 14(4): 210–219.

134. Sitler G. 2003. Noninvasive monitoring in neonatal and pediatric care. In *Perinatal and Pediatric Respiratory Care*, 2nd ed., Czervinske MP, and Barnhart SL, eds. Philadelphia: Saunders. 130–138.

135. Whitaker K. 2001. *Comprehensive Perinatal and Pediatric Respiratory Care*, 3rd ed. Albany, New York: Delmar Thomson Learning, 278–280.

136. Nugent J. 1983. Acute respiratory care of the newborn. *Journal of Obstetric, Gynecologic, and Neonatal Nursing* 12(3 supplement): S31–S44.

137. Doenges ME, Moorhouse MF, and Murr AC. 2006. Maternal postpartal concepts and newborn concepts. In *Nursing Care Plans: Guidelines for Individualizing Client Care Across the Life Span*, 7th ed. Philadelphia: FA Davis on CD-ROM.

138. Sconyers S, Ogden B, and Goldberg H. 1987. The effect of body position on the respiratory rate of infants with tachypnea. *Journal of Perinatology* 7(2): 118–121.

139. American Academy of Pediatrics Committee on Fetus and Newborn and Canadian Paediatric Society Fetus and Newborn Committee. 2006. Prevention and management of pain and stress in the neonate: An update. *Pediatrics* 118(5): 2231–2241.

140. Coleman MM, Solarin K, and Smith C. 2002. Assessment and management of pain and distress in the neonate. *Advances in Neonatal Care* 2(3): 123–136.

141. Gibbins S, and Stevens B. 2003. The influence of gestational age on the efficacy and short-term safety of sucrose for procedural pain relief. *Advances in Neonatal Care* 3(5): 241–249.

142. Henry PR, Haubold K, and Dobrzykowski TM. 2004. Pain in the healthy full-term neonate: Efficacy and safety of interventions. *Newborn and Infant Nursing Reviews* 4(2): 106–113.

143. Prince WL, et al. 2004. Treatment of neonatal pain without a gold standard: The case for caregiving interventions and sucrose administration. *Neonatal Network* 23(4): 33–45.

144. Cunha-Goncalves D, et al. 2007. Inflation lung mechanics deteriorates markedly after saline instillation and open endotracheal suctioning in mechanically ventilated healthy piglets. *Pediatric Pulmonology* 42(1): 10–14.

145. Clifton-Koeppel R. 2006. Endotracheal tube suctioning in the newborn: A review of the literature. *Newborn and Infant Nursing Reviews* 6(2): 94–99.

146. American Academy of Pediatrics Committee on Nutrition. 1985. Nutritional needs of low birth weight infants. *Pediatrics* 75(5): 976–986.

147. Bell EF. 2011. Nutritional support. In *Assisted Ventilation of the Neonate*, 5th ed., Goldsmith JP, and Karotkin EH, eds. Philadelphia: Saunders, 466–483.

148. Greenleaf AM. 2007. Gastric and transpyloric tubes. In *Atlas of Procedures in Neonatology*, 4th ed., MacDonald MG, and Ramasethu J, eds. Philadelphia: Lippincott Williams & Wilkins, 291–298.

149. McGuire W, and McEwan P. 2004. Systematic review of transpyloric versus gastric tube feeding for preterm infants. *Archives of Diseases in Childhood. Fetal and Neonatal Edition* 89(3): F245–F248.

150. Premji SS, et al. 2002. Evidenced-based feeding guidelines for very low-birth-weight infants. *Advances in Neonatal Care* 2(1): 5–18.

151. Parker P, Stroup S, and Greene H. 1981. A controlled comparison of continuous versus intermittent feeding in the treatment of infants with intestinal disease. *Journal of Pediatrics* 99(3): 68–71.

152. Pereira GR, and Lemons JA. 1981. Controlled study of transpyloric and intermittent gavage feeding in the small preterm infant. *Pediatrics* 67(1): 68–71.

153. Newell SJ. 2000. Enteral feeding of the micropremie. *Clinics in Perinatology* 27(1): 221–234.

154. Edward WH, Conner JM, and Soll RF. 2001. The effect of Aquaphor original emollient ointment on nosocomial sepsis rates and skin integrity of birth weight 501–1,000 grams. *Pediatric Research* 49: 388A.

155. Lund CH, et al. 2001. Neonatal skin care: Clinical outcomes of the AWHONN/NANN evidenced-based clinical practice guideline. *Journal of Obstetric, Gynecologic, and Neonatal Nursing* 30(1): 41–51.

156. Nurses' Association of the American College of Obstetricians and Gynecologists. 1992. *Neonatal Skin Care.* OGN Nursing Practice Resource, 1–9.

157. Fox MD. 2011. Wound care in the neonatal intensive care unit, *Neonatal Network* 30(5): 291–303.

158. Als H. 1984. *Guidelines for the Practical Implementation of Individualized Care and Intervention in the NICU.* Boston: Children's Hospital.

159. Carpenito-Moyet LJ. 2004. *Nursing Diagnosis: Application to Clinical Practice,* 10th ed. Philadelphia: Lippincott, 405–416, 534–544.

160. Gardener AL, and Goldson E. 2006. The neonate and the environment: Impact on development. In *Handbook of Neonatal Intensive Care,* 6th ed., Merenstein GB, and Gardner SL, eds. Philadelphia: Mosby, 295–318.

161. Sizun J, and Westrup B. 2004. Early developmental care for preterm neonates: A call for more research. *Archives of Disease in Childhood. Fetal and Neonatal Edition* 89(5): F384–F388.

162. Loo KK, et al. 2003. Using knowledge to cope with stress in the NICU: How parents integrate learning to read the physiologic and behavioral cues of the infant. *Neonatal Network* 22(1): 31–37.

163. Ludington-Hoe SM, et al. 2003. Safe criteria and procedure for kangaroo care with intubated preterm infants. *Journal of Obstetric, Gynecologic, and Neonatal Nursing* 32(5): 579–588.

164. McFarland GK, and McFarlane EA. 1997. *Nursing Diagnosis and Intervention: Planning for Patient Care,* 3rd ed. Philadelphia: Mosby, 692–698, 826–833.

165. Zaichkin J, ed. 2010. *Newborn Intensive Care: What Every Parent Needs to Know,* 3rd ed. Elk Grove Village, Illinois: American Academy of Pediatrics.

Notes

NOTES

5 Pulmonary Function Evaluation in the Critically Ill Neonate

Jay S. Greenspan, MD
Thomas L. Miller, PhD
Thomas H. Shaffer, PhD

The ability to assess pulmonary function in neonates is not new. It has been possible for years to measure respiratory pressure, airflow, and volume and to calculate pulmonary mechanics, energetics, and functional residual capacity (FRC). In the past, because of difficulties in taking these measurements and the time required to interpret the data, these values have not been clinically useful. However, recent advances in computer-assisted technology as well as miniaturization of equipment allow simple and rapid pulmonary function assessment and real-time monitoring of the critically ill neonate at the bedside.

An understanding of the indications for and information obtained from pulmonary function profiles of critically ill neonates is essential to nursing care. When pulmonary function measurements are performed carefully, the results are reproducible and accurate and can have important implications for ventilatory management, assessment of interventions, and evaluation of new technologies.

The indications for and benefits of pulmonary function evaluation in the critically ill neonate vary with length of gestation, postnatal age, and clinical condition. A pulmonary function assessment in a neonate at risk for pulmonary disease can provide insight into the type and progression of a pulmonary abnormality, assess the response to therapeutic interventions, diagnose unsuspected pathology, and possibly suggest a prognosis. Pulmonary function should be monitored routinely in infants at risk for respiratory disease, in those with acute changes in respiratory status, and in those being evaluated for new respiratory problems or therapeutic interventions. The fundamentals and basic interpretation

of pulmonary function monitoring, as well as some of the information learned through a pulmonary function assessment, are discussed in this chapter.

THE PULMONARY FUNCTION PROFILE

The pulmonary function profile represents all available pulmonary information obtainable on a particular infant. Because not all tests can be performed on a given infant, this profile needs to be tailored for each patient. A basic pulmonary function profile typically includes measurement of (1) pulmonary mechanics (compliance, resistance, time constant), (2) energetics (work of breathing), and, when possible, (3) lung volume, or FRC.

State-of-the-art equipment has made rapid evaluation at the bedside possible for even the sickest infants. The basic pulmonary function measurements should, therefore, be included in a pulmonary profile of any infant with lung disease, along with an assessment of respiratory rate, oxyhemoglobin saturation, and a physical examination. Although these pulmonary function evaluations generally provide accurate and reproducible results, their utility depends on consistent preparation, positioning, and monitoring.

MEASUREMENTS AND DATA ACQUISITION

Ventilation is the result of changes in pressure, flow, and volume over time. Mechanical ventilators drive inspiration using positive pressure to expand the chest. During spontaneous breathing, the contraction of the diaphragm and expansion of the rib cage drive inspiration. In both situations, expiration is passive.

To provide effective ventilation under either artificial or spontaneous conditions, respiratory effort must

FIGURE 5-1
Normal tidal flow-volume relationship.

Note even flow on inspiration (lower portion of the loop) and expiration (upper portion) as gas is inhaled and exhaled through normal airways.

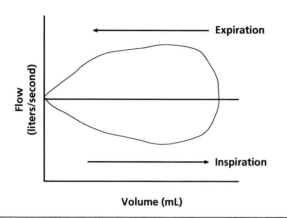

FIGURE 5-2
Schematic of a pneumotachograph, which attaches to a face mask or endotracheal tube to measure flow.

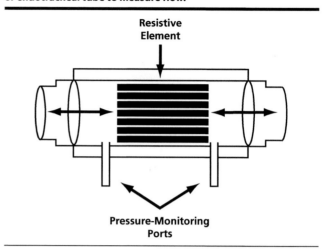

be sufficient to overcome the intrinsic properties of the lung that oppose air movement: the elastic and resistive components or the mechanics of the respiratory system (see Chapter 11). Surface tension, lung tissue, the chest wall, and the abdomen all contribute resistance to air movement. By monitoring changes in pressure and flow in the respiratory system, the caregiver can quantify these components.

Pulmonary mechanics can be tested under two conditions: (1) during active, uninterrupted breathing (dynamic mechanics) and (2) during interrupted breathing, produced by briefly occluding the airway at one or more points in the cycle (static mechanics). The techniques discussed in this section refer to measuring dynamic mechanics, this being the most common and practical technique in clinical use.

Monitoring Flow

Flow measurements are obtained by placing a flow sensor between a ventilated infant's endotracheal or tracheostomy tube and the ventilator circuit or, for a spontaneously breathing infant, by attaching the flow sensor to a face mask. Flow sensors have standard connectors on both ends, allowing them to be connected to standard ventilation equipment such as an endotracheal tube, a face mask, or a ventilator circuit.

Using a computerized pulmonary function monitoring system allows sampling of the flow signal identified by the sensor many times per second and integrating it with time to calculate tidal volume. The monitoring system can also graphically display the relationship of flow and volume for a breath as a flow-volume loop

(Figure 5-1). Flow-volume loops are useful in evaluating the infant for flow restrictions caused by tracheobronchomalacia or bronchospasm.

The most direct method of monitoring flow is **pneumotachography.** A pneumotachograph consists of a tube containing an element that creates resistance to flow, with pressure-monitoring ports on both sides of the resistive element (Figure 5-2). The resistive element can be a series of smaller tubes or a mesh screen. As air moves through the pneumotachograph during inspiration and expiration, a pressure difference that is proportional to the flow rate is created across the resistive element.

Another technique for measuring flow is hot-wire **anemometry.** Instead of a resistive element, as in pneumotachography, the anemometer contains a filament, or hot wire. The filament is maintained at a constant temperature regardless of the amount of flow moving across it. To maintain a constant temperature, voltage is supplied to the filament as gas flow changes. The change in voltage correlates with flow. As with pneumotachography, the flow signal is integrated with time to yield tidal volume.

Independent, self-contained pulmonary function evaluation systems most often incorporate a pneumotachograph for flow measurement. However, because anemometers are less expensive and do not require as much hardware (pressure transducers and tubing) as a pneumotachograph, mechanical ventilators now include these flow sensors to provide valuable real-time assessment data. Changes in tidal volume can be monitored with other parameters to detect changes in the infant's condition or to signal the need for interventions such as

FIGURE 5-3
Typical scalar tracing showing pressure, flow, and volume for consecutive breaths.

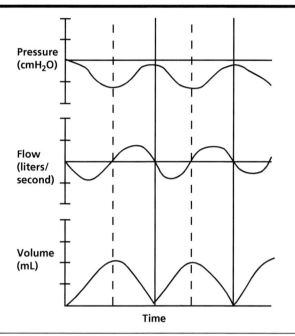

FIGURE 5-4
Typical pressure-volume loop for a single breath.

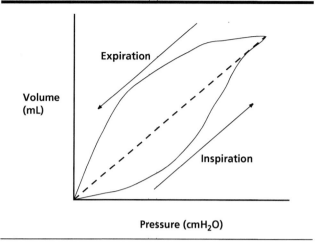

suctioning. Because anemometers have less dead space than pneumotachographs, they can be used to monitor an infant for long periods without compromising ventilation.

Monitoring Pressure

Airway pressure monitoring, including peak inflating and end-distending pressure, as well as mean airway pressure, is an integral part of managing mechanical ventilation. For most ventilation schemes, the pressure sensor is placed at the airway opening, and the positive pressure value is displayed on the ventilator. The pulmonary function monitoring offered by mechanical ventilators is limited to airway opening pressure; other pressure readings are needed to appropriately determine mechanical properties of the lung. Ideally, **transpulmonary pressure** is measured during a thorough pulmonary function evaluation and is required for spontaneous breathers, whose airway opening pressure is negligible.

Transpulmonary pressure is the pressure across the lung, from the airway opening to the pleural space. Airway opening pressure is sampled at a port on the ventilatory circuit connector closest to the patient. Intrapleural pressure is not sampled directly but can be safely and accurately estimated by monitoring esophageal pressure.[1] Specially designed esophageal balloons or water-filled catheters are made for this application.

A catheter is passed into the esophagus until the tip is in the distal third. Pressure signals can be viewed in real time for proper esophageal balloon placement and during data sampling.

A typical computer display is shown in Figure 5-3. Transpulmonary pressure, flow, and volume can be viewed on a single screen to monitor breathing during data sampling and to assess the quality of the pressure and flow signals before data sampling begins. Pressure can also be graphically displayed in relation to volume, plotted in a pressure-volume loop (Figure 5-4).

Real-Time Monitoring versus Sampling and Breath Analysis

The current generation of ventilators and pulmonary function monitoring devices provide a real-time display of pulmonary profile parameters. These systems are limited, however, in that they generally rely on airway opening pressures and display data for each breath one breath at a time. The more precise alternative is to utilize pulmonary function testing systems that incorporate esophageal balloons to generate transpulmonary pressures and sample multiple breaths to produce mean values from a period of respiration.

With pulmonary function testing systems, pressure and flow signals are sampled by a self-contained unit separate from other respiratory devices.[2] Sampling usually takes less than 60 seconds, depending on the infant's respiratory rate, and data from all breaths are averaged to produce a pulmonary function report. Each breath is analyzed for artifact caused by air leaks or excessive patient movement and can be reviewed manually by the clinician, who can further check the quality of the

FIGURE 5-5
Change in compliance at different lung volumes.

Individual breaths have low compliance (flattening of the compliance curve) at low or high lung volumes. The greatest changes in compliance occur at the points on the curve known as inflection points.

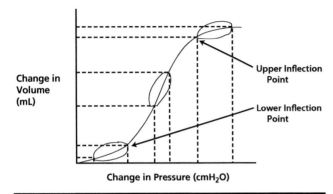

Change in Volume (mL)

Upper Inflection Point

Lower Inflection Point

Change in Pressure (cmH₂O)

breaths sampled. Breaths with significant artifact can be eliminated from the calculations.

With both real-time monitoring and data sampling, the pressure and flow signals are integrated with time and each other, and a number of pulmonary function parameters can be quantified and calculated. These calculated parameters include tidal volume, respiratory rate, minute ventilation, inspiratory and expiratory times, peak inspiratory and expiratory flows, peak pressure changes, as well as mechanics and energetics.[3]

MECHANICS AND ENERGETICS

Indices of pulmonary mechanics are calculated from the pressure and flow data sampled during each breath. An important distinction must be made between real-time pulmonary function data from a ventilator or monitoring system and mechanics calculated from a data sampling system that incorporates an esophageal balloon for transpulmonary pressure assessment. As noted earlier, real-time monitoring systems used with mechanically ventilated infants rely on airway opening pressures alone, thus measuring the total mechanics of the airways, lung, and chest wall. Systems that utilize transpulmonary pressure as the difference between airway opening pressure and esophageal pressure calculate pulmonary mechanics of the airways and lungs without including the chest wall. It is also noteworthy that mechanics in a spontaneously breathing infant (i.e., one not receiving mechanical ventilation) require an esophageal pressure reading. In these patients, esophageal pressures are almost always negative, and airway opening pressures are generally at or near zero.

Pulmonary Compliance

Pulmonary compliance describes the elastic properties of the lung. It is defined as the unit change in volume per unit change in pressure and is expressed in mL/cmH₂O. When the change in volume (tidal volume) is expressed in terms of the change in transpulmonary pressure, the resulting measurement is lung compliance. Surface tension and lung tissue properties contribute to lung compliance. If there is a large amount of interstitial fluid in the lungs, lung tissue becomes less compliant. This is true in both the acute and chronic phases of respiratory distress syndrome.

Without the use of an esophageal balloon, the chest wall and the abdomen also contribute to the calculated compliance value. In that case, the calculated value represents total compliance of the respiratory system. However, the difference between respiratory system and lung compliance measurements in neonates is generally minimal because the neonatal chest wall is highly compliant and therefore does not contribute to an appreciable reduction in respiratory compliance values.[4] The chest wall can adversely affect compliance when there is chest wall edema or if the infant is paralyzed. Also, a distended abdomen displaces the diaphragm upward and resists movement during inspiration, decreasing compliance.

Pulmonary compliance depends on lung volume. The lungs of a newborn premature infant with surfactant deficiency typically have a low volume as a result of atelectasis.[5] The transpulmonary pressure required to inflate these lungs would be high in relation to the change in volume, yielding low compliance values. Conversely, an overdistended lung, such as occurs in an infant with air trapping or one who is on excessively high ventilator pressures, will also have poor pulmonary compliance because the lungs are stretched to capacity and cannot easily accommodate additional volume.[6] Figure 5-5 illustrates this relationship between compliance and lung volume and identifies the lower and upper inflection points where compliance changes dramatically as a result of under- and overexpansion, respectively.

Pulmonary compliance is also related to the size of the infant's lungs. In this regard, larger lungs (an adult versus an infant, for instance) will move more volume per change in pressure than smaller lungs. To appropriately compare compliance values from an infant on different days, or between infants, some means of normalizing for lung size is required. Dividing the measured pulmonary compliance by the infant's weight is the simplest method of normalization. Pulmonary compliance is then expressed as mL/cmH$_2$O/kg. Other means of normalization include dividing the measured compliance by body length or dividing the measured compliance by FRC. Normalization utilizing FRC is sometimes referred to as the "specific compliance."[7]

There is a difference between dynamic and static compliance. Compliance, as defined in this chapter, is the unit change in volume per unit change in pressure. Graphically, it is represented as the slope of a line between any two points on a pressure-volume curve (see Figure 5-4). Dynamic compliance is obtained by measuring volume and pressure changes over the entire breath. Static compliance is measured by holding inflation at different points during inspiration for pressure and volume readings. The difference between the two is technique, as well as the respiratory rate dependence of dynamic compliance. When the airway is occluded during testing under static conditions, airway and alveolar pressures have time to equilibrate throughout the lung. When dynamic mechanics are measured, the changes in volume and pressure are influenced by respiratory rate and airway resistance.[7–9] Lung segments that expand more slowly than others may cause overall lower dynamic compliance values. Dynamic compliance is therefore respiratory rate dependent.[10]

Pulmonary Resistance

Airflow in the respiratory system is also subject to resistance, which is generated primarily by the airways and to a lesser extent by the lung parenchyma. With measurements made without the use of esophageal pressure, the chest wall also contributes to the resistance value. Pulmonary resistance is typically measured by assessing transpulmonary pressure and dividing by flow. Airway resistance is affected by several factors, including the radius and length of the airway, the viscosity of gas in the airways, the flow, and the driving pressure required to generate that flow.[6]

The relationship between these factors and resistance was first described by Poiseuille in the following formula:[11]

$$Flow = \frac{P \pi r^4}{8 h l}$$

In this equation, P is driving pressure, r is the airway radius, h is viscosity, and l represents length. This formula illustrates the relationship between airway length, size, and resistance. The exponential relationship between airway size and resistance is critically important. A reduction in airway size by one-half would cause airway resistance to increase 16-fold, not merely to double.

Resistance is proportional to airway length. If an infant has fewer airways, as can be seen in those with pulmonary hypoplasia resulting from diaphragmatic hernia, airway resistance may be lower than in an infant with normal lungs.

Endotracheal tubes introduce a new source of resistance into the respiratory system. By necessity, these tubes are smaller than the infant's upper airway, and the smaller tube size dictates an increase in resistance.[12] To decrease the impact of tube length on resistance, endotracheal tubes are usually shortened by several centimeters after the infant is intubated.

Endotracheal tubes can also add to resistance by altering the pattern of airflow. Poiseuille's formula is used to describe resistance and flow under laminar conditions (in the absence of turbulence). Resistance is increased in the presence of turbulent flow. Normally, airflow is closest to laminar in distal airways, but some turbulence is present in the trachea and larger airways. Excessive turbulence can be generated when high flow rates are used to deliver air through an endotracheal tube.

For infants on mechanical ventilation, the additional resistance generated by the tube has little impact on ventilation. Intubated infants weaning from ventilation, however, may not be able to generate enough pressure and flow to overcome this additional resistance.

Respiratory Time Constant

Inspiration and expiration do not occur at constant rates. The rate at which tidal volume is inhaled or exhaled depends on both the elastic and resistive properties of the lungs. The time constants, calculated by multiplying compliance and resistance, reflect these properties. A time constant is measured in seconds and reflects how long inspiration or expiration takes. By definition, one time constant reflects the amount of time needed to move 63 percent of the tidal volume.[13] Three time constants are needed to move 95 percent of tidal volume because the time constant is exponential.

Knowledge of an infant's time constants can be useful in some cases of neonatal lung disease.[14] Infants with airway diseases such as tracheobronchomalacia generally have disproportionately high airway resistance relative to compliance. In these infants, the expiratory time constant is long, reflecting the elevated resistance and relatively good compliance. If such an infant is on a high ventilator rate, the expiratory time allowed by the ventilator may be less than is needed, as indicated

FIGURE 5-6
Pulmonary function testing circuit to determine functional residual capacity by the helium dilution technique.

The infant can be connected to the circuit from a ventilator or when breathing spontaneously. The drop in helium concentration following connection of the infant to the closed breathing circuit (gray line) is proportional to lung volume.

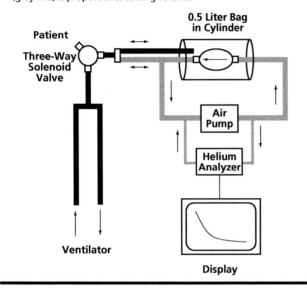

by the time constant. When this occurs, the infant is at risk for air trapping.

Work of Breathing

The amount of work required to overcome the elastic and resistive forces of the lung is termed the *resistive work of breathing*, which is one measure of pulmonary energetics. The work of breathing (WOB) indicates how much energy is required to generate a breath, either by the infant breathing spontaneously or by the ventilator during assisted ventilation. When compliance is poor or resistance is high, the WOB will be high. *Work* is defined as force multiplied by distance and is normalized to weight.

EXPANDING THE PULMONARY FUNCTION PROFILE

Many other tests are available to expand the pulmonary function profile. Some of these, such as plethysmography and occlusion methods, can be substituted for some of the techniques previously discussed to produce similar measures of lung function.[15–20] More advanced procedures are designed to test pulmonary drive, strength and endurance, distribution of ventilation, perfusion, pulmonary blood flow, and diffusion.[21–27] Still other tests can assess lung activity outside the range of normal tidal breathing, as in forced expiratory flows, or in unusual circumstances, such as in

bronchoprovocation tests.[28–37] Although many of these tests are very useful in certain circumstances, their utility in evaluating the acutely ill neonate is limited, and they are not discussed here.

Two additional techniques that can be easily used and that add valuable information to assessment in the neonatal population are briefly described below. These are measures of FRC and thoracoabdominal motion.

Functional Residual Capacity

FRC is defined as the volume of gas remaining in the lungs at the end of expiration and essentially represents the volume of gas in communication with the airways. As an important indicator of lung status that can be utilized alone to alter management strategies, this measurement is particularly useful as a complement to other measures of pulmonary function. In this regard, compliance, resistance, and other measures of lung function can be markedly altered by changes in FRC.

FRC can be assessed through several techniques. The **helium dilution technique** is a simple method of determining FRC that can be used for even the sickest infant.[5,38–41] This technique requires the infant's airway to be connected, at the end of a normal expiration, to a reservoir of known volume and helium concentration. The drop in helium concentration over 30–90 seconds is proportional to the lung volume at the time of connection, which can be easily calculated (Figure 5-6).

Several parameters can affect the accuracy of the measurement. Leaks around the face mask or endotracheal tube, oxygen consumption over the 30–90 seconds of equilibration, and prolonged lung time constants can all affect measurements.[42] In addition, the calibration and inaccuracies of the helium analyzer can complicate measurements. Also, many critically ill infants do not tolerate changes in ventilation or oxygen concentration for prolonged periods of time, necessitating a rapid method of testing. Many of these issues have been addressed within the mathematical equations used to calculate FRC by the latest generation of computerized equipment. Accurate FRC measurement is now possible at the bedside of even the most critically ill neonate.

FRC can also be measured in newborns by gas washout techniques. With the **nitrogen washout technique**, the infant breathes 100 percent oxygen continuously, and the expired gas is sampled for nitrogen content.[43] The integration of the nitrogen concentration curve of the exhaled gas can be utilized to determine the FRC. Problems with this technique arise from the necessity of breathing 100 percent oxygen, inaccuracies when the

FIGURE 5-7
Measurement of thoracoabdominal motion.

Elastic bands wrapped around the thorax and abdomen contain small wires that sense the expansion and contraction of these body compartments. The information from the bands is integrated in a device that calculates the phase angle between the waveforms.

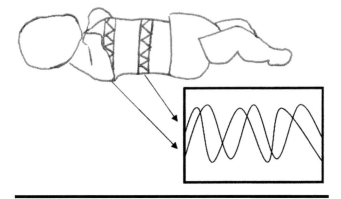

FIGURE 5-8
Sample pressure-volume loops.

A. Pressure-volume loop representing the ideal range for a tidal volume. **B.** Insufficient PEEP allows end-expiratory lung volume to fall below the lower inflection point of the pressure-volume relationship. **C.** Excessive inspiratory pressure or gas trapping can cause lung volume to surpass the upper inflection point of the pressure-volume relationship.

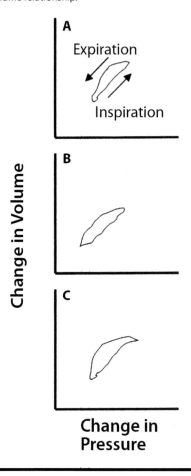

infant is already breathing high oxygen concentrations, and difficulties with gas leaks. An alternative to nitrogen washout is washout of an inert tracer gas, sulfur hexafluoride.[44–46] This technique uses the same principles as nitrogen washout, but the infant can breathe any respiratory gas mixture, and the system is not as sensitive to leaks in the circuit. As with the helium dilution technique, computerization has permitted these methods to be employed at the neonate's bedside.

Thoracoabdominal Motion

An additional, noninvasive evaluation technique that can add valuable information to the pulmonary function profile is an assessment of thoracoabdominal motion. Inductive plethysmography utilizes elastic bands placed around the thorax and the abdomen that feed information on the expansion and contraction of each body cavity into a device that calculates the phase angle between the motions of the two compartments (Figure 5-7).[19,47] Ideally, the phase angle between the rib cage and the abdomen is around zero as the chest and abdomen expand together during inspiration; however, in a preterm neonate, the phase angle is generally not that low. With increased levels of respiratory distress, the phase angle increases, identifying a greater degree of asynchrony between body compartments during inspiration. Therefore, improvements (i.e., reductions) in phase angle can be used to track improvements in respiratory proficiency. When phase angle is measured repeatedly, it is important that body position and level of airway pressure support remain constant because

these factors influence phase angle independent of lung status.[48,49]

INTERPRETING BASIC PULMONARY FUNCTION DATA

Careful monitoring of ventilatory pressures, flow rates, and lung volumes permits the caregiver to maximize the lung-protective goal of positive pressure–supported respiration. In both ventilated and spontaneously breathing infants, pulmonary function data can provide the information to optimize lung function. The display screen on a pulmonary function monitoring device generally lists the basic values for tidal volume, pulmonary resistance, pulmonary compliance, and

FIGURE 5-9
Sample flow-volume loops.

A. Normal flow-volume loop. **B.** Gross structural or mucus-associated flow limitations can be seen by flow abnormalities in both the inspiratory and expiratory phases of respiration. **C.** Airway collapse can be seen on the expiratory limb of this flow-volume loop, which has a normal inspiratory limb.

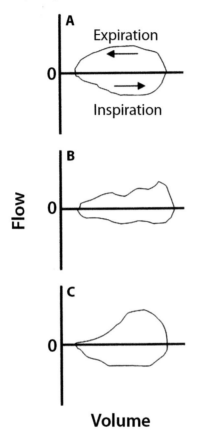

respiratory time constants. These data can be interpreted against normative values for infants of the same gestational age or age of life. Interpretation of basic respiratory values can indicate such respiratory concerns as surfactant insufficiency (indicated by poor compliance) or airway abnormalities (indicated by elevated resistance).[50] However, a greater appreciation of the infant's respiratory prognosis can be gained by interpretation of the pressure-volume and flow-volume relationships, which are displayed on the monitoring device as loops on an X-Y axis.

PRESSURE-VOLUME LOOPS

The benefit of visualizing the pressure-volume relationship is most pronounced in mechanically ventilated infants. Information from the graphic display of lung compliance through the range of a tidal volume

can be used to determine optimal settings for pressure support (Figure 5-8). Modern ventilators provide this information in real-time displays and show the effects of ventilator pressure changes on lung mechanics almost immediately. With the use of esophageal pressure measurement, these data can be monitored periodically and used to adjust positive airway pressure settings in spontaneously breathing infants as well.

End-Distending Pressure

Positive end-expiratory pressure (PEEP) in the ventilated infant or continuous positive airway pressure in the spontaneously breathing infant are used to maintain alveolar recruitment. The objective in determining the ideal end-distending pressure is to maintain lung volume just above the lower inflection point of the lung's pressure-volume relationship. Loop B in Figure 5-8 illustrates the effects of an insufficient PEEP setting where the lower inflection point can be identified. In this instance, the PEEP setting on the ventilator should be increased to minimize atelectasis-related trauma from the repeated opening and closing of lung units.[51]

Overexpansion

Whereas spontaneously breathing infants will regulate the depth of their own tidal volumes, mechanically ventilated infants are at the mercy of the ventilator settings. Beyond the upper inflection point of the lung's pressure-volume relationship, compliance is markedly decreased as the parenchymal tissue nears its capacity for expansion. If ventilator-delivered breaths are too large or in instances of gas trapping, this upper inflection point can be reached. This phenomenon is also identifiable on pressure-volume loops (Figure 5-8, loop C), and ventilator settings should be adjusted to minimize lung injury from overexpansion.[52–54]

FLOW-VOLUME LOOPS

Prematurity and positive pressure ventilation can have a pronounced impact on lung function, as well as on the airways that serve as conduits to deliver respiratory gases to and from the lung. Disruptions in normal airway function can be identified by visualizing the flow-volume relationship on the pulmonary function monitor display.

Flow-volume loops show gas flow through the airways and lung throughout the range of a tidal volume during both inspiration and expiration. A normal flow volume loop (Figure 5-9, loop A) should appear smooth and grossly similar between the inspiratory and expiratory phases of respiration. Alterations in this basic waveform can be indicative of airway conduction abnormalities that should be addressed. Airway deformations resulting from factors such as increased airway secretions or gross structural abnormalities can be visualized on a flow-volume loop as an erratic tracing such as the one in loop B of Figure 5-9.

The forces associated with mechanical ventilation can alter the properties of the infant airway in ways that promote airway collapse during expiration, a symptom of tracheobronchomalacia.[55,56] An alteration in airway function can also be identified on a flow-volume loop where there is a discrepancy between the inspiratory and expiratory phases of respiration. In the case of altered airway stability, the inspiratory limb appears normal, but flow diminishes abruptly during expiration as the airway collapses (Figure 5-9, loop C).

Nursing Implications

The high-risk neonate presents special challenges in diagnosis, treatment, and follow-up. An integrated clinical-physiologic approach utilizing state-of-the-art pulmonary function monitoring coupled with appropriate therapeutic measures of respiratory management can help the clinician meet these challenges. Bedside pulmonary function monitoring is an important tool for the team caring for these infants. The data that can be obtained and documented by the nurse at the bedside can be integrated into every aspect of the nursing care plan. By using pulmonary function monitoring and understanding and analyzing the results, nurses add another dimension to their assessment skills, positively influencing appropriate intervention for the neonate.

With real-time monitoring, pulmonary function data can be utilized much like arterial blood chemistry: to assess status, effect change, alter management, and guide prognosis. A complete understanding of the capabilities and limitations of these data is important to all the infant's caregivers. For instance, identifying and understanding abnormalities in ventilator-generated breaths—such as excessive tidal volume, prolonged inspiratory pause, significant gas leak, or gas trapping—can allow more rapid changes in management strategy. If the bedside team must wait for the periodic blood gas results to identify problems, thousands of suboptimal breaths might be delivered to the infant in the interim. Instead, the bedside team can utilize readily available pulmonary function profiles to make important changes in clinical care that can positively affect outcomes.

Ensuring Accurate Pulmonary Function Data

The expertise of the intensive care nurse is invaluable in ensuring the validity of the pulmonary function data. Although the tests are noninvasive, physical manipulation of the infant is often required; this is especially true in spontaneously breathing patients. During a pulmonary evaluation, the nurse assures good positioning, maintains a stable airway, and monitors for changes in the infant's status. To assure accurate and reproducible pulmonary function data for the infant's record, the infant must be prepared consistently for pulmonary evaluation in the following ways:

1. **Address feeding concerns:**
   - Delay recording pulmonary function data until one hour after feeding.
   - If using an esophageal balloon in an infant receiving gavage feedings, aspirate the stomach contents with a syringe. Remove nasogastric and orogastric tubes to allow placement of the balloon catheter.

2. **Quiet the infant (applies to spontaneous breathers):**
   - Consider sedation with chloral hydrate in older infants, particularly those with bronchopulmonary dysplasia (BPD). Sedation facilitates passage of the esophageal balloon and permits sampling of quiet breathing. Chloral hydrate causes transient decreases in respiratory rate and tidal volume, but otherwise does not have a significant effect on pulmonary function.
   - If chloral hydrate is not used, the nurse can hold an irritable infant during testing. Holding does not affect test results as long as the infant can breathe freely.

3. **Maintain proper head and neck position:**
   - If feasible, place the infant supine, positioning the head in the midline and the neck in the neutral position. If the neck is flexed or hyperextended, the upper airway may be narrowed, creating artificially high airway resistance even for intubated infants.
   - Assess the effect of neck and head position by monitoring flow-volume loops on-line before recording data. If significant airway obstruction is present, the flow-volume loop will show inspiratory or expiratory flow restriction.
   - In a nonintubated infant, avoid excessive compression of the face mask to the face; compression alters airway resistance measurements.

THE ROLE OF PULMONARY FUNCTION DATA

MANAGEMENT OF ACUTE LUNG DISEASE

The pulmonary function profile varies with the infant's diagnosis. Soon after birth, preterm infants present with low lung compliance and reduced FRC, while airway resistance is relatively normal.[57,58] Reductions in compliance and lung volume are related to both high alveolar surface tension and atelectasis.

When these infants are treated with surfactant, FRC and oxygenation improve within 2 hours of treatment, but a significant improvement in compliance may not be seen for 12 hours following surfactant administration.[5,59,60] Pulmonary function evaluation of the preterm infant may help to determine (1) the frequency of surfactant replacement therapy, (2) the need for other pulmonary interventions such as high-frequency ventilation or inspired nitric oxide therapy, and (3) the pulmonary process and prognosis.[57,61]

During the first few weeks of life, pulmonary mechanics may worsen as new problems develop. Sequential testing of pulmonary mechanics in very low birth weight (VLBW) neonates shows a decrease in compliance and an increase in pulmonary resistance between one and two weeks of life.[58,62] These measurements return to week 1 values by week 4. Although not universally observed in all preterm infants, this "worsening" during the second week probably has a multifactorial etiology. Pulmonary problems at this time can result from sepsis and pneumonia, a patent ductus arteriosus, or the inflammation seen in early stages of chronic lung disease.

In ventilator dependent, low birth weight neonates at two weeks of age, airway reactivity and bronchospasm may represent a new problem, and airway management can be a challenge. Pulmonary function analysis can again be utilized to diagnose bronchospasm and to evaluate the effectiveness of interventions such as administration of a bronchodilator.[28,29]

Tracheobronchomalacia can be diagnosed by examining flow-volume loops for evidence of airway collapse on expiration. Infants with airway collapse have very high expiratory resistance values and prolonged time constants. By monitoring real-time flow-volume loops while adjusting PEEP levels, the nurse can minimize expiratory collapse.

The pulmonary function profile improves slowly over weeks in premature infants recovering from respiratory distress syndrome. Airway reactivity may present a significant management challenge, but pulmonary function assessments can be used to identify the infant's response to changes in ventilator settings or to bronchodilator administration. Pulmonary mechanics can remain abnormal even after the infant has been weaned from mechanical ventilation and oxygen.

Like that of a preterm infant, the pulmonary function profile of a term infant with respiratory compromise also differs with the diagnosis. Infants with congenital diaphragmatic hernia may present with reduced compliance and FRC resulting from a combination of lung hypoplasia and lung compression caused by displaced abdominal viscera. Airway resistance in these patients may be low because of the decreased number of airways in the affected lung regions. Infants with meconium aspiration syndrome also show reduced lung compliance and FRC. Airway resistance may be high in these infants because of the presence of debris in the airways.

Abnormal pulmonary function values may indicate the need for alternate therapies for these infants, such as extracorporeal membrane oxygenation (ECMO). In particular, knowledge of low FRC, which may predict impending respiratory failure, may facilitate timely initiation of treatment or transfer to a tertiary center for the appropriate treatment. For infants on ECMO, pulmonary function testing has been used to monitor lung recovery and to assess readiness to wean from ECMO back to conventional ventilation.

The role of pulmonary analysis in predicting lethal lung hypoplasia and the response to newer modalities such as nitric oxide and liquid ventilation therapies is currently being evaluated.

MANAGEMENT OF CHRONIC LUNG DISEASE

Although much has been learned about BPD during the 25 years since its initial description, chronic lung disease remains a significant complication of prematurity. Substantial advances in understanding its pathophysiology and pathogenesis are reflected in new therapeutic interventions.

Largely, current research is directed toward prevention. New approaches for surfactant replacement therapy, high-frequency ventilation, inhaled nitric oxide therapy, antioxidant and anti-inflammatory administration, and other pharmacologic strategies to minimize lung injury are being explored.

Much of the current research in neonatal pulmonology focuses on biologic pathways for lung maturation and mechanisms that can hasten lung healing. Ongoing studies of inflammatory products, growth factors, and cytokines may lead to new therapies that will favorably influence the fibroproliferative phase of BPD.

Although advances in neonatal care have given infants weighing <750 g a better than 60 percent chance of survival, the incidence of BPD has increased at the same time.[63] In the extremely immature neonate, the initial respiratory disease progresses to BPD in as many as 55 percent of cases.[63,64] BPD continues to remain a significant medical and social problem, not only in infancy, but through the first year of life. These infants create a large emotional and financial burden for their parents, caregivers, and society with their prolonged initial hospitalization, home care, increased need for rehospitalization, and associated problems.

Preparation for Discharge

One approach to controlling costs, managing care, and minimizing the need for intense, prolonged treatment of infants with BPD is to determine a plan of care well before discharge. Successful discharge planning begins at the time of admission. There is a need for objective data to define pulmonary morbidity, evaluate potential therapies and interventions, and integrate the infant's pulmonary status into the discharge plan. Even though an infant may be breathing room air for several weeks, significant pulmonary morbidity may still exist.

Pulmonary function evaluation at discharge can assess for the presence of residual parenchymal dysfunction, airway reactivity, and increased WOB. It is possible for such abnormalities to go unrecognized in the unstressed infant at the time of discharge, but to be exacerbated by intercurrent illness or additional stressors at home, such as a smoky environment and cold or less humidified air.

An understanding of the susceptibility of infants with BPD to ongoing pulmonary problems promotes more effective anticipatory guidance and may suggest prophylactic therapy. It is not unusual, for instance, to suggest on a discharge evaluation that a bronchodilator be available for infants who seem to respond well to this therapy. In addition, the infant's nutritional status may be related to the WOB, and estimates of calorie requirements can be correlated with pulmonary function analysis.

Once a discharge pulmonary function evaluation is obtained, a teaching plan can be developed, and parents can learn how to handle this aspect of their infant's care at home. In addition, the infant's pulmonary needs can be fully ascertained, social services can be integrated, and home care can be coordinated in a timely fashion.

Rehospitalization

BPD severity ranges widely. The most severe form, occurring in 0.5–19 percent of all VLBW infants, is seen in those who require oxygen and/or ventilator treatment for more than three months.[65] The morbidity in this group is higher than that of infants with chronic lung disease who do not require such treatment.

To reduce costs, many institutions transfer BPD-affected infants to a rehabilitation hospital soon after they are weaned from the ventilator. In 1993, Bachrach and colleagues documented savings of $60,000 per patient transferred to a rehabilitation hospital.[66]

With the aid of pulmonary function evaluations, early diagnosis of lung injury and prediction of the severity and chronicity of the infant's disease can enhance goal setting for these infants, help reduce hospitalization, and facilitate early transfer to a rehabilitative facility. Such a program could markedly decrease lengths of stay and reduce hospital costs, without an increase in morbidity or mortality. The focus could then shift from acute care needs to training for home care and technological support for home oxygen therapy, facilitating effective and efficient discharge planning.

SUMMARY

Respiratory insufficiency is a primary or secondary diagnosis in more than 80 percent of the infants admitted to intensive care. These high-risk neonates present special challenges in diagnosis, treatment, and follow-up. It is difficult to accurately determine the nature of an infant's respiratory dysfunction on the basis of physical examination and arterial blood gases alone. In addition, responses to therapies vary dramatically among infants who are considered to have similar disease processes.

A more detailed analysis of the pathophysiology of the pulmonary disease is essential if appropriate therapies are to be instituted and managed optimally. Pulmonary function monitoring, with its ability to describe and quantify neonatal lung disease, offers such an analysis. Although the basic tools of history and physical assessment remain the mainstay of infant evaluation, modern pulmonary function assessment techniques facilitate a more physiologic approach, which can reduce morbidity, mortality, and cost.

REFERENCES

1. Beardsmore CS, et al. 1980. Improved esophageal balloon technique for use in infants. *Journal of Applied Physiology* 49(4): 735–742.
2. Bhutani VK, et al. 1988. Evaluation of neonatal pulmonary mechanics and energetics: A two factor least mean square analysis. *Pediatric Pulmonology* 4(3): 150–158.

3. Bancalari E. 1986. Pulmonary function testing and other diagnostic laboratory procedures. In *Neonatal Pulmonary Care*, 2nd ed., Thibeault DW, and Gregory GA, eds. Norwalk, Connecticut: Appleton-Century-Crofts, 49–73.

4. Comroe JHJ. 1962. *The Lung: Clinical Physiology and Pulmonary Function Tests*, 2nd ed. Chicago: Year Book.

5. Goldsmith LS, et al. 1991. Immediate improvement in lung volume after exogenous surfactant: Alveolar recruitment versus increased distention. *Journal of Pediatrics* 119(3): 424–428.

6. Fisher JB, et al. 1988. Identifying lung overdistention during mechanical ventilation by using volume-pressure loops. *Pediatric Pulmonology* 5(1): 10–14.

7. Polgar G. 1986. Mechanical properties of lung and chest wall. In *Neonatal Pulmonary Care*, 2nd ed., Thibeault DW, and Gregory GA, eds. Norwalk, Connecticut: Appleton-Century-Crofts, 195–233.

8. Guslits BG, et al. 1987. Comparison of methods of measurement of compliance of the respiratory system in children. *American Review of Respiratory Disease* 136(3): 727–729.

9. Migdal M, et al. 1987. Compliance of the total respiratory system in healthy preterm and full-term newborns. *Pediatric Pulmonology* 3(4): 214–218. (Published erratum in *Pediatric Pulmonology*, 1987, 3[5]: 383.)

10. Wanner A, et al. 1974. Relationship between frequency dependence of lung compliance and distribution of ventilation. *Journal of Clinical Investigation* 54(5): 1200–1213.

11. West JB. 2008. Mechanics of breathing. In *Respiratory Physiology: The Essentials*. Philadelphia: Lippincott Williams & Wilkins, 95–122.

12. LeSouef PN, England SJ, and Bryan AC. 1984. Total resistance of the respiratory system in preterm infants with and without an endotracheal tube. *Journal of Pediatrics* 104(1): 108–111.

13. Woolcock AJ, Vincent NJ, and Macklem PT. 1969. Frequency dependence of compliance as a test of obstruction in the small airways. *Journal of Clinical Investigation* 48(6): 1097–1106.

14. Mammel MC, et al. 1989. Determining optimum inspiratory time during intermittent positive pressure ventilation in surfactant-depleted cats. *Pediatric Pulmonology* 7(4): 223–229.

15. Auld PA, et al. 1963. Measurement of thoracic gas volume in the newborn infant. *Journal of Clinical Investigation* 42: 476–483.

16. Ashutosh K, et al. 1974. Impedance pneumograph and magnetometer methods for monitoring tidal volume. *Journal of Applied Physiology* 37(6): 964–966.

17. Beardsmore CS, et al. 1989. Measurement of lung volumes during active and quiet sleep in infants. *Pediatric Pulmonology* 7(2): 71–77.

18. Beardsmore CS, Stocks J, and Silverman M. 1982. Problems in measurement of thoracic gas volume in infancy. *Journal of Applied Physiology* 52(4): 995–999.

19. Duffty P, et al. 1981. Respiratory induction plethysmography (Respitrace): An evaluation of its use in the infant. *American Review of Respiratory Disease* 123(5): 542–546.

20. Grunstein MM, et al. 1987. Expiratory volume clamping: A new method to assess respiratory mechanics in sedated infants. *Journal of Applied Physiology* 62(5): 2107–2114.

21. Greenspan JS, et al. 1992. Increased respiratory drive and limited adaptation to loaded breathing in bronchopulmonary dysplasia. *Pediatric Research* 32(3): 356–359.

22. Motoyama EK. 1977. Pulmonary mechanics during early postnatal years. *Pediatric Research* 11(3 part 1): 220–223.

23. Motoyama EK, et al. 1987. Early onset of airway reactivity in premature infants with bronchopulmonary dysplasia. *American Review of Respiratory Disease* 136(1): 50–57.

24. Bose CL, et al. 1986. Measurement of cardiopulmonary function in ventilated neonates with respiratory distress syndrome using rebreathing methodology. *Pediatric Research* 20(4): 316–320.

25. Duara S, et al. 1985. Preterm infants: Ventilation and P_{100} changes with CO_2 and inspiratory resistive loading. *Journal of Applied Physiology* 58(6): 1982–1987.

26. Duara S, et al. 1991. Metabolic and respiratory effects of flow-resistive loading in preterm infants. *Journal of Applied Physiology* 70(2): 895–899.

27. Sly PD, Lanteri C, and Bates JH. 1990. Effect of the thermodynamics of an infant plethysmograph on the measurement of thoracic gas volume. *Pediatric Pulmonology* 8(3): 203–208.

28. Greenspan JS, DeGiulio PA, and Bhutani VK. 1989. Airway reactivity as determined by a cold air challenge in infants with bronchopulmonary dysplasia. *Journal of Pediatrics* 114(3): 452–454.

29. Greenspan JS, Wolfson MR, and Shaffer TH. 1991. Airway responsiveness to low inspired gas temperature in preterm neonates. *Journal of Pediatrics* 118(3): 443–445.

30. Morgan WJ. 1988. Evaluation of forced expiratory flow in infants. In *Neonatal Pulmonary Function Testing: Physiological, Technical, and Clinical Considerations*, 2nd ed., Bhutani VK, Shaffer TH, and Vidyasagar D, eds. Ithaca, New York: Perinatology Press, 107–123.

31. Prendiville A, Green S, and Silverman M. 1987. Paradoxical response to nebulized salbutamol in wheezy infants, assessed by partial expiratory flow-volume curves. *Thorax* 42(2): 86–91.

32. Stefano JL, et al. 1986. Inductive plethysmography—A facilitated postural calibration technique for rapid and accurate tidal volume determination in low birth weight premature newborns. *American Review of Respiratory Disease* 134(5): 1020–1024.

33. Taussig LM. 1977. Maximal expiratory flows at functional residual capacity: A test of lung function for young children. *American Review of Respiratory Disease* 116(6): 1031–1038.

34. Taussig LM, et al. 1982. Determinants of forced expiratory flows in newborn infants. *Journal of Applied Physiology* 53(5): 1220–1227.

35. Tepper RS, et al. 1986. Expiratory flow limitation in infants with bronchopulmonary dysplasia. *Journal of Pediatrics* 109(6): 1040–1046.

36. Tepper RS, et al. 1986. Physiologic growth and development of the lung during the first year of life. *American Review of Respiratory Disease* 134(3): 513–519. (Published erratum in *American Review of Respiratory Disease*, 1987, 136[3]: 800.)

37. Tepper RS, and Reister T. 1993. Forced expiratory flows and lung volumes in normal infants. *Pediatric Pulmonology* 15(6): 357–361.

38. Fox WW. 1988. Measurement of functional residual capacity in infants using the helium dilution method. In *Neonatal Pulmonary Function Testing: Physiological, Technical, and Clinical Considerations*, Bhutani VK, Shaffer TH, and Vidyasagar D, eds. Ithaca, New York: Perinatology Press, 81–90.

39. Antunes MJ. 1992. Decreased functional residual capacity predates requirement for ECMO and lung opacification during ECMO. *Pediatric Research* 31(4 part 2): 192A.

40. Antunes MJ, et al. 1995. Prognosis with preoperative pulmonary function and lung volume assessment in infants with congenital diaphragmatic hernia. *Pediatrics* 96(6): 1117–1122.

41. Antunes MJ, et al. 1994. Continued pulmonary recovery observed after discontinuing extracorporeal membrane oxygenation. *Pediatric Pulmonology* 17(3): 143–148.

42. Fox WW, Schwartz JG, and Shaffer TH. 1979. Effects of endotracheal tube leaks on functional residual capacity determination in intubated neonates. *Pediatric Research* 13(1): 60–64.

43. Gerhardt T, et al. 1985. A simple method for measuring functional residual capacity by N_2 washout in small animals and newborn infants. *Pediatric Research* 19(11): 1165–1169.

44. Bjorklund LJ, et al. 1996. Changes in lung volume and static expiratory pressure-volume diagram after surfactant rescue treatment of neonates with established respiratory distress syndrome. *American Journal of Respiratory and Critical Care Medicine* 154(4 part 1): 918–923.

45. Jonmarker C, et al. 1985. Measurement of functional residual capacity by sulfur hexafluoride washout. *Anesthesiology* 63(1): 89–95.

46. Gustafsson PM, et al. 2003. Method for assessment of volume of trapped gas in infants during multiple-breath inert gas washout. *Pediatric Pulmonology* 35(1): 42–49.

47. Stick SM, et al. 1992. Validation of respiratory inductance plethysmography ("Respitrace") for the measurement of tidal breathing parameters in newborns. *Pediatric Pulmonology* 14(3): 187–191.

48. Locke R, et al. 1991. Effect of nasal CPAP on thoracoabdominal motion in neonates with respiratory insufficiency. *Pediatric Pulmonology* 11(3): 259–264.

49. Wolfson MR, et al. 1992. Effect of position on the mechanical interaction between the rib cage and abdomen in preterm infants. *Journal of Applied Physiology* 72(3): 1032–1038.

50. Shaffer TH, Wolfson MR, and Greenspan JS. 1991. Pulmonary function testing in the critically ill neonate. In *Fetal and Neonatal Physiological Measurements*, Lafeber HN, ed. Amsterdam: Excerpta Medica, 100–205.

51. Amato MB, et al. 1998. Effect of a protective-ventilation strategy on mortality in the acute respiratory distress syndrome. *New England Journal of Medicine* 338(6): 347–354.

52. Goldstein I, et al. 2001. Mechanical ventilation-induced air-space enlargement during experimental pneumonia in piglets. *American Journal of Respiratory and Critical Care Medicine* 163(4): 958–964.

53. Rouby JJ, et al. 1993. Histologic aspects of pulmonary barotrauma in critically ill patients with acute respiratory failure. *Intensive Care Medicine* 19(7): 383–389.

54. Bjorklund LJ, et al. 1997. Manual ventilation with a few large breaths at birth compromises the therapeutic effect of subsequent surfactant replacement in immature lambs. *Pediatric Research* 42(3): 348–355.

55. Bhutani VK, Ritchie WG, and Shaffer TH. 1986. Acquired tracheomegaly in very preterm neonates. *American Journal of Diseases of Children* 140(5): 449–452.

56. Penn RB, Wolfson MR, and Shaffer TH. 1988. Effect of ventilation on mechanical properties and pressure-flow relationships of immature airways. *Pediatric Research* 23(5): 519–524.

57. Goldman SL, et al. 1983. Early prediction of chronic lung disease by pulmonary function testing. *Journal of Pediatrics* 102(4): 613–617.

58. Greenspan JS, Abbasi S, and Bhutani VK. 1988. Sequential changes in pulmonary mechanics in the very low birth weight (≤1,000 grams) infant. *Journal of Pediatrics* 113(4): 732–737.

59. Couser RJ, et al. 1990. Effects of exogenous surfactant therapy on dynamic compliance during mechanical breathing in preterm infants with hyaline membrane disease. *Journal of Pediatrics* 116(1): 119–124.

60. Davis JM, et al. 1988. Changes in pulmonary mechanics after the administration of surfactant to infants with respiratory distress syndrome. *New England Journal of Medicine* 319(8): 476–479.

61. Gerhardt T, et al. 1987. Serial determination of pulmonary function in infants with chronic lung disease. *Journal of Pediatrics* 110(3): 448–456.

62. Abbasi S, and Bhutani VK. 1990. Pulmonary mechanics and energetics of normal, non-ventilated low birthweight infants. *Pediatric Pulmonology* 8(2): 89–95.

63. Collaborative European Multicenter Study Group. 1988. Surfactant replacement therapy for severe neonatal respiratory distress syndrome: An international randomized clinical trial. *Pediatrics* 82(5): 683–691.

64. Abbasi S, Bhutani VK, and Gerdes JS. 1993. Long-term pulmonary consequences of respiratory distress syndrome in preterm infants treated with exogenous surfactant. *Journal of Pediatrics* 122(3): 446–452.

65. Avery ME, et al. 1987. Is chronic lung disease in low birth weight infants preventable? A survey of eight centers. *Pediatrics* 79(1): 26–30.

66. Bachrach SJ, et al. 1993. Early transfer to a rehabilitation hospital for infants with chronic bronchopulmonary dysplasia. *Clinical Pediatrics* 32(9): 535–541.

Notes

Notes

6 Blood Gas Analysis

Debbie Fraser, MN, RNC-NIC

Blood gas analysis is one of the major tools in assessing the respiratory status of the newborn. To adequately use this information, one must have a basic understanding of gas transportation and acid-base physiology. These topics are addressed in this chapter to provide a basis for applying these principles to the interpretation of neonatal blood gases. Common terminology is defined in Table 6-1.

TRANSPORT OF OXYGEN AND CARBON DIOXIDE

OXYGEN

Oxygen is used in aerobic reactions throughout the human body and is supplied to the tissues through the efforts of the respiratory and cardiovascular systems. The lungs are responsible for bringing an adequate supply of oxygen to the blood. Control of this process occurs mainly in response to the effect of carbon dioxide (CO_2) levels on receptors in the large arteries and the brain. At moderate to severe levels of hypoxemia, peripheral chemoreceptors take the dominant role in increasing ventilation, resulting in increased oxygen intake and lower than normal partial pressure of carbon dioxide in arterial blood ($PaCO_2$).[1]

The cardiovascular system regulates the oxygen supply by altering cardiac output in response to the metabolic rate of peripheral tissues. Distribution of oxygen to specific tissues is determined by local metabolic activity. Oxygen transport is affected by:[2]

- partial pressure of oxygen in inspired air
- alveolar ventilation
- ventilation-to-perfusion matching
- arterial pH and temperature
- cardiac output
- blood volume
- hemoglobin
- hemoglobin's affinity for oxygen

Oxygen transport to the tissues can be divided into a three-phase process, involving oxygen diffusion from the alveoli to the pulmonary capillaries (external respiration) (phase 1), gas transport in the bloodstream (phase 2), and diffusion of oxygen from the capillaries to the cells (internal respiration) (phase 3). The first two phases are discussed below.

Oxygen diffuses from the alveoli to the pulmonary capillaries. Oxygen enters the lung during inspiration and diffuses across the alveolar-capillary membrane, depending on the concentration gradient of oxygen in the alveolus and the capillary (Figure 6-1). Factors that interfere with oxygenation at this point include a decrease in minute ventilation, ventilation-perfusion mismatch, and alterations in the alveolar-capillary membrane.[1]

Once in the blood, oxygen must be transported to the tissues. A small amount of oxygen (about 2–5 percent) is dissolved in the plasma; 95–98 percent is bound to hemoglobin. The total volume of oxygen carried in the blood is termed the *arterial oxygen content* and reflects both the oxygen combined with hemoglobin and the amount dissolved in the plasma.

The smaller, dissolved portion of oxygen is measured as the partial pressure of oxygen (PaO_2). *Partial pressure* refers to the force the gas exerts in the blood. Through simple diffusion, gases move from an area of higher pressure to an area of lower pressure. PaO_2 is the most

TABLE 6-1
Terminology Associated with Blood Gas Analysis

Term	Definition
Acid	Donator of H+ ions
Base	Acceptor of H+ ions
Buffer	Weak acid and strong base pair that accept or donate hydrogen ions to maintain a balanced pH
pH	Negative logarithm of hydrogen ion
$\neq$ H+	pH more acid
$\emptyset$ H+	pH more alkaline
Acidemia	Blood pH below 7.35
Alkalemia	Blood pH above 7.45
Acidosis	Process causing acidemia
Alkalosis	Process causing alkalemia

FIGURE 6-1
Oxygen diffusion across the alveolar-capillary membrane.

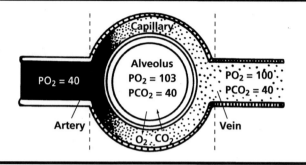

From: Cherniack RM. 1972. *Respiration in Health and Disease,* 2nd ed. Philadelphia: Saunders. Reprinted by permission.

important factor in determining the amount of oxygen bound to hemoglobin. As PaO_2 increases, more oxygen diffuses into the red blood cells, where it combines with hemoglobin to form oxyhemoglobin.

Each hemoglobin molecule contains four atoms of iron and therefore can combine with four molecules of oxygen. When fully combined with oxygen, 1 g of hemoglobin carries 1.34 mL of oxygen.[1] The combination of oxygen and hemoglobin is expressed as *oxygen saturation:* a measure of the hemoglobin sites filled divided by the sites available (Figure 6-2).

Oxygen-hemoglobin saturation is plotted on an S-shaped curve known as the oxyhemoglobin dissociation curve (see Figure 4-10); this curve is based on adult hemoglobin at normal temperature and blood pH. Normal hemoglobin is 60 percent saturated at a PaO_2 of 30 mmHg and 90 percent saturated at a PaO_2 of 60 mmHg. At a PaO_2 of 90 mmHg, 95 percent of hemoglobin is saturated with oxygen.[3]

At the low PaO_2 values seen on the steep slope of the curve in Figure 4-10, a small increase in PaO_2 results in a large increase in oxygen saturation. Conversely, on the flat upper portion of the curve, a large increase in PaO_2 results in only a small increase in saturation. Hemoglobin cannot be more than 100 percent saturated, but PaO_2 can exceed 100 mmHg. At a PaO_2 of >100 mmHg, O_2 saturation cannot reflect PaO_2. For this reason, PaO_2 is a more sensitive indicator of high oxygen levels in the blood than is the measurement of saturation.[4]

Several factors change the affinity of hemoglobin for oxygen, shifting the curve to the left or to the right (see Figure 4-10). Alkalosis, hypocarbia, hypothermia, decreased amounts of 2,3-diphosphoglycerate (2,3-DPG), and the presence of fetal hemoglobin all shift the curve to the left.[1] An organic phosphate, 2,3-DPG is produced as a by-product of red cell metabolism. It binds with hemoglobin and decreases its oxygen affinity.

With a shift to the left, there is an increased affinity between oxygen and hemoglobin; therefore, hemoglobin more easily picks up oxygen and doesn't release it until the PaO_2 level falls. This can impede oxygen release to the tissues, but enhances uptake of oxygen in the lungs.[2]

Acidosis, hypercapnia, hyperthermia, increased 2,3-DPG, and the presence of mature, or adult, hemoglobin move the curve to the right.[1] A shift to the right causes oxygen to bind less tightly to hemoglobin and to release from hemoglobin at higher levels of PaO_2, thereby enhancing oxygen unloading at the tissue level.[2]

Tip: An easy way to remember how shifts in the curve affect oxygen delivery is to think of it this way: left on the hemoglobin, right into the tissues.

CARBON DIOXIDE

Body cells produce CO_2 as a by-product of metabolism. Carbon dioxide diffuses from the cells down a concentration gradient, from areas of high partial pressure of CO_2 to areas of low partial pressure of CO_2. A small amount (8 percent) travels dissolved in the plasma; another small portion (2 percent) is transported in the plasma bound to proteins, forming carbamino compounds.[1] The remainder is transported within the red blood cells.

In red blood cells, about 10 percent of the CO_2 forms carbamino compounds by combining with amino acids contained in the globin portion of the hemoglobin. The remaining 80 percent is acted upon by carbonic anhydrase, which combines carbon dioxide and water to form carbonic acid (H_2CO_3) and then undergoes hydrolysis and forms bicarbonate (HCO_3^-) and hydrogen ions

FIGURE 6-2
Oxygen saturation.

Saturation is equal to the percentage of hemoglobin that is carrying oxygen. Hemoglobin can be carrying either four molecules of oxygen (oxygenated) or none (deoxygenated).

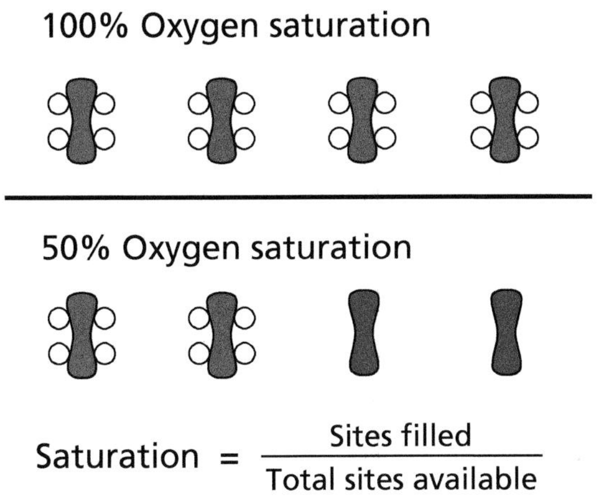

100% Oxygen saturation

50% Oxygen saturation

$$Saturation = \frac{Sites\ filled}{Total\ sites\ available}$$

FIGURE 6-3
Carbon dioxide transport.

A schematic representation of the three major mechanisms for carbon dioxide transport in blood. dCO_2 = the carbon dioxide molecules dissolved in plasma; this is the carbon dioxide that determines the partial pressure. $HbCO_2$ = carbon dioxide chemically combined to amino acid components of hemoglobin molecules; usually referred to as carbamino-CO_2. HCO_3^- = intra-red blood cell carbonic anhydrase mechanism produces bicarbonate ions.

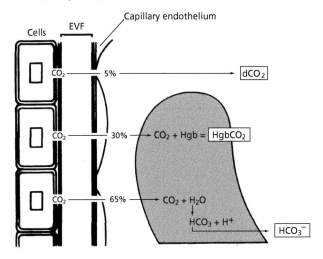

Key: EVF = extracellular volume fraction; Hgb = hemoglobin.

From: Shapiro BA, Peruzzi WT, and Kozelowski-Templin R. 1994. Respiratory acid-base balance. In *Clinical Application of Blood Gases.* Philadelphia: Mosby, 26. Reprinted by permission.

(H^+). The hydrogen ions are buffered by desaturated hemoglobin, and HCO_3^- is transported out of the erythrocytes into the plasma (Figure 6-3).[1] As oxygen is unloaded from hemoglobin along the tissue capillaries, more CO_2 can be transported because of the enhanced ability of deoxygenated hemoglobin to form carbamino compounds.[1]

ACID-BASE HOMEOSTASIS

Normal function of the body's cells depends on maintaining a biochemical balance within a narrow range of free H^+ concentration. Free H^+ is constantly released in the body as waste products from the metabolism of proteins and fats. The measurement of free H^+ present in the body in very low concentrations is expressed as *pH*, which is the negative logarithm of the H^+ concentration—that is, the more H^+ present in a solution, the lower the pH or the more acidic the solution. Conversely, the fewer H^+ present, the higher the pH or the more alkaline the solution. A pH of 7 is neutral, that is, neither alkaline nor acidic. A pH range of 7.35–7.45 is normal for cellular reactions in the human body.

Most of the acids formed by metabolism come from the interaction of carbon dioxide and water, which forms H_2CO_3, as illustrated in the following equation:

$$CO_2 + H_2O \rightarrow H_2CO_3 \rightarrow H^+ + HCO_3^-$$

Carbonic anhydrase, an enzyme, accelerates this reaction. Carbonic acid is referred to as a volatile acid

because it is transformed back into CO_2 in the lungs and exhaled, allowing the respiratory system to control the majority of acid-base regulation. Sulfuric, phosphoric, and other organic acids are nonvolatile acids that are eliminated in the renal tubules.

Changes in CO_2 affect pH by altering the amount of HCO_3^- in the body. Changes in pH caused by changes in CO_2 tension are therefore termed *respiratory*. Hyperventilation causes a lower partial pressure of carbon dioxide (PCO_2), lower H_2CO_3 concentration, and increased pH. Hypoventilation has the opposite effect. Remember that concentrations of CO_2, H_2CO_3, and H^+ move in the opposite direction of pH:

$$\uparrow PCO_2 \rightarrow \uparrow H_2CO_3 \rightarrow \uparrow H^+ \rightarrow \downarrow pH$$

$$\downarrow PCO_2 \rightarrow \downarrow H_2CO_3 \rightarrow \downarrow H^+ \rightarrow \uparrow pH$$

Metabolic acids are formed in the body during the metabolism of protein, anaerobic metabolism resulting in the formation of lactic acid and keto acids, which are formed when glucose is unavailable as a fuel source. The kidneys provide the most important route by which metabolic acids can be excreted and buffered.

FIGURE 6-4
The chloride shift.

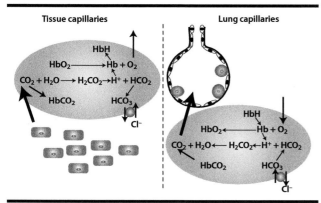

Courtesy of William Diehl-Jones.

FIGURE 6-5
Mechanisms of renal bicarbonate excretion/retention.

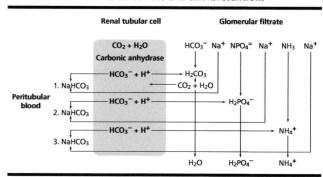

From: Shapiro BA, Peruzzi WT, and Kozelowski-Templin R. 1994. *Clinical Application of Blood Gases,* 5th ed. Philadelphia: Mosby, 7. Reprinted by permission.

Hydrogen excretion takes place through the active exchange of sodium ions (Na^+) for H^+. The kidneys are also responsible for plasma levels of HCO_3^-, the most important buffer of H^+ (discussion follows). Therefore, pH changes that occur because of changes in bicarbonate concentrations are termed *metabolic*.

Tip: Remember the following equations:

$$\uparrow HCO_3^- \rightarrow \uparrow pH$$

$$\downarrow HCO_3^- \rightarrow \downarrow pH$$

THE HENDERSON-HASSELBALCH EQUATION

The concentration of H^+ resulting from the dissociation of H_2CO_3 is determined by an interrelationship between bases, buffers, and blood acids. In blood gas analysis, the Henderson-Hasselbalch equation is used to calculate HCO_3^- if pH and PCO_2 are known.[3] This equation describes the fixed relationship between H_2CO_3, HCO_3^-, and H_2CO_3 concentration. When the equation is used in the clinical situation, H_2CO_3 is replaced by the amount of dissolved CO_2 in the blood, as shown in the following equation:[3]

$$pH = pK + log \ \frac{[HCO_3^-]}{[s \times PCO_2]}$$

in which pK (a constant) = 6.1 and s (solubility of CO_2) = 0.0301. It is important to remember that this is a calculated bicarbonate value, not one that is measured.

BUFFER SYSTEMS

Buffer systems are a combination of a weak acid and a strong base, which work by accepting or releasing hydrogen ions to maintain acid-base balance. The body has three primary buffers: plasma proteins, hemoglobin,

and bicarbonate.[5] Of these, HCO_3^- is the most important system and is regulated by the kidney. Bicarbonate ions are formed from the hydroxylation of CO_2 by water inside red blood cells, catalyzed by carbonic anhydrase. Once formed, HCO_3^- enters the plasma in exchange for chloride ions (Cl^-) through an active transport mechanism known as the chloride shift, which is depicted in Figure 6-4. In blood gas analysis, bicarbonate and base deficit/excess are used in determining the nonrespiratory portion of the acid-base equation. Some centers provide both values in blood gas results; others report either HCO_3^- levels or base excess/deficit.

Bicarbonate is expressed in milliequivalents per liter (mEq/liter). The normal range is 22–26 mEq/liter.[1] Base excess or base deficit is reported in mEq/liter, with a normal range of −4 to +4.[3] Negative values indicate a deficiency of base or an excess of acid (metabolic acidosis); positive values indicate alkalosis. Clinically, the base excess or deficit is calculated from the Siggaard-Andersen nomogram (Appendix A).

The kidney has several mechanisms for controlling excretion of H^+ and retention of HCO_3^-. These are illustrated in Figure 6-5 and include the following:[5]

- Resorption of filtered HCO_3^- (H^+ is excreted in the renal tubular cells in exchange for Na^+, which combines with HCO_3^- to form sodium bicarbonate, which enters the blood.)
- Excretion of acids (One example is phosphoric acid, which is formed from the combination of H^+ and hydrogen phosphate.)
- Formation of ammonia (NH_3) (Elevated acid levels in the body result in the formation of NH_3, which combines with H^+ to form ammonium, which is excreted in the urine.)

FIGURE 6-6
Normal 20:1 bicarbonate:carbon dioxide ratio.

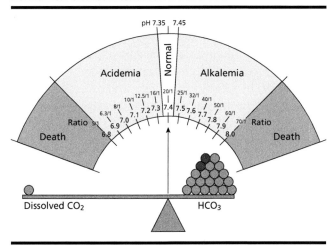

From: Jacob SW, and Francone CA. 1970. *Structure and Function in Man,* 2nd ed. Philadelphia: Saunders. Reprinted by permission.

An acid-base ratio of 1:20—that is, 1 part carbonic acid to 20 parts bicarbonate—is needed to maintain a pH of 7.4.[3] It is the ratio of PCO_2 to HCO_3^- that determines the pH; therefore, abnormalities can be compensated for by adding or subtracting on one side of the scale or the other. This is demonstrated in Figure 6-6.

If buffers cannot normalize the pH, compensatory mechanisms are activated. Healthy lungs are able to compensate for acid-base imbalances within minutes by altering the respiratory rate or volume to regulate CO_2 levels. The kidneys have a slower but more sustained response, either retaining or excreting HCO_3^- in response to changes in blood pH. The kidneys are also able to excrete additional H^+ in combination with phosphate and ammonia. Renal compensatory responses are outlined in Table 6-2. In the neonate, compensatory mechanisms may be limited by respiratory disease and the inability of the immature neonatal kidney to conserve HCO_3^-.

DISORDERS OF ACID-BASE BALANCE

Classification and interpretation of blood gas values are based on a set of normal values, such as the ones shown in Table 6-3. Because of immaturity and the presence of fetal hemoglobin, values for the term and preterm infant differ from those of the adult. In addition, the exact values accepted as normal vary from institution to institution and in the literature.[3,6]

The terms applied to acid-base disorders can be a source of confusion. *Acidemia* and *alkalemia* refer to measurements of blood pH; *acidosis* and *alkalosis* refer to underlying pathologic processes.

As previously discussed, a blood pH <7.35 is said to be acidemic; a pH >7.45 is alkalemic. The PCO_2 and HCO_3^- levels, respectively, determine the respiratory and metabolic contributions to the acid-base equation.

During a disturbance of acid-base balance, the body can attempt to return the pH to a normal level in one of two ways:

1. **Correction** occurs when the body alters the component responsible for the abnormality. If CO_2 levels are increased, for example, the body attempts to correct the problem by increasing the excretion of it. The neonate is often unable to correct an acid-base disturbance because of the limitations of immaturity (such as diminished response of chemoreceptors and decreased lung compliance).

TABLE 6-2
Renal Response to Acid-Base Imbalance

Imbalance	Response
Metabolic acidosis	Phosphate and ammonia buffers are used to increase H^+ excretion.
Respiratory acidosis	H^+ excretion and HCO_3^- reabsorption are increased.
Metabolic alkalosis	HCO_3^- reclamation from the urine is decreased. H^+ excretion decreases when serum Na^+ and K^+ are normal. If hyponatremia is present, Na^+ is reabsorbed, requiring H^+ excretion and HCO_3^- retention. If hypokalemia is present, K+ is reabsorbed in place of H^+.
Respiratory alkalosis	H^+ excretion and HCO_3^- reabsorption decrease.

Adapted from: Shapiro BA, Peruzzi WT, and Kozelowski-Templin R. 1994. *Clinical Application of Blood Gases.* Philadelphia: Mosby, 8–9.

TABLE 6-3
Normal Arterial Blood Gas Values

Value	Normal Range
pH	7.35–7.45
$PaCO_2$	35–45 mmHg
PaO_2 term infant	50–70 mmHg
preterm infant	45–65 mmHg
HCO_3^-	22–26 mEq/liter
Base excess	–2 to +2 mEq/liter
O_2 saturation	92–94%

Adapted from: Malley WJ. 2005. *Clinical Blood Gases,* 2nd ed. Philadelphia: Saunders, 4; and Durand DJ, Phillips B, and Boloker J. 2003. Blood gases: Technical aspects and interpretation. In *Assisted Ventilation of the Neonate,* 4th ed., Goldsmith JP, and Karotkin EH, eds. Philadelphia: Saunders, 290. Reprinted by permission.

TABLE 6-4
Causes of Acid-Base Imbalances in Neonates

	↑PaCO$_2$	
Respiratory Acidosis		**Metabolic Alkalosis**
Hypoventilation		Gain of bases
Asphyxia		Bicarbonate administration
Apnea		Acetate administration
Upper airway obstruction		Loss of acids
Decreased lung tissue		Vomiting, gastric suctioning
Respiratory distress syndrome		Diuretic therapy
Pneumothorax		Hypokalemia, hypochloremia
Pulmonary interstitial emphysema		
Ventilation-to-perfusion mismatching		
Meconium aspiration		
Pneumonia		
Pulmonary edema		
Transient tachypnea		
Persistent pulmonary hypertension		
of the newborn		
Cardiac disease		
↓pH ────────────────────────────────		↑pH
Metabolic Acidosis		**Respiratory Alkalosis**
Increased acid formation		Hyperventilation
Hypoxia due to lactic acidosis		Iatrogenic mechanical
Inborn errors of metabolism		hyperventilation
Hyperalimentation		Central nervous system
Loss of bases		response to:
Diarrhea		Hypoxia
Renal tubular acidosis		Maternal heroin addiction
Acetazolamide administration		
	↑PaCO$_2$	

2. **Compensation** occurs when the body normalizes the pH by altering the blood gas component not responsible for the abnormality. If metabolic acidosis is present, for example, the lungs will excrete more CO_2 to normalize the pH. If respiratory acidosis is present, the kidneys will excrete more H^+ and conserve HCO_3^- in an attempt to compensate for the respiratory problem. Compensation is also limited in the neonate because of immaturity.

Respiratory Acidosis

Respiratory acidosis results from the formation of excess H_2CO_3 as a result of increased PCO_2: (↑ PCO_2 → ↑ H_2CO_3 → ↑ H^+ → ↓ pH). Blood gas findings are a low pH, high PCO_2, and normal bicarbonate levels.

Respiratory acidosis is caused by insufficient alveolar ventilation secondary to lung disease. Compensation occurs over three to four days as the kidneys increase the rates of H^+ excretion and HCO_3^- reabsorption. Compensated respiratory acidosis is characterized by a low-normal pH (7.35–7.40), with increased CO_2 and HCO_3^- levels as a result of the kidney retaining HCO_3^- to compensate for elevated CO_2 levels.

Respiratory Alkalosis

Respiratory alkalosis results from alveolar hyperventilation, which leads to a deficiency of H_2CO_3. Blood gas findings are a high pH, low PCO_2, and normal HCO_3^-.

Respiratory alkalosis is caused by hyperventilation, usually iatrogenic.[7] To compensate, the kidneys decrease H^+ secretion by retaining chloride and excreting fewer acid salts. Bicarbonate reabsorption is also decreased. The pH will be high normal (7.40–7.45), with low CO_2 and HCO_3^- levels.

Metabolic Acidosis

Metabolic acidosis results from a deficiency in the concentration of HCO_3^- in extracellular fluid. It also occurs when there is an excess of acids other than H_2CO_3. Blood gas findings are a low pH, low HCO_3^-, and normal PCO_2.

Metabolic acidosis can be caused by any systemic disease that increases acid production or retention or by problems leading to excessive base losses. Examples are hypoxia leading to lactic acid production, renal disease, or loss of bases through diarrhea.[7] If healthy, the lungs will compensate by blowing off additional CO_2 through hyperventilation. If renal disease is not significant, the kidneys will respond by increasing the excretion of acid salts and the reabsorption of HCO_3^-. The pH will be low normal (7.35–7.40), with low levels of CO_2 and HCO_3^- ions.

Metabolic Alkalosis

Metabolic alkalosis results from an excess concentration of HCO_3^- in the extracellular fluid. Blood gas findings are high pH, high HCO_3^- level, and normal PCO_2.

Metabolic alkalosis is caused by problems leading to increased loss of acids, such as severe vomiting, gastric suctioning, or increased retention or intake of bases, such as occurs with excessive administration of sodium bicarbonate. The lungs compensate by retaining CO_2 through hypoventilation. The pH will be high normal (7.40–7.45), with high levels of CO_2 and HCO_3^- ions.

Table 6-4 lists common causes of acid-base disturbances in the neonate.

BLOOD GAS SAMPLING

Blood gas analysis provides the basis for determining the adequacy of alveolar ventilation and perfusion. The accuracy of this test depends a great deal on the skill and knowledge of both the person drawing the sample and the person providing the analysis. It is therefore crucial that those performing and interpreting this test understand appropriate techniques and potential sources of error.

Regardless of the type of sample obtained, attention should be given to the following factors:

1. **Infection control/universal precautions.** All types of blood gas sampling carry the risk of transmission of infection to the infant through the introduction of organisms into the bloodstream. In addition, the potential exposure of the clinician to the infant's blood demands the use of appropriate precautions.

2. **Bleeding disorders.** The potential for bruising and excessive bleeding should be kept in mind, particularly if an arterial puncture is being considered.

3. **Steady state.** Ideally, blood gases should measure the infant's condition in a state of equilibrium. After changing ventilator settings or disturbing the infant, a period of 20–30 minutes should be allowed for arterial blood to reach a steady state.[1] The length of time needed to reach steady state varies from infant to infant.

INTRAPARTUM TESTING

Fetal Scalp Sampling

Scalp blood pH sampling in the fetus has been shown to be a useful tool for evaluating fetal well-being in the presence of suspect fetal heart tracings.[8,9] Values are similar to umbilical cord gases obtained at delivery (Table 6-5). The accuracy of fetal scalp pH is diminished in the presence of scalp edema or caput succedaneum.[10]

A pH value of 7.25 or greater is classified as normal. Values of 7.20–7.25 are borderline and should be repeated in 30 minutes, and those below 7.20 are considered indicative of fetal acidosis.[11] Despite its clinical value, scalp sampling is not widely practiced because it is technically difficult and invasive for both the mother and the fetus.[10]

Serum lactate has been used in research settings as a method of evaluating fetal well-being. The development of hand-held microvolume devices to measure blood lactate levels has made the use of lactate levels a promising alternative to fetal scalp pH testing. A randomized controlled trial comparing fetal scalp pH to fetal lactate levels found no difference in the predictive value of the two tests, but noted that measuring serum lactate provided quicker results and fewer sampling errors than did measuring scalp pH.[12] A more recent randomized controlled trial again found there was no significant difference between lactate and pH analysis in predicting acidemia at birth.[13]

TABLE 6-5
Normal Fetal Blood Gas Values

Value	Umbilical Artery	Umbilical Vein	Fetal Scalp
pH	≥7.20	≥7.25	≥7.25
PCO$_2$ (mmHg)	40–50	≤40	≤50
PO$_2$ (mmHg)	18 ± 2	30 ± 2	≥20
Base excess (mEq/liter)	0 to –10	0 to –5	<–6

From: Martin RW, and McColgin SG. 1990. Evaluation of fetal and neonatal acid-base status. *Obstetrics and Gynecology Clinics of North America* 17(1): 225. Reprinted by permission.

Continuous Intrapartum Fetal Pulse Oximetry

The intermittent nature of fetal scalp sampling combined with the technical difficulties in obtaining accurate specimens has prompted the development of techniques to more continuously monitor fetal well-being. As an adjunct to fetal heart rate monitoring, it is now possible to continuously monitor fetal oxygenation using pulse oximetry. Studies evaluating this technology have largely focused on whether fetal oximetry can clarify the condition of the fetus in the face of a nonreassuring fetal heart rate tracing, potentially reducing the rate of unnecessary cesarean section deliveries.[14]

Cord Blood Gases

Cord blood gases provide an accurate assessment of the fetus's condition at the time of delivery, but do not predict long-term outcomes.[15] Table 6-5 lists normal umbilical cord blood gas values.

Blood from the umbilical artery represents fetal status because this is blood returning from the fetus. Umbilical venous blood provides a measure of placental status. For example, in cases of cord compression, the placenta is functioning normally. Therefore, the venous gas is normal, and the arterial gas reflects a lower pH and increased PCO$_2$. With decreased placental perfusion, the pH in the venous gas drops, as does the arterial pH.[9]

ARTERIAL SAMPLING

Arterial blood can be obtained from the neonate either from an indwelling line or through intermittent sampling of a peripheral artery. The choice of sample site depends on the clinical situation. An indwelling arterial catheter should be placed when it is anticipated that the neonate will require frequent arterial blood sampling. Many criteria are used to determine the need for an indwelling line: These include gestational age, disease process, and the percentage of oxygen required

FIGURE 6-7
Blood gas algorithm.

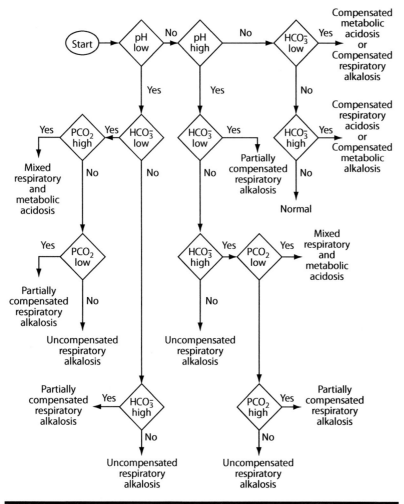

From: Chatburn RL, and Carlo WA. 1988. Assessment of neonatal gas exchange. In *Neonatal Respiratory Care*, Carlo WA, and Chatburn RL, eds. St. Louis: Mosby, 56. Reprinted by permission.

by the neonate. Common sites for neonatal arterial sampling include the following:

1. **Umbilical artery.** The umbilical artery is usually readily accessible for line placement for three to four days and is often usable for up to two weeks after birth.[6] Polyvinyl chloride (PVC) or silastic catheters are available in a variety of sizes, with 3.5 and 5.0 French being the most commonly used. A Cochrane Review of umbilical catheter materials suggests that catheters constructed of silastic material may be less thrombogenic than PVC catheters.[16] The umbilical arterial catheter (UAC) should be positioned either between T6 and T10 or between L3 and L4. The distance for insertion of a high line can be estimated by measuring the distance between the infant's umbilicus and shoulder tip and adding 2 cm. The following formula, based on the infant's birth weight, can also be used:[6]

$$3 \times Weight\ (in\ kg) + 9$$

A meta-analysis examining catheter position found a lower incidence of peripheral vascular complications associated with high line positioning. Recommendations from this review included the exclusive use of the high position for catheter placement.[17] Some caution is warranted, however, given recent studies suggesting that sampling from umbilical arterial lines, especially those in a high position, may result in disruptions in cerebral blood flow and oxygenation.[18,19] Other UAC complications include hemorrhage, ischemic organ damage, infection, and thrombus formation.[6,20,21] UAC placement is unsuccessful in 10–15 percent of infants.[6]

2. **Peripheral arterial lines** (radial, posterior tibial). These peripheral arteries can be accessed at any time beyond delivery with a small-gauge intravascular catheter. Risks for these lines include arteriospasms, tissue necrosis, thrombus formation, infection, and hemorrhage.[21]

3. **Intermittent arterial samples.** Intermittent samples can be obtained from the radial, posterior tibial, or dorsalis pedis arteries. The femoral and brachial arteries are not recommended for sampling because of poor collateral circulation, close proximity of nerves, and the risk of complications such as nerve damage or circulatory impairment.[6,22] See Figure 4-12 for a depiction of the radial site.

4. **Continuous blood gas monitoring.** Technological developments over the past 10–15 years have resulted in the development of devices that allow continuous monitoring of arterial blood gases, usually through an indwelling UAC. Studies evaluating these devices have generally been positive, demonstrating good correlation with intermittently drawn arterial gases.[23–26] Of the values measured, pH, partial pressure of oxygen (PO$_2$), and PCO$_2$. PO$_2$

TABLE 6-6
Compensated Acid-Based Imbalances

Primary Problem	pH	PCO$_2$	HCO$_3$$^-$
Respiratory acidosis	Low normal	High	High
Respiratory alkalosis	High normal	Low	Low
Metabolic acidosis	Low normal	Low	Low
Metabolic alkalosis	High normal	High	High

values were found to be the least accurate, but still within acceptable accuracy limits, in one study.[27]

See Chapter 4 for additional information on blood gas sampling techniques and considerations.

CAPILLARY SAMPLING

Capillary blood can be "arterialized" by warming the skin to increase local blood flow. Samples can then be obtained from the outer aspects of the heel (see Figure 4-13) or from the side of a finger or toe. Transitional events during the first few hours of life and poor perfusion at any time diminish the accuracy of capillary gas measurements. Opinion is mixed as to the reliability of capillary blood gas values as estimators for arterial values. Some studies have found good correlation between arterial and capillary pH and PCO$_2$.[28–32] Others question the validity of capillary PCO$_2$ values and suggest caution when basing treatment decisions on capillary blood gas values.[33] Escalante-Kanashiro and Tantalean-Da-Fieno examined 75 paired arterial and capillary samples and found good correlation between pH (0.85), PCO$_2$ (0.86), and oxygen (0.65). Neither tissue perfusion nor temperature significantly affected correlations, but the presence of hypotension did.[34]

Other research has also demonstrated a poor correlation between PO$_2$ and PaO$_2$.[6,35] Given that finding, treatment decisions are not normally based on capillary PO$_2$ alone.

ERRORS IN BLOOD GAS MEASUREMENT

In examining blood gases, the clinician should be aware of potential sources of error that can affect the quality of the results:[6,36,37]

- **Temperature.** Most blood gas machines report results for 37°C (98.6°F). Hypothermia or hyperthermia can alter true arterial gas values.
- **Hemoglobin.** Calculated oxygen saturations are based on adult hemoglobin, not on fetal or mixed hemoglobins.

- **Dilution.** Heparin in a gas sample lowers the PCO$_2$ and increases the base deficit without altering the pH.
- **Air bubbles.** Room air has a PCO$_2$ close to 0 and a PO$_2$ of 150 mmHg. Therefore, air bubbles in the sample decrease the PaCO$_2$ and increase the PaO$_2$ unless the PaO$_2$ is >150 mmHg.

INTERPRETING BLOOD GASES

The blood gas report contains many pieces of information that must be examined and interpreted. Although oxygenation and acid-base status are interrelated, it is usually easier to consider these separately. The order in which to evaluate these parameters is a matter of personal preference, but it is important to use an organized, step-by-step approach to simplify the process and ensure that nothing is overlooked.

The following steps offer a systematic way of evaluating neonatal blood gases. Figure 6-7 illustrates the first five of these steps and is a useful way of visualizing the decision-making process.

Step 1: Assess the pH. A pH >7.45 is alkalotic, and a pH <7.35 is acidotic. When pH and either PCO$_2$ or HCO$_3$$^-$ are abnormal, the abnormal factor defines the origin of the imbalance. A normal pH should be further evaluated because compensation can normalize the pH while primary acid-base imbalances are present.

Step 2: Assess the respiratory component. A PCO$_2$ >45 mmHg lowers the pH. A PCO$_2$ <35 mmHg raises the pH.

Step 3: Assess the metabolic component. An HCO$_3$$^-$ value <22 mEq/liter lowers the pH. An HCO$_3$$^-$ value >26 mEq/liter raises the pH.

> *Tip:* For primary abnormalities, remember the following:
>
> *Abnormal pH and PCO$_2$ = respiratory alkalosis (PaCO$_2$ <35 mmHg) or acidosis (PaCO$_2$ >45 mmHg)*
>
> *Abnormal pH and HCO$_3$$^-$ = metabolic acidosis (HCO$_3$$^-$ <22 mEq/liter) or alkalosis (HCO$_3$$^-$ >26 mEq/liter)*

Mixed problems: In some cases, abnormalities in both the metabolic and the respiratory systems may be present. This is more common in acidosis than in alkalosis. If both PCO$_2$ and HCO$_3$$^-$ are abnormal, consider the patient's history to determine which problem came first or is more severe.

Step 4: Assess the compensation status. When the pH is abnormal, with one of the acid-base components (PCO_2 or HCO_3^-) being abnormal and the other normal, the gas is said to be uncompensated.[1] When both acid-base parameters are abnormal in opposite directions, the body is beginning to compensate for the primary abnormality. When the pH reaches the normal range, the gas is compensated.

When the pH is normal and respiratory and metabolic parameters are abnormal in opposite directions (e.g., one is acidotic and one alkalotic), it may be unclear which is the primary abnormality. Because the body does not normally compensate beyond the minimum acceptable pH, the pH usually leans in the direction of the primary problem. A pH of <7.4 in a compensated gas would result from a primary acidosis with an alkalotic compensation, and a pH >7.4 would result from a primary alkalosis with an acidotic compensation.[1] Table 6-6 outlines the common findings in compensated gases.

Step 5: Complete the acid-base classification. Add the information from the blood gas analysis to the clinical assessment of the infant's condition and knowledge of the pathophysiology of the infant's disease process to determine a course of action. Remember, a blood gas result that is abnormal on paper may be quite acceptable given the infant's gestational age or disease process. For example, a pH as low as 7.25 may be considered acceptable in a preterm infant. A pH of 7.45 may be desirable if a term infant has persistent pulmonary hypertension of the newborn (PPHN).

Step 6: Evaluate the oxygenation. Three pieces of information are routinely used to determine oxygenation: PaO_2, oxygen saturation, and the presence of cyanosis. The arterial blood gas value provides information about the pulmonary component of oxygenation, specifically the PaO_2.

- **PaO_2.** Normal values for PaO_2 in the term infant are 50–70 mmHg; in the preterm infant, they are 45–65 mmHg (fetal hemoglobin results in higher saturations at lower oxygen levels).[6]

Hypoxia (inadequate tissue oxygen supply) may result from a number of factors, including heart failure, anemia, abnormal hemoglobin affinity for oxygen, and a decreased PaO_2. Hypoxemia (low PaO_2) results from lung disease or cyanotic congenital heart disease.[3] A PaO_2 value <45–50 mmHg is associated with vasoconstriction of pulmonary vasculature and vasodilation of the ductus arteriosus.[38] Low PaO_2 levels are implicated in the etiology of PPHN.

Hyperoxemia (PaO_2 >90–100 mmHg) should also be avoided, especially in the preterm infant, for whom high levels of oxygen in the blood are associated with retinal injury.[38]

Note: When interpreting neonatal PaO_2 values, it may be important to identify whether the sample is preductal or postductal in origin. (See Chapter 2 for a discussion of preductal and postductal gases.)

- **Oxygen saturation.** Although oxygen saturation levels may be reported as part of an arterial blood gas result, they are more commonly obtained from an oximeter. Saturations reported as part of the blood gas result may be measured or calculated from a nomogram. Calculated saturations predict saturation based on the pH and PaO_2 and have limited clinical value.[1]

Measured oxygen saturation is usually a good indicator of reduced arterial oxygen content. Because of the shape of the oxyhemoglobin dissociation curve, saturation is not a good indicator of hyperoxemia or pulmonary deterioration.[1] PaO_2 readings of >100 mmHg occur on the flat upper portion of the curve; therefore, there is little change in oxygen saturation.

Concern regarding the incidence of retinopathy of prematurity (ROP) has prompted recommendations to maintain oxygen saturation at lower levels than those previously accepted. Tin and associates found that infants whose oxygen saturation (SpO_2) levels were maintained at between 70 and 90 percent were four times less likely to develop ROP requiring treatment than those given oxygen to maintain an SpO_2 of 88–98 percent.[39] This is substantiated by the results of a survey of 142 U.S. NICUs that demonstrated that beyond the first two weeks of life, an SpO_2 of <93 percent was associated with a significant decrease in the incidence of Stage 3 or greater ROP and the need for retinal ablation.[40] Chow and colleagues used research data to craft a practice guideline for their institution recommending that oxygen saturation levels be maintained between 85 and 93 percent. Implementation of this policy along with an education program for staff significantly decreased the rate of ROP observed in their NICU.[41]

- **Cyanosis.** Peripheral cyanosis is defined as a blue discoloration of the skin. It may be difficult to assess in dark-skinned infants. Central cyanosis is a blue discoloration of the mucous membranes and is a more reliable indicator of hypoxemia than peripheral cyanosis.

Cyanosis results from an increased amount of uncombined, or desaturated, hemoglobin. It is normally seen when the quantity of desaturated hemoglobin in the capillaries exceeds 5 g/100 mL.[1] This corresponds to a PaO_2 of about 40 mmHg. Because cyanosis depends on the quantity of desaturated hemoglobin, an anemic infant may not look cyanotic despite having a low PO_2, and an infant with polycythemia may appear cyanotic despite adequate oxygenation because of an increase in total hemoglobin.

Step 7: Formulate a plan. By following steps 1–6, the nurse can interpret blood gas values. A plan should then be formulated to accomplish the following:

• **Correct acid-base imbalances.** Correction of acid-base imbalances is achieved, where possible, through treatment of the underlying cause. Treatment suggestions for the four primary acid-base imbalances follow.

• **Respiratory acidosis.** Increase alveolar ventilation to remove CO_2 by applying nasal continuous positive airway pressure (CPAP) or mechanical ventilation. For infants already on mechanical ventilation, increase the tidal volume, rate, peak inspiratory pressure, or positive end-expiratory pressure (PEEP) to facilitate CO_2 removal (see Chapter 7). Sodium bicarbonate is not recommended for treating respiratory acidosis because it reacts with acids to form CO_2.

• **Respiratory alkalosis.** For mechanically ventilated infants, reduce the tidal volume, rate, or pressure on the ventilator.

• **Metabolic acidosis.** Where possible, treat the cause of the acidosis (e.g., correct hypovolemia, decrease the protein load in total parenteral nutrition). If the acidosis is severe, sodium bicarbonate can be administered at a dose of 2 mEq/kg or according to the following formula:

Base deficit × Weight (in kg) × 0.3

The amount of HCO_3^- calculated by this formula should theoretically correct half of the base deficit and should be administered slowly over 30–60 minutes. Fluid replacement may also be of benefit in treating metabolic acidosis by helping the infant metabolize lactic acid.[6]

Note: After fluid replacement, the infant may show a transient deterioration in acid-base status resulting from improved transport of acid from the peripheral to the central circulation.

• **Metabolic alkalosis.** Treat the cause by removing acetate from intravenous fluids, reducing diuretic doses, and replacing lost gastrointestinal secretions. Treat hyponatremia, hypokalemia, and hypochloremia.

• **Correct hypoxemia.** Hypoxemia secondary to ventilation-to-perfusion mismatching can be improved by administering supplemental oxygen. In addition, oxygenation can be improved by increasing the mean airway pressure in an infant on mechanical ventilation. Chapter 7 discusses mean airway pressure.

CASE STUDIES

The following case studies illustrate how the steps for interpreting blood gases might be applied for various infants.

CASE 1

An infant born at 31 weeks gestation is two hours old with the following physical findings: respiratory rate 94 breaths per minute, heart rate 162 beats per minute, temperature 36.5°C (97.7°F), and grunting with moderate retractions.

Capillary blood gas results are as follows:
• pH   7.30
• PCO_2 56 mmHg
• HCO_3^- 26 mEq/liter
• PO_2 40 mmHg

The steps for analysis indicate the following:
1. The pH is low, indicating acidosis.
2. The PCO_2 is high, indicating a respiratory problem.
3. The metabolic component (HCO_3^-) is normal.
4. No compensation is present (pH is not normal).
5. This is uncompensated respiratory acidosis.
6. Oxygenation is adequate.
7. Treatment should be aimed at improving alveolar ventilation. Depending on the infant's clinical status and chest x-ray findings, treatment could consist of nasal CPAP or intermittent positive pressure ventilation.

CASE 2

A 26-week-gestational-age infant is receiving total parenteral nutrition (TPN) with 3.5 g/kg of protein and 15 g/kg of glucose. The infant's urine output is 7 mL/kg/hour, and the baby's weight has dropped 30 g over the past 24 hours. Capillary refill is sluggish.

Capillary blood gas results are as follows:
• pH   7.24

- PCO_2 36 mmHg
- HCO_3^- 15 mEq/liter
- PO_2 50 mmHg

The steps for analysis indicate the following:

1. The pH is low, indicating acidosis.
2. The respiratory component (PCO_2) is normal.
3. The HCO_3^- is low, indicating a metabolic problem.
4. There is no compensation (pH is not normal).
5. This is uncompensated metabolic acidosis.
6. Oxygenation is adequate.
7. Consider giving volume to compensate for hypovolemia and to help metabolize lactic acids, or reduce the amount of protein in the TPN feedings to lower the metabolic acid load.

Case 3

A 28-week-gestational-age infant is on mechanical ventilation for respiratory distress syndrome. Settings are a rate of 40 breaths per minute, tidal volume of 5 mL/kg, PEEP +4, and fractional concentration of oxygen in inspired gas (FiO_2) 0.50.

Arterial blood gas results are as follows:

- pH   7.48
- $PaCO_2$ 27 mmHg
- HCO_3^- 22 mEq/liter
- PaO_2 95 mmHg

The steps for analysis indicate the following:

1. The pH is high and shows an alkalemia.
2. The PCO_2 is low, indicating respiratory alkalosis.
3. The metabolic component (HCO_3^-) is normal.
4. There is no compensation (pH is not normal).
5. This is uncompensated respiratory alkalosis.
6. The PO_2 is too high.
7. Reduce alveolar ventilation. Assess the infant's chest expansion and spontaneous respirations to determine whether the tidal volume or the ventilator rate should be lowered. Reduce the FiO_2, ensuring that the oxygen saturation remains within the desired range.

Case 4

A three-week-old infant underwent bowel surgery three days ago. On continuous gastric suction, the infant is receiving TPN with sodium and potassium acetate.

Capillary blood gas results are as follows:

- pH   7.51
- PCO_2 43 mmHg
- HCO_3^- 34 mEq/liter
- PO_2 52 mmHg

The steps for analysis indicate the following:

1. The pH is high, showing an alkalemia.

2. The respiratory component (PCO_2) is high normal.
3. The HCO_3^- is high, leading to metabolic alkalosis.
4. There is no compensation.
5. This is uncompensated metabolic alkalosis.
6. The PO_2 is adequate.
7. Consider eliminating the acetate in the TPN in favor of chloride salts. Ensure that the serum sodium and potassium are adequate.

Case 5

An infant born at 26 weeks gestational age is now three weeks old and receiving mechanical ventilation for chronic lung disease. The infant is on full nasogastric feedings.

Capillary blood gas results are as follows:

- pH   7.37
- PCO_2 49 mmHg
- HCO_3^- 34 mEq/liter
- PO_2 52 mmHg

The steps for analysis indicate the following:

1. The pH is normal.
2. The PCO_2 is high, suggesting respiratory acidosis.
3. The HCO_3^- is high, suggesting a metabolic alkalosis.
4. The pH is normal with abnormal CO_2 and HCO_3^-; therefore, there is compensation. The pH is low normal; therefore, it is compensated acidosis. The high HCO_3^- does not fit with acidosis, but the high PCO_2 does.
5. This is compensated respiratory acidosis that fits with the clinical history of chronic lung disease.
6. Oxygen levels are satisfactory.
7. This infant's kidneys have become efficient at conserving HCO_3^- and excreting H^+, so treatment is not necessary. Keep in mind that further changes in the infant's condition (atelectasis, pneumonia, or metabolic causes of acidosis) will likely exceed the infant's ability to compensate and result in acidosis.

Case 6

A term infant, with Apgar scores of 4 at one minute and 6 at five minutes and born through thick meconium, is pale, with retractions and grunting respirations. Temperature is 35.8°C (96.4°F).

Capillary blood gas results are as follows:

- pH   7.25
- PCO_2 49 mmHg
- HCO_3^- 16 mEq/liter
- PO_2 35 mmHg

The steps for analysis indicate the following:

1. The pH is low, indicating an acidosis.

2. The PCO_2 is high, suggesting a respiratory acidosis.

3. The HCO_3^- is low, suggesting a metabolic acidosis.

4. No compensation is present.

5. This is a mixed respiratory and metabolic acidosis that is uncompensated.

6. The PO_2 is low.

7. Warm the infant slowly. Improve the alveolar ventilation, and provide supplemental oxygen. Do not administer HCO_3^- unless ventilation is improved.

Summary

Interpretation of a blood gas requires a systematic approach based on an understanding of the physiology of gas transport and acid-base balance. Such an approach permits timely and appropriate interventions aimed at providing optimal care for the compromised infant.

References

1. Malley WJ. 2005. *Clinical Blood Gases: Assessment and Intervention, 2nd ed.* Philadelphia: Saunders.

2. Delivoria-Papadopoulos M, and McGowan JE. 2004. Oxygen transport and delivery. In *Fetal and Neonatal Physiology*, Polin RA, Fox WW, and Abman SH, eds. Philadelphia: Saunders, 880–889.

3. Parry WH, and Zimmer J. 2006. Acid-base homeostasis and oxygenation. In *Handbook of Neonatal Intensive Care, 6th* ed., Merenstein GB, and Gardner SL, eds. Philadelphia: Mosby, 210–222.

4. Bradshaw WT, Turner BS, and Pierce JR. 2006. Physiologic monitoring. In *Handbook of Neonatal Intensive Care, 6th* ed., Merenstein GB, and Gardner SL, eds. Philadelphia: Mosby, 117: 139–156.

5. Heuther S. 2001. The cellular environment: Fluids and electrolytes, acids and bases. In *Pathophysiology: The Biologic Basis for Disease in Adults and Children*, 4th ed., McCance KL, and Heuther SE, eds. Philadelphia: Mosby, 102–111.

6. Durand DJ, Phillips BL, and Boloker J. 2003. Blood gases: Technical aspects and interpretation. In *Assisted Ventilation of the Neonate*, 4th ed., Goldsmith JP, and Karotkin EH, eds. Philadelphia: Saunders, 279–292.

7. Davis ID, and Avner ED. 2001. Fluid, electrolytes and acid-base homeostasis. In *Neonatal-Perinatal Medicine*, 7th ed., Fanaroff AV, and Martin RJ, eds. Philadelphia: Mosby, 619–634.

8. Morgan BL, et al. 2002. Correlation between fetal scalp blood samples and intravascular blood pH, pO_2 and oxygen saturation measurements. *Journal of Maternal-Fetal and Neonatal Medicine* 11(5): 325–328.

9. Martin RW, and McColgin SG. 1990. Evaluation of fetal and neonatal acid-base status. *Obstetrics and Gynecology Clinics of North America* 17(1): 223–233.

10. Greene KR. 1999. Scalp blood gas analysis. *Obstetrics and Gynecology Clinics of North America* 26(4): 641–656.

11. Clark SL, and Miller FC. 1984. Scalp blood sampling—FHR patterns tell you when to do it. *Contemporary OB/GYN* 23: 47.

12. Westgren M, et al. 1998. Lactate compared with pH analysis at fetal scalp blood sampling: A prospective randomised study. *British Journal of Obstetrics and Gynaecology* 105(1): 29–33.

13. Wiberg-Itzel E, et al. 2008. Determination of pH or lactate in fetal scalp blood in management of intrapartum fetal distress: Randomised controlled multicentre trial. *BMJ* 336(7656): 1284–1287.

14. McNamara HM, and Dildy GA 3rd. 1999. Continuous intrapartum pH, pO_2, pCO_2, and SpO_2 monitoring. *Obstetrics and Gynecology Clinics of North America* 26(4): 671–693.

15. Aarnoudse YG, Yspeert-Gerards J, and Huisjes HJ. 1985. Neurological follow-up in infants with severe acidemia. Abstract No 297. Presented at Society for Gynecologic Investigation, Phoenix, Arizona, March. Cited in Martin RW, and McColgin SG. 1990. Evaluation of fetal and neonatal acid-base status. *Obstetrics and Gynecology Clinics of North America* 17(1): 223–233.

16. Barrington KJ. 2000 Umbilical artery catheters in the newborn: Effects of catheter materials (Cochrane Review). In *The Cochrane Library* Issue 2, Oxford Update Software.

17. Barrington KJ. 2002. Umbilical artery catheters in the newborn: Effects of position of the catheter tip. *The Cochrane Database of Systematic Reviews* (2): CD000505.

18. Lott JW, Connor GK, and Phillips JB. 1996. Umbilical artery catheter blood sampling alters cerebral blood flow velocity in preterm infants. *Journal of Perinatology* 16(5): 341–345.

19. Roll C, et al. 2000. Umbilical artery catheter blood sampling decreases cerebral blood volume and oxygenation in very low birthweight infants. *Acta Paediatrica* 89(7): 862–866.

20. Rodriguez RJ, Martin RJ, and Fanaroff AA. 2001. Respiratory distress syndrome and its management. In *Neonatal-Perinatal Medicine: Diseases of the Fetus and Infant*, 7th ed., Fanaroff AV, and Martin RJ, eds. Philadelphia: Mosby, 1001–1011.

21. Gomella T, et al. 2004. *Neonatology: Management, Procedures, On-Call Problems, Diseases and Drugs*, 5th ed. New York: Appleton and Lange, 166.

22. Pape KE, Armstrong DL, and Fitzhardinge PM. 1978. Peripheral median nerve damage secondary to brachial arterial blood gas sampling. *Journal of Pediatrics* 93(5): 852–856.

23. Morgan C, et al. 1999. Continuous neonatal blood gas monitoring using a multiparameter intra-arterial sensor. *Archives of Disease in Childhood, Fetal and Neonatal Edition* 80(2): F93-F98.

24. Widness JA, et al. 2000. Clinical performance of an in-line point-of-care monitor in neonates. *Pediatrics* 106(3): 497–504.

25. Rais-Bahrami, et al. 2002. Continuous blood gas monitoring using an in-dwelling optode method: Comparison to intermittent arterial blood gas sampling in ECMO patients. *Journal of Perinatology* 22(6): 472–474.

26. Meyers PA, et al. 2002. Clinical validation of a continuous intravascular neonatal blood gas sensor introduced through an umbilical artery catheter. *Respiratory Care* 47(6): 682–687.

27. Ganter M, and Zollinger A. 2003. Continuous intravascular blood gas monitoring: Development, current techniques, and clinical use of a commercial device. *British Journal of Anaesthesia* 91(3): 397–407.

28. Gandy G, et al. 1964. The validity of pH and PCO_2 measurements in capillary samples of sick and healthy newborn infants. *Pediatrics* 34: 192–197.

29. Bannister A. 1969. Comparison of arterial and arterialized capillary blood in infants with respiratory distress. *Archives of Disease in Childhood* 44(238): 726–728.

30. Harrison AM, et al. 1997. Comparison of simultaneously obtained arterial and capillary blood gases in pediatric intensive care unit patients. *Critical Care Medicine* 25(11): 1904–1908.

31. Kirubakaran C, Gnananayagam JE, and Sundaravalli EK. 2003. Comparison of blood gas values in arterial and venous blood. *Indian Journal of Pediatrics* 70(10): 781–785.

32. Yildizdas D, et al. 2004. Correlation of simultaneously obtained capillary, venous, and arterial blood gases of patients in a paediatric intensive care unit. *Archives of Disease in Childhood* 89(2): 176–180.

33. Courtney SE, et al. 1990. Capillary blood gases in the neonate: A reassessment and review of the literature. *American Journal of Diseases of Children* 144(2): 168–172.

34. Escalante-Kanashiro R, and Tantalean-Da-Fieno J. 2000. Capillary blood gases in a pediatric intensive care unit. *Critical Care Medicine* 28(1): 224–226.

35. American Association for Respiratory Care. 1994. AARC clinical practice guideline: Capillary blood gas sampling for neonatal and pediatric medicine. *Respiratory Care* 39(12): 1180–1183.

36. Fan LL, et al. 1980. Potential errors in neonatal blood gas measurements. *Journal of Pediatrics* 97(4): 650–652.

37. Gayed AM, Marino ME, and Dolanski EA. 1992. Comparison of the effects of dry and liquid heparin on neonatal arterial blood gases. *American Journal of Perinatology* 9(3): 159–161.

38. Hay WW Jr, Thilo E, and Curlander JB. 1991. Pulse oximetry in neonatal medicine. *Clinics in Perinatology* 18(3): 441–472.

39. Tin W, et al. 2001. Pulse oximetry, severe retinopathy, and outcome at one year in babies of less than 28 weeks gestation. *Archives of Disease in Childhood. Fetal and Neonatal Edition* 84(2): F106–F110.

40. Anderson CG, Benitz WE, and Madan A. 2004. Retinopathy of prematurity and pulse oximetry: A national survey of recent practices. *Journal of Perinatology* 24(3): 164–168.

41. Chow LC, et al. 2003. Can changes in clinical practice decrease the incidence of severe retinopathy of prematurity in very low birth weight infants? *Pediatrics* 111(2): 339–345.

NOTES

7 Principles of Mechanical Ventilation

Thomas R. Harris, MD
Debbie Fraser, MN, RNC-NIC

The use of mechanical ventilation to treat newborns with respiratory distress dates back almost 60 years, with the eventual predominant method consisting of continuous flow, time-cycled, pressure-limited, intermittent mandatory ventilation.[1,2] Over the years, mechanical ventilators have changed significantly; however, the fundamental principles underlying ventilation remain unchanged. The use of mechanical ventilation has markedly improved the survival and outcomes of both premature and ill term neonates. Survival among these infants has further improved with the introduction of adjunct therapies such as surfactant replacement, inhaled nitric oxide, and antenatal steroids. Despite these improvements, concern remains over the potential harmful effects of both the pressure and the volume generated by mechanical ventilation.

Effective mechanical ventilation of the neonate requires up-to-date knowledge and a working understanding of certain basics, including (1) key concepts of pulmonary physiology and flow mechanics; (2) select laws that govern gas pressure, flow, and volume; (3) equations that define relationships between elements of pulmonary function or components of gas laws; (4) the predominant pathophysiologic mechanisms involved in neonatal respiratory diseases, the natural or expected courses of these diseases, and the pathophysiology of their associated complications; (5) the capabilities, advantages, and potential disadvantages of the different modes of mechanical ventilation and of the machines that deliver them; and (6) the specific effects of altering various ventilator control settings on cardiopulmonary function in general and on gas exchange (as reflected in blood gas values) in particular.

Safe and effective mechanical ventilation of the neonate also requires the formulation of rational treatment strategies based on physiologic principles and close monitoring of their implementation to detect early deviations from the expected results. Caregivers must be constantly aware of the potential for complications, especially in infants at high risk for them. Such anticipation allows for proactive initiation of preventive and/or ameliorative measures.

This chapter discusses the history and language of mechanical ventilation in the neonate. It deals with the application of positive pressure mechanical ventilation in the form of intermittent mandatory ventilation (IMV) at conventional and rapid rates to neonates in respiratory failure. From time to time, comparisons are made with the newer modes of mechanical ventilation, including patient-triggered and high-frequency ventilation; however, these subjects receive extensive coverage in Chapters 9 and 12, respectively. Brief commentary is given on the rather subjective indications for mechanical ventilation, followed by delineation of the essential characteristics of IMV and the differences among pressure-cycled, volume-cycled, and time-cycled infant ventilators capable of delivering IMV. A conceptual framework is offered for a working understanding of the basic components of the positive pressure being delivered and how the different ventilator control settings can be rationally manipulated to influence an infant's level of ventilation and oxygenation as reflected in blood gas values (see also Chapter 6).

Examples are given of how key physiologic principles can be applied on a practical level to a wide range of clinical situations when using IMV to support infants. Ways in which the gas laws and the Laplace relationship apply when providing IMV support to infants under special circumstances are also addressed. The most common neonatal lung diseases and their associated complications (described in detail in Chapters 2 and 10, respectively) that lead to respiratory failure and subsequent need for mechanical ventilation are categorized into three major groups based on their predominant pathophysiology. Finally, generally accepted ventilator strategies are outlined for the safe and effective application of IMV, at conventional or rapid rates, for each of these three categories of lung disease, and reasons for setting ventilator-control variables within one specific range rather than another are provided. Embedded within and throughout this chapter are two philosophic principles already alluded to. The first is the importance of an anticipatory, preventive medicine approach to mechanical ventilation of the neonate. The second is the necessity of making all changes with moderation to avoid bouncing from one extreme to the other—and thus inadvertently thwarting homeostasis.

HISTORICAL PERSPECTIVE

Donald and Lord first described the use of patient-controlled ventilation for newborns in 1953.[3] At that time, use of mechanical ventilation was reserved for treating moribund patients with intractable respiratory failure because success was limited (less than 10 percent survived) and the procedure was technically difficult.[4–7] In 1962, several centers began providing ventilation to newborns with respiratory insufficiency. Reports of these early attempts at ventilation stimulated further debate about the efficacy of this treatment.[8,9] In the milieu of health care in the 1960s, the use of mechanical ventilation was not an accepted method of treatment for infants with respiratory distress syndrome (RDS) despite the early success of Donald and Lord and the promising results of Thomas and coworkers.[3,4] The first neonatal randomized trials of mechanical ventilation took place in the late 1960s.[10–12] Two of the first three trials involved the use of a negative-pressure, body-enclosing respirator.[11,12] The other trial examined the more conventional form of ventilation using endotracheal intubation.[10] The years 1970 and 1971 were watershed ones for mechanical ventilation of the newborn. Kirby and colleagues described IMV; Smith, Daily, and associates published their series "Mechanical Ventilation of Newborn Infants" in *Anesthesiology*; and Gregory and coworkers reported their data on continuous positive airway pressure (CPAP).[5–7,13,14]

Further studies by Reynolds refined the approach to neonatal mechanical ventilation by suggesting that prolonged inspiratory time and lower peak inspiratory pressure (PIP) would improve oxygenation and decrease the likelihood of sequelae.[15–17] Mannino and colleagues showed improved survival with fewer sequelae in infants treated with early mechanical ventilation without prior application of CPAP, compared with infants receiving conventional management of RDS, which at that time consisted of hood oxygen and CPAP.[18] The criteria for initiating mechanical ventilation changed. The use of CPAP as an initial treatment for severe RDS and meconium aspiration syndrome leading to respiratory failure gave way to use of IMV for initial therapy in many centers.[19,20]

CRITERIA FOR MECHANICAL VENTILATION

The main purpose of attaching any baby in respiratory failure to a mechanical ventilator is to reduce his work of breathing while overcoming alveolar atelectasis and achieving adequate pulmonary gas exchange.[1] The ventilator supplies the mechanical, or bellows, function of the diaphragm and other (intercostal and accessory) muscles that normally generate the force to move gas into and out of the lungs. It is now recognized that these goals must be achieved using minimal pressure, volume, and flow while avoiding atelectasis.[1] The association of mechanical ventilation with complications such as air leaks, chronic lung disease, and respiratory infections has made the avoidance of prolonged intubation imperative.[21]

There remains considerable debate among neonatal clinicians over what constitutes respiratory failure and, consequently, over criteria for intubation and placement of an infant on mechanical ventilation. These disagreements are understandable given the fact that application of a noninvasive form of distending airway pressure such as nasal CPAP may not only improve the level of oxygenation in a baby with RDS, but also actually reduce his or her work of breathing. The reason is that CPAP slows the baby's spontaneous respiratory rate as well as the rate of gas flow during inspiration and expiration, thereby reducing his need to generate large and rapid intrapleural pressure swings to achieve adequate airflow and gas exchange. If all that was needed was to better oxygenate an infant who was not yet tiring of the work of breathing or who was not experiencing intractable apnea, it would be preferable to initiate a noninvasive form of CPAP rather than mechanical ventilation.

The decision to intubate and ventilate a neonate is based on a number of factors, including gestational age, underlying pathophysiology, chest x-ray, clinical findings, and blood gas results. Indications for endotracheal intubation and mechanical ventilation have not been uniformly defined and, over time, have become less clear. General criteria include:[22]

- A rising PCO_2 with pH falling below 7.25
- Severe hypoxemia (PaO_2 <50 mmHg) (No consensus has been reached on the level of inspired O_2 the infant requires that would dictate the need for the initiation of mechanical ventilation.)
- Severe apnea

More recently, clinicians, in a move toward providing gentle ventilation[23] and in recognition of heightened concern over the toxic effects of oxygen free radicals,[24] have suggested modifying these criteria by lowering the minimally acceptable pH to 7.20[25] before resorting to intubation and mechanical ventilation in cases of early RDS. Respiratory acidosis severe enough to lower pH below 7.20 or 7.15 due to partial pressures of carbon dioxide in arterial blood ($PaCO_2$s) in the 60–80 mmHg range represents a valid indicator for intubating and placing the infant on mechanical ventilation. However, if a portion of the acidosis is metabolic in nature, with a base excess of –4 or –5 mEq/liter and the $PaCO_2$ still below 55 mmHg (indicating a mixed acidosis rather than strictly a respiratory acidosis), the cautious clinician is probably justified in undertaking a trial of nasal CPAP rather than going directly to intubation and mechanical ventilation.

COMPONENTS OF CONVENTIONAL MECHANICAL VENTILATION

All mechanical ventilators are basically force generators capable of producing a pressure gradient between the airway opening and the alveoli, allowing gas to flow down that gradient into the lungs, while at the same time improving gas distribution in relation to pulmonary blood flow.[26] Infant ventilators have other capabilities, of course, such as delivering adjustable concentrations of enriched oxygen and a constant, minimal amount of distending airway pressure, or positive end-expiratory pressure (PEEP). But it is the mechanical ventilator's generation of variously configured waveforms of pressure, or applied force, over time and its ability to thereby

deliver adjustable volumes of gas per unit time that make mechanical ventilators unique when contrasted with CPAP or extracorporeal membrane oxygenation (see Chapter 13). This unique capability of force generation is essential, even life saving, in providing acute respiratory support to neonates suffering from any form of respiratory distress that compromises their ability to ventilate the lungs.

IMV, as the name implies, provides intermittent mandatory positive pressure breaths superimposed on a continuous flow of gas through the ventilator circuit. Prior to development of the Baby Bird ventilator in the early 1970s (conceived by Robert Kirby, an anesthesiologist, with the clinical expertise of Robert deLemos, a neonatologist, but assembled into a workable machine by Jimmy Schultz, a respiratory therapist using components from a Bird Mark V ventilator), any infant on intermittent positive-pressure ventilation (IPPV) who attempted to breathe out of phase with the inspiratory flow cycle of the machine ended up rebreathing exhaled stale gas.[14] With IMV, the constant flow through the circuit provides fresh gas at all times for the infant to breathe; it also provides background CPAP using a flow or threshold resistor, impeding circuit outflow. When the expiratory limb of the circuit is closed completely and then reopened in a repetitive, precisely timed fashion, a predetermined amount of mechanical ventilation is provided to combine with the baby's own spontaneous breathing. Another advantage of IMV comes with weaning, when the number of mandatory breaths provided by the machine can be gradually decreased while allowing the baby's spontaneous breathing to increase.

POSITIVE PRESSURE VENTILATOR CLASSIFICATIONS

Positive pressure ventilators are most commonly classified according to their method of terminating inspiration and thus are divided into pressure-cycled, volume-cycled, and time-cycled machines.[27–30] Newer ventilators have been introduced that can function as either volume-controlled or pressure-controlled, time-cycled ventilators (Babylog [Dräger Medical Inc., Lübeck, Germany], VIP Bird [Cardinal Health, Dublin, Ohio]). Microprocessors have also been developed that allow ongoing modifications in pressure, flow, and volume throughout the respiratory cycle, making modes such as proportional assist ventilation and respiratory muscle loading possible.[31]

- **Pressure-cycled ventilators** deliver a volume of gas until a preset pressure is reached within the ventilator circuit or patient interface (also lending this type

FIGURE 7-1
Typical pressure waveform generated by a conventional ventilator in IMV mode during a complete respiratory cycle or mandatory breath, superimposed on PEEP, or background CPAP.

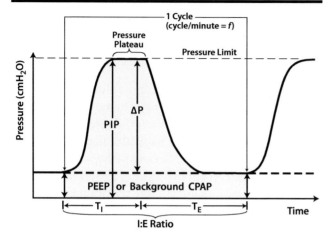

Key: CPAP = continuous positive airway pressure; PEEP = postiive end-expiratory pressure; PIP = peak inspiratory pressure; ΔP = airway pressure gradient; T_I = inspiratory time; T_E = expiratory time
Mean airway pressure is the solid blue area under the curve.

of machine the name *pressure-preset ventilator*). The delivered volume from the machine is determined by the rate of internal gas flow (a control setting) and the duration of inspiration. Although the peak pressure delivered to the infant remains constant, the actual volume of gas delivered to the alveoli is variable, depending on: (1) the compliance of the ventilator circuit, including the humidifier; (2) the compliance of the infant's lungs; (3) the resistance to gas flow through the circuit, endotracheal (ET) tube, and the infant's airways; and (4) the presence or absence of air leakage around the ET tube.[10] Thus, the volume of gas delivered to the patient on inspiration may vary tremendously from breath to breath. In cases of sudden decreases in lung compliance (e.g., development of a pneumothorax) or increases in upper airway resistance (e.g., mucus plugging), preset cycling pressure will be reached prematurely, shutting off inspiration and shortening "time-of-flow" to the point of causing ineffective alveolar ventilation (even though the infant is receiving "controlled" mechanical ventilation).

- **Volume-cycled ventilators** deliver a constant tidal volume of gas from the machine into the patient circuit during the inspiratory phase, regardless of the pressure generated, unless pressure limits are set. Inspiration is terminated when a preset volume has been delivered, lending this type of machine the name *volume-preset ventilator*. The relative distribution of that volume into the circuit, humidification apparatus, and patient tubing versus the volume actually delivered to the patient's alveoli depends on the relative compliance and resistance of the circuit versus that of the infant's upper airway and lungs. In cases of nonhomogeneous lung disease, portions of the lung that are obstructed or atelectatic require higher opening pressure. With volume preset ventilators, most of the volume reaching the lung is preferentially delivered to areas of the lung that are open, resulting in an increased potential for overdistention. Furthermore, because the preset volume is delivered into the patient circuit irrespective of the pressure it takes to deliver it, the first place a sizable portion of the inspiratory gas flow may escape is out of a leak around the ET tube (i.e., taking the path of least resistance).

- **Time-cycled ventilators** utilize electronic timers to terminate the machine's inspiratory phase. Time-cycled ventilators may be pressure limited; but unlike with pressure-cycled machines, gas flow to the patient does not cease when the preset pressure is reached. Rather, flow tapers off to hold the preset peak pressure steady (forming a pressure plateau, as shown in Figure 7-1, at the preset peak pressure and pressure limit). Any excess flow, which otherwise would drive pressure over the preset limit, is simply vented from the circuit. The volume actually delivered to the patient by time-cycled machines depends again on compliance and resistance factors, as well as on the chosen inspiratory time, gas flow rate, and preset pressure limit.[30] Actual volume delivered to the infant's lungs using time-cycled ventilators has been shown to be more consistant than that provided by pressure-cycled ventilators, and the performance of time-cycled machines is comparable to that of volume-cycled machines in this regard.[28]

Knowing how the various types of infant ventilators apply pressure and deliver volume, and especially understanding how the machine(s) you employ perform these tasks, is the first step toward applying safe and effective mechanical ventilation in IMV mode (or any other ventilation mode) to newborn infants. The second step is gaining a working knowledge of the various components of the positive pressure force an infant ventilator delivers and learning how to adjust these ventilator control settings (variables) to allow additional gas flow per unit time in support of the infant's own spontaneous breathing and achievement of adequate gas exchange.

Managing Mechanical Ventilation

A graph displaying how the pressure waveform generated during a mandatory breath is altered when ventilator settings are adjusted in one direction or the other provides a useful visual reference to help clinicians keep all the components and variables straight. Figure 7-1 depicts a typical pressure waveform generated by a conventional ventilator in IMV mode during a complete respiratory cycle or mandatory breath, superimposed on background CPAP, or PEEP. The discussion that follows individually addresses the pressure components (PIP and PEEP), time intervals (inspiratory and expiratory time [T_I and T_E]), timing derivative (inspiratory:expiratory [I:E] ratio), airway pressure gradient (ΔP), and pressure composite (mean airway pressure [Paw]), all of which are graphically illustrated in Figure 7-1.

Peak Inspiratory Pressure

Peak inspiratory pressure PIP is the maximum level of pressure generated during the inspiratory phase of the ventilator cycle, signified graphically as the apex of the pressure waveform shown in Figure 7-1. The higher the PIP setting on a time-cycled, pressure-limited ventilator, the more gas delivered to the patient (all other determining factors being equal). The difference between PIP and PEEP, known as the airway pressure gradient (ΔP), is the primary determinant of the tidal volume delivered by a pressure-limited ventilator.[31]

To select an appropriate PIP, the clinician must consider the infant's gestational age, weight, lung compliance and resistance, and the type and severity of the disease process. The safest PIP setting is the lowest level needed to achieve adequate ventilation. When treating respiratory failure caused by RDS, initial PIP settings may range between 18 and 24 cmH_2O. Opening or reopening areas of collapsed lung requires PIP levels that exceed the lung unit's critical opening pressure. However, when PIP levels approach 25 cmH_2O on conventional or rapid-rate IMV, it is time to consider switching to a high-frequency mode of ventilation (see Chapter 12).

Positive End-Expiratory Pressure or Background CPAP

PEEP is the residual positive pressure remaining in the patient circuit at the end of expiration, even when there is no flow in the circuit between positive pressure breaths during intermittent IPPV. When dealing with IMV, however, PEEP is better conceived as *background CPAP*.[32] That is because the same continuous flow of fresh gas through the circuit that distinguishes IMV from IPPV also produces the back pressure against which the baby exhales, just as when an infant is attached to any CPAP apparatus and is breathing spontaneously. The pneumatic-splinting effect of background CPAP (or PEEP) during IMV prevents collapse of alveoli at end expiration (discussed later in this chapter in the section on the Laplace relationship).

As is the case for PIP, the selection of an appropriate PEEP depends on the size of the patient and the underlying disease process. Although PEEP contributes greatly to the maintenance of normal lung volume, it is probably not reasonable to assume it contributes much to lung volume recruitment.[33] The levels of background CPAP commonly used during IMV (i.e., 4–6 cmH_2O) are well below the critical opening pressure of most atelectatic alveoli, although partially collapsed units may respond to noninvasive CPAP if it is applied relatively early in the course of RDS.

T_I, T_E, AND I:E RATIO

T_I (or I-time), T_E (or E-time), and I:E ratio are fairly self-explanatory control variables. They do require attention, however, because they may be set differently on different infant ventilators and because either T_I or I:E ratio must be repeatedly adjusted as the ventilator rate is changed. When using a time-cycled machine, the T_I is selected along with the rate, and the combination of these two variables automatically determines the T_E and the I:E ratio. The usual setting range for T_I is 0.3–0.5 second, for T_E, 0.6–1.2 seconds, and for I:E ratio, 1:2–1:3. Both slow-rate, long T_I (or reverse I:E ratio) IMV and rapid-rate, short T_I IMV (sometimes called high-frequency mechanical ventilation or high-frequency positive pressure ventilation) have been used as alternative modes for treatment of RDS because both allow PIP (thought to be the major culprit in producing barotrauma and subsequent bronchopulmonary dysplasia) to be reduced.[17,34,35] However, if not administered with extreme precision and timing, especially in the recovery phase of RDS, both modalities can result in problems with insufficient time for exhalation. Without enough time to exhale, air trapping,

FIGURE 7-2
Effects of low versus high ventilator flow rates on pressure waveforms.

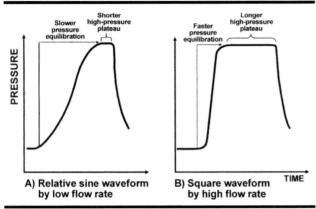

Adapted from: Spitzer AR, and Clark RH. 2011. Positive-pressure ventilation in the treatment of neonatal lung disease. In *Assisted Ventilation of the Neonate*, 5th ed., Goldsmith JP, and Karotkin EH, eds. Philadelphia: Saunders, 167. Reprinted by permission.

inadvertent PEEP, lung overexpansion, volutrauma, air leak, diminished pulmonary capillary blood flow with increased intrapulmonary shunting, reduced venous return and cardiac output, and increased risk for intraventricular hemorrhage can occur.[36] This unfortunate sequence is discussed further later in this chapter under the headings **Mean Airway Pressure, Controlling Blood Gases during IMV, Compliance,** and **Time Constants.**

Airway Pressure Gradient

The airway pressure gradient is the difference between PIP and PEEP (i.e., PIP – PEEP = ΔP) and represents the pressure gradient between the machine and the patient's lower airway or the gradient down which all air flows to the patient's lungs during inspiration. If there is no difference in pressure between the outside air (i.e., the patient circuit if the infant is on a ventilator) and the alveoli, the result is no airflow. ΔP represents the main motor for bulk flow ventilation of the type generated by conventional mechanical ventilation. ΔP exactly parallels pulse pressure in blood pressure measurements: Pulse pressure is the difference between systolic and diastolic blood pressures and largely determines stroke volume. Just as stroke volume multiplied by heart rate yields cardiac output, so ΔP multiplied by ventilator rate approximates alveolar ventilation. That is because the inspiratory volume delivered by the machine roughly equals tidal volume (V_T), and V_T minus dead-space volume multiplied by breathing rate determines minute volume, or alveolar ventilation. The contribution of ΔP

to alveolar ventilation becomes even more important during high-frequency ventilation, where V_T is exponentially related to minute ventilation or CO_2 excretion per unit time (see Chapter 12).

Mean Airway Pressure

Mean airway pressure (or Paw) defines the mean pressure delivered to the proximal airways from the beginning of one inspiration to the beginning of the next, averaged over a series of respiratory cycles. Paw is determined by calculating the area beneath the pressure curves of both inspiration and expiration and then dividing that area by its appropriate time interval.[37] Paw is represented diagrammatically by the total area beneath the pressure waveform (see Figure 7-1) and is monitored electronically by integration of repeated airway pressure measurements made multiple times per second throughout a number of cycles. Thus, Paw is the composite measure of all pressures transmitted to the airways by a mechanical ventilator.[38] Paw is not a variable that can be set on a conventional ventilator. Rather, it is determined by the PIP, PEEP, I:E ratio, and flow.

The ideal Paw can be defined, but only for the individual patient, given the fact that results are largely dependent on the type and severity of the disease process being treated.[37] The less compliant or stiffer the lungs, the higher the level of Paw the patient can tolerate without adverse cardiovascular effects. This is true because lungs with low compliance allow less transmission of airway pressure to the capillary bed on the outside walls of the alveoli and to the interstitial, interpleural, or intrathoracic spaces. Finding the optimal Paw is similar to finding optimal PEEP when treating adults with IPPV.[39] In both cases, the clinician seeks out the maximum level of PEEP or Paw that yields improving values for lung mechanics (e.g., lung compliance) and gas exchange (e.g., PaO_2, $PaCO_2$) without causing significant deterioration in measured cardiovascular parameters (such as central venous pressure and/or cardiac output). Paw is the major determinant of oxygenation when applying all modalities of mechanical ventilation (including IMV) to most forms of neonatal lung disease. Paw levels above 11–12 cmH_2O while on IMV are generally considered an indication to switch to a high-frequency mode of ventilation where higher levels of Paw can be more safely applied.

Flow Rate

In most ventilators capable of delivering IMV, flow rate is the rate of continuous gas flow through the patient circuit and also what determines inspiratory flow rate during mandatory breaths. Flow rate determines the ability of the ventilator to deliver the set PIP, I:E ratio, and respiratory rate.[31] Flow rates may be categorized as either low flow (0.5–3 liters/minute) or high flow (4–10 liters/minute or more).[29] When IMV is being applied to infants, the circuit flow rate is usually set somewhere between 4 and 10 liters/minute.[29] The minimal acceptable flow rate is considered to be at least two times an infant's minute ventilation, or two times 210 mL/kg/minute.[40] With a low flow rate (Figure 7-2A), it takes longer to reach pressure equilibration at the set PIP. If the flow rate is too low relative to minute ventilation, dead space ventilation and CO_2 levels increase because effective airway opening pressure is not being adequately maintained.[29] At the other extreme, flow rates as high as 10 to 12 liters/minute find use in delivering high levels of PIP, in producing a waveform resembling a square wave (Figure 7-2B), when reversing the I:E ratio, or when delivering high-pressure, rapid-rate IMV. In these cases, the high inspiratory flow rate allows for quick delivery of the volume needed to reach the preset PIP (i.e., quick equilibration of PIP between the circuit and the baby's alveoli). Be aware, however, that forcing high-pressure gas into noncompliant lungs is a setup for barotrauma, overdistention of the more compliant terminal gas-exchange units (i.e., the respiratory bronchioles and alveolar ducts), and volutrauma in premature babies with RDS. Slower flow rates generate less turbulence and a waveform that more resembles a sine wave (Figure 7-2A), thereby better mimicking the normal infant respiratory pattern and providing a smoother, gentler increase in pressure during inspiration.[28]

VENTILATOR RATE OR FREQUENCY

Ventilator rate, or frequency, refers to the number of breaths delivered per minute by the ventilator during IMV (the baby's spontaneous breaths are not included). Along with inspiratory volume (or V_T if one subtracts anatomic dead space), ventilator rate is a primary determinant of alveolar ventilation during conventional mechanical ventilation. IMV can be classified as slow rate (<40 breaths per minute), medium rate (40–60 breaths per minute), and rapid rate (>60 breaths per minute).[29] As a rapid-rate IMV range is reached or exceeded, during use of a conventional ventilator, the following changes can be anticipated in the pressures generated, volumes delivered, and other ventilator-control variables:[41,42]

1. Paw increases.

2. If the ventilator rate is increased markedly while the I:E ratio is kept constant, the preset PIP may not be reached because the marked increase in ventilator rate may shorten T_I to the point at which it is insufficient to permit achieving the preset PIP level.

3. If T_I is left unchanged, the I:E ratio will be reversed because T_E will become progressively shorter. Eventually, this will prevent complete emptying of the last breath delivered before the next mandatory breath comes in.

4. Once the rate exceeds 25–30 breaths per minute when using most conventional ventilators, inspiratory volume delivered to the circuit (and therefore V_T) will progressively decrease.

5. Minute volume (and therefore alveolar ventilation) will continue to increase, but only up to a rate of about 75 breaths per minute. At higher rates, both minute volume delivered and the patient's alveolar ventilation actually fall off. Thus, rate increases beyond 75 breaths per minute are counterproductive when using conventional ventilators at unconventional rates.

CONTROLLING BLOOD GASES DURING IMV

TO CONTROL VENTILATION: ADJUSTING A CONVENTIONAL VENTILATOR

In its strictest definition, ventilation is synonymous with CO_2 excretion, or the process of blowing off carbon dioxide. Clinically, the degree of CO_2 excretion is reflected in $PaCO_2$ arterial blood gas values. While IMV is being applied, alveolar ventilation is roughly the product of V_T multiplied by cycling frequency ($V_T \times$ rate). Tidal volume, in turn, is determined largely by the ΔP down which gas flows from the machine to the most distal airways, or the difference between PIP and PEEP. Thus, the two main ways to control the $PaCO_2$ on a conventional ventilator are to make changes in (1) ΔP and (2) ventilator rate. Only through their impact on ΔP do any of the other ventilator control variables alter $PaCO_2$ levels or the degree of alveolar ventilation. The following examples should make this clear:

- Increasing the preset PIP level increases ventilation and lowers $PaCO_2$, but only because any increase in PIP widens the pressure difference (increases ΔP).
- Decreasing PIP has the opposite effect—narrowing the difference between PIP and PEEP and thus reducing ventilation and increasing $PaCO_2$ (reduces ΔP).

FIGURE 7-3
Compliance and its relationship to initial level of lung expansion.

A, B, and C are pressure-volume loops representing single breaths taken or ventilator cycles delivered when the starting level of lung expansion was low, normal, and high, respectively.

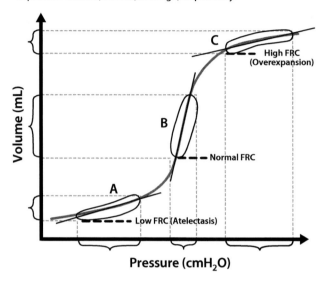

Key: FRC = funtional residual capacity

Adapted from: Keszler M, and Abubakar MK. 2011. Physiologic principles. In *Assisted Ventilation of the Neonate,* 5th ed., Goldsmith JP, and Karotkin EH, eds. Philadelphia: Saunders, 22. Reprinted by permission.

- Increasing PEEP while administering IMV has a negative impact on ventilation because increasing PEEP reduces ΔP.
- In contrast, a drop in the level of PEEP increases ΔP, thereby increasing ventilation and lowering $PaCO_2$.
- Increasing both PIP and PEEP settings by the same amount while administering IMV has no influence on ventilation (although it has a great deal of influence on the level of oxygenation, as seen below) because ΔP is not changed in the process.
- Decreasing both PIP and PEEP settings by the same amount should likewise have no effect on ventilation because ΔP is not changed in the process. However, the resulting sudden fall in Paw may lead to rapid loss of lung volume, negatively affecting both oxygenation and ventilation by reducing the surface area available for gas exchange.

Clinical Pearls
- If PIP is raised so high that it causes overexpansion of a significant number of already inflated alveoli, the result is hyperinflation rather than hyperventilation, and $PaCO_2$ goes up rather than down. Hyperinflation places the infant near the top on the flat portion of the

compliance curve (Figure 7-3C) where large pressure changes produce little or no volume change.
- Hyperventilation also has its risks if taken to the extreme. In the past, moderately aggressive hyperventilation has proved useful in the treatment of persistent pulmonary hypertension of the newborn (PPHN).[43] In this approach, $PaCO_2$ levels are intentionally lowered, resulting in an improved level of oxygenation. Once hypoxemia is overcome, the vicious cycle (depicted in Chapter 2, Figure 2-6 summarizing the pathogenesis of PPHN) is broken and the pulmonary vasoconstriction reversed. However, if $PaCO_2$ drops precipitously and excessively (to <18 mmHg) due to overaggressive use of rapid-rate IMV or high-frequence ventilation, the infant will experience a rapid fall in blood pressure and a significant reduction in cerebral blood flow to a degree capable of producing cerebral ischemia and/or infarction, periventricular leukomalacia, and subsequent cerebral palsy.[44,45]
- If background CPAP (or PEEP) is lowered to such a degree that airway pressure at end expiration falls below the closing pressure of a significant number of lung units, then $PaCO_2$ will begin to rise due to subsequent gas trapping behind collapsed proximal airways.[29]
- Normally, changes in the I:E ratio have no noticeable effect on the level of ventilation. However, if the I:E ratio is excessively reversed (i.e., if the T_I is set so that it is considerably longer than the T_E), the T_E may not permit complete emptying of expiratory volume, thereby causing gas trapping and reduction in alveolar ventilation.
- At the other extreme, if the T_I is shortened much below 0.25 second when applying rapid-rate IMV, it is quite likely, even in early, severe RDS, that there will be insufficient time for full pressure equilibration, preventing the preset PIP from being reached. This means that the full tidal-volume breath will not be delivered and that alveolar ventilation will subsequently decrease (see also the section on TIME CONSTANTS later in this chapter). In summary, then, CO_2 retention is likely to occur at both extremes of I:E ratio settings!
- Increasing the ventilator rate much above 60 breaths per minute with a conventional ventilator accomplishes little or no further increase in alveolar ventilation.[40,41] Increasing the circuit flow rate and increasing the preset level of PIP may provide some help in this regard. However, by making such

compensatory setting changes, the clinician delivers more of a square-wave inspiratory waveform and applies higher levels of distending airway pressure. This defeats the original purpose of switching to rapid-rate IMV—namely, to reduce the risk of barotrauma and eventual bronchopulmonary dysplasia (BPD).[34]

From a design standpoint, the underlying problem the clinician faces when attempting to apply high-frequency ventilation with a conventional IMV machine is that a large percentage of the inspiratory volume delivered is invariably lost in the relatively compliant circuit and large-volume humidifier chamber found on most conventional ventilators.[41] Keeping the humidifier filled to the brim may help a little, but the hard reality remains: These machines were not designed to be run at high-frequency rates.

To Control Oxygenation: Adjusting a Conventional Ventilator

It has become abundantly clear through the groundbreaking studies of Herman and Reynolds in London and Boros and coworkers in St. Paul, Minnesota, that when ventilating premature infants with IMV for respiratory failure caused by RDS, Paw is the major determinant of oxygenation.[17,37,38,46] The same holds true in most cases when applying all of the newer mechanical ventilation modalities, including high-frequency jet ventilation (HFJV) and high-frequency oscillatory ventilation (HFOV), to patients with RDS or other forms of diffuse, homogeneous lung disease.

There are essentially five different ways to increase Paw (Figure 7-4). These five approaches correspond to five control variables, or settings, found on most infant ventilators. To increase Paw:
1. Increase the inspiratory flow rate.
2. Raise PIP.
3. Reverse the I:E ratio (i.e., prolong the T_I while shortening the T_E).
4. Increase PEEP or background CPAP.
5. Increase the ventilator rate or cycling frequency.

Although Paw can be increased in any of these five ways, it would be a mistake to conclude that it doesn't really matter which of the five ventilator control variables one uses alone or in combination to increase Paw and thereby improve oxygenation. For one thing, the different ventilator setting changes that affect increases in Paw produce different degrees of PaO_2 increases per unit of Paw increase (or $\Delta PaO_2/\Delta Paw$).[36]

FIGURE 7-4
Five ventilator adjustments that can increase Paw.

1. Speed up inspiratory flow rate (i.e., circuit flow)
2. Increase PIP
3. Reverse the I:E ratio or prolong T_I
4. Increase PEEP
5. Increase ventilator rate or cycling frequency

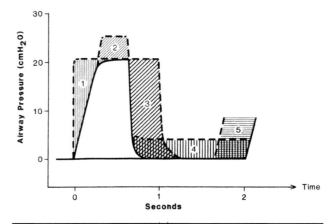

Adapted from: Reynolds EOR. 1974. Pressure waveform and ventilator settings for mechanical ventilation in severe hyaline membrane disease. *International Anesthesiology Clinics* 12(4): 259. Reprinted by permission.

For example, when treating newborns with RDS, for the same change in Paw produced by increases in PEEP or PIP, you get three times or two and a half times more rise in PaO_2, respectively, than if you raise Paw by lengthening the T_I. The explanation for these differences in efficiency at improving oxygenation among the control variables rests with their physiologic or pathophysiologic effects, which affect oxygenation by mechanisms other than increases in Paw. For example, in one study of RDS patients, increasing Paw by increasing the T_I quite likely resulted in overdistention of a significant number of normal lung units, triggering intrapulmonary right-to-left shunting and venous admixture, which then blunted the overall increase in PaO_2.[36]

A second reason it really matters which one of several available options the clinician chooses to use to raise Paw is that specific ventilator setting changes that increase Paw are also powerful means of achieving other desirable goals besides improving oxygenation—goals related to degree of ventilation and avoidance of complications. The following examples should make this clear:

• Raising PEEP to increase Paw also reduces ΔP and, in turn, the degree of alveolar ventilation, as explained previously. If a strategy of permissive hypercapnia is already being used, it may not be desirable to let

$PaCO_2$ rise any higher than it already is in the patient at this point.

Conversely, raising PIP to increase Paw and improve both oxygenation and ventilation brings with it substantial risks, especially if the preset PIP is held high in the pressure plateau by way of a prolonged T_I (see Figure 7-1). Instead of just recruiting collapsed lung units, raising PIP could further expand (or overexpand) lung units that are already open. If the predominant outcome is overexpansion, that increases the risk for pulmonary complications such as air leaks, barotrauma, volutrauma, and eventual BPD, as well as the risk for cardiovascular complications such as obstructed venous return to the heart, elevated cerebral venous pressure, reduced cerebral blood flow, and the potential for both intraventricular hemorrage and hemorrhagic cerebral infarction.[44,45]

- Although reversing the I:E ratio by extending the T_I also raises Paw, remember that the associated shortening of the T_E may result in gas trapping—unless, of course, the rate is reduced concurrently.

Which ventilator control variable(s) the clinician elects to increase or prolong to improve oxygenation by increasing Paw depends on what else she wishes to accomplish or avoid, given the patient's underlying condition, status, and level of support. Sometimes, when faced with two concurrent types of pathophysiology or two conflicting objectives, there is no clear choice. In such situations, focus on the parameter furthest from the norm, and change the setting that will best move that parameter back in the desired direction toward the middle ground and homeostasis. If the clinical situation allows some leeway, consider first reducing the most damaging factor(s) being applied, such as very high PIP with prolonged T_I or high FiO_2. That approach reduces the risk of the treatment causing acute or long-term complications.

In certain situations, further increases in Paw may have a paradoxic or negative effect on oxygenation.[46,47] Such is the case, for example, when treating premature infants with severe RDS complicated by pulmonary interstitial emphysema (PIE). At this point, the lungs are already overexpanded (although most of the air is in the wrong places). Further increases in PIP and/or Paw only make matters worse by perpetuating the air leak and further reducing pulmonary blood flow. In this difficult situation, a switch to HFJV, which allows for lower PIP while still providing adequate ventilation, reduction in the amount of ongoing air leak, and lower distal mean airway pressures may be indicated.[48-50]

Clinical Pearls

- Raising the level of PEEP to increase Paw loses its effectiveness in improving oxygenation once moderately high levels of PEEP (5–6 cmH_2O) have been reached. Further increases in PEEP beyond this point do not predictably alter oxygenation and may, in fact, lower rather than raise its level.[46]

- As is the case with high levels of PIP, very high levels of Paw may cause a series of adverse consequences, including (1) overinflation of already well-ventilated lung units; (2) compression of the pulmonary capillaries coursing through the intra-alveolar septa, thereby impeding capillary blood flow and diverting blood through the extra-alveolar vessels that now act as right-to-left shunts (contributing to venous admixture); (3) reduction of venous blood return to the heart; and (4) reduction of cardiac output and oxygen delivery to the tissues.[51]

KEY CONCEPTS OF PULMONARY MECHANICS AND THEIR CLINICAL APPLICATIONS

This section addresses key concepts of pulmonary mechanics and explains how to apply them in clinical practice. See also Chapter 1 and citation material for in-depth reviews of the topics that follow.[29,40,47,52,53]

COMPLIANCE

Understanding Compliance

Compliance describes the property of elasticity or distensibility of a material or structure or the ease with which it can be stretched. When determining lung compliance (C_L), or how easy it is to stretch the lung, consider that this is a structure that has volume. To increase the volume of the lung (to stretch the lung), pressure over time (force) is applied to the structure. C_L is measured by inflating the lungs in a series of step changes in volume and recording the pressure required to hold open the lungs at each volume step. Mathematically, compliance is expressed as unit change in volume per unit change in pressure, or:

$$Compliance\ (liters/cmH_2O) = \frac{\Delta Volume\ (liters)}{\Delta Pressure\ (cmH_2O)}$$

The step-wise measurements for determining C_L described above are made under static conditions, meaning that there is no movement of air into or out of the lungs when the lungs are being held at each ramp up in volume for successive measurements of pressure (see also Chapter 5). The purpose here is to measure just the elastic properties of the lung while eliminating the component of pressure-force required to overcome airway resistance (discussed below) during lung inflation. When limited to describing just the elastic properties (or elastance) of the lungs, compliance becomes an expression of the elastic recoil force of the lungs. Mathematically speaking, compliance can also be defined as the reciprocal of elastic recoil or:

Compliance = 1/Elastic Recoil

As Figure 7-3 shows, total compliance of the respiratory system (i.e., lung compliance plus chest wall compliance) expressed graphically describes an S-shaped curve. If ventilating at a low level of lung expansion to begin with, as represented by pressure-volume loop A in Figure 7-3, a substantial increase in pressure produces little increase in volume. Thus, the slope (represented by the straight line through the loop) of that portion of the compliance curve is relatively flat, meaning that compliance is low. In the midportion of the compliance curve, where tidal volume breathing normally takes place, pressure-volume loop B reflects a large volume increase resulting from a very small pressure increase. In this situation, the slope of the compliance curve is steep, almost vertical, so compliance is high. At the high end of the compliance curve approaching total lung capacity, a tidal volume breath (loop C) results in little additional lung volume despite a marked increase in pressure difference. Again, the slope of that portion of the compliance curve is relatively flat, meaning that compliance is low. Thus, it should be clear from the overall *S* shape of the compliance curve in Figure 7-3 that compliance is reduced in any condition associated with either low or excessively high lung volume.

Turning this concept around, changes or local differences in lung compliance represent the major determinants of overall lung volume and the distribution of volume, respectively. By adding the factor of time to the equation, we can say that changes or local differences in lung compliance largely determine the degree of ventilation and distribution of ventilation, respectively (when the mode of delivery is by bulk flow convection, as is generally the case during conventional mechanical ventilation).

Clinical Applications of the Compliance Concept

Examples illustrating application of the compliance concept in clinical practice follow:

- Because chest wall compliance is essentially a non-factor in the neonate because of the softness of the infant's thoracic cage, and because the major factor determining lung compliance is alveolar surface tension, the infant with primary surfactant deficiency or RDS will experience a radical reduction in alveolar surface tension and a rise in respiratory system compliance when exogenous surfactant is instilled into the lungs. The rapid rise in compliance that accompanies surfactant instillation means that the previously high peak pressures applied by a conventional ventilator will now deliver considerably larger tidal volumes than before treatment. Thus, shortly after instilling the surfactant, the caregiver will need to reduce high levels of distending airway pressure, if used, to avoid overinflation of the lungs. Major improvement may come in a matter of minutes, not hours, requiring immediate reductions in FiO_2, PIP, and ventilator rate (in that order).

- Now picture what might happen if most of the prescribed exogenous surfactant bolus was instilled down the right main stem bronchus rather than uniformly throughout the bronchial tree. Obviously, compliance would improve more on the right than on the left, increasing the likelihood of unequal distribution of ventilation. In a worst-case scenario, subsequent tidal volume breaths might soon be delivered almost entirely into the right lung, overexpanding it and increasing the risk for a right-sided air leak and eventual reduction in right lung ventilation. Reduced ventilation could result either from extrinsic restriction secondary to a right-sided tension pneumothorax or simply from ongoing hyperinflation of that right lung, driving it up onto the flat portion of the compliance curve (see Figure 7-3C). Either way, the right lung compliance would eventually drop to a level comparable to that on the left, self-correcting the original problem of iatrogenic ventilation inequality. But in the process, the infant would undoubtedly pay a very high price.

AIRWAY RESISTANCE

Understanding Airway Resistance

Resistance is the result of friction between moving parts. In relation to breathing, there are two main types of resistance. *Tissue*, or *viscous, resistance* is frictional

FIGURE 7-5
Resistance to airflow through a single-tube delivery system under two flow conditions: laminar and turbulent.

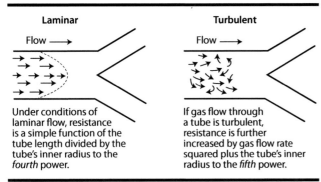

Laminar	Turbulent
Flow ⟶	Flow ⟶
Under conditions of laminar flow, resistance is a simple function of the tube length divided by the tube's inner radius to the *fourth* power.	If gas flow through a tube is turbulent, resistance is further increased by gas flow rate squared plus the tube's inner radius to the *fifth* power.

Adapted from: Widdicombe J, and Davies A. 1983. Lung ventilation. In *Respiratory Physiology*. London: Hodder Arnold, 46. Reprinted by permission.

resistance generated by tissue elements moving past one another within the lungs and thorax as their shape is altered. *Airway,* or *flow, resistance* is frictional resistance to fast-flowing molecules of gas bumping against the inner walls of the nasal passages, trachea, bronchi, and bronchioles. Together, airway and lung tissue resistance make up *total pulmonary resistance.*

Resistance to airflow is an inherent property of the lungs. It is expressed mathematically as the change in pressure per unit change in flow, or:

$$\frac{Resistance}{(cmH_2O/liter/second)} = \frac{\Delta Pressure\ (cmH_2O)}{\Delta Flow\ (liters/second)}$$

In contrast to compliance, resistance is dynamic rather than static. Resistance exists only when things are moving for a period of time. To overcome airway resistance and achieve gas flow, additional pressure, beyond that required simply to stretch the elastic elements of the lung and chest wall, must be applied over time. In contrast to changes in compliance, increases or decreases in resistance will affect the rate of lung inflation (i.e., the time it takes to achieve a certain percentage of tidal volume delivery), but will not alter the ultimate lung volume. That assumes, of course, that there is an adequate inspiratory time for full tidal volume delivery.

A number of factors determine resistance to flow through a single-tube system including (1) the flow rate, or velocity, of the airflow; (2) the viscosity and density of the gas breathed (not a significant factor when breathing various mixtures of air and oxygen); (3) the length of the conducting airway or tube; and (4) the inner diameter (or radius) of the airway or tube. The radius of the tube is by far the most important determinant of airway

resistance in a single-tube system (such as through an ET tube; see discussion in the **Clinical Applications of the Airway Resistance Concept** section that follows).

Likewise, in a multitube system such as the human bronchial tree, the radii of all the various tubes (more accurately quantified as the total cross-sectional area of the airways) at each level of the lung is the most important determinant of airway resistance. Airway resistance drops off exponentially when measured at deeper and deeper levels within the lung because total cross-sectional area of all the airways increases exponentially when moving from proximal to distal levels of the lung. Thus, airway resistance and total cross-sectional area are mirror images of each other, with the highest resistance occurring within the distal trachea and segmental bronchi where cross-sectional area is the least, and lowest resistance occurring within the terminal bronchioles and alveolar ducts where total cross-sectional area is greatest.

Also important in determining airway resistance is whether the flow is laminar (streaming smoothly) or turbulent (swirling irregularly) (Figure 7-5). As illustrated, laminar flow is characterized by gas molecules moving in organized layers that run parallel to the axis of the airway. The individual layers move with increasing velocity the closer they are to the center of the airway because the moving gas molecules are less and less likely to bump into the airway wall. The changing velocities of laminar flow layers across the diameter of the airway are called *velocity profiles,* which form a "cone-" or "spike-shaped" front. Turbulent flow, in contrast, lacks organization of the moving molecules, and the front is roughly square in shape. Under normal breathing conditions, turbulent flow exists in the trachea and large proximal bronchi, whereas laminar flow predominates in the smaller, more distal bronchioli and alveolar ducts.

Clinical Applications of the Airway Resistance Concept

Examples illustrating practical application of the airway resistance concept in clinical practice follow.

• During spontaneous breathing, inspiratory airway resistance is less than expiratory resistance because the airways widen during inspiration (due to the surrounding, slightly negative intrathoracic pressure caused by descent of the diaphragm and lifting of the ribs), whereas the airways narrow during exhalation (due to the switchover to positive intrathoracic pressure during exhalation). This explains the ball-valve mechanism that leads to the gas trapping seen in infants who have aspirated particulate matter such as meconium. Gas trapping occurs behind bronchi that are only partially occluded with meconium because air can get by the obstruction during inspiration as the airways dilate, but is blocked from escaping during expiration when they narrow. Once on mechanical ventilation, moderately high PEEP or background CPAP levels can keep the bronchi dilated even during exhalation and actually help alleviate gas trapping.

- For an infant on a ventilator, it is essential also to consider resistance to the flow of gas through the circuit and its interface, namely, the ET tube and its adapter. As early as 1968, Cave and Fletcher pointed out that turbulent flow is produced in standard 2.5 mm inside diameter (ID) ET tubes whenever flow rate exceeds 3 liters/minute and in 3 mm ID ET tubes whenever flow rate exceeds 7.5 liters/minute. Any increase in flow rate above these critical levels produces disproportionately large increases in airway resistance. For example, when employing a small (2.5 mm ID) ET tube, increasing the circuit flow rate from 5 to 10 liters/minute raises airway resistance from 32 to 84 cmH$_2$O/liter/second, more than two and one-half times its original value.[54] These data obviously have major implications when it comes to mechanical ventilation of tiny premature infants requiring small ET tubes and when a choice of low, medium, or high flow rate (as defined earlier in the section) must be made. It is not always a simple choice, however, because high inspiratory flow rates are generally needed when delivering high PIPs and/ or supporting seriously ill infants with rapid-rate IMV.

The effect of local differences in airway resistance on distribution of ventilation and speed of gas delivery to individual lung segments is clearly illustrated in Figure 7-6. Although compliance of the two segments shown is the same (i.e., $c_1 = c_2$), airway resistance to the segment on your left is greater than to the segment on your right (i.e., $r_1 > r_2$) because of partial airway occlusion from particulate matter of the one segment. In addition, because flow preferentially takes the path of least resistance, considerably more flow is delivered to the unobstructed segment. Furthermore, flow delivery is slower to the partially obstructed segment because it has the longer time constant (i.e., $r_1c_1 > r_2c_2$; see also **Time Constants** later in this section).

FIGURE 7-6
Partial airway occlusion and its effect on airway resistance, distribution of ventilation, time constants, and thus speed of tidal volume delivery and degree of inflation.

Variable airway resistance caused by mucus secretions or meconium aspiration may lead to unequal distribution of ventilation and different degrees of local inflation.

Two schematic clusters of alveoli in an infant with uneven airway obstruction. The speed of equalization of proximal airway and alveolar pressures during inspiration (and expiration) depends on the time constant, which is the product of resistance (*r*) and compliance (*c*). Unobstructed alveoli can be preferentially ventilated by applying a short inspiratory cycle at a comparatively high peak airway pressure.

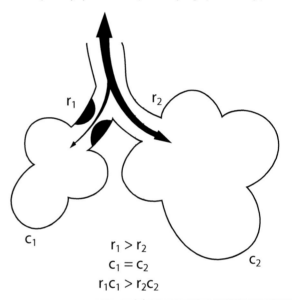

From: Reynolds O. 1979. Ventilator therapy. In *Neonatal Pulmonary Care*, Thibeault DW, and Gregory GA, eds. Reading, Massachusetts: Addison-Wesley, 233. Reprinted by permission.

ELASTIC RECOIL

Understanding Elastic Recoil

Elastic recoil refers to the natural tendency of stretched objects to return, or recoil, to their original unstretched, or resting, state or volume. During the expiratory phase of breathing, when the inspiratory muscles in the diaphragm and intercostal spaces relax, the elastic elements in the tissues of the chest wall, abdominal wall, and lungs that were stretched during inspiration are free to recoil to their original length (Figure 7-7). Surface tension at the gas-liquid interfaces of the alveoli also contributes to the collapsing force during exhalation. If left unopposed, expiratory elastic recoil plus surface-tension forces would reduce lung volume well below resting volume, or functional residual capacity (FRC), resulting in a severe drop in lung compliance and a marked increase in the work of breathing (WOB).

FIGURE 7-7
Elastic recoil during the expiratory phase of breathing.

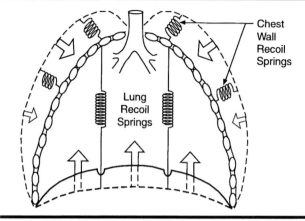

From: Keszler M, and Abubakar MK. 2011. Physiologic principles. In *Assisted Ventilation of the Neonate*, 5th ed., Goldsmith JP, and Karotkin EH, eds. Philadelphia: Saunders, 23. Reprinted by permission.

Fortunately, other elastic recoil forces within the chest wall work to prevent further collapse. Once lung volume drops below FRC, elastic elements within the chest cage begin to resist being stretched in the opposite direction, providing a recoil force that works to reexpand the lungs (which are coupled to the chest wall through the parietal and visceral pleural surfaces). One can witness this balancing of elastic recoil forces during surgery if the chest is opened while the patient is temporarily disconnected from the anesthesia machine providing positive pressure: The lungs collapse and the ribs literally spring outward.

When present in sufficient quantity, surfactant also helps to balance lung-collapsing and chest-expanding forces at the FRC level by reducing surface tension by more than 50 percent at rest volume level. Furthermore, surfactant resists compression to lung volumes below FRC level by acting to lower surface tension to near zero, further ensuring alveolar stability, even during forced exhalation.[40] Premature infants are in double jeopardy when it comes to achieving a balance between the elastic recoil forces tending toward collapse and those resisting further collapse because they often suffer from primary surfactant deficiency or RDS and, as a result of immaturity, invariably have nonrigid chest cages prone to collapsing (as evidenced by substernal and intercostal retractions during labored breathing).

Clinical Applications of the Elastic Recoil Concept

Examples illustrating practical clinical applications of the elastic recoil concept follow.

- Since 1971, and even after the availability of artificial surfactant, the primary mode of treating RDS has been the application of distending airway pressure as a means of providing a so-called pneumatic splint that literally props open the alveoli from inside through the entire respiratory cycle.[5] This distending pressure has been delivered as PEEP during IPPV; as CPAP via ET tube, tight-fitting face mask, or nasal prongs; and as background CPAP during IMV. Figure 7-8 shows how distending airway pressure works to stabilize small and/or surfactant-deficient alveoli.

- Because elastic recoil provides the force or pressure gradient over time down which exhaled gas flows, it is rightfully considered the internal force generator, or "motor," of passive exhalation. When describing the function of most conventional infant ventilators, the term *passive* implies that the machine is only passively involved during the expiratory phase of the respiratory cycle, relying on the elastic recoil of the baby's own lungs and chest cage to provide the force for exhalation. Only the SensorMedics 3100A high-frequency oscillator (Viasys Healthcare, Conshohocken, Pennsylvania) employs an *active* exhalation, whereby the oscillating diaphragm forcefully displaces gas within the circuit away from the patient. The vacuum created as gas is pulled away from the patient during active exhalation may produce choke points in the proximal airways when the intra-airway pressure drops below the closing pressure of the proximal airways. This, in turn, can result in gas trapping and significant risk for lung overexpansion. To overcome this potential problem while ventilating with this high-frequency oscillator, the clinician must consistently use higher Paw levels than with other modes of mechanical ventilation to ensure that proximal airways stay open during active exhalation.[50]

TIME CONSTANTS

Understanding Time Constants

Time constants are a measure of how long it takes the lungs to fill with a tidal volume breath during inspiration (inspiratory time constant) or to empty that breath during expiration (expiratory time constant). Stated another way, time constants measure how long it takes during inspiration for the pressure gradient between the proximal airway and the alveoli to equilibrate or, during expiration, for the alveolar and patient-circuit pressure difference to equilibrate. When the pressures equilibrate,

FIGURE 7-8
The Laplace relationship and its influence on preterm infants' elastic recoil and functional residual capacities.

Diagrammatic illustration of the Laplace relationship and the effects of surfactant film (**A**) and alveolar radius (**B**) on wall or surface tension. The degree (reflected in the size of the *open arrows*) of airway or intra-alveolar pressure (P) needed to counteract the tendency of alveoli to collapse (represented by the *solid arrows*) is directly proportional to double the wall or surface tension (ST) and inversely proportional to the size of the radius (r). Distending airway pressure applied during assisted ventilation can be likened to a "pneumatic splint."

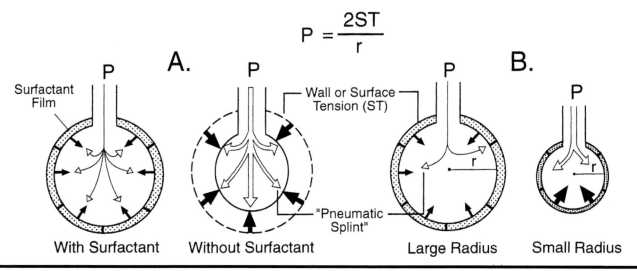

From: Keszler M, and Abubakar MK. 2011. Physiologic principles. In *Assisted Ventilation of the Neonate*, 5th ed., Goldsmith JP, and Karotkin EH, eds. Philadelphia: Saunders, 23. Reprinted by permission.

ΔP becomes zero, and flow ceases. At this point, the full tidal volume has been delivered.

Because the time necessary for the lungs to fill or empty depends primarily on the resistance and compliance of the respiratory system, time constants are mathematically represented as the product of the two. Thus:

Time Constant *(seconds)* = **Resistance** *(cmH₂O/liter/second)* × **Compliance** *(liters/cmH₂O)*

One inspiratory time constant of the respiratory system, by convention, is a measure of the time in seconds necessary for the alveolar pressure to reach 63 percent of the total change in pressure (ΔP, or PIP minus PEEP) delivered by the machine. For example, in an infant with normal airway resistance and normal lung compliance, one time constant is approximately 0.15 second.[55] Infants with RDS who have markedly decreased compliance (approximately one-sixth of normal) have a much shorter time constant, measured to be around 0.02 second.[52] As you can see from the time constant curves in Figure 7-9A, three time constants achieve 95 percent, four achieve 98 percent, and five achieve 99 percent equilibration. Furthermore, knowing the exact volume the ventilator delivers at the particular PIP and PEEP settings chosen plus having the results of online pulmonary function tests (see Chapter 5) that measured the baby's lung compliance and airway resistance permit calculation of the percentage of volume delivered during each successive time constant (Figure 7-9B). The exact same rules that govern ΔP equilibration also apply to step changes in volume, and so the percentages of volume delivered during each successive time constant are identical to the percentages of equilibration.

Patients receiving mechanical ventilation are at risk for incomplete tidal volume delivery and/or incomplete emptying of previously inspired volume whenever the lung condition for which they are being ventilated involves increased airway resistance without comparable reduction in lung compliance or whenever there is a mismatch between the inspiratory or expiratory time constants and the T_I or T_E settings on the ventilator.

Clinical Applications of the Time Constants Concept

Examples illustrating some practical clinical applications of the time constants concept follow.

- Consider, for example, the inspiratory time constant of an infant with moderate meconium aspiration syndrome (MAS). Assume that, because of increased airway resistance, his or her time constants are double those of a healthy infant. Accepting again that the normal infant's inspiratory time constant is 0.15 second,[55] the baby with MAS would have an

FIGURE 7-9
Inspiratory time constants curves.

Inspiratory time constants measure how long it takes during inspiration for the pressure gradient between the proximal airway and the alveoli to equilibrate (**A**), or how long it takes to deliver increasing percentages (**B**).

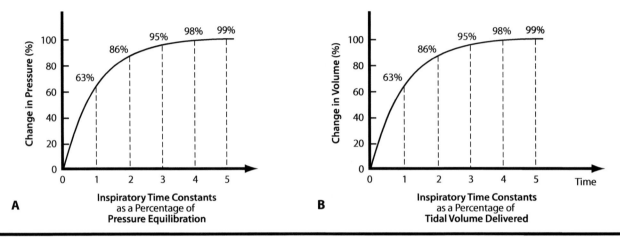

A Inspiratory Time Constants as a Percentage of Pressure Equilibration

B Inspiratory Time Constants as a Percentage of Tidal Volume Delivered

Adapted from: Carlo WA, and Martin RJ. 1986. Principles of neonatal assisted ventilation. *Pediatric Clinics of North America* 33(1): 221. Reprinted by permission.

inspiratory time constant of 0.30 second. To get 99 percent equilibration of a ΔP that we will further assume to be 25 cmH_2O (reflecting typical IMV ventilator settings of 30/5), it would be necessary to set the inspiratory time at 1.5 seconds (equals five time constants) to achieve the goal of 99 percent pressure equilibration (Figure 7-9A) and, therefore, full tidal volume delivery. However, using a 1.5-second T_I and still maintaining a 1:4 I:E ratio (so as to allow adequate time for emptying in a condition notorious for gas trapping), the ventilator rate could be no greater than eight breaths per minute (60 seconds/7.5 seconds = 8).

- Alternatively, choosing a rate of 30 breaths per minute and keeping the PIP, PEEP, and I:E ratio settings the same as before, the T_I would be 0.4 second, or just under two time constants. This means (Figure 7-9A) that less than 86 percent of the prescribed ΔP would have time to equilibrate (i.e., instead of 25 cmH_2O, around 21 cmH_2O, which is equivalent to settings of 26/5 rather than 30/5). Furthermore, less than 86 percent of the desired tidal volume would have time to be delivered (Figure 7-9B).
- Finally, choosing instead to achieve full ΔP equilibration and full tidal volume delivery by setting the T_I back to 1.5 seconds and still maintaining a rate of 30 breaths per minute would produce a T_E of only 0.5 second (i.e., one time constant), producing a reversed I:E ratio of 5:1. Such settings would surely result in

gas trapping due to insufficient time for expiratory emptying (Figure 7-10). And gas trapping brings with it a number of physiologic and pathophysiologic changes:[56]

- Lung volume increases, as reflected in a rise in measured FRC levels or in depression of the diaphragm below nine and a half posterior ribs, as seen on anteroposterior chest x-ray.[57]
- There is a buildup of pressure (or back pressure) in the alveoli and distal airways that persists through end expiration. Weigl appropriately named this pressure buildup "inadvertent PEEP," reflecting the fact that the additional end-expiratory pressure is usually unintentional and unrecognized by the clinician, existing as it does inside the lung and not out in the distal circuit where so-called proximal airway pressure is generally measured.[58,59]
- Work of breathing increases even while alveolar ventilation decreases.[56]
- Finally, the risk of occurrence of complications associated with alveolar overdistention (similar to those resulting from excessively high levels of PIP and Paw, as discussed earlier) increases.

Understanding and Applying Gas Laws

An understanding of gas laws is useful in applying IMV effectively in the clinical setting. See the classic reviews of the topics that follow.[40,53] Boyle's law states that pressure (P) multiplied by volume (V) is a constant. In other words, if pressure goes up, volume goes down, and the product of the two remains the same. Think of a known quantity of gas as so many molecules of the gaseous substance uniformly distributed within an enclosed space and producing a measurable pressure within that space. If that space is compressed to half its original volume (e.g., from 4 down to 2 square inches of volume), then the measured pressure within the container will double: If the pressure was originally 3 pounds per square inch (psi), it will increase to 6 psi. Thus, P1 × V1 (or 4 × 3) equals P2 × V2 (or 2 × 6), and the product of pressure and volume remains the same (12) before and after the change. Of course, the total number of gas molecules within the enclosed space has not changed (barring any air leak), but after the change, the molecules are compressed closer together because the enclosed space was made smaller. Pressure is simply a measure of the degree of compression of gas molecules, randomly bouncing off each other with increasing frequency the closer they are brought together.

Charles's law brings in the factor of temperature (T). It states that the volume of a given mass (specific number of molecules) of gas held at constant pressure varies directly with the absolute temperature (C° + 273) (i.e., volume is proportional to absolute temperature). The greater the temperature, the more the gas molecules will be put in motion to bounce off each other with increasing frequency, causing expansion of the space (increased volume) if pressure inside the space is held constant.

The general gas equation combines the gas laws of Boyle and Charles to show the interaction, or relationship, between all three factors: pressure, volume, and temperature. Thus:

$$\frac{P1 \times V1}{T1} = \frac{P2 \times V2}{T2}$$

Understanding the general gas equation helps answer the following questions relevant to mechanical ventilation of the newborn: What happens clinically when cold gas is inspired or delivered via a ventilator and warmed by the body (at constant pressure) upon entry into the lungs? What happens to lung volume and alveolar pressure when gas within the bronchial tree and alveoli is compressed through forced exhalation against a closed airway (Valsalva maneuver) or against a closed exhalation valve of a ventilator?

The general gas equation explains the temporary advantages and potential disadvantages of delivering cold, nonhumidified gas to a sick newborn during air transport using a time-cycled transport ventilator (as is usually the case). The good news is that the cold air

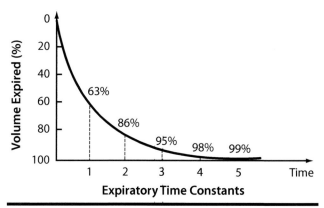

FIGURE 7-10
Expiratory time constants curve.

Adapted from: Hansen TN. 2003. Respiratory physiology. In *Contemporary Diagnosis and Management of Neonatal Respiratory Diseases,* 3rd ed., Weisman LE, and Hansen TN, eds. Newtown, Pennsylvania: Handbooks in Health Care, 17. © Handbooks in Health Care. www.hhcbooks.com. Reprinted by permission.

expands as it warms inside the lungs, culminating in delivery of a larger tidal volume with the same pressure settings that were being used to ventilate the infant in the referring hospital. Furthermore, the ΔP being generated (and thus the tidal volume delivered) grows larger as the transport vehicle climbs in altitude because the outside reference pressure falls (as barometric pressure falls with altitude), thereby increasing the difference between P1 and P2. The bad news is implicit in the following question: What if the clinician doesn't make the appropriate adjustments to the ventilator settings, and the infant's fragile lungs simply can't tolerate the additional pressure and volume delivered due to these changes?

The general gas equation also helps to explain the inherent danger for the infant who is fighting the ventilator. If an infant on IMV exhales spontaneously just as the exhalation valve closes to initiate the inspiratory cycle of a mandatory breath, intra-alveolar pressure may increase substantially because gas is being compressed (from both directions) at a time of no exit.

UNDERSTANDING AND APPLYING THE LAPLACE RELATIONSHIP

The Laplace relationship states that the pressure exerted by a spherical liquid surface enclosing a volume of gas (and thus forming a two-dimensional spherical gas-liquid interface) equals twice the surface tension (ST) divided by the radius (r) of the sphere, or:[40,53]

$$P = {}^{2ST}/r$$

FIGURE 7-11
Surface tension.

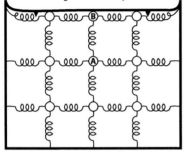

B. Molecules at the surface have no forces attracting them from above, so surface has a tension along its horizontal plane.

C. Surface forces are resolved towards the center of a curvature when the surface is curved.

A. Molecules in liquid mutually attract each other in all directions.

Adapted from: Widdicombe J, and Davies A. 1983. *Respiratory Physiology*. Baltimore: University Park Press, 10. Reprinted by permission.

Before explaining some practical, clinical applications of the Laplace relationship, let's first explore the physical nature of ST.

- Molecules in *solids* are very tightly packed, attract each other strongly, move about very little, and seldom escape from the surface into the surrounding air. Molecules in a *liquid*, such as water, are also closely packed and powerfully attracted to each other, but are much freer to move about and thus frequently escape into the air above the surface to exert a water vapor pressure in the gaseous phase of 47 mmHg at body temperature. Molecules in *gas* are widely dispersed to begin with and are moving rapidly (at velocities of about 500 m/second) so that they are only weakly attracted to one another.
- When liquid interfaces with gas, forming a flat liquid surface, the molecules of liquid at the surface are attracted to other molecules essentially from one side only, namely, from the underlying liquid, because there are so few gaseous molecules above the surface to attract them. This makes the surface molecules of the liquid act like a skin, producing a liquid surface tension along a horizontal plane. This ST force tends to draw in, or constrict, the gas-liquid interface toward a least-possible surface area. When the liquid surface is curved, as in a bubble, the molecules in the surface skin are pulled toward the center of the bubble, tending to make the bubble smaller (Figure 7-11).
- When we attempt to counteract the tendency of small, surfactant-deficient alveoli to collapse by

applying a pneumatic splint to their inside surface in the form of positive distending pressure, we are in fact applying the "P" represented on the left side of the Laplace relationship.

- Conversely, the right side of the Laplace relationship explains why it takes more distending airway pressure to inflate smaller units than larger ones. It also explains why high pressures (especially if held at the pressure plateau) go preferentially to those lung units already expanded (with longer time constants because they have higher compliance), causing their overexpansion, rather than going to smaller, atelectatic segments for alveolar recruitment purposes. Figure 7-8 represents the opposing forces on both sides of the Laplace relationship and illustrates how surfactant acts in the exact opposite direction as surface tension, namely, increasing its effectiveness in lowering ST the smaller the alveoli become.

NEONATAL LUNG DISEASE CATEGORIES AND STRATEGIES FOR VENTILATOR MANAGEMENT

It is possible to separate out three different pathophysiologic mechanisms that define three distinct categories of neonatal lung defects or diseases: (1) atelectatic, (2) restrictive, and (3) obstructive. The clinician approaches each of these three with quite different ventilator strategies.

ATELECTATIC LUNG DISEASE

In atelectatic lung disease, often called *diffuse* or *homogeneous* lung disease, the alveoli tend to collapse (become atelectatic) as a result of primary surfactant deficiency or secondary surfactant inactivation. RDS is the most common such disease in the newborn period. Other examples include capillary leak syndrome following asphyxial, infectious, or toxic insult to the pulmonary capillaries (and vessels of other organ systems) and heart failure leading to pulmonary edema.

From a ventilator management point of view, the basic problem in atelectatic lung disease is one of maintaining an adequate pressure gradient across the alveolar walls to reopen and keep open the alveoli until the lungs recover and initiate or restart surfactant production. On mechanical ventilation, this alveolar wall pressure gradient is provided by means of distending airway pressure applied to the inside of the alveoli. In the past, severe cases of atelectatic lung disease were sometimes treated using a "high-volume" strategy as follows:

- When using conventional IMV, the high-volume strategy entailed starting with a high peak pressure and holding it in pressure plateau for an appreciable length of time (i.e., T_I up to 0.5 second) to recruit or reexpand collapsed alveoli. Once surfactant was administered and lung volume began to normalize, it was then possible to back off the high levels of PIP and FiO_2 while increasing PEEP just a little to maintain the high lung volume. PEEP, or background CPAP, was maintained until natural surfactant production got underway (usually beginning around 48 hours into treatment), making the pneumatic splint no longer necessary.
- The high-volume strategy was originally developed for use with HFOV[60] and then later modified for HFJV.[61] When switching from IMV to HFOV, the clinician begins with Paw levels that are 2–3 cmH_2O higher than those last used on IMV. When switching from IMV to HFJV, the clinician sets (1) the PIP on the jet at about the same level as that last used on IMV, (2) the PIP on the in-tandem conventional ventilator to 1–2 cmH_2O lower than that on the jet (to avoid stacking of breaths), (3) the rate of the IMV sigh breaths at 4 or 5/minute, and then (4) the PEEP (as displayed on the jet but regulated through the in-tandem conventional ventilator) to whatever level is needed (usually around 10–12 cmH_2O) to provide a Paw just slightly less than what was being provided when the infant was last on IMV.
- Recognition of the detrimental effect of high peak inspiratory pressures on the alveoli has led to a much more gentle approach to ventilation such that high-volume strategies are seldom used with conventional mechanical ventilation.[62]

Restrictive Lung Disease

A number of clinical conditions affecting the newborn are categorized as restrictive in nature because the primary defect involves restriction of alveolar expansion (with or without restriction of pulmonary blood flow). Restrictive defects can be further subdivided into intrinsic and extrinsic etiologies, with the former restriction due to processes within the lung structures themselves and the latter restriction due to processes that are extrapulmonary (or outside the lungs), but then impinge on the lungs. Examples of intrinsic lung defects include congenital hypoplastic lungs; congenital malformations of the lung such as cystic adenomatoid malformation, pulmonary sequestration, and pulmonary lymphangiectasia; and PIE. Examples of extrinsic lung defects include

congenital diaphragmatic hernia (which also produces hypoplastic lungs, worse on the ipsilateral than the contralateral side), tension pneumothorax, pleural effusion, abdominal distention, and so on. When treating restrictive lung disease, it is preferable to employ a so-called low-volume strategy:

- When using conventional mechanical ventilation, rapid-rate IMV is the preferred mode of treatment for restrictive lung defects. This approach entails delivery of small tidal volume breaths at rapid rates to ensure adequate minute ventilation without overexpanding or overpressurizing the alveoli. Higher peak pressures are required, but they are maintained for relatively short periods during inspiration. This limits the volume delivered and provides fairly equal distribution of ventilation. Relatively high PEEP levels are also required to maintain any ground won in reexpanding compressed lung tissue, thereby slowly overcoming the restriction. However, increases in PEEP have a one-to-one effect of raising Paw, and they also diminish ΔP, thereby reducing the degree of alveolar ventilation.
- Dealing with bilateral tension PIE complicating severe RDS creates a treatment dilemma. On the one hand, high levels of PIP and relatively long T_I are needed to maintain a high level of Paw to overcome atelectasis caused by the surfactant deficiency. On the other hand, high peak pressure held for prolonged periods holds wide open the hole in the ruptured bronchiole or marginal alveolus with each mandatory breath, facilitating ongoing air leakage. This is where HFJV is particularly effective due to its ability to achieve adequate ventilation at lower distending airway pressures and shorter T_I (20 milliseconds, or just 0.02 second) than those provided by any other mode of ventilatory support.

Obstructive or Nonhomogeneous Lung Disease

The most common purely obstructive lung disorder encountered in newborn infants is meconium aspiration syndrome. Other nonhomogeneous lung diseases include bronchial or lobar pneumonia, transient tachypnea of the newborn, and unilateral PIE. In MAS, the airways are partially or totally obstructed with particulate matter and offer increased resistance to airflow and increased work of breathing for the infant. Beyond airways that are partially obstructed, there is air trapping and local overdistention, whereas beyond bronchi or bronchioles that are totally occluded, there is segmental atelectasis. On chest x-ray, one sees patchy areas of infiltration or atelectasis alongside radiolucent areas of emphysema. Overall lung expansion appears increased, but alveolar ventilation is frequently reduced. When $PaCO_2$ values begin to climb much over 45 mmHg within four to six hours of age, the baby will predictably slip into respiratory failure and require mechanical ventilation.[63]

The treatment of obstructive lung disease is rarely simple and most often requires a rather complicated, yet flexible strategy. You might call this the "First do no harm" strategy aimed at avoiding air leaks:

- Provide ample time for gas emptying during passive exhalation by choosing a slower rate (starting at about 30 breaths per minute and never exceeding 40 breaths per minute) and an I:E ratio of at least 1:3.
- Higher PIP settings will be needed to overcome the increased airway resistance, and high circuit flow rates will be needed to achieve pressure equilibration at these higher PIP levels within the relatively short T_I dictated by the 1:3 or 1:4 I:E ratio.
- It is also very important to maintain middle-range levels of PEEP (5–7 cmH_2O) to splint open the airways during expiration and hopefully avoid the ball-valve mechanism for air trapping.[64]

Clinical Pearls

- It is essential for clinicians to anticipate the natural course of the disease they are treating as well as the expected response to the mode of ventilation and strategy they choose as appropriate given what they believe to be the disease's predominant pathophysiology.
- It is also important that clinicians anticipate even the blood gas results, making an educated guess of what they will be *before* receiving the values back from the laboratory. This helps practitioners hone their clinical skills in anticipating both direction and magnitude of changes in blood gas results after making similar ventilator setting changes under somewhat similar circumstances in the future. Besides, correctly predicting the results can raise a clinician's value in colleagues' eyes.
- If the infant responds as anticipated, the clinician should be able to make subsequent oxygen concentration and ventilator changes as usual.[65] She should also be able to confirm the infant's anticipated worsening or improvement with blood gas and oxygen saturation values that stay within acceptable ranges determined previously.

- If the infant does not respond as anticipated or if the mode of ventilation thought to be appropriate is not getting the job done, the clinician should be willing to rethink the situation. Be open to reconsidering the predominant pathophysiology operative at the moment and then the appropriateness of the strategy that has been applied up to this point. Consider the need to switch to a different strategy or to alter the mode of ventilation itself. If subsequent ventilator-setting changes do not take the infant in the desired direction at the anticipated rate of improvement, be ready to rethink and possibly change the course of treatment.
- Finally, the clinician should attempt to use the minimum amount of all treatment modalities (including enriched oxygen, ΔP, and Paw) possible while still achieving one or more specific but limited goals. Because of their developmental immaturity, most infants are oscillating systems that are prone to vacillating from one extreme to the other. To help infants move toward balance, make small changes that serve to dampen that oscillation and better maintain homeostasis.

REFERENCES

1. Donn SM, and Sinha SK. 2002. Newer techniques of mechanical ventilation: An overview. *Seminars in Neonatology* 7(5): 401–407.
2. McGettigan MC, et al. 1998. New ways to ventilate newborns in acute respiratory failure. *Pediatric Clinics of North America* 45(3): 475–509.
3. Donald I, and Lord J. 1953. Augmented respiration studies in atelectasis neonatorum. *Lancet* 1(6749): 9–17.
4. Thomas DV, et al. 1965. Prolonged respirator use in pulmonary insufficiency of the newborn. *JAMA* 193: 183–190.
5. Gregory GA, et al. 1971. Treatment of the idiopathic respiratory distress syndrome with continuous positive airway pressure. *New England Journal of Medicine* 284(24): 1333–1340.
6. Daily WJR, et al. 1971. Mechanical ventilation of newborn infants. Part III: Historical comments and development of a scoring system for selection of infants. *Anesthesiology* 34(2): 119–126.
7. Smith PC, and Daily WJ. 1971. Mechanical ventilation of newborn infants. Part IV: Technique of controlled intermittent positive-pressure ventilation. *Anesthesiology* 34(2): 127–131.
8. Swyer PR. 1969. An assessment of artificial respiration in the newborn. In *Problems of Neonatal Intensive Care Units, Report of the 59th Ross Conference on Pediatric Research*, Lucey JF, ed. Columbus, Ohio: Ross Laboratories.
9. Harrison VC, Hesse H de V, and Klein M. 1968. The significance of grunting in hyaline membrane disease. *Pediatrics* 41(3): 549–559.
10. Reid DH, Tunstall ME, and Mitchell RG. 1967. A controlled trial of artificial respiration in the respiratory-distress syndrome of the newborn. *Lancet* 1(7489): 532–533.
11. Silverman WA, et al. 1967. A controlled trial of management of respiratory distress syndrome in a body-enclosing respirator. Part I: Evaluation of safety. *Pediatrics* 39(5): 740–748.
12. Sinclair JC, Engel K, and Silverman WA. 1968. Early correction of hypoxemia and acidemia in infants of low birth weight: A controlled trial of oxygen breathing, rapid alkali infusion, and assisted ventilation. *Pediatrics* 42(4): 565–589.
13. Daily WJR, Sunshine P, and Smith PC. 1971. Mechanical ventilation of newborn infants. Part V: Five years experience. *Anesthesiology* 34(2): 132–138.
14. Kirby RR, et al. 1971. A new pediatric volume ventilator. *Anesthesia and Analgesia* 50(4): 533–537.

15. Reynolds EOR. 1971. Effects of alterations in mechanical ventilator settings on pulmonary gas exchange in hyaline membrane disease. *Archives of Disease in Childhood* 46(246): 152–159.

16. Reynolds EOR. 1974. Pressure waveform and ventilator settings for mechanical ventilation in severe hyaline membrane disease. *International Anesthesiology Clinics* 12(4): 259–280.

17. Herman S, and Reynolds EOR. 1973. Methods for improving oxygenation in infants mechanically ventilated for severe hyaline membrane disease. *Archives of Disease in Childhood* 48(8): 612–617.

18. Mannino F, et al. 1976. Early mechanical ventilation in RDS with a prolonged inspiration. *Pediatric Research* 10(1): 464A.

19. Rhodes PG, et al. 1983. Minimizing pneumothorax and bronchopulmonary dysplasia in ventilated infants with hyaline membrane disease. *Journal of Pediatrics* 103(4): 634–637.

20. Stark AR, and Frantz ID. 1986. Respiratory distress syndrome. *Pediatric Clinics of North America* 33(3): 533–544.

21. Halliday HL. 2004. What interventions facilitate weaning from the ventilator? A review of the evidence from systematic reviews. *Paediatric Respiratory Reviews* 5(supplement A): S347–S352.

22. Truog WE, and Golombek SG. 2005. Principles of management of respiratory problems. In *Avery's Neonatology: Pathophysiology & Management of the Newborn*, MacDonald MG, Mullett MD, and Seshia MMK, eds. Philadelphia: Lippincott Williams & Wilkins, 600–621.

23. Wung JT, et al. 1985. Management of infants with severe respiratory failure and persistence of fetal circulation without hyperventilation. *Pediatrics* 76(4): 488–494.

24. White CW. 1988. Pulmonary oxygen toxicity: Cellular mechanisms of oxidant injury and antioxidant defense. In *Bronchopulmonary Dysplasia*, Bancalari E, and Stocker JT, eds. Washington, DC: Hemisphere, 22–41.

25. Carlo WA, Martin RJ, and Fanaroff AA. 2002. Assisted ventilation and complications of respiratory distress. In *Neonatal-Perinatal Medicine: Diseases of the Fetus and Newborn*, Fanaroff AA, and Martin RJ, eds. St. Louis: Mosby, 1011–1025.

26. Downes JJ. 1971. Mechanical ventilation of the newborn (editorial). *Anesthesiology* 34(2): 116–118.

27. Kirby RR. 1979. Design of mechanical ventilators. In *Neonatal Pulmonary Care*, Thibeault DW, and Gregory GA, eds. Menlo Park, California: Addison-Wesley, 154–167.

28. Yoder BA, et al. 1986. Design of mechanical ventilators. In *Neonatal Pulmonary Care*, 2nd ed., Thibeault DW, and Gregory GA, eds. Norwalk, Connecticut: Appleton-Century-Crofts, 281–305.

29. Spitzer AR, Greenspan JS, and Fox WW. 2003. Positive-pressure ventilation: Pressure-limited and time-cycled ventilators. In *Assisted Ventilation of the Neonate*, 4th ed., Goldsmith JP, and Karotkin EH, eds. Philadelphia: Saunders, 149-169.

30. Simbruner G, and Gregory GA. 1981. Performance of neonatal ventilators: The effects of changes in resistance and compliance. *Critical Care Medicine* 9(7): 509–514.

31. Spitzer AR. 2005. Positive pressure ventilation: The use of mechanical ventilation in the treatment of neonatal lung disease—General principles. In *Intensive Care of the Fetus and Neonate*, Spitzer AR, ed. Philadelphia: Elsevier Mosby, 623–654.

32. Harris TR. 1981. Physiologic principles. In *Assisted Ventilation of the Neonate*, Goldsmith JP, and Karotkin EH, eds. Philadelphia: Saunders, 44.

33. Gregory GA. 1986. Continuous positive airway pressure. In *Neonatal Pulmonary Care*, 2nd ed., Thibeault DW, and Gregory GA, eds. Norwalk, Connecticut: Appleton-Century-Crofts, 349–366.

34. Bland RD, et al. 1980. High frequency mechanical ventilation in severe hyaline membrane disease: An alternative treatment? *Critical Care Medicine* 8(5): 275–280.

35. Heicher DA, Kasting DS, and Harrod JR. 1981. Prospective clinical comparison of two methods for mechanical ventilation of neonates: Rapid rate and short inspiratory time versus slow rate and long inspiratory time. *Journal of Pediatrics* 98(6): 957–961.

36. Stewart AR, Finer NN, and Peters KL. 1981. Effects of alterations of inspiratory and expiratory pressures and inspiratory/expiratory ratios on mean airway pressure, blood gases, and intracranial pressure. *Pediatrics* 67(4): 474–481.

37. Boros SJ, et al. 1977. The effect of independent variations in inspiratory-expiratory ratio and end expiratory pressure during mechanical ventilation in hyaline membrane disease: The significance of mean airway pressure. *Journal of Pediatrics* 91(5): 794–798.

38. Boros SJ. 1979. Variations in inspiratory:expiratory ratio and airway pressure wave form during mechanical ventilation: The significance of mean airway pressure. *Journal of Pediatrics* 94(1): 114–117.

39. Suter PM, Fairley B, and Isenberg MD. 1975. Optimum end-expiratory airway pressure in patients with acute pulmonary failure. *New England Journal of Medicine* 292(6): 284–289.

40. Hansen TN. 1998. Respiratory physiology. In *Contemporary Diagnosis and Management of Neonatal Respiratory Diseases*, 2nd ed., Hansen TN, Cooper TR, and Weisman LE, eds. Newtown, Pennsylvania: Handbooks in Health Care, 6–49.

41. Boros SJ, et al. 1984. Using conventional infant ventilators at unconventional rates. *Pediatrics* 74(4): 487–492.

42. Gonzalez F, et al. 1986. Rapid mechanical ventilation effects on tracheal airway pressure, lung volume, and blood gases of rabbits. *American Journal of Perinatology* 3(4): 347–351.

43. Drummond WH, et al. 1981. The independent effects of hyperventilation, tolazoline, and dopamine on infants with persistent pulmonary hypertension. *Journal of Pediatrics* 98(4): 603–611.

44. Greisen G, and Trojaborg W. 1987. Cerebral blood flow, $PaCO_2$ changes, and visual evoked potentials in mechanically ventilated, preterm infants. *Acta Paediatrica Scandinavica* 76(3): 394–400.

45. Graziani LJ, et al. 1992. Mechanical ventilation in preterm infants: Neurosonographic and developmental studies. *Pediatrics* 90(4): 515–522.

46. Fox WW, et al. 1977. The PaO_2 response to changes in end-expiratory pressure in the newborn respiratory distress syndrome. *Critical Care Medicine* 5(5): 226–229.

47. Harris TR, and Wood BR. 1996. Physiologic principles. In *Assisted Ventilation of the Neonate*, 3rd ed., Goldsmith JP, and Karotkin EH, eds. Philadelphia: Saunders, 21–68.

48. Carlo WA, et al. 1984. Decrease in airway pressure during high-frequency jet ventilation in infants with respiratory distress syndrome. *Journal of Pediatrics* 104(1): 101–107.

49. Gonzalez F, et al. 1987. Decreased gas flow through pneumothoraces in neonates receiving high-frequency jet versus conventional ventilation. *Journal of Pediatrics* 110(3): 464–466.

50. Harris TR, and Bunnell JB. 2004. *RT 501: Towards a Working Understanding of High-Frequency Ventilation*. PowerPoint presentation on CD-ROM. Available at no cost by e-mail request to either author: trhhere@aol.com or bbl@bunl.com.

51. Hansen TN. 1998. Positive pressure ventilatory support. In *Contemporary Diagnosis and Management of Neonatal Respiratory Diseases*, 2nd ed., Hansen TN, Cooper TR, and Weisman LE, eds. Newtown, Pennsylvania: Handbooks in Health Care, 245–260.

52. Carlo WA, and Martin RJ. 1986. Principles of neonatal assisted ventilation. *Pediatric Clinics of North America* 33(1): 221–237.

53. Widdicombe J, and Davies A. 1983. *Respiratory Physiology*. Baltimore: University Park Press.

54. Cave P, and Fletcher G. 1968. Resistance of nasotracheal tubes used in infants. *Anesthesiology* 29(3): 588–590.

55. Wood B. 2003. Physiologic Principles. In *Assisted Ventilation of the Neonate*, 4th ed., Goldsmith JP, and Karotkin EH, eds. Philadelphia: Saunders, 15–40.

56. Donahue LA, and Thibeault DW. 1979. Alveolar gas trapping and ventilator therapy in infants. *Perinatology-Neonatology* 3(3): 35–37.

57. Cartwright DW, Willis MM, and Gregory GA. 1984. Functional residual capacity and lung mechanics at different levels of mechanical ventilation. *Critical Care Medicine* 12(5): 422–427.

58. Weigl J. 1973. The infant lung: A case against high respiratory rates in controlled neonatal ventilation. *Respiratory Therapy* 3(1): 57–62.

59. Simbruner G. 1986. Inadvertent positive end-expiratory pressure in mechanically ventilated newborn infants: Detection and effect on lung mechanics and gas exchange. *Journal of Pediatrics* 108(4): 569–595.

60. Clark RH, and Null DM. 1993. High-frequency oscillatory ventilation. In *Neonatology for the Clinician*, Pomerance JJ, and Richardson CJ, eds. East Norwalk, Connecticut: Appleton & Lange, 289–309.

61. Keszler M, et al. 1997. Multicenter controlled clinical trial of high-frequency jet ventilation in preterm infants with uncomplicated respiratory distress syndrome. *Pediatrics* 100(4): 593–599.

62. Kaempf JW, et al. 2003. Implementing potentially better practices to improve neonatal outcomes after reducing postnatal dexamethasone use in infants born between 501 and 1250 grams. *Pediatrics* 111(4 part 2): e534–e541.

63. Vidyasagar D, Harris V, and Pildes RS. 1975. Assisted ventilation in infants with meconium aspiration syndrome. *Pediatrics* 56(2): 208–213.

64. Fox WW, et al. 1975. The therapeutic application of end-expiratory pressure in meconium aspiration syndrome. *Pediatrics* 56(2): 214–217.

65. Chatburn DW, Carlo WA, and Lough MD. 1983. Clinical algorithm for pressure-limited ventilation of neonates with respiratory distress syndrome. *Respiratory Care* 28(12): 1579–1585.

NOTES

8 Noninvasive Ventilation for Neonates

Debra Bingham, DrPH, RN
Debbie Fraser, MN, RNC-NIC

Over the past 20 years, there has been increasing attention given to the role of mechanical ventilation in the development of chronic lung disease (CLD) in low birth weight infants. In an attempt to reduce the exposure of the premature lung to the potentially damaging forces (volume and pressure) associated with mechanical ventilation, there has been renewed interest in the role of noninvasive ventilation (NIV) in premature infants.

Noninvasive ventilation is an umbrella term encompassing several types of devices or ventilation strategies. NIV describes devices that provide both continuous positive airway pressure (CPAP) across the respiratory cycle and mechanical "breaths" or phasic increases in airway pressure.[1] Devices that provide CPAP alone are sometimes included in the category of noninvasive ventilation.[2] Others consider CPAP a separate ventilation strategy.[1] For the purpose of this chapter, CPAP will be included in the discussion of noninvasive ventilation. Where the content is only applicable to CPAP, this is noted.

TYPES OF NIV

CPAP

CPAP is defined as the application of positive pressure to the airways of a spontaneously breathing patient throughout the respiratory cycle. The use of CPAP in adults with respiratory diseases was described as early as the 1930s.[3] But it wasn't until the early 1970s that George Gregory, an anesthesiologist working in an NICU, first wrote about its use for neonates with idiopathic respiratory distress syndrome (RDS).[4]

The terms *CPAP* and *PEEP* (positive end-expiratory pressure) are sometimes confused or used interchangeably, but the two mean different things. CPAP is considered a mode of ventilation, while PEEP refers to a level of pressure. During CPAP therapy, the specified amount of pressure is delivered continuously during both the inspiratory and expiratory phases of breathing. During mechanical ventilation, PEEP is generated at the end of exhalation, between delivered breaths and not across the respiratory cycle.

CPAP can be delivered by a variety of devices employing two types of flow: continuous and variable. In the U.S., continuous flow devices are most common and include neonatal ventilators, which provide an ongoing flow of fresh gas while limiting the outflow of gases to deliver the set pressure, and bubble CPAP, which generates pressure when the expiratory tubing is submerged in a chamber of water. The level of water determines the level of pressure generated.

Variable flow devices utilize specialized prongs or masks and flow generators or drivers to maintain the desired airway pressure. With variable flow CPAP, pressure is generated by changing the flow rate of gases during inspiration and expiration to maintain a constant airway pressure or resistance to the flow of gases leaving the nasal prongs or mask.[5,6]

BUBBLE CPAP

A simple and inexpensive way of generating pressure is to submerge the expiratory tubing in fluid to achieve the desired level of pressure. For example, at Columbia Hospital of New York (CHONY), CPAP is delivered by emptying a one-liter bottle of 0.25 percent acetic acid

FIGURE 8-1
Simple, inexpensive CPAP pressure generation system.

One-liter solution bottle contains 7 cm of 0.25 percent acetic acid; exhalation tube is immersed to 5 cm.

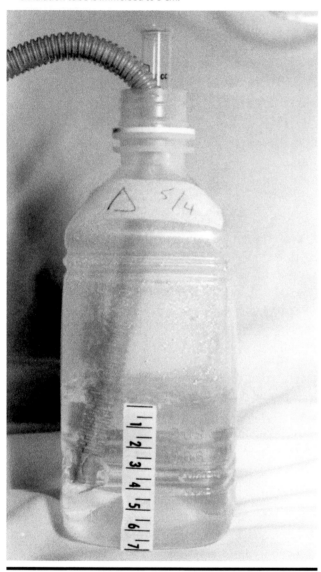

solution to a level of 7 cm and submerging the expiratory end of the CPAP tubing 5 cm into the remaining solution to generate pressure of +5 cm water pressure. The tubing is secured at the neck of the container by a 10 mL syringe with the cap and plunger removed (Figure 8-1). It is not necessary to use acetic acid if it is not available. NICUs that have used sterile water have not reported any problems with overgrowth of bacteria within the outlet bottles.

This simple pressure-generation system is inexpensive, readily available, easily replaced and maintained, as long as heaters and a gas source is available, and does not limit the number of patients who can be on CPAP at any time. Leaving no more than 7 cm of solution in the container eliminates the risk of delivering more than 7 cm of CPAP. Commercial bubble CPAP systems are also available.

Bubble CPAP produces vibrations similar to high-frequency ventilation. These vibrations have been measured at a frequency of 15–30 Hz.[7] It has been speculated that the additive effects of these vibrations may account for the positive findings in studies comparing bubble CPAP to ventilator-delivered CPAP.[8,9] Other researchers have found that the bubbling has no additive effect on oxygenation[10] and that the bubbling effects are dampened by the time the flow reaches the nasal prongs.[11]

HIGH-FLOW NASAL CANNULA

Nasal cannulae have been used as a method of delivering oxygen to newborns for a number of years. Until recently, the flow rates used with nasal cannulae have been limited by the ability to adequately humidify inspired gases. In the past, higher flow rates resulted in drying and erosion of the nasal tissues. The development of humidification systems has led to increased use of higher flow rates that deliver variable amounts of positive pressure to the infant's lungs. The amount of pressure reaching the infant's lungs will vary according to the type of cannula, the flow rate, and the infant's weight.[1] One study demonstrated that a cannula with an external diameter of 0.3 cm and a flow rate of 2 liters/minute generated a mean pressure of 9 cmH_2O.[12] Another study by Kubicka and colleagues enrolled 27 infants and placed them on high-humidity, high-flow nasal cannula (HFNC) using a catheter with a 0.2 cm outer diameter. They found a linear relationship between flow rate and pressures as long as the infant's mouth was closed. When the mouth was open, no pressure was detected. The highest pressure achieved was 4.5 cmH_2O with a flow rate of 8 liters/minute. They concluded that HFNC was not equivalent to CPAP.[13]

Some concern has been raised in using HFNC as a method of delivering positive pressure. Because the nasal cannula has no method of pressure monitoring and no safety release valve, it is essentially delivering unknown levels of pressure.[1,14] To date, the American Association for Respiratory Care continues to recommend against the use of flow rates greater than 2 liters/minute.[15] Additionally, some studies using HFNC have found increased rates of Gram-negative sepsis.[16,17] Graham and

FIGURE 8-2
Phasic ventilation.

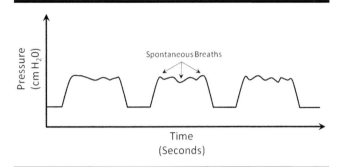

TABLE 8-1
Primary Effects of Some Types of NIV

Prevention of atelectasis
Conservation of surfactant
Increased functional residual capacity
Increased airway diameter
Improved diaphragmatic excursion
Decreased intrapulmonary shunting
Decreased respiratory rate and improved respiratory synchrony
Improved lung growth

associates speculate that the increased rate of sepsis may be the result of damage to the nasal mucosa.[16]

The system most commonly used, Vapotherm (Vapotherm, Stevensville, Maryland), was recalled in January of 2006 because some infants had developed pneumonia or sepsis caused by Ralstonia, which was traced back to the Vapotherm catheters. The Vapotherm was re-released in January of 2007.[5] A second device, the HFNC System (Fisher & Paykel RT329, Salter Labs, Arvin, California) is also available in some markets.

NASAL INTERMITTENT POSITIVE PRESSURE VENTILATION (NIPPV)

NIPPV combines with ventilator breaths delivered at a set peak pressure.[18] These increases in airway pressure, can either be delivered at set time intervals (nonsynchronized) known as *nasal intermittent positive pressure ventilation (NIPPV)* or can be triggered by the infant's respiratory efforts (synchronized). Synchronized nasal intermittent positive pressure ventilation (SNIPPV) has been studied more extensively than nonsynchronized NIPPV.

In NIPPV the peak inspiratory pressure, rate, and inspiratory time are all set by the operator.[6] There are no studies reported that delineate the optimal settings for NIPPV. A review of the topic done by Owen and coworkers notes that rates of 10–25 breaths per minute and PEEP levels of 3–6 cmH$_2$O are the parameters most commonly used in the available research studies.[18]

It is unclear by what mechanism NIV confers its proposed benefits to the neonatal lung. For example, it is not known whether breaths are transmitted to the lungs or simply act on the upper airway. In a review of phasic NIV, Moretti and colleagues note that studies have demonstrated variable transmission of breaths with more transmission during synchronous than asynchronous breaths.[19] Other theories explaining the physiologic

benefits of phasic NIV include increased pharyngeal dilation, increased respiratory drive, increased tidal volume and minute ventilation, and reduced asynchrony between the chest and abdomen.[18–22] It is also speculated that SNIPPV may be creating inadvertent PEEP, thereby allowing further recruitment of alveoli, resulting in a higher functional residual capacity (FRC).[20,23]

NASAL BILEVEL POSITIVE AIRWAY PRESSURE

Bilevel CPAP provides continuous positive pressure at two separate CPAP levels (Figure 8-2). The baseline CPAP level is normally set at 4–6 cmH$_2$O, while a second flow meter is set to deliver "sighs" or periods of elevated pressure, usually 2–4 cmH$_2$O higher than the baseline CPAP. A rate is set to determine the frequency of the sighs, and each sigh is usually 0.5–2 seconds long. The Infant Flow SiPAP device (CareFusion, Yorba Linda, California) and the BiPAP system (Respironics, Murrysville, Pennsylvania) are examples of bilevel CPAP devices. As with NIPPV, mechanisms suitable to detect the onset of a neonatal breath are lacking and therefore, at present, no synchronized bilevel CPAP devices are available.

The advantage of bilevel CPAP is thought to come from a higher mean airway pressure and recruitment of unstable alveoli during the sigh breaths. To date, only a few studies have examined SiPAP use in infants. Migliori and colleagues conducted an observational study, which demonstrated that SiPAP provided better gas exchange than conventional CPAP.[24] Ancora and associates retrospectively examined the use of SiPAP after surfactant to prevent the need for reintubation. They found that fewer infants in the SiPAP group required mechanical ventilation compared to historical controls.[25] Finally, an RCT done by Lista and coworkers compared SiPAP with CPAP for initial support in preterm infants with RDS and found that the infants in the SiPAP group had a shorter duration of mechanical ventilation, shorter length of hospital stay, and less oxygen dependence.[26]

TABLE 8-2
Comparison of the Effects of Surfactant and CPAP on the Lung and Alveoli

Characteristic	Effect of Surfactant	Effect of CPAP
Functional residual capacity	Increases	Increases
Alveolar collapse	Prevents at low transpulmonary pressures	Prevents
Intrapulmonary shunting	Decreases	Decreases
Lung compliance	Increases	Increases
Distribution of ventilation	Improves	Improves
Alveolar surface tension	Decreases	Conserves surfactant thereby decreasing surface tension
Surfactant	N/A	Conserves
Transpulmonary pressure	N/A	Increases

NASAL NEURALLY ADJUSTED VENTILATORY ASSIST (NAVA)

NAVA technology has recently been approved by the FDA for both invasive and noninvasive ventilatory support.[27] With NAVA, a 5.5 French feeding tube with attached electrodes is positioned in the esophagus at the level of the diaphragm. Nerve impulses in the diaphragm are detected by the electrodes and used to trigger a positive pressure breath. NAVA can be used in small infants and is not affected by the infant's movements or by the air leaks. NAVA devices are currently very expensive and require further research before widespread use.[27]

BENEFITS OF NIV

NIV, including CPAP, has a number of primary effects (Table 8-1). They include preventing atelectasis, conserving surfactant, decreasing intrapulmonary shunting, increasing FRC, increasing compliance, increasing airway diameter and "splinting" the airways and the diaphragm, regularizing respirations and decreasing asynchrony, decreasing respiratory rate, improving lung growth, and mimicking the effects of surfactant. It is important to note that not all NIV devices have been shown to have the same benefits and, in some cases, limited research is available for devices other than CPAP. Much of the work delineating the benefits of CPAP was done during its early use, but more recent studies and reviews of both conventional and bilevel CPAP have confirmed these benefits.[8,28]

PREVENTION OF ATELECTASIS

Some degree of atelectasis is found in most neonatal respiratory dysfunction, and it results in respiratory distress. For the neonate, the primary benefit of NIV is prevention of atelectasis. NIV provides the pressure necessary to mechanically stabilize the air sacs, preventing their collapse.

Prevention of atelectasis is critical because it is much easier to maintain an expanded alveolus than to reexpand it. CPAP not only prevents alveolar collapse, but also recruits additional alveoli for gas exchange.[8]

CONSERVATION OF SURFACTANT

Surfactant production is low in the premature infant, and available surfactant may be quickly depleted, leading to alveolar collapse. When the alveoli collapse, decreasing the surface area, surfactant is consumed at an even higher rate.[6] CPAP acts to stabilize the alveolar wall mechanically until production of surfactant is adequate. When used effectively, CPAP mimics the effects of surfactant (Table 8-2).

The early application of NIV is important in decreasing or preventing the loss of existing surfactant. In addition, NIV reduces the chance of damage to Type II pneumocytes that can be caused by the inspiratory pressures generated by mechanical ventilation.

DECREASE IN INTRAPULMONARY SHUNTING

Physiologic shunting within the lung occurs when the web of blood vessels cannot exchange carbon dioxide and oxygen within the collapsed alveolus. When gas exchange does not occur over a widespread area, hypoxia and hypercarbia result. With NIV, shunting of blood decreases, which lessens the ventilation-to-perfusion mismatch and results in improved gas exchange and increased arterial oxygen tension.[29]

INCREASE IN FUNCTIONAL RESIDUAL CAPACITY

FRC is the air remaining in the lungs after exhalation. It provides an important reserve of air because gas exchange continues between breaths. In many infants with respiratory illness, FRC is greatly diminished, decreasing activity tolerance and increasing the chance of hypoxia. CPAP increases a neonate's ability to adjust to episodes of increased respiratory demand, such as nursing care, medical procedures, feeding, or activity.[30]

INCREASE IN COMPLIANCE

Improving FRC generally improves compliance as well. NIV keeps the alveoli partially distended, preventing total collapse and making reexpansion during breathing easier. However, lung compliance can decrease if too much distending pressure is applied and the alveoli become overdistended, especially in the presence of a normal lung.[31]

INCREASE IN AIRWAY DIAMETER, AIRWAY AND DIAPHRAGM "SPLINTING"

Through the mechanical action of distending pressure, NIV stabilizes and slightly distends the airways, acting as a splint to keep them open. This increase in airway diameter lowers resistance during both inspiration and exhalation.[30] Airway collapse is lessened or prevented, and premature infants exhibit a reduction in obstructive and mixed apnea.[29,32]

REGULARIZATION OF RESPIRATIONS AND IMPROVED SYNCHRONY

Neonates' breathing patterns become more regular on NIV. Premature infants are prone to periods of irregular breathing and apnea because of their flexible chest structure, immature respiratory drive, and lack of musculature. A neonate on CPAP benefits from the mechanical effects of the distending pressure, which help stabilize the chest wall and reduce thoracic distortion.[30] Elgellab and associates demonstrated that CPAP improves thoracoabdominal synchrony and reduces the work of breathing.[33]

DECREASE IN RESPIRATORY RATE AND MINUTE VENTILATION

Most newborns on NIV experience a decrease in their respiratory rate, which decreases minute ventilation (minute ventilation = tidal volume × respiratory rate). In spite of the decrease in minute ventilation, the $PaCO_2$ remains stable or falls, demonstrating that alveolar ventilation is adequate. This likely occurs as a result of an increase in tidal volume and from the recruitment of additional alveoli seen in infants on CPAP.[33,34]

IMPROVEMENT IN LUNG GROWTH

CPAP has been shown to promote lung growth in animal models. Zhang, Garbutt, and McBride found that use of CPAP with immature animals was associated with increases in lung volume, lung weight, and total lung protein and DNA.[35] This strain-induced lung growth may support the practice some NICUs have of using nasal prong CPAP as the primary means of providing respiratory support to infants. These NICUs rarely if ever use nasal cannulas or oxyhoods for ongoing or postextubation care.

DECREASED LUNG INFLAMMATION

Animal studies of bubble CPAP suggest that markers of acute lung inflammation are decreased in preterm lambs compared to lambs receiving mechanical ventilation.[36]

SECONDARY EFFECTS OF NIV-CPAP

Local changes in cardiac, renal, and cerebral blood flow distribution have been reported as a result of applying distending pressure to the airway. Again, the effects discussed below will vary depending on the device used. These changes, which vary greatly among the studies reporting them, are influenced by the infant's disease process, the NIV delivery system, and the amount of pressure generated.

CARDIAC

The effects of NIV on the infant's cardiac system are directly related to the amount of pressure used. High levels of pressure may impede venous return and have a detrimental effect on cardiac output. In contrast, pressure levels that are appropriate for the newborn's size and lung condition will restore normal intrathoracic pressure and improve overall cardiac function.[37]

Neonates with hyaline membrane disease often demonstrate right-to-left shunting through the foramen ovale and left-to-right shunting through the ductus arteriosus. This shunting contributes significantly to the hypoxemia, pulmonary fluid retention, and morbidity seen in many newborns with this disease. The effects of distending pressure on cardiac function were studied in premature lambs, and some beneficial effects were found. Shunting through the foramen ovale was decreased, which improved oxygenation. Right ventricular output was increased without significant change in left ventricular output or pulmonary vascular resistance. Left-to-right ductal flow also decreased.[38] These physiologic responses to distending pressure improve cardiac output and oxygenation.

RENAL

Much of the impact of NIV on the renal system results from changes in cardiac output. If the infant's blood pressure decreases with the application of distending pressure, urinary output, glomerular filtration, and sodium and potassium excretion will be decreased.[39] Renal blood flow is either reduced or redistributed. The water- and sodium-retaining hormone systems— antidiuretic hormone and aldosterone—are stimulated, producing an antidiuretic effect.[40,41] These changes are reversed when the distending pressure is withdrawn.

NEUROLOGIC

Some studies suggest that distending pressure increases intracranial pressure.[42,43] This was especially true in older studies when CPAP is delivered by a head box.[44,45] In the face of the lower systemic blood pressure seen in infants on distending pressure, there is a drop in cerebral perfusion pressure, which may decrease the risk of intraventricular hemorrhage.[42] Again, the amount of pressure applied and the infant's lung compliance appear to play important roles in determining the degree of the effect. Higher levels of distending pressure, coupled with less compliant lungs, are associated with higher intracranial pressures and decreased cerebral perfusion pressure.

COMPARISON OF METHODS OF PROVIDING NIV

Studies comparing various types of NIV have yielded conflicting results. Stefanescu and associates studied 162 extremely low birth weight (ELBW) infants and found no difference in extubation rates between the Infant Flow continuous positive airway pressure system (IF-CPAP) and ventilator-generated CPAP, but infants on variable flow did have fewer days on oxygen and shorter lengths of stay than those on standard CPAP.[46] Likewise, in a study of 140 infants born between 24 and 29 weeks, Gupta and coworkers also found no difference in extubation failure rates between the group of infants receiving variable flow via the Infant Flow Driver system CPAP, and those receiving bubble CPAP.[47] Boumecid and colleagues found increased tidal volumes and improved synchrony with the variable-flow CPAP compared to ventilator-generated CPAP in infants with mild respiratory distress.[48] Liptsen and associates compared bubble CPAP to variable-flow CPAP in 18 infants with birth weights <1,500 g and found that the variable-flow CPAP resulted in less asynchrony and less work of breathing than bubble CPAP.[49] Courtney and coworkers found that lung recruitment was superior with variable-flow CPAP than continuous flow. They speculated that this may be a result of the more consistent mean airway pressures seen with variable-flow CPAP.[50] Finally, in a study of 24 preterm infants, Pandit and colleagues found that infants receiving continuous-flow CPAP had increased work of breathing (13–29 percent higher) over those same infants when they were receiving variable-flow CPAP.[51]

Several studies have been published that compare a high-flow nasal cannula nasal prong CPAP. Sreenan and associates examined the use of HFNC compared to nasal prong CPAP for the management of apnea of prematurity and found that when the HFNC (flow rates of up to 2.5 liters/minute) was used to generate an esophageal pressure of +6 cmH_2O and compared to nasal prong CPAP of +6 cmH_2O, there were no differences between the groups in the frequency of apnea.[52] In a similar study, Saslow and coworkers found no differences in work of breathing in two groups of infants with birth weights of <2 kg, one group receiving NIV via HFNC (3, 4, and 5 liters/minute) and one group receiving NIV via nasal prong CPAP of +6 cmH_2O.[53] When comparing HFNC to a variable-flow CPAP device, Campbell and colleagues found that infants receiving HFNC had significantly higher rates of reintubation than infants receiving variable-flow nasal prong CPAP.[54] However, when Shoemaker and associates compared HFNC to continuous flow CPAP in 101 infants born at 26.5–29.5 weeks gestation, they found a lower rate of extubation failure (18 vs 40 percent) with the early application of HFNC. No differences in the rates of adverse outcomes were noted in this study.[17]

In a review of the HFNC studies, Dani and associates concluded that, although some studies have demonstrated benefits of HFNC in preventing reintubation, methodologic issues in these studies render the data inconclusive.[55] In his review, de Klerk concluded that HFNC should not be regarded as a type of CPAP, but rather as another form of respiratory support.[5]

Several studies have been published that compare either NIPPV or SNIPPV to conventional CPAP. Earlier studies generally used nonsynchronized NIPPV, but more recent studies have focused on NIPPV synchronized (SNIPPV) to the infant's inspiratory efforts. This change requires some degree of caution in interpreting the research data in this area. No studies have compared NIPPV to SNIPPV.[18]

Two meta-analyses have been published examining the role of NIPPV in preventing extubation failure and in treating apnea of prematurity.[56,57] Both of these reviews report on three studies where NIPPV was compared to CPAP after extubation.[58–60] In each of these studies, NIPPV was found to be superior to CPAP in preventing reintubation. The same meta-analyses evaluated two studies that examined the role of NIPPV in treating apnea of prematurity and found that, though NIPPV may have an advantage over conventional CPAP, the data were not conclusive.[21,61]

Several studies done since the early 2000s have added support to the efficacy of NIPPV. Using an unblended crossover design, Migliori and coworkers studied 20 infants using two cycles of nasal prong CPAP alternating with NIPPV. These researchers found that during NIPPV, infants had higher transcutaneous oxygen levels ($TcPO_2$s), lower levels of carbon dioxide, and a decreased respiratory rate.[24] A 2007 study of 84 neonates 28–33 weeks of age with RDS done by Kugelman and colleagues found that infants randomized to NIPPV were less likely to require ventilation than the CPAP group (25 vs 49 percent) and were less likely to develop bronchopulmonary dysplasia (BPD) (5 vs 33 percent).[62] In a randomized study of 63 infants <1,251 g, Moretti and associates compared SNIPPV to nasal prong CPAP after extubation and found that 94 percent of infants on SNIPPV were successfully extubated compared to 61 percent of those receiving nasal prong CPAP.[63] Recently, Lista and coworkers compared nasal prong CPAP and bilevel CPAP in infants 28–34 weeks gestational age and found that those on nasal prong CPAP required a longer duration of respiratory support and oxygen therapy and a longer hospital stay than those receiving NIPPV.[26]

Other studies did not find any difference in tidal volume or minute ventilation when comparing nasal prong CPAP and SNIPPV.[64,65]

INDICATIONS FOR NIV

There are three primary indications for the use of NIV: (1) respiratory distress of any origin (except congenital diaphragmatic hernia), (2) weaning from mechanical ventilation, and (3) apnea and bradycardia of the premature newborn.

TREATMENT FOR NEONATAL RESPIRATORY DISTRESS

NIV can be very effective in stabilizing the respiratory system while the underlying disease process is evaluated and treated. Common neonatal respiratory problems successfully treated with NIV include RDS, meconium aspiration syndrome, pulmonary edema, transient tachypnea of the newborn (TTN), and BPD. Of these conditions, the use of NIV in the treatment of RDS has received the most attention in the research literature. However, most of the initial studies on CPAP and RDS were done prior to the availability of exogenous surfactant. A meta-analysis of these early studies concluded that the early application of CPAP improved survival in infants <1,500 g.[66] More recently, attention

has been given to the use of NIV in preventing or reducing the severity of BPD. Studies addressing this issue are described below.

The importance of early application of NIV to prevent atelectasis and minimize the downward spiral of acute respiratory distress leading to respiratory failure, must be emphasized. Treatment with NIV is most effective when applied promptly after respiratory distress is recognized. Early application of NIV reduces both the need for intermittent positive pressure ventilation and the duration of respiratory assistance—even in very low birth weight (VLBW) infants.[66]

WEANING FROM MECHANICAL VENTILATION

CPAP has been shown to facilitate weaning from mechanical ventilation and prevent extubation failure. Mechanical ventilation can be harmful even at low settings. The longer an infant is on a mechanical ventilator, the greater the potential for damage to the lungs.[67] Extubation failures are stressful to the neonate and increase the risk of repeated episodes of atelectasis and reintubation. However, extubation of the relatively stable infant can be considered sooner when oxygen and PEEP can be delivered via NIV.

Espagne and Hascoët showed that when combined with the administration of caffeine, application of nasal prong CPAP resulted in an extubation success rate of 81 percent in their study population of 71 infants, 26.9–31.9 weeks gestational age.[68] A systematic review looking at the use of CPAP after extubation included nine trials published between 1982 and 2005 and found that CPAP applied immediately after extubation was effective in preventing failure of extubation and adverse events including apnea, respiratory acidosis, and increasing oxygen requirements.[66]

TREATMENT FOR APNEA AND BRADYCARDIA

There are three types of apnea in the neonate: central, obstructive, and mixed. Most neonatal apneas have an obstructive component. Obstructive apnea and mixed apnea are the most responsive to the application of NIV because of its mechanical effect of chest wall stabilization and splinting of the airways and diaphragm. It is thought that CPAP could improve the infant's respiratory drive by stimulating the pulmonary stretch receptors.[69] Central apnea seems to show little or no response to CPAP.[70–72] Overall, the evidence supporting CPAP's effectiveness is less clear than that examining extubation failure. A Cochrane review of CPAP for treatment of apnea in neonates found only one trial that met the inclusion criteria for review and concluded that more study was required.[73]

Studies specifically examining NIPPV in the management of apnea of prematurity also showed mixed results. Ryan, Finer, and Peters showed no difference between CPAP and NIPPV in the management of apnea.[61] Lin and colleagues found a more significant reduction in apnea in infants treated with NIPPV than to CPAP.[21] In a meta-analysis, de Paoli, Davis, and Lemyre found that SNIPPV may be more beneficial than nasal prong CPAP in reducing apnea.[57] This was confirmed in the Cochrane review comparing NIPPV to nasal prong CPAP for the treatment of apnea of prematurity.[56]

NIV AND BRONCHOPULMONARY DYSPLASIA

BPD results from a complex interaction of factors including incomplete lung development and lung injury and inflammation. Over the years, several definitions of BPD have been used in the literature. In 2000, a consensus conference was held at the National Institutes of Health that resulted in a definition of BPD that included the need for supplemental oxygen for a minimum of 28 days with the amount of oxygen required at 36 weeks postmenstrual age (in infants <32 weeks at birth) determining the severity of disease.[74] Contributing factors to a diagnosis of BPD include prematurity, mechanical ventilation, barotrauma and volutrauma, pulmonary oxygen toxicity, patent ductus arteriosus, and infection. Intubation with mechanical ventilation has been identified as a major contributing factor to the development of BPD.[9]

Interest in the use of NIV to prevent BPD dates back to the 1980s. In 1987, Avery and associates published a retrospective study in which they compared survival and the incidence of CLD (defined as an oxygen requirement greater than room air at 28 days of age) at eight tertiary neonatal centers. Data were collected between 1982 and 1984 and were adjusted for differences in birth weight, sex, and race. Overall survival rates did not vary significantly among the centers, but the incidence of CLD was much lower at Columbia Presbyterian Medical Center's Babies Hospital (now known as the Children's Hospital of New York at New York Presbyterian Medical Center) than at any of the other seven centers. The main differences in practices between Columbia and the other centers were the early use of nasal prong CPAP, reduced dependence on mechanical ventilation and intubation, permissive hypercapnia (up to 60 mmHg), and the avoidance of muscle relaxants at Columbia.[75]

In 1994 (nearly ten years later and in the post surfactant era), the International Neonatal Network, in a preliminary analysis of 5,390 infants from 99 hospitals, found that Columbia/CHONY continued to have the lowest adverse event rate, with an adverse event defined as oxygen dependence at 36 weeks postconceptional age, major cerebral damage before discharge, or death.[76]

In 2000, Van Marter and coworkers revisited the issue of variations in respiratory management among NICUs and subsequent differences in the incidence of chronic lung disease (defined as supplemental oxygen at 36 weeks gestational age). The incidence of CLD at Columbia/CHONY was again significantly lower than at the two comparison hospitals (4 percent vs 22 percent).[77]

In 2001, in a historic cohort study, de Klerk and de Klerk documented the results of applying a primarily CPAP-based system of respiratory support, closely modeled on the CHONY system, to a Level III NICU in South Auckland, New Zealand. The study compared the CPAP group with the more conventionally managed historic cohort. The infants ranged in weight from 1,000 to 1,500 g. CLD, defined as the need for supplemental oxygen at 28 days of age, decreased (11 percent in the historic cohort vs 0 percent in the CPAP group). The number of infants requiring mechanical ventilation decreased (65 percent vs 14 percent), as did the number of infants receiving surfactant (40 percent vs 12 percent).[78] In a follow-up prospective study within the same NICU, continuing the use of the CPAP-based Columbia/CHONY model, Meyer, Mildenhall, and Wong looked at infants weighing <1,000 g and compared their outcomes with those within the Australia and New Zealand Neonatal Network. The investigators noted a reduction in the use of mechanical ventilation, significantly less surfactant use, shorter periods of supplemental oxygen, and a significantly lower requirement for oxygen at 28 days (25 percent vs 63.8 percent) and for oxygen or respiratory support at 36 weeks (19.1 percent vs 45.4 percent).[79] In a retrospective study, Narendran and colleagues examined the application of bubble CPAP shortly after delivery in 79 infants with birth weights of 401–1,000 g. They found that early CPAP significantly reduced the intubation rate, days on mechanical ventilation, and postnatal steroid use in this population. Although there was a reduction in CLD at 28 days of life, when CLD was defined as any form of respiratory support at 36 weeks gestation there was no difference between the groups.[80] A recent study evaluating the introduction of bubble CPAP for VLBW infants with RDS found that, with bubble CPAP, fewer infants needed mechanical ventilation for more than six days (13.6 vs 26.3 percent of historical controls). However, there was no difference in the rate of BPD after the practice change.[81]

Given the harmful effects of mechanical ventilation, several studies have investigated whether or not nasal prong CPAP can be used instead of intubation and ventilation in low birth weight infants. Kamper and associates found that using an "early CPAP and permissive hypercapnia" approach when caring for ELBW infants results in lower incidences of chronic lung disease than conventional treatment.[82] CPAP has been shown to reduce days on ventilation, supplemental oxygen, and BPD.[78,79,83–90]

While the role of NCPAP in the delivery room is receiving increasing attention, study results have been mixed. In a randomized controlled trial published in 2004, Finer and coworkers found that 80 percent of ELBW infants placed on nasal prong CPAP in the delivery room required mechanical ventilation by one week of age.[91] The CPAP or intubation (COIN) trial was a large multicenter study that set out to determine the role of CPAP in decreasing the rates of BPD and death in preterm infants. Six hundred and ten infants born at 25–28 weeks gestational age were randomly assigned to CPAP (+8 cmH$_2$O) or intubation and ventilation at five minutes of age. At 36 weeks gestational age, 33.9 percent of the CPAP infants (104) had died or had BPD, compared to 38.9 percent (118) of the intubated group. At 28 days of life, there was a lower risk of death or need for oxygen in the CPAP group (53.7 percent compared to 64.7 percent); 46 percent of the CPAP group required intubation. These investigators concluded that nasal prong CPAP does not reduce the rate of death or BPD in preterm infants.[92] These findings are similar to those of Sandri and colleagues, who studied the use of CPAP in 230 infants 28–31 weeks gestational age. In this study, CPAP was applied when the infant's FiO$_2$ reached 40 percent. There was no difference in the need for mechanical ventilation or in long-term outcomes. The CPAP group did have an increased incidence of pneumothorax.[93]

Surfactant and NIV

Currently, the administration of surfactant requires at least a brief period of mechanical ventilation. Attempts to avoid mechanical ventilation have meant that many of the infants in the previously described studies did not receive surfactant. This may account for the lack of effect shown in some of these studies. Surfactant has been clearly shown to be of benefit to low birth weight infants.[94] So many practitioners are moving to an approach first reported in Sweden.[95] This approach, dubbed INSURE, involves elective intubation, administration of surfactant, and extubation to NIV. The initial study of the INSURE method demonstrated a 50 percent reduction in the number of neonates requiring mechanical ventilation.[95] Using the same approach, Bhandari and associates found that infants who were intubated, given surfactant, and extubated to SNIPPV had significantly fewer deaths and BPD than infants maintained on conventional ventilation. There were no differences in other morbidities or developmental follow-up scores between the two groups.[23] In a randomized controlled trial of infants 27–32 weeks gestational age assigned to either early CPAP or intubation, surfactant, two minutes of manual ventilation, and extubation, Rojas and associates found that the infants receiving surfactant initially has less need for subsequent intubation and mechanical ventilation ($p <.05$), fewer air leaks, and less BPD ($p <.05$) than infants initially placed on CPAP.[96]

A systematic review examining the use of surfactant combined with extubation to nasal prong CPAP found a decreased need for mechanical ventilation, fewer air leaks, and a decreased rate of BPD in the group receiving early surfactant than in those receiving surfactant later.[94] Geary and coworkers report on their experience with implementing several practice changes including surfactant with nasal prong CPAP treatment at delivery, lowered oxygen saturation goals, and early amino acid administration. They compared two groups of ELBW infants, one born between 2001 and 2002, and the other born during 2004 and 2005. Implementation of these practice changes resulted in improved morbidity and growth.[97]

On the other hand, Sandri and associates found that INSURE did not offer an advantage over early NCPAP and selective surfactant in decreasing the need for mechanical ventilation or in reducing the incidence of BPD.[98] A large multi-centered study (SUPPORT trial) examined early NCPAP with intubation and surfactant in ELBW infants and found that BPD rates did not differ between the two groups. There were no differences in the rate of air leaks, necrotizing enterocolitis, intraventricular hemorrhage, or retinopathy of prematurity.[99] However, this study did not control for the temperature of the gas, level of humidity, and the type and size of nasal prongs that were used. These are important factors to control because cooler, less humidified gases may alter the infant's body temperature and increase cold stress and affect secretions. In addition, some prongs make the work of infant breathing harder. For example, it is a matter of simple physics that longer prongs with a narrow internal diameter will increase resistance and make the work of breathing harder.

A new method for administering surfactant developed by Kribs and colleagues in Germany may eliminate the need for intubation for surfactant and provide further support for the use of NCPAP at delivery. In their study, infants were stabilized on NCPAP and then given surfactant via an intratracheal catheter.[100]

ADMINISTRATION OF PRESSURE

Since the use of CPAP began, researchers have been seeking the "optimal" level of PEEP that relieves respiratory distress while causing the fewest complications. At present, no studies have been published that define the optimal levels of distending pressure for NIV. An analysis of data from the 2003 systematic review of nasal prong CPAP trials found no benefit for CPAP levels of <5 cmH$_2$O;[66] 5 cmH$_2$O has been the starting pressure most often recommended in the literature.[29]

Low levels of PEEP (0–3 cmH$_2$O) generally do little lung damage and do not cause overinflation, but may not be high enough to overcome atelectasis. In a meta-analysis of CPAP for the prevention of extubation failure, it was found that CPAP <5 cmH$_2$O was ineffective.[66] In a study of infants with mild RDS, it was found that infants had the highest end expiratory lung volumes and tidal volumes and the lowest respiratory rates at pressures of 8 cmH$_2$O.[33] At high levels of PEEP (>8 cmH$_2$O), complications such as decreased lung compliance, air leak, impaired venous return, and increased PaCO$_2$ can occur.[29]

Manipulating the amount of gas flow changes the amount of pressure delivered to the neonate (pressure = flow × resistance). A minimum flow of 5 liters/minute is necessary to generate sufficient pressure and flush carbon dioxide from the system. A maximum flow of 10 liters/minute minimizes the risk of too much distending pressure to the lungs and excessive airflow into the abdomen via the esophagus. Also, flow is a very important component of CPAP because the continuous flow of inspired gas does part of the work of breathing.[101]

It is important to maintain consistent distending pressure. A loss of pressure forces the infant to increase the work of breathing. That can lead to decreased FRC and compliance and increase symptoms of respiratory distress.

DELIVERING NIV

When CPAP was first used in neonates, it was given through an endotracheal tube.[4] Since that time, a variety of nasal prongs (short, long, single prong, and binasal prongs) and face masks have been developed for neonatal use. There is a dearth of studies comparing various delivery devices.[102]

ENDOTRACHEAL TUBE CPAP

Delivering CPAP by endotracheal tube ensures delivery of a specified amount of pressure directly to the lungs. If the infant deteriorates, mechanical ventilation can begin immediately because the infant is already intubated. However, CPAP delivered by endotracheal tube has some serious drawbacks. The endotracheal tube is longer and narrower than the neonate's trachea. Resistance is increased in tubes with longer lengths and smaller diameters.[103] CPAP delivered by endotracheal tube is analogous to breathing through a straw. Work of breathing becomes much harder, and fatigue may lead to apnea or symptoms of respiratory distress.

Because endotracheal CPAP is delivered directly to the lungs, it leaves no way for the neonate to "pop off" excess pressure, whether delivered deliberately or inadvertently. The risks of increased levels of PEEP have already been described. Other drawbacks of endotracheal CPAP include laryngeal, tracheal, and vocal cord irritation or damage, increased risk of infection, need for sterile endotracheal suctioning technique, delay of feedings, and undetected endotracheal tube malpositioning.

NASOPHARYNGEAL CPAP

Nasopharyngeal CPAP involves the insertion of one tube or a set of longer prongs through the nares to rest in the pharynx. Although this method avoids the risks associated with endotracheal tubes, it shares the significant problem of increased resistance. To facilitate their passage and decrease trauma, these tubes are narrower than the airway. Because they are also long enough to reach the pharynx, they force the neonate to work harder to breathe.

In addition, these tubes cause moderate to large amounts of secretions. Clearing these secretions to keep the system patent and effective can be difficult and time-consuming. Retropharyngeal abscess secondary to nasopharyngeal CPAP is reported rarely, but remains a potentially serious complication.[104]

FACE MASKS

Face masks were once a common method of applying positive pressure. However, with these masks, it was difficult to obtain a seal between the face and the mask that was tight enough to generate positive pressure and yet not damage the skin. During early use, neonatal face mask devices were associated with cerebellar hemorrhage.[105] Additional concerns with face masks include the loss of PEEP during suctioning and reports of gastric distention, especially at high flow rates. Soft silicone masks are now available and provide a better seal without excessive pressure on the face. Currently, there are no published data on the efficacy of these newer masks, and comparisons between face masks and nasal prongs have yet to be reported.[106]

In a recent review of nasal prong CPAP, Diblasi notes that, because face masks do not obstruct or narrow the nares, these devices may offer an advantage over binasal prongs. However, this has not yet been tested in research studies.[107] Additionally, face masks can be alternated with nasal prongs to reduce the nasal irritation seen in some infants. Further study is needed to address the use of face masks to provide NIV.

NASAL PRONGS

Nasal prongs are an easy and effective way to deliver NIV. De Paoli and colleagues found that although it remains to be determined which short binasal prongs are the most effective, the evidence suggests that short binasal prongs are more effective in preventing reintubation than are nasopharyngeal tubes.[108] There is limited research comparing the various types of binasal prongs. One study comparing Argyle prongs (Sherwood Medical, St. Louis, Missouri) to Hudson prongs (Hudson RCI, Temecula, California) in premature infants of different birth weights found that both types of prongs were effective in delivering CPAP, but nasal irritation occurred earlier in infants <1,000 g on Argyle prongs. Infants weighing between 1,000 g and 1,500 g in this study had more episodes of prong displacement with the Argyle prongs than the Hudson prongs.[109]

Several types of nasal prongs are commercially available for neonates, and each NICU has developed strategies for keeping them in place. Systems that require constant readjustment of nasal prongs, especially for the active infant, have earned NIV the reputation of being hard to work with and not very useful. Careful selection of prong type decreases staff labor and increases NIV effectiveness. The best prongs have the following characteristics:

- They are short, wide, and thin walled, to maximize airflow and decrease resistance.
- They are very soft and flexible, to minimize trauma.
- They are available in a variety of sizes, to ensure a good fit for all neonates.
- They can be easily and firmly secured, even on active neonates, to provide continuous therapy with minimal staff effort.
- Their design minimizes the chance of tissue damage or irritation. Prongs that are set on a bridge do not rest on the face. Prongs that must be set firmly against the nose to generate sufficient pressure may predispose infants to nasal septum breakdown; they should not be used.
- They have tubing that is lightweight and flexible, to allow the infant to be positioned comfortably and the NIV system to be adjusted to him, rather than vice versa.

Nasal prong CPAP has the lowest incidence of pneumothorax of the CPAP delivery types, an incidence that is comparable to that of spontaneous pneumothorax. Another major advantage of nasal prong CPAP is the speed with which the system can be applied and removed. If the equipment is at hand, a trained professional can set up and apply CPAP in only a few minutes, with minimal risk to the infant. The nasal prongs are easy to remove for suctioning and then to replace. The infant's mouth is left free for feedings, pacifiers, or hygiene.

It is also easy to take a stable baby off nasal prong CPAP for a trial. Simply remove the prongs from the nares, and observe the infant for signs of increasing distress. Weaning a chronically ill child from CPAP may be done using an on/off schedule that takes only a few minutes to perform and can be cut short if distress occurs.

Note: Do not discontinue CPAP, even briefly, by shutting off the gas flow and leaving the prongs in place. Because newborns are obligate nose breathers, either the prongs must be removed from the nares or a supply of fresh gas must be provided.

CONTRAINDICATIONS TO **NIV**

NIV will not benefit all infants requiring respiratory support and in some cases may worsen the infant's condition. At present, the delivery of surfactant requires intubation. Although infants may be intubated, given surfactant, and extubated to NIV, it has been shown that infants with surfactant deficiency who benefit from

FIGURE 8-3
Benign abdominal distention ("CPAP belly") seen in some infants receiving nasal prong CPAP.

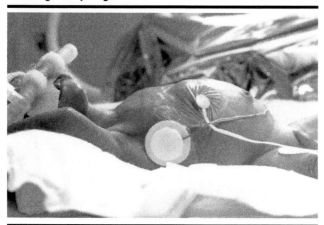

From: Jones DB, and Deveau D. 1991. Nasal prong CPAP: A proven method for the reduction of chronic lung disease. *Neonatal Network* 10(4): 7–15. Reprinted by permission.

surfactant should be treated with exogenous surfactant prior to initiating NIV.[94] However, this study should be considered along with the evidence that was previously discussed; infants who received the Columbia/CHONY nasal-prong CPAP system early (within a minute or two of life) may not have as great a need for surfactant because these infants may have less early-onset atelectasis.

Other contraindications to NIV include congenital anomalies of the airways and lungs and gastrointestinal tract, shock and sepsis, severe apnea, nasal trauma, and the presence of air leak syndromes.[6,110]

COMPLICATIONS OF NIV

Although less invasive than mechanical ventilation, NIV has a number of possible complications. The incidence and severity of these unintended effects is dependent on the size of the infant, the type of equipment used, the duration of NIV, and the level of distending pressure applied. Reported complications include abdominal distention, feeding disturbances and nasal injury, air leaks, decreased venous return, and decreased cardiac output.[8,28]

ABDOMINAL DISTENTION

A neonate on nasal prong CPAP may have some gastric and intestinal distention, or "CPAP belly" (Figure 8-3). It is unclear whether the distention is caused by the baby swallowing air, the amount of pressure in the system, decreased gut motility, or a combination of these factors. Research conducted by Jaile-Marti

and associates has shown that CPAP belly is benign and can usually be differentiated from distention caused by necrotizing enterocolitis.[111] The clinical characteristics of a benign CPAP belly are a softly distended abdomen without skin discoloration and stable vital signs. The presence of bowel loops may be a sign of necrotizing enterocolitis or may just be from the CPAP. It is important to recognize that significant abdominal distention will place upward pressure on the diaphragm and may result in respiratory compromise.[42] One study of NIPPV identified an increased rate of gastrointestinal perforation in the study group.[112] But the Cochrane review of NIPPV found no incidence of gastric perforation in the three included studies.[58–60,113]

Research by Havranek, Madramootoo, and Carver suggests that caution in evaluating infants on nasal prong CPAP is warranted. These researchers studied 18 infants between 21 and 33 weeks gestation, comparing pre- and postprandial intestinal blood flow when the infants were receiving nasal prong CPAP to their blood flow off nasal prong CPAP. They found that both the mean velocity and peak systolic velocity were significantly lower when the infants were on CPAP. The authors postulate that altered intestinal blood flow may impact feeding tolerance.[114] Research on bubble CPAP in ELBW infants does not suggest an increased risk of necrotizing enterocolitis following gastric distention caused by CPAP.[80]

NASAL IRRITATION OR SKIN BREAKDOWN

Yong, Chen, and Boo identify nasal septal irritation as a known side effect of NIV.[115] A study by Robertson and coworkers found that up to 20 percent of infants in a study of variable-flow CPAP experienced nasal injury. Injuries included necrosis of the columella nasi, flaring of nostrils, and snubbing of the nose.[116] Septal injury is usually the result of a combination of friction, pressure, and excessive moisture. It has been speculated that injury to the nasal septum may be the cause of some cases of newborn septicemia.[117] The most common cause of nasal trauma is incorrect positioning of the prongs.[6] Prevention and management of nasal trauma is discussed in the section on nursing care.

AIR LEAKS

Early studies of nasal prong CPAP in preterm infants reported an increased risk of pneumothorax and pneumomediastinum.[118,119] More recent studies show mixed results. In the COIN trial, infants randomized to early CPAP had a significantly higher incidence of pneumothorax (9 percent vs 3 percent).[92] But a study done by Rojas and colleagues showed a significantly lower risk of air leak in infants receiving CPAP after surfactant and brief ventilation than in those receiving CPAP alone (2 percent vs 9 percent).[96] The systematic review of six studies in which infants received early surfactant administration and extubation to nasal prong CPAP showed lower rates of air leaks compared to infants given surfactant and continued mechanical ventilation.[94]

CARDIAC COMPROMISE

Cardiac compromise during administration of NIV can occur if pressure levels are high enough to impede venous return.[37] A study designed to measure the impact of nasal prong CPAP on cardiac output in preterm infants found decrease in stroke volume or cardiac output when levels of CPAP between 3.5 and 5.3 cmH$_2$O were used.[120]

CARE OF INFANTS RECEIVING NIV

Caring for an infant receiving NIV poses challenges for care providers. The success of this therapy is largely dependent on keeping the prongs or face mask in the correct position and carefully assessing the infant for the effectiveness of the therapy as well as for the development of complications. Although infants receiving NIV may be less critically ill than some infants receiving mechanical ventilation, appropriate training and nurse:patient ratios remain critical in ensuring patient well-being. All infants receiving NIV should have continuous cardiorespiratory and oxygen saturation monitoring. Blood gases should be evaluated as indicated by the infant's clinical condition.[121]

RESPIRATORY ASSESSMENT

A system-by-system evaluation of the neonate's response to NIV should be performed regularly to determine the effectiveness of the treatment and to guide care. There are several methods to employ when evaluating an infant's respiratory response and the effectiveness of NIV (Table 8-3). Even in a high-tech hospital environment, skill in physical assessment is important. Many decisions about the management of neonates on NIV are based on observation and physical examination. Infants make many physical adjustments in both method and rate of breathing in an effort to maintain homeostasis *before* technological tools indicate a change in respiratory status.

For example, after a visual assessment of the neonate's retractions, respiratory rate, and overall work of

TABLE 8-3
Evaluation of Respiratory Status

Visual Observation (at rest and when awake)
- Respiratory rate
- Retractions (upper and lower chest)
- Nasal flaring
- Overall work of breathing
- Comparison of upper and lower chest movement (synchronized, lag on inspiration, or seesaw)

Auditory/Auscultation
- Breath sounds
- Grunting (inspiratory or expiratory)

Machine-based Monitoring
- Oximetry
- Blood gas analysis
- Radiography
- Transcutaneous monitoring

breathing, the nurse may conclude that the infant is not breathing comfortably. She may determine that the prongs being used are too small and that air is leaking around them. The decision to change the size of the prongs can be made before any deterioration is evidenced in the infant's oxygen saturation, blood gas values, and/ or x-ray film. All three are often late indications of the degree of respiratory distress.

During a trial off NIV, the infant may become tachypneic and show increased work of breathing by retracting and nasal flaring. The decision to restart the NIV should be based on the neonate's clinical response, even if the oxygen saturation level, blood gas values, and x-ray film remain unchanged. Just as the nurse does not wait for an infant to become hypothermic before initiating interventions to maintain a neutral thermal environment, so must she use physical assessment skills to decide to resume CPAP.

The Silverman-Andersen Retraction Score is available to help quantitate the nurse's visual assessments of the neonate (Chapter 4).[122] The index can be particularly useful for the nurse who is learning to evaluate respiratory distress. Signs that NIV is effective include a decrease in the infant's work of breathing and improvement in oxygen saturations and blood gases. The infant may remain tachypneic despite a decrease in work of breathing.[121]

How frequently the infant's respiratory status should be evaluated depends on the severity of the condition. In most situations, an evaluation every three to four hours is adequate as long as continuous oxygen saturation monitoring is maintained. When evaluating respiratory status, make visual observations of the infant's breathing when at rest and compare these to his breathing when awake or agitated. Visual observations are early indicators of how well the NIV is working, as well as of the severity and progression of the respiratory disease. When the immersion technique for generating pressure is used, the bubbling sounds may interfere with auscultation of breath sounds.

Airway Care

The percentage of humidity being delivered in the NIV system is an important component of airway care, but one that is often overlooked. As close as possible to 100 percent humidity is optimal. Gas temperatures higher than 36.5°C (97.7°F) have been shown to reduce the severity of CLD and the incidence of pneumothorax.[123] One indicator of adequate humidity is the amount of "rain out" in the system. When 100 percent humidity and the gas temperature required to maintain it are being delivered, condensation in the NIV tubing is inevitable. The tubing will need to be emptied every two to three hours or so. If no "rain out" occurs, the percentage of humidity is probably too low.

The critical importance of providing adequate humidity in the system must be emphasized. If the humidity of the gas being administered is not adequate, the infant's mucous membranes become extremely dry, making it difficult to suction the nasopharynx without causing irritation and bleeding. If bleeding occurs, scabs form that may block off part of the airway and cause pain and trauma to the infant whenever suctioning takes place. In addition, without adequate humidity, the infant's secretions will be thicker and more tenacious, making them more difficult to remove and decreasing the effectiveness of the NIV system. Every three hours, the nurse should evaluate and document the temperature of the gas so that appropriate adjustments can be made. High gas temperatures may burn or damage the mucosa of the nasopharynx or lungs. The administration of too cold or too hot gas adversely affects the infant's body temperature. Body temperature outside the neutral thermal range has a negative impact on the infant's respiratory status, including oxygen consumption, blood vessel size, and oxygen saturation. Provision of inadequately humidified gas causes the infant to use energy to warm and humidify the inspired air at the expense of thermoregulation.

When a mouth leak occurs, the unidirectional flow of air through the nose alters the normal humidification process. In a study of adults using nasal prong CPAP for sleep apnea, when participants breathed through their open mouths, nasal resistance and congestion increased considerably. Increasing the amount of humidity relieved congestion and reduced resistance.[124] According to Poiseuille's law of laminar flow, resistance is inversely proportional to the radius to the fourth power. In other words, if the radius of a tube is halved, resistance is increased 16 times. Thus, an airway blocked by thick secretions, edema, and/or scabs has increased resistance, leading to increased work of breathing and increased signs of respiratory distress. More frequent suctioning is required, but the need for frequent suctioning leads to additional trauma in the area, and a vicious cycle begins.

The airway should be assessed for patency every two to three hours and nares suctioned as necessary.[121] If the infant experiences repeated apnea and bradycardia or shows a gradual decline in oxygen saturation levels, one of the first considerations is to determine whether secretions are blocking the airway. If the infant's nasopharynx is dry and difficult to suction, the use of a few drops of normal saline before suctioning can help lubricate the area and reduce trauma. If the nasal passages are dry or the secretions are extremely thick and tenacious, the humidity of the gas being delivered may need to be reevaluated and increased. It is very important not to suction any more frequently than necessary to avoid creating edema in the nasal passages.

To retrieve secretions that pool in the naso- and oropharynx, it is important to measure suction depth before inserting the catheter. Usually a distance one and one-half times the distance from the pinna to the nares is sufficient. Using a slow, steady insertion, twist, and removal technique is more effective and less traumatic than rapid repeated insertions.

The size of suction catheter needed depends on the size of the infant. If the catheter is too small, suctioning will not be effective, and the infant will have difficulty breathing. If the catheter is too large, it may cause trauma to the area. The larger the catheter, the more effective the yield. Most infants can be suctioned effectively with a #8 French catheter (Figure 8-4).

Care of the Nasal Septum

Meticulous attention to the nasal septum is an important aspect of nursing care for infants on CPAP. There are three main culprits associated with nasal septal breakdown: pressure, friction, and excessive moisture. Increased pressure on the nasal septum decreases circulation in the area, leading to pressure necrosis. Friction causes loss of skin or mucosal integrity.

FIGURE 8-4
A Velcro mustache and nasal suctioning (on room air CPAP).

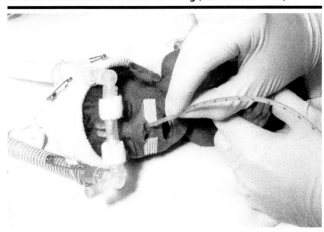

FIGURE 8-5
Correct size and positioning of nasal prongs for CPAP.

This 18-day-old, 35-week gestation infant remains on CPAP for retractions and tachypnea after extracorporeal membrane oxygenation for congenital diaphragmatic hernia.

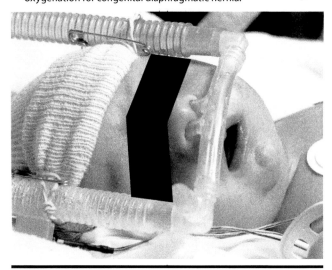

From: Jones DB, and Deveau D. 1991. Nasal prong CPAP: A proven method for the reduction of chronic lung disease. *Neonatal Network* 10(4): 7–15. Reprinted by permission.

Use of creams or hydrocolloid barriers in the area of the columella traps moisture, softening the skin and making it more susceptible to injury. They should be used cautiously and only in special circumstances.

Six components are key in helping the nurse maintain the integrity of the infant's nasal septum: (1) the type and size of nasal prongs used, (2) the hat used to anchor and position the tubing and prongs, (3) proper positioning of the neonate and the prongs, (4) use of lightweight tubing, (5) use of a Velcro mustache, and (6) avoidance of creams or routine use of hydrocolloid barriers.

The nurse must frequently assess and document the position of the nasal prongs and the condition of the nasal septum. If an infant begins to show redness of the columella, the nurse must increase the frequency of visual assessments of the area and reassess all six components individually. Occurrence of an injury does not contraindicate the use of CPAP. Prong size and placement can be adjusted to avoid further injury and permit healing while CPAP therapy is continued.

Type and Size of Prongs

The type and size of the nasal prongs used in administering CPAP are the most important component in preventing nasal septum breakdown. Prongs should fit the nares snugly without putting pressure on the nasal septum. Nasal prongs should be large enough to fill the nostrils completely without force, and part of the prong should remain outside the nose (Figure 8-5).[125] This keeps the bridge of the prongs from pressing into the septum. If the prongs are too small, not only will they allow pressure to escape, compromising the effective delivery of CPAP, but they are also more likely to cause

friction damage as they slide in and out of the nose. Also, the space between the prongs may be too narrow, pinching the septum.

Choosing large prongs that fit snugly helps keep the prongs in place, saving nursing time and decreasing the incidence of nasal irritation; the larger the prongs, the lower the airway resistance. Prong size varies based on the manufacturer's recommendations, the infant's size, and the infant's physical features. For the newborn weighing <700 g, the nostrils may need to be dilated slightly with a cotton swab lubricated in saline to allow a larger prong to fit. Some dilation of the nares occurs during nasal CPAP therapy, but in our clinical experience, the dilation is temporary and diminishes over time, often disappearing before the infant's discharge home.

Hat

A hat that is snug and stationary on the neonate's head serves as an effective anchor for the CPAP delivery system. If the hat moves around, the prongs will move around as well. *Note:* The hats that are provided with commercial prongs do not always fit well or may lose their shape over time and slide off the infant's head. A two- or three-inch- (and occasionally four-inch-) wide stockinette works best. The size of the neonate's head determines the width of the stockinette. Neonates

FIGURE 8-6
Stockinette hat with CPAP tubing secured to the rim.

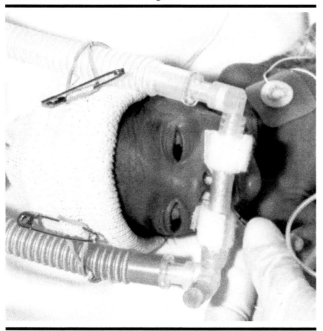

FIGURE 8-7
The use of a chest pad to facilitate prone positioning of a 13-day-old infant.

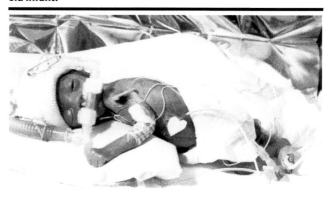

weighing <1,000 g usually require a two-inch-wide stockinette; those weighing >1,000 g usually need three-inch-wide material.

The length of the stockinette varies as well; 11 inches usually provides enough length to form a two- to three-inch-deep rim and secure the hat at the crown. The rim is made by folding the stockinette twice; the CPAP tubing is secured to the rim (Figure 8-6). A tie or rubber band on the stockinette at the crown of the head helps prevent the hat from slipping down. A more stable double-layered hat may be made by twisting a length of stockinette tubing midway and folding one end back over the other to make a two-layered sack. The open end can then be folded back to make a secure, wide rim.

As the hat loosens with use, the nurse will have more difficulty keeping the CPAP prongs in their proper position. After 24–36 hours, the hat will be stretched out and need to be replaced. Although a snug hat is important, the hat should not be so tight that it leaves ridges in the infant's skin, possibly decreasing perfusion to the area. The wider the brim, the more evenly the pressure of the tubing will be distributed.

Position the hat so that it rests along the lower part of the neonate's ears and across the forehead. Make sure that the infant's earlobes are lying flat, not folded. Clean behind the neonate's earlobes at least daily. If intravenous or arterial lines need to be placed in the

scalp while the infant is on CPAP, a hole may be cut in the hat to facilitate visualization of the site.

Infant Positioning

Labile infants in severe respiratory distress are usually positioned prone or on one side or the other using a small neck roll and supportive nesting rolls and elevating the head of the bed approximately 30 degrees. Keeping the head and neck aligned in the "sniffing" position of mild extension optimizes the airway.[106] Although the prone position is thought to enhance oxygenation, a Cochrane review on positioning for acute respiratory distress found no evidence that the prone position is better than supine or side-lying for nonventilated preterm infants.[126] Using a pad under the infant's chest is a simple way to position the baby prone (Figure 8-7). Rolls or other creative devices can be employed to facilitate positioning. Swaddling is effective in minimizing movement and can help to prevent tension on the hat or CPAP tubing. An infant on CPAP can easily be placed in a parent's arms or held skin-to-skin; however, overall handling should be limited to decrease the amount of stress on the infant.

Tubing

Lightweight respiratory tubing should be used. In-line water collection bottles should be avoided because the additional weight they add to the tubing can pull the prongs toward the nasal septum. Tubing that twists in one direction or the other makes it more difficult to keep the prongs in the nostrils and the tubing resting lightly on the infant's cheeks. The tubing should be adjusted so that it does not press into the infant's cheeks (see Figure 8-6).

Anchor the tubing to the hat using Velcro or safety pins and rubber bands. No matter which method is used, the primary consideration is that the tubing be held securely in place with enough room to make necessary fine adjustments up and down. When using safety pins (see Figure 8-6), point them toward the crown of the infant's head rather than the face. Pass the pins through all thicknesses of the hat rim, being careful not to injure the infant's scalp. Catching all layers of the rim makes a more secure attachment and keeps the hat from being pulled out of shape.

Mustache on the Philtrum

No matter how well the hat fits, how lightweight the tubing is, how the baby is positioned, or the size and type of prongs used, it is difficult in some infants to keep the prongs off the septum. For these infants, a Velcro mustache (see Figure 8-4) placed over a piece of occlusive dressing (such as Tegaderm) or ultrathin hydrocolloid has been used effectively at CHONY and St. Luke's–Roosevelt Hospital Center to maintain the prongs in the proper position. Be sure to size and position the mustache correctly so that the Velcro does not rub against the septum. The moisture in the humidified gas and in nasal and oral secretions will cause the mustache to loosen over time. When that happens, it will need to be removed and replaced so that it does not accidentally dislodge and irritate surrounding tissue or the eyes.

Creams and Barriers

Hydrocolloid barriers are often used under tape to protect the skin of premature infants. However, hydrocolloids do not protect the nasal septum from injury and may actually increase breakdown of the septum by trapping moisture around the nares.[43] For mild redness or difficulty in maintaining a seal around the nose, a thin layer of a product such as DuoDERM (Convarec, Skillman, New Jersey) can be used with caution, but should be changed every 12 hours to allow a full assessment of the nares.[43,127]

Pressure Delivery Monitoring

The opening and closing of the infant's mouth can cause the amount of pressure being delivered in the system to fluctuate. To maintain consistent pressure delivery, some units apply a chin strap (Figure 8-8). The strap, made from a strip of soft gauze or stockinette, allows the jaw to be pulled gently forward to keep the mouth closed at rest. Even a firm chin strap permits the infant to cry or yawn and allows excess pressure in the circuit to escape if necessary. No increase in aspiration

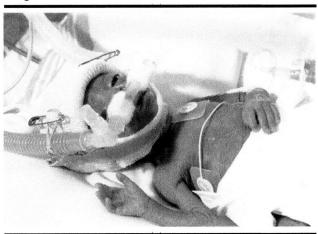

FIGURE 8-8
A chin strap on a 13-day-old infant born at 27 weeks gestation and 588 g.

of stomach contents has been documented in infants with chin straps. A pacifier can also be used to minimize pressure loss.[125]

A sudden loss of all pressure is recognized by lack of bubbling in the solution bottle, an alarm from the pressure monitor, an alarm from the ventilator, a drop in oxygen saturation, or apnea and bradycardia. The loss of pressure may be caused by a leak in the system, such as disconnected tubing, dislocated prongs, or a mechanical malfunction. A system check is warranted to see where the breakdown has occurred. If it is determined that the level of PEEP needs to be adjusted, it is advisable to remove the prongs from the infant's nares before making any changes. Test the system before replacing the prongs. With a bubble CPAP system, vigorous bubbling usually indicates excessive gas flow.

Feeding

Decisions regarding whether to feed a neonate on NIV are based on his respiratory and physiologic status. There is no contraindication to feeding a stable infant receiving NIV.[43] At least one study has shown that gastric emptying time is reduced on CPAP, perhaps because of pressure on the stomach from the diaphragm.[128]

When a neonate is on nasal prong CPAP, tube feeding is given via an orogastric tube. Tube feedings may be given intermittently or maintained as a continuous feeding, depending on the infant's condition. To help reduce the amount of distention, the stomach should be gently aspirated every three to four hours using an orogastric tube and a syringe.[43] After aspirating the stomach, remove the tube and document the amount of air obtained. Leaving the orogastric tube indwelling

FIGURE 8-9
Sample Nasal prong CPAP quality improvement tool.

Date: _____   Unit: _____   Assessment Performed by: _____

Instructions: Record the medical record number of the infant whose CPAP is being evaluated.

- Mark No for any of the following criteria not met.
- Mark N/A if the criterion is not applicable for this infant at this time.

Quality Criteria	Medical Record No.		Medical Record No.		Medical Record No.	
1. Complete provider order in chart (type of CPAP, flow, pressure, and % O_2)	☐ No		☐ No		☐ No	
2. Provider order the same as what infant is receiving	☐ No		☐ No		☐ No	
3. CPAP connected to blended air/oxygen gas supply	☐ No		☐ No		☐ No	
4. Flow between 5 and 10 liters/minute	☐ No		☐ No		☐ No	
5. Humidifier temperature and settings set to maintain humidification as close as possible to 100%	☐ No		☐ No		☐ No	
6. Tubing temperature at 37°C (98.6°F)	☐ No		☐ No		☐ No	
7. Humidifier chamber contains water	☐ No		☐ No		☐ No	
8. Neck roll size and position effectively keeping airway in mild extension	☐ No		☐ No		☐ No	
9. Neck roll removed if infant is lying prone	☐ No	☐ N/A	☐ No		☐ No	
10. Oxygen saturation probe preductal if infant requires more than 21% oxygen	☐ No	☐ N/A	☐ No	☐ N/A	☐ No	☐ N/A
11. Hat fits snugly with large, wide brim	☐ No		☐ No		☐ No	
12. Nasal prongs fit nares snugly	☐ No		☐ No		☐ No	
13. Nasal prongs not touching the nasal columella (Crossbar between prongs is 2–3 mm clear of columella and septum.)	☐ No		☐ No		☐ No	
14. Nasal prongs not twisted, rotated, or causing lateral septal pressure	☐ No		☐ No		☐ No	
15. Septum intact	☐ No		☐ No		☐ No	
16. Corrugated tubing twisted so it is not touching the infant's face	☐ No		☐ No		☐ No	
17. Corrugated tubing fixed to hat in alignment with prongs	☐ No		☐ No		☐ No	
18. Mustache adhering completely to skin, of appropriate size, clear of eyes, not touching nares or mouth	☐ No		☐ No		☐ No	
19. Chin strap in place and effectively keeping mouth closed at rest	☐ No	☐ N/A	☐ No		☐ No	
20. Head, neck, and body alignment developmentally appropriate	☐ No		☐ No		☐ No	
21. Excess rain out (efferent tubing) drained	☐ No		☐ No		☐ No	
22. Infant receiving 5 cmH$_2$O	☐ No		☐ No		☐ No	
For Bubble CPAP Only:						
a. Tape measure 7 cm mark at base of bottle	☐ No	☐ N/A	☐ No	☐ N/A	☐ No	☐ N/A
b. Tape measure 0 cm mark at water level	☐ No	☐ N/A	☐ No	☐ N/A	☐ No	☐ N/A
c. Tubing securely fixed at 5 cm under water	☐ No	☐ N/A	☐ No	☐ N/A	☐ No	☐ N/A
d. Gas bubbling continuously	☐ No	☐ N/A	☐ No	☐ N/A	☐ No	☐ N/A
23. CPAP system changed according to protocol	☐ No		☐ No		☐ No	
24. Nasal/oral suctioning intervals documented in the nurses' notes every 3 hours during the 24 hours prior to the survey	☐ No	☐ N/A	☐ No	☐ N/A	☐ No	☐ N/A
25. Respiratory therapy notes and nurses' notes show no discrepancies during the 24 hours prior to the survey	☐ No		☐ No		☐ No	
26. All electrical equipment used in CPAP delivery system has current biomed sticker	☐ No		☐ No		☐ No	

may lead to unwanted irritation and vagal stimulation without any clinical benefit. An indwelling tube may even increase the amount of air the baby swallows. If the neonate is receiving bolus gavage feedings, aspirate the stomach before feeding him.

Continuous or transpyloric feeding may be of benefit for infants with feeding intolerance.[1] If the neonate is receiving continuous feedings and has some abdominal distention, the feeding may be interrupted and air and stomach contents aspirated gently with a syringe. Any milk aspirated is returned to the stomach, and the continuous feeding is restarted.

Infants on nasal prong CPAP may nipple feed if they are clinically stable. An older, more stable infant who can tolerate short periods off CPAP may be nipple fed without the CPAP, but most infants need CPAP during feeding if they need it at other times. An infant who has passed the acute stage of respiratory illness and is otherwise stable may also be given the opportunity to suckle at the breast. Kangaroo care provides an excellent opportunity for a mother and her premature infant to explore the beginnings of the breastfeeding relationship.

EQUIPMENT MAINTENANCE

Changing the Equipment

Because of the high moisture level within an effectively humidified circuit, the NIV equipment should be changed according to the manufacturer's recommendations and unit policy. When changing the equipment of a labile or VLBW infant, it is often necessary for two people to work together. All of the new equipment should be connected and checked to be sure that it is functioning before the old system is removed. Infants weighing <1,000 g are often dependent on NIV and may experience apnea and bradycardia immediately when taken off the system. These usually resolve quickly when the NIV is replaced.

Troubleshooting

Frequent apnea and bradycardia or a decrease in oxygenation in the infant on NIV requires an examination of the equipment to look for any leaks in the system. The baby is checked for hyper- or hypoflexion of the neck, which could cause narrowing of the trachea. If no external mechanical problem is identified, the neonate should be suctioned gently and quickly to check for blockage of the airway by secretions. The most common blockage location is in the nasopharynx.

Depending on the equipment being used, excessive bubbling, an increase in pressure, or increased

TABLE 8-4
Indications for Mechanical Ventilation in Neonates at CHONY

- Marked retractions on CPAP
- Frequent, prolonged apnea on CPAP
- PaO_2 <50 mmHg with FiO_2 0.8–1.0
- $PaCO_2$ >65 mmHg (after stabilization)
- Cardiovascular collapse
- Unrepaired congenital diaphragmatic hernia

Adapted, courtesy of Columbia Presbyterian Medical Center, New York.

abdominal distention can be caused by excessive flow rates. The range of flow for all babies is between 5 and 10 liters/minute. Most infants require a flow of 6–8 liters/minute. If the flow is set too low, carbon dioxide may be retained in the system.

STAFF COMPETENCY VALIDATION AND QUALITY IMPROVEMENT

Competency validation of staff caring for infants on NIV helps ensure the delivery of high-quality, consistent care. Regular quality improvement surveys should be done to document that the standard of care is being met and to identify any deficiencies. Figure 8-9 depicts one data collection tool that can be used for this purpose. *Note:* This tool can be easily modified to document validation of clinical competence in caring for infants on a variety of NIV devices.

Each case of nasal septal erosion should be reported, evaluated, and analyzed. These data are useful in determining if there is a need for improvement strategies within the unit and among the clinical staff. Some of the variables reviewed are staffing patterns, nursing assignments, staff competency review, introduction of new products into the unit, and evaluation and scrutiny of the entire NIV setup. Multiple factors affect the incidence of nasal septal damage, making it an excellent routine multidisciplinary quality improvement surveillance activity.

CPAP FAILURE CRITERIA

Although CPAP may be used successfully by an experienced staff on even very ill, labile infants, there are limitations to its application. Determining when an infant receiving NIV needs intubation and mechanical ventilation is dependent on a number of factors. It is important for the clinician to consider the infant's gestational age, weight, and underlying medical condition. No specific parameters have been determined by research, but De Paoli and associates suggest the following as indications for intubation: significant episodes of apnea, a PCO_2 exceeding 60 mmHg, and the need for more than 60 percent oxygen to achieve acceptable oxygen saturations.[14] The risk:benefit ratio of any decision involving an invasive procedure must be carefully considered. Table 8-4 outlines the criteria for mechanical ventilation used at CHONY.

WEANING FROM CPAP

There are no evidence-based guidelines that identify the optimal approach to weaning infants from NIV. The postdelivery age at which infants are ready to be weaned from NIV can vary greatly. For example, a term infant with TTN may require CPAP for only a few hours, but an infant weighing <1,000 g may remain on room-air CPAP for several weeks because of apnea, bradycardia, and a high potential for atelectasis. The need for supplemental oxygen in the absence of cyanotic heart disease is a sign of lingering respiratory disease. Generally, weaning is initiated when the work of breathing normalizes, oxygen requirements are minimal, and the infant is not having significant apneic and bradycardic episodes. Another sign that the infant may be ready to be weaned from NIV is tolerance of short periods off of support, such as during weighing or position changes, without an increase in work of breathing or oxygen requirements.

When phasic NIV has been used, the backup rate is normally decreased, and then the infant is switched to CPAP. The CPAP pressures are then gradually weaned until they reach 4 or 5 cmH_2O. Depending on the etiology of the respiratory distress, infants may be weaned from CPAP to nasal cannula.

During a trial off CPAP, careful attention needs to be paid to maintaining a clear airway, supporting thermoregulation, and reducing energy expenditure during the trial. The initial trial-off period may last for from one to several hours. There may be some initial tachypnea as the infant adjusts to the loss of pressure support. But if this period passes without apnea, bradycardia, decreased in oxygen saturation, or other signs of worsening distress, then the trial is considered successful. Any infant taken off NIV who does not breathe comfortably and at a regular rate, or who has frequent apnea and bradycardia is not ready to be weaned from NIV.

SUMMARY

Noninvasive ventilation is a safe, effective, and relatively inexpensive method of providing ventilatory support to infants in mild to moderate respiratory distress. Early application of NIV is especially beneficial to treat symptoms and to prevent further deterioration. There is growing evidence supporting the use of NIV as a strategy to decrease the incidence and severity of BPD in low birth weight infants.

It is important to recognize that not all NIV devices have been shown to have the same benefits and, in some cases, limited research is available for devices other than CPAP. Regardless of the NIV delivery system used, careful patient assessment, attention to detail, and evidence-based practice grounded in known physiologic principles remain important nursing responsibilities. The successful use of NIV is dependent on the appropriate selection and application of equipment and on vigilant monitoring of the infant.

ACKNOWLEDGMENTS

The authors wish to acknowledge the outstanding work of Dianne Deveau, MS, RNC, on the previous edition of this chapter. We want to thank Rose de Klerk, RN, for her early contributions to this revised chapter. Their contributions remain evident throughout this revision, and their clinical skills and devotion to the infants in their care are of a standard to which we can all aspire.

Our thanks go also to Jen Tien Wung, MD, for his continued commitment to and enthusiasm in the care of these most vulnerable of patients. We thank him for sharing his clinical expertise and knowledge with us and for supporting our professional development. The nasal prong CPAP system described in this chapter is based on his work.

REFERENCES

1. Courtney SE, and Barrington KJ. 2007. Continuous positive airway pressure and noninvasive ventilation. *Clinics in Perinatology* 34(1): 73–92.

2. Soll RF. 2007. A review on noninvasive ventilation: The Cochrane Systematic Reviews 2006. *Journal of Perinatology* 27(Supplement 1): S21–S25.

3. Barach AL. 1936. The therapeutic use of helium. *JAMA* 107(16): 1273–1280.

4. Gregory GA, et al. 1973. Treatment of idiopathic respiratory distress syndrome with continuous positive airway pressure. *New England Journal of Medicine* 284(24): 1333–1340.

5. de Klerk A. 2008. Humidified high-flow nasal cannula: Is it the new and improved CPAP? *Advances in Neonatal Care* 8(2): 98–106.

6. Davis PG, Morley CJ, and Owen LS. 2009. Non-invasive respiratory support of preterm neonates with respiratory distress: Continuous positive airway pressure and nasal intermittent positive pressure ventilation. *Seminars in fetal and Neonatal Medicine* 14(1): 14–20.

7. Lee KS, et al. 1998. A comparison of underwater bubble continuous positive airway pressure with ventilator-derived continuous positive airway pressure in premature neonates ready for extubation. *Biology of the Neonate* 73(2): 69–75.

8. Donn SM, and Sinha SK. 2003. Invasive and noninvasive neonatal mechanical ventilation. *Respiratory Care* 48(4): 426–439.

9. Ramanathan R, and Sardesai S. 2008. Lung protective ventilatory strategies in very low birth weight infants. *Journal of Perinatology* 28(Supplement 1): S41–S46.

10. Morley CJ, et al. 2005. Nasal continuous positive airway pressure: Does bubbling improve gas exchange? *Archives of Disease in Childhood. Fetal and Neonatal Edition* 90(4): F343–F344.

11. Kahn DJ, et al. 2007. Unpredictability of delivered bubble nasal continuous positive airway pressure: Role of bias flow magnitude and nares-prong air leaks. *Pediatric Research* 62(3): 343–347.

12. Locke RG, et al. 1993. Inadvertent administration of positive end-distending pressure during nasal cannula flow. *Pediatrics* 91(1): 135–138.

13. Kubicka ZJ, Limauro J, and Darnall RA. 2008. Heated, humidified high-flow nasal cannula therapy: Yet another way to deliver continuous positive airway pressure? *Pediatrics* 121(1): 82–88.

14. De Paoli AG, Morley C, and Davis PG. 2003. Nasal CPAP for neonates: What do we know in 2003? *Archives of Disease in Childhood. Fetal and Neonatal Edition* 88(3): F168–F172.

15. American Association for Respiratory Care. 2002. Selection of an oxygen delivery device for neonatal and pediatric patients—2002 revision and update. Retrieved January 4, 2010, from http://www.rcjournal.com/cpgs/pdf/06.02.707.pdf.

16. Graham PL III, et al. 2006. Risk factors for late onset Gram-negative sepsis in low birth weight infants hospitalized in the neonatal intensive care unit. *The Pediatric Infectious Disease Journal* 25(2): 113–117.

17. Shoemaker MT, et al. 2007. High flow nasal cannula versus nasal CPAP for neonatal respiratory disease: a retrospective study. *Journal of Perinatology* 27(2): 85–91.

18. Owen LS, Morley CJ, and Davis PG. 2007. Neonatal nasal intermittent positive pressure ventilation: What do we know in 2007? *Archives of Disease in Childhood. Fetal and Neonatal Edition* 92(5): F414–F418.

19. Moretti C, et al. 1999. Comparing the effects of nasal synchronized intermittent positive pressure ventilation (nSIPPV) and nasal continuous positive airway pressure (NCPAP) after extubation in very low birth weight infants. *Early Human Development* 56(2-3): 167–177.

20. Khalaf MN, et al. 2001. A prospective randomized, controlled trial comparing synchronized nasal intermittent positive pressure ventilation versus nasal continuous positive airway pressure as modes of extubation. *Pediatrics* 108(1): 13–17.

21. Lin CH, et al. 1998. Efficacy of nasal intermittent positive pressure ventilation in treating apnea of prematurity. *Pediatric Pulmonology* 26(5): 349–353.

22. Kiciman NM, et al. 1998. Thoracoabdominal motion in newborns during ventilation delivered by endotracheal tube or nasal prongs. *Pediatric Pulmonology* 25(3): 175–181.

23. Bhandari V, et al. 2007. A randomized controlled trial of synchronized nasal intermittent positive pressure ventilation in RDS. *Journal of Perinatology* 27(11): 697–703.

24. Migliori C, et al. 2005. Nasal bilevel vs. continuous positive airway pressure in preterm infants. *Pediatric Pulmonology* 40(5): 426–430.

25. Ancora G, et al. 2010. Role of bilevel positive airway pressure in the management of preterm newborns who have received surfactant. *Acta Paediatrica* 99(12): 1807–1811.

26. Lista G, et al. 2010. Nasal continuous positive airway pressure (CPAP) vs bi-level nasal CPAP in preterm babies with respiratory distress syndrome: A randomized control trial. *Archives of Disease in Childhood. Fetal and Neonatal Edition* 95(2): F85–F89.

27. DiBlasi RM. 2011. Neonatal noninvasive ventilation techniques: Do we really need to intubate? *Respiratory Care* 56(9): 1273–1294.

28. Polin RA, and Sahni R. 2002. Newer experience with CPAP. *Seminars in Neonatology* 7(5): 379–389.

29. Davis PG, and Morley CJ. 2008. Noninvasive respiratory support: An alternative to mechanical ventilation in preterm infants. In *The Newborn Lung*, Bancalari E, ed. Philadelphia: Saunders, 361–376.

30. Locke R, et al. 1991. Effect of nasal CPAP on thoracoabdominal motion in neonates with respiratory insufficiency. *Pediatric Pulmonology* 11(3): 259–264.

31. Bancalari E, and del Moral T. 2006. Continuous positive airway pressure: Early, late, or stay with synchronized intermittent mandatory ventilation? *Journal of Perinatology* 26(supplement 1): S33–S37.

32. Miller MJ, et al. 1990. Effects of nasal CPAP on supraglottic and total pulmonary resistance in preterm infants. *Journal of Applied Physiology* 68(1): 141–146.

33. Elgellab A, et al. 2001. Effects of nasal continuous positive airway pressure (NCPAP) on breathing pattern in spontaneously breathing premature newborn infants. *Intensive Care Medicine* 27(11): 1782–1787.

34. Durand M, McCann E, and Brady JP. 1983. Effect of continuous positive airway pressure on the ventilatory response to CO2 in preterm infants. *Pediatrics* 71(4): 634–638.

35. Zhang S, Garbutt V, and McBride JT. 1996. Strain-induced growth of the immature lung. *Journal of Applied Physiology* 81(4): 1471–1476.

36. Jobe AH, et al. 2002. Decreased indicators of lung injury with continuous positive expiratory pressure in preterm lambs. *Pediatric Research* 52(3): 387–392.

37. Sherman TI, et al. 2003. Physiologic effects of CPAP: Application and monitoring. *Neonatal Network* 22(6): 7–16.

38. Cotton RB, et al. 1980. Effect of positive-end-expiratory-pressure on right ventricular output in lambs with hyaline membrane disease. *Acta Paediatrica Scandinavica* 69(5): 603–606.

39. Fewell JE, and Norton JB Jr. 1980. Continuous positive airway pressure impairs renal function in newborn goats. *Pediatric Research* 14(10): 1132–1134.

40. Annat G, et al. 1983. Effect of PEEP ventilation on renal function, plasma renin, aldosterone, neurophysins and urinary ADH, and prostaglandins. *Anesthesiology* 58(2): 136–141.

41. Hall SV, Johnson EE, and Hedley-Whyte J. 1974. Renal hemodynamics and function with continuous positive-pressure ventilation in dogs. *Anesthesiology* 41(5): 452–461.

42. Upadhyay A, and Deorari AK. 2004. Continuous positive airway pressure—a gentler approach to ventilation. *Indian Pediatrics* 41(5): 459–469.

43. Bonner KM, and Mainous RO. 2008. The nursing care of the infant receiving bubble CPAP therapy. *Advances in Neonatal Care* 8(2): 78–95.

44. Gabriele G, et al. 1977. Continuous airway pressure breathing with the head-box in the newborn lamb: Effects on regional blood flows. *Pediatrics* 59(6): 858–864.

45. Aidinis SJ, Lafferty J, and Shapiro HM. 1976. Intracranial responses to PEEP. *Anesthesiology* 45(3): 275–286.

46. Stefanescu BM, et al. 2003. A randomized, controlled trial comparing two different continuous positive airway pressure systems for the successful extubation of extremely low birth weight infants. *Pediatrics* 112(5): 1031–1038.

47. Gupta S, et al. 2009. A randomized controlled trial of post-extubation bubble continuous positive airway pressure versus Infant Flow Driver continuous positive airway pressure in preterm infants with respiratory distress syndrome. *Journal of Pediatrics* 154(5): 645–650.

48. Boumecid H, et al. 2007. Influence of three nasal continuous positive airway pressure devices on breathing pattern in preterm infants. *Archives of Disease in Childhood. Fetal and Neonatal Edition* 92(4): F298–F300.

49. Liptsen E, et al. 2005. Work of breathing during nasal continuous positive airway pressure in preterm infants: A comparison of bubble vs variable-flow devices. *Journal of Perinatology* 25(7): 453–458.

50. Courtney SE, et al. 2001. Lung recruitment and breathing pattern during variable versus continuous flow nasal continuous positive airway pressure in premature infants: An evaluation of three devices. *Pediatrics* 107(2): 304–308.

51. Pandit PB, et al. 2001. Work of breathing during constant- and variable-flow nasal continuous positive airway pressure in preterm neonates. *Pediatrics* 108(3): 682–685.

52. Sreenan C, et al. 2001. High-flow nasal cannulae in the management of apnea of prematurity: A comparison with conventional nasal continuous positive airway pressure. *Pediatrics* 107(5): 1081–1083.

53. Saslow JG, et al. 2006. Work of breathing using high-flow nasal cannula in preterm infants. *Journal of Perinatology* 26(8): 476–480.

54. Campbell DM, et al. 2006. Nasal continuous positive airway pressure from high flow cannula versus infant flow for preterm infants. *Journal of Perinatology* 26(9): 546–549.

55. Dani C, et al. 2009. High flow nasal cannula therapy as respiratory support in the preterm infant. *Pediatric Pulmonology* 44(7): 629–634.

56. Lemyre B, Davis PG, and de Paoli AG. 2002. Nasal intermittent positive pressure ventilation (NIPPV) versus nasal continuous positive airway pressure (NCPAP) for apnea of prematurity. *Cochrane Database of Systematic Reviews* (1): CD002272.

57. De Paoli AG, Davis PG, and Lemyre B. 2003. Nasal continuous positive airway pressure versus nasal intermittent positive pressure ventilation for preterm neonates: A systematic review and meta-analysis. *Acta Paediatrica* 92(1): 70–75.

58. Barrington KJ, Bull D, and Finer NN. 2001. Randomized trial of nasal synchronized intermittent mandatory ventilation compared with continuous positive airway pressure after extubation of very low birth weight infants. *Pediatrics* 107(4): 638–641.

59. Friedlich P, et al. 1999. A randomized trial of nasopharyngeal-synchronised intermittent mandatory ventilation versus nasopharyngeal continuous positive airway pressure in very low birth weight infants after extubation. *Journal of Perinatology* 19 (6 part 1): 413–418.

60. Khalaf MN, et al. 1999. A prospective randomized, controlled trial comparing synchronized nasal intermittent positive pressure ventilation (SNIPPV) versus nasal continuous positive airway pressure (NCPAP) as mode of extubation. *Pediatric Research* 45: 204A.

61. Ryan CA, Finer NN, and Peters KL. 1989. Nasal intermittent positive-pressure ventilation offers no advantages over nasal continuous positive airway pressure in apnea of prematurity. *American Journal of Diseases of Children* 143(10): 1196–1198.

62. Kugelman A, et al. 2007. Nasal intermittent mandatory ventilation versus nasal continuous positive airway pressure for respiratory distress syndrome: A randomized, controlled, prospective study. *Journal of Pediatrics* 150(5): 521–526.

63. Moretti C, et al. 2008. Nasal flow-synchronized intermittent positive pressure ventilation to facilitate weaning in very low-birthweight infants: Unmasked randomized controlled trial. *Pediatrics International* 50(1): 85–91.

64. Aghai ZH, et al. 2006. Synchronized nasal intermittent positive pressure ventilation (SNIPPV) decreases work of breathing (WOB) in premature infants with respiratory distress syndrome (RDS) compared to nasal continuous positive airway pressure (NCPAP). *Pediatric Pulmonology* 41(9): 875–881.

65. Ali N, et al. 2007. Effects of non-invasive pressure support ventilation (NI-PSV) on ventilation and respiratory effort in very low birth weight infants. *Pediatric Pulmonology* 42(8): 704–710.

66. Ho JJ, et al. 2002. Continuous distending pressure for respiratory distress syndrome in preterm infants. *Cochrane Database of Systematic Reviews* (2): CD002271.

67. Gau GS, Ryder TA, and Mobberley MA. 1987. Iatrogenic epithelial change caused by endotracheal intubation of neonates. *Early Human Development* 15(4): 221–229.

68. Espagne S, and Hascoët JM. 2002. Noninvasive ventilation of premature infants. *Archives de Pédiatrie* 9(10): 1100–1103.

69. Speidel BD, and Dunn PM. 1976. Use of nasal continuous positive airway pressure to treat severe recurrent apnoea in very preterm infants. *Lancet* 2(7987): 658–660.

70. Martin RJ, et al. 1977. The effect of low continuous positive airway pressure on the reflex control of respiration in the preterm infant. *Journal of Pediatrics* 90(6): 976–981.

71. Miller MJ, Carlo WA, and Martin RJ. 1985. Continuous positive airway pressure selectively reduces obstructive apnea in preterm infants. *Journal of Pediatrics* 106(1): 91–94.

72. Kattwinkel J, et al. 1975. Apnea of prematurity. Comparative therapeutic effects of cutaneous stimulation and nasal continuous positive airway pressure. *Journal of Pediatrics* 86(4): 588–592.

73. Henderson-Smart DJ, Subramaniam P, and Davis PG. 2001. Continuous positive airway pressure versus theophylline for apnea in preterm infants. *Cochrane Database of Systematic Reviews* (4): CD001072.

74. Jobe AH, and Bancalari E. 2001. Bronchopulmonary dysplasia. *American Journal of Respiratory Critical Care Medicine* 163(7): 1723–1729.

75. Avery ME, et al. 1987. Is chronic lung disease in low birth weight infants preventable? A survey of eight centers. *Pediatrics* 79(1): 26–30.

76. Tarnow-Mordi W. 1994. International comparisons of hospital performance. *International Neonatal Network Newsletter* No. 4.

77. Van Marter LJ, et al. 2000. Do clinical markers of barotrauma and oxygen toxicity explain interhospital variation in rates of chronic lung disease? *Pediatrics* 105(6): 1194–1201.

78. de Klerk AM, and de Klerk R. 2001. Nasal continuous positive airway pressure and outcomes in preterm infants. *Journal of Paediatrics and Child Health* 37(2): 161–167.

79. Meyer M, Mildenhall L, and Wong M. 2004. Outcomes for infants weighing less than 1000 grams cared for with a nasal continuous positive airway pressure-based strategy. *Journal of Paediatrics and Child Health* 40(1-2): 38–41.

80. Narendran V, et al. 2003. Early bubble CPAP and outcomes in ELBW preterm infants. *Journal of Perinatology* 23(3): 195–199.

81. Nowadzky T, Pantoja A, and Britton JR. 2009. Bubble continuous positive airway pressure, a potentially better practice, reduces the use of mechanical ventilation among very low birth weight infants with respiratory distress syndrome. *Pediatrics* 123(6): 1534–1540.

82. Kamper J, et al. 1993. Early treatment with nasal continuous positive airway pressure in very-low-birth-weight infants. *Acta Paediatrica* 82(2): 193–197.

83. Jacobsen T, et al. 1993. "Minitouch" treatment of very-low-birth-weight infants. *Acta Paediatrica* 82(11): 934–938.

84. Gittermann MK, et al. 1997. Early nasal continuous positive airway pressure treatment reduces the need for intubation in very low birth weight infants. *European Journal of Pediatrics* 156(5): 384–388.

85. Lindner W, et al. 1999. Delivery room management of extremely low birth weight infants: Spontaneous breathing or intubation? *Pediatrics* 103(5 Part 1): 961–967.

86. Joris N, Sudre P, and Moessinger A. 2000. Early application of CPAP in newborns with gestational age below 34 weeks lowers intubation rate and shortens oxygen therapy without altering mortality and morbidity. *Schweizerische Medizinische Wochenschrift* 130(49): 1887–1893.

87. Aly H, et al. 2004. Does the experience with the use of nasal continuous positive airway pressure improve over time in extremely low birth weight infants? *Pediatrics* 114(3): 697–702.

88. Miksch RM, et al. 2008. Outcome of very low birthweight infants after introducing a new standard regime with the early use of nasal CPAP. *European Journal of Pediatrics* 167(8): 909–916.

89. Kirchner L, et al. 2005. Is the use of early nasal CPAP associated with lower rates of chronic lung disease and retinopathy of prematurity? Nine years of experience with the Vermont Oxford Neonatal Network. *Journal of Perinatal Medicine* 33(1): 60–66.

90. te Pas AB, and Walther FJ. 2007. A randomized, controlled trial of delivery-room respiratory management in very preterm infants. *Pediatrics* 120(2): 322–329. (Published erratum in *Pediatrics*, 2007, 120[4]: 936.)

91. Finer NN, et al. 2004. Delivery room continuous positive airway pressure/ positive end-expiratory pressure in extremely low birth weight infants: A feasibility trial. *Pediatrics* 114(3): 651–657.

92. Morley CJ, et al. 2008. Nasal CPAP or intubation at birth for very preterm infants. *New England Journal of Medicine* 358(7): 700–708. (Published erratum in *New England Journal of Medicine*, 2008, 358[14]: 1529.)

93. Sandri F, et al. 2004. Prophylactic nasal continuous positive airways pressure in newborns of 28–31 weeks gestation: Multicentre randomised controlled clinical trial. *Archives of Disease in Childhood. Fetal and Neonatal Edition* 89(5): F394–F398.

94. Stevens TP, et al. 2007. Early surfactant administration with brief ventilation vs. selective surfactant and continued mechanical ventilation for preterm infants with or at risk for respiratory distress syndrome. *Cochrane Database of Systematic Reviews* (4): CD003063.

95. Bohlin K, et al. 2007. Implementation of surfactant treatment during continuous positive airway pressure. *Journal of Perinatology* 27(7): 422–427.

96. Rojas MA, et al. 2009. Very early surfactant without mandatory ventilation in premature infants treated with early continuous positive airway pressure: A randomized, controlled trial. *Pediatrics* 123(1): 137–142.

97. Geary CA, et al. 2008. Improved growth and decreased morbidities in <1000 g neonates after early management changes. *Journal of Perinatology* 28(5): 347–353.

98. Sandri F, et al. 2010. Prophylactic or early selective surfactant combined with NCPAP in very preterm infants. *Pediatrics* 125(6): e1402–e1409.

99. Finer NN, et al., 2010. SUPPORT Study Group of the Eunice Kennedy Shriver NICHD Neonatal Research Network. Early CPAP versus surfactant in extremely preterm infants. *New England Journal of Medicine* 362(21): 1970–1979.

100. Kribs A, et al. 2010. Surfactant without intubation in preterm infants with respiratory distress: First multi-center data. *Klinische Padiatrie* 222(1): 13–17.

101. Katz JA, Kraemer RW, and Gjerde GE. 1985. Inspiratory work and airway pressure with continuous positive airway pressure delivery systems. *Chest* 88(4): 519–526.

102. Wisewell TE, and Srinivasan P. 2003. Continuous airway pressure. In *Assisted Ventilation of the Neonate*, 4th ed., Goldsmith JP, and Karotkin EH, eds. Philadelphia: Saunders, 127–147.

103. Wall MA. 1980. Infant endotracheal tube resistance: Effects of changing length, diameter, and gas density. *Critical Care Medicine* 8(1): 38–40.

104. Jones SW, and King JM. 1993. Retropharyngeal abscess secondary to nasopharyngeal CPAP in a preterm neonate (letter). *Archives of Disease in Childhood* 68(5 Special No.): 620.

105. Pape KE, Armstrong DL, and Fitzhardinge PM. 1976. Central nervous system pathology associated with mask ventilation in the very low birthweight infant: a new etiology for intracerebellar hemorrhages. *Pediatrics* 58(4): 473–483.

106. Morley C, and Davis P. 2004. Continuous positive airway pressure: Current controversies. *Current Opinion in Pediatrics* 16(2): 141–145.

107. Diblasi RM. 2009. Nasal continuous positive airway pressure (CPAP) for the respiratory care of the newborn infant. *Respiratory Care* 54(9): 1209–1235.

108. De Paoli AG, et al. 2008. Devices and pressure sources for administration of nasal continuous positive airway pressure (NCPAP) in preterm neonates. *Cochrane Database of Systematic Reviews* (1): CD002977.

109. Rego MA, and Martinez FE. 2002. Comparison of two nasal prongs for application of continuous positive airway pressure in neonates. *Pediatric Critical Care Medicine* 3(3): 239–243.

110. Hutchison AA, and Bignall S. 2008. Non-invasive positive pressure ventilation in the preterm neonate: Reducing endotrauma and the incidence of bronchopulmonary dysplasia. *Archives of Disease in Childhood. Fetal and Neonatal Edition* 93(1): F64–F68.

111. Jaile-Marti J, et al. 1992. Benign gaseous distension of the bowel in premature infants treated with nasal continuous airway pressure: A study of contributing factors. *American Journal of Roentgenology* 158(1): 125–127.

112. Garland JS, et al. 1985. Increased risk of gastrointestinal perforations in neonates mechanically ventilated with either face mask or nasal prongs. *Pediatrics* 76(3): 406–410.

113. Davis PG, Lemyre B, and de Paoli AG. 2001. Nasal intermittent positive pressure ventilation (NIPPV) versus nasal continuous positive airway pressure (NCPAP) for preterm neonates after extubation. *Cochrane Database of Systematic Reviews* (3): CD003212.

114. Havranek T, Madramootoo C, and Carver JD. 2007. Nasal continuous airway pressure affects pre- and postprandial intestinal blood flow velocity in preterm infants. *Journal of Perinatology* 27(11): 704–708.

115. Yong SC, Chen SJ, and Boo NY. 2005. Incidence of nasal trauma associated with nasal prong versus nasal mask during continuous positive airway pressure treatment in very low birthweight infants: A randomised control study. *Archives of Disease in Childhood. Fetal and Neonatal Edition* 90(6): F480–F483.

116. Robertson NJ, et al. 1996. Nasal deformities resulting from flow driver continuous positive airway pressure. *Archives of Disease in Childhood. Fetal and Neonatal Edition* 75(3): F209–F212.

117. Ronnestad A, et al. 2005. Septicemia in the first week of life in a Norwegian national cohort of extremely premature infants. *Pediatrics* 115(3): e262–e268.

118. Hall RT, and Rhodes PG. 1975. Pneumothorax and pneumomediastinum in infants with idiopathic respiratory distress syndrome receiving continuous positive airway pressure. *Pediatrics* 55(4): 493–496.

119. Ogata ES, et al. 1976. Pneumothorax in the respiratory distress syndrome: incidence and effect on vital signs, blood gases, and pH. *Pediatrics* 58(2): 177–183.

120. Moritz B, et al. 2008. Nasal continuous positive airway pressure (n-CPAP) does not change cardiac output in preterm infants. *American Journal of Perinatology* 25(2): 105–109.

121. Askin DF. 2007. Noninvasive ventilation in the neonate. *Journal of Perinatal & Neonatal Nursing* 21(4): 349–358.

122. Silverman WA, and Andersen DH. 1956. A controlled clinical trial of effects of water mist on obstructive respiratory signs, death rate and necropsy findings among premature infants. *Pediatrics* 17(1): 1–10.

123. Tarnow-Mordi WO, et al. 1989. Low inspired gas temperature and respiratory complications in very low birth weight infants. *Journal of Pediatrics* 114(3): 438–442.

124. Richards GN, et al. 1996. Mouth leak with nasal continuous positive airway pressure increases nasal airway resistance. *American Journal of Respiratory Critical Care Medicine* 154(1): 182–186.

125. Bohlin K, et al. 2008. Continuous positive airway pressure and surfactant. *Neonatology* 93(4): 309–315.

126. Wells DA, Gillies D, and Fitzgerald DA. 2005. Positioning for acute respiratory distress in hospitalized infants and children. *Cochrane Database of Systematic Reviews* (2): CD003645.

127. McCoskey L. 2008. Nursing Care Guidelines for prevention of nasal breakdown in neonates receiving nasal CPAP. *Advances in Neonatal Care* 8(2): 116–124.

128. Gounaris A, et al. 2004. Gastric emptying in very-low-birth-weight infants treated with nasal continuous positive airway pressure. *Journal of Pediatrics* 145(4): 508–510.

NOTES

NOTES

9 Synchronized and Volume-Targeted Ventilation

Martin Keszler, MD

Mechanical ventilation has improved to the point where few infants now die of acute respiratory failure. Early mortality is now predominantly from other complications of extreme prematurity, such as infection and hemorrhage. This development has shifted the clinical focus from reducing mortality to reducing the still unacceptably high incidence of chronic lung disease. Although high-frequency ventilation has shown promise in this regard, inconsistent results and continued concerns about the hazards of inadvertent hyperventilation have limited its acceptance as first-line therapy in infants with uncomplicated respiratory distress syndrome (RDS).[1] At the same time, with improved technology, synchronized (also known as patient-triggered) ventilation has become widely available. Even more promising is the advent of volume-targeted modalities of conventional ventilation that, for the first time, allow effective control of delivered tidal volume for neonatal ventilation. This chapter briefly reviews the basic modes of synchronized ventilation, describes the concept of volume-targeted ventilation, and discusses the clinical application of both.

SYNCHRONIZED VENTILATION

The standard type of mechanical ventilation used in newborn infants before the introduction of synchronized modes was known as intermittent mandatory ventilation (IMV). IMV is a time-cycled, pressure-limited mode of ventilation that provides a set number of "mandatory" mechanical breaths. The patient is able to breathe spontaneously at any time, using the fresh gas flow available in the ventilator circuit, which at the same time provides positive end-expiratory pressure (PEEP). Unfortunately,

the infant's random respiratory rate frequently leads to asynchrony between the infant and the ventilator.

High airway pressures, poor oxygenation, and large fluctuations in intracranial pressure result from instances when the ventilator inspiratory cycle occurs just as the infant is breathing out. Heavy sedation and muscle paralysis were often employed to suppress the infant's spontaneous respiratory effort and prevent him from "fighting the ventilator." These interventions resulted in greater dependence on respiratory support, lack of respiratory muscle training, generalized edema, and inability to assess the infant's neurologic status.

The advantages of synchronizing the infant's spontaneous effort with the ventilator cycle, instead of using muscle relaxants, seem intuitively obvious (Table 9-1). However, the introduction of synchronized ventilation into clinical practice in neonates lagged far behind its use in adults because of technological challenges imposed by the small size and rapid respiratory rates of preterm newborns.

TYPES OF TRIGGERING DEVICES

The ideal triggering device must be sensitive enough to be activated by a small preterm infant, yet relatively immune from auto-triggering. It must also have a sufficiently rapid response time to match the short inspiratory times and rapid respiratory rates seen in small premature infants. Variable leakage of gas around uncuffed endotracheal tubes (ETTs) adds another significant problem. Table 9-2 lists the types of triggering devices used in clinical care and their relative advantages and disadvantages. Clinical and laboratory experience has shown that flow triggering using a flow sensor at the

TABLE 9-1
Generally Accepted Benefits of Synchronized Mechanical Ventilation

Elimination of asynchrony
Avoidance of muscle paralysis
Decreased need for sedation
Reduction of airway pressures
Decreased risk of barotrauma and intraventricular hemorrhage
Facilitation of respiratory muscle training
Facilitation of weaning

TABLE 9-2
Comparison of Triggering Methods

Method	Advantages	Disadvantages
Pressure	No added dead space	Poor sensitivity
		Long trigger delay
		High work of breathing
Airflow	Most sensitive	Added dead space
Pneumatic capsule	Rapid response	Positioning is critical
	No extra dead space	
Impedance	No added dead space	Poor sensitivity
		Artifacts

airway opening (at the ETT adapter) is ultimately the best compromise.[2,3] At this time, all infant ventilators in common use utilize this triggering mode. An attractive new concept is to use the electrical activity of the diaphragm to trigger the ventilator. This technique requires the placement of an esophageal probe to sense the diaphragmatic contraction and modulate the inspiratory pressure of the ventilator. It is unaffected by leak around endotracheal tubes and has a very rapid response time. However, currently its availability is limited to a single device, and the triggering function cannot be separated from the proportional assist component, which may not function optimally in preterm infants with immature respiratory control (see below).

POTENTIAL PITFALLS OF FLOW TRIGGERING

Although flow triggering is the most widely used method, there are potential problems with this mode of triggering. The interposition of the flow sensor adds approximately 0.5–1 mL of dead space to the breathing circuit, which may become proportionally more significant with the tiniest of infants. Claure and colleagues describe introducing a small, fixed leak into the circuit, which makes it possible to effectively wash out the dead space of the flow sensor.[4] If this approach proves to be practical in the clinical setting, it would eliminate one drawback of flow triggering.

The second problem is susceptibility to auto-triggering in the presence of significant leakage around the ETT. Any substantial leakage of flow during the expiratory phase is (mis)interpreted by the device as inspiratory effort, triggering the ventilator at an excessively rapid rate. When recognized, the problem can be corrected by decreasing trigger sensitivity. Unfortunately, the magnitude of the leak often changes quite rapidly, requiring frequent adjustment. Furthermore, making the trigger less sensitive increases the effort needed to trigger the device and increases the trigger delay; both highly undesirable. One device, the Dräger Babylog 8000 plus

(Dräger Medical, Inc., Lübeck, Germany), offers an elegant solution to this problem. The Babylog 8000 plus utilizes a proprietary leak compensation technology that allows the device to instantaneously derive the leak flow throughout the ventilator cycle and mathematically subtract this flow from the measured value. This effectively eliminates the leak-related problem of auto-triggering and allows the trigger sensitivity to remain at the most sensitive value, preserving rapid response time and minimal work to trigger the device.

SYNCHRONIZED VENTILATION MODES

Considerable confusion exists in the terminology used to describe various modalities of respiratory support. Device manufacturers often use different terms to describe essentially identical modes. In basic terms, ventilator breaths can be time or flow cycled (onset of inspiration and expiration) and pressure or volume limited. Triggering can occur at a fixed rate set by the user or at a variable rate determined by the patient. Detailed discussion of the terminology is beyond the scope of this chapter. The interested reader is referred to in-depth reviews of the subject.[5] The following sections briefly define the terminology for modes used primarily in newborns.

Synchronized Intermittent Mandatory Ventilation

The synchronized intermittent mandatory ventilation (SIMV) mode provides a preset number of mechanical breaths as in standard IMV, but the breaths are synchronized with the infant's spontaneous respiratory effort, if present. Spontaneous breaths in excess of the preset number are not supported, resulting in uneven tidal volumes (V_T) and potentially a high work of breathing (WOB), especially during weaning. This is an important issue, particularly in extremely small and immature infants with correspondingly narrow ETTs. The high airway resistance of a narrow ETT, the infant's limited muscle strength, and the mechanical disadvantage conferred by the infant's excessively compliant chest wall typically result in small, ineffective V_T. Because anatomic dead space is fixed, a very small V_T that largely is dead-space gas being recirculated contributes little to effective alveolar ventilation (alveolar ventilation = minute ventilation – dead-space ventilation). To maintain adequate alveolar minute ventilation with the limited number of mechanical breaths provided by the ventilator in SIMV mode, relatively large V_T is required.

Assist/Control

Like SIMV, assist/control (A/C) is a time-cycled, pressure-limited mode, but unlike in SIMV, in A/C, every spontaneous breath that exceeds the trigger threshold is supported by the ventilator. This approach delivers more uniform V_T and lowers the WOB. The clinician still sets a ventilator rate for mandatory breaths, which provides a minimum rate in case of apnea. This rate should normally be set slightly below the infant's spontaneous rate so as not to preempt spontaneous breaths. Because the infant controls the effective ventilator rate, weaning is accomplished by lowering the peak inspiratory pressure, rather than the ventilator rate. This approach decreases the amount of support provided to each breath, allowing the infant gradually to take over the WOB. One reason for the apparent reluctance to adopt this mode appears to be this slightly less intuitive weaning strategy.

Pressure Support Ventilation

Pressure support ventilation (PSV) is a flow-, rather than time-, cycled, pressure-limited mode that supports every spontaneous breath (just as A/C does). However, PSV also terminates each breath when inspiratory flow declines to a preset threshold, usually 10–20 percent of peak flow. This feature eliminates inspiratory hold (prolonged inspiratory time, which keeps the lungs at peak inflation) and thus presumably provides more optimal synchrony. In some devices, PSV can be used to support spontaneous breathing between low-rate SIMV to overcome the problems associated with the patient's inadequate spontaneous respiratory effort and high ETT resistance. However, with some devices, PSV is used as a stand-alone technique, much like A/C.

Proportional Assist Ventilation

Proportional assist ventilation (PAV) is an interesting technique not currently available in the U.S. Based on elastic and resistive unloading of the respiratory system, PAV aims to overcome the added workload imposed by poor lung compliance and high airway and ETT/

ventilator circuit resistance.[6] The ventilator develops inspiratory pressure in proportion to patient effort—in essence, it is a positive feedback system. The concept assumes a mature respiratory control mechanism and a closed system. Unfortunately, neither of these assumptions is valid in the preterm infant with an uncuffed ETT. For example, the common problem of periodic breathing would be accentuated by the ventilator, with less support being generated with hypopnea and an excessively high level of assistance provided when the infant becomes agitated. Also, because the system responds to inspiratory flow and volume, a large leak around the ETT would be interpreted as a large inspiration and given a correspondingly high level of inspiratory pressure, potentially leading to a dangerously large V_T. Limited clinical data are available on the use of PAV in preterm infants.

Neurally Adjusted Ventilatory Assist

Neurally adjusted ventilatory assist (NAVA) utilizes the electrical activity of the diaphragm to trigger and modulate inspiratory gas flow. Similar to PAV, it assumes a mature respiratory control center. Like PAV, it is a positive feedback control mechanism, providing higher pressure when the infant breathes vigorously and less or no support when the infant hypoventilates or becomes apneic. As such, it may not be suitable for preterm infants, who are notorious for their periodic breathing. Although the available backup rate will adequately deal with apnea, the potential to accentuate periodic breathing is an issue that requires careful evaluation.

Choosing a Synchronized Mode

Despite years of routine use, there is no clear consensus regarding the relative merits of A/C and SIMV, the two most widely used modalities of synchronized ventilation. Information documenting the superiority of one mode over the other is limited. There are no large prospective trials with important clinical outcomes, such as incidence of air leak, chronic lung disease, or length of ventilation. However, short-term clinical trials have demonstrated smaller and less variable V_T, less tachypnea, more rapid weaning from mechanical ventilation, and smaller fluctuations in blood pressure with A/C than with SIMV.[7-10]

There are important physiologic considerations, as outlined earlier, why SIMV may not provide optimal support in very premature infants. However, many clinicians still prefer SIMV, especially for weaning from mechanical ventilation. This preference is based on the assumption, unsupported by data, that fewer mechanical

FIGURE 9-1
Interaction of patient and ventilator pressures to generate delivered V_T with different modes of synchronized ventilation.

The V_T is the result of the combined inspiratory effort of the patient (negative intrapleural pressure on inspiration) and the positive pressure generated by the ventilator. This combined effort (the baby "pulling" and the ventilator "pushing") results in the transpulmonary pressure, which together with the compliance of the respiratory system, determines the V_T.

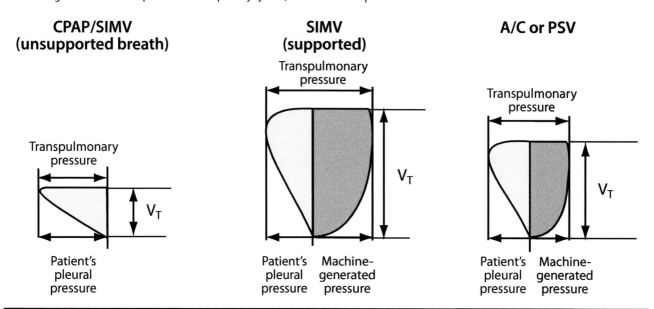

breaths are less damaging and on the belief that weaning of ventilatory rate is necessary before extubation. It has been unequivocally demonstrated that lung injury is most directly caused by excessive V_T, irrespective of the pressure required to generate that V_T.[11–13] A rate of 60 breaths per minute, compared with rates of 20–40 breaths per minute, was shown to result in less air leak with unsynchronized IMV.[14] This finding lends further support to the putative advantage of A/C, with its smaller V_T and higher mechanical breath rate, over SIMV.

Some clinicians also believe that supporting every breath does not provide the infant with an opportunity for respiratory muscle training. This concern is also unfounded and highlights some clinicians' limited understanding of the patient-ventilator interaction during synchronized ventilation. As Figure 9-1 illustrates, with synchronized ventilation, V_T is the result of the inspiratory effort of the patient (negative intrapleural pressure on inspiration) combined with the positive pressure generated by the ventilator. This combined effort (the baby "pulling" and the ventilator "pushing" the gas) results in the transpulmonary pressure, which, together with the compliance of the respiratory system, determines the V_T. Thus, as ventilator inspiratory pressure is decreased during weaning, the infant gradually assumes a greater proportion of the work of breathing;

in the process, the respiratory muscles are trained. Ultimately, the ventilator pressure is decreased to the point where it is overcoming only the added resistance of the ETT and circuit. At that point, the infant is ready for extubation.

Finally, extensive experience with high-frequency ventilation (HFV) makes it clear that lowering pressure amplitude and leaving the rate unchanged is an effective way of reducing ventilator support to the point of extubation. Although we cannot make a direct parallel between A/C and HFV, it is reasonable to accept that a larger number of smaller breaths with A/C need not be detrimental. But a definitive large study comparing the relative merits of SIMV and A/C is lacking.

CLINICAL TRIALS OF SYNCHRONIZED VENTILATION

Despite widespread acceptance of synchronized mechanical ventilation in newborn intensive care, there is a surprising paucity of information on the impact of this modality on major outcomes, such as mortality, chronic lung disease, and length of hospitalization. A number of small studies have shown improvement in short-term physiologic outcomes (Table 9-3), but demonstrating "bottom line" long-term outcome improvement has been elusive.[15] Unfortunately, the only available studies suffer from important design and device

TABLE 9-3
Demonstrated Short-Term Benefits of Synchronized Ventilation

Reference	Population	Mode	Benefit
Berenstein et al., 1994[37]	30 NB	SIMV	Higher and more consistent V_T
Cleary et al., 1995[38]	10 NB <32 weeks <12 hours	SIMV	Improved ventilation and oxygenation
Jarreau et al., 1996[39]	6 NB with RDS	A/C	Decreased work of breathing
Quinn et al., 1998[40]	59 NB <32 weeks	A/C	Decreased catecholamine levels
Smith et al., 1997[41]	17 NB with RDS	SIMV	Less tachypnea

Key: A/C = assist/control ventilation; NB = newborn; RDS = respiratory distress syndrome; SIMV = synchronized intermittent mandatory ventilation.

limitations, leaving clinicians with the unsatisfactory situation of using an "unproven" therapy day after day.

In the first large clinical trial, Bernstein and associates compared SIMV and IMV in a prospective randomized multicenter study of 327 infants ventilated with the Infant Star ventilator with Star Sync module (Grasby capsule abdominal movement sensor) (Infrasonics, Inc., San Diego, California).[16] Compared with IMV, there was a shorter duration of mechanical ventilation among infants >2,000 g on SIMV, less need for sedation for infants 1,000–1,499 g on SIMV, a lower mean airway pressure at one hour postentry in all age groups on SIMV, as well as a shorter time to regain birth weight when ventilated for >14 days on SIMV. The researchers further showed less need for oxygen at 36 weeks corrected gestational age (CGA) among infants weighing <1,000 g and less need for oxygen at 36 weeks CGA for all infants <2,000 g during SIMV. There was no difference between SIMV and IMV in the primary endpoints—survival, air leak, and overall length of mechanical ventilation—in this rather heterogeneous group. Had the investigators chosen bronchopulmonary dysplasia (BPD) at 36 weeks CGA as their primary outcome, they would have been able to report a significant improvement in their entire study population (reduction from 42 percent to 28 percent, *p* <.05) (result reanalyzed based on the published data). A much smaller single-center randomized trial by Chen and coworkers using the same device enrolled 77 neonates with RDS and meconium aspiration syndrome (MAS) requiring mechanical ventilation. Premature infants with RDS on SIMV had a significantly shorter duration of ventilation, less need for reintubation, a lower incidence of severe intraventricular hemorrhage (IVH) (grades 3 and 4), and a lower

incidence of BPD than those on IMV. No differences were seen in the small number of MAS infants.[17]

Baumer and colleagues, in a large randomized trial, compared A/C with IMV in 924 preterm infants with RDS. A/C was provided using the SLE 2000 (airway pressure trigger) (SLE Ltd., South Croydon, United Kingdom) in the large majority of patients and the Draeger Babylog 8000 (airway flow trigger) in the rest. Some centers lacked prior experience with triggered ventilation. This trial showed no difference in chronic lung disease, pneumothorax, duration of ventilation, or risk of IVH between the two groups. The author and colleagues concluded that there was no observed benefit from the use of A/C, particularly in infants <28 weeks gestational age.[18] It is important to interpret the results in light of the device used in the majority of patients. The SLE 2000 uses airway pressure to sense patient effort. Pressure triggering has been shown to result in failure to trigger in a large proportion of infants <1,000 g.[3] There was a nonsignificant trend to a higher incidence of air leak in infants <1,000 g in the triggered group. Given the long trigger delay of pressure-triggered ventilators, it is tempting to speculate that the increased air leak incidence resulted from late cycling of the ventilator at a time the infant was already starting to exhale. The author and colleagues appropriately stated in their discussion that these results apply to the SLE 2000 device and to the population studied and may not be generalizable to other situations.[18]

Beresford and associates enrolled 386 preterm infants with birth weights of 1–2 kg in a randomized trial of IMV or triggered ventilation with the SLE 2000 (pressure trigger) ventilator. Infants in the trigger group were ventilated using A/C, then weaned using SIMV, whereas those in the control group had their ventilator rate adjusted manually to match each infant's own respiratory rate initially and were then weaned. Chronic lung disease, death, pneumothorax, IVH, number of ventilator days, and length of oxygen dependency were similar in the two groups. It could be concluded that careful manual synchronization of ventilator set rate with the infant's breathing is as effective as automatic synchronization by the ventilator when using pressure trigger.[19] How practical manual synchronization is outside of a study protocol remains an open question, however. Once again, the issue of the relative ineffectiveness of the pressure-triggered device adds uncertainty regarding interpretation of the data.

Clearly, the two studies using a rapidly acting surface trigger device (the Infant Star) had better results than the two trials that used the pressure-triggered device, the SLE 2000. Ventilator studies should be interpreted with caution, and the conclusions drawn from them should be considered specific to the devices and strategies employed. These conflicting results highlight the difficulties involved in conducting ventilator studies where many different devices are used and experience with their use differs among participating centers. The characteristics of the sensing and triggering device are crucial to its performance in synchronizing infant and machine breaths, especially in the tiniest infants. Meta-analysis is an important tool to use in evaluating research to arrive at evidence-based practice, but lumping together studies using different ventilation devices and approaches to ventilation may obscure the important differences and confuse, rather than clarify, the issues.

VOLUME-TARGETED VENTILATION

The most recent—and in many ways most promising—advance in neonatal ventilation is the advent of volume-targeted ventilatory modes. The recognition that volume, rather than pressure, is the critical determinant of ventilator-induced lung injury,[12,13] along with mounting evidence that hypocarbia is associated with neonatal brain injury,[20–22] has rekindled interest in directly controlling V_T. Traditional volume-controlled ventilation is difficult in small neonates because of the unpredictable loss of V_T to gas compression in the circuit, stretching of the tubing, and variable leakage around uncuffed ETTs. Nonetheless, one publication did demonstrate feasibility of volume-controlled ventilation in infants <1,500 g, at least under carefully controlled study conditions. The study suggested that, when a proximal flow sensor is used to accurately measure exhaled tidal volume and the set V_T is manually adjusted at frequent intervals to maintain the desired exhaled V_T, it is possible to achieve effective volume control. The patients randomized to the volume control mode reached an arbitrary primary endpoint of *either* mean airway pressure of <8 cmH$_2$O *or* an alveolar-arterial oxygen difference (AaDO$_2$) <100, though the duration of mechanical ventilation and oxygen supplementation was not different.[23] However, monitoring of proximal tidal volume and frequent manual adjustment of set tidal volume are not routinely practiced with volume-controlled ventilation. For this reason, a number of modifications of time-cycled, pressure-limited ventilation designed to target a set tidal volume using microprocessor-directed adjustments of peak pressure or inspiratory time have recently been developed. Each of the available modes has advantages and disadvantages. The most widely available modes of volume-targeted ventilation are discussed below.

VOLUME-TARGETED VENTILATION MODES

Pressure-Regulated Volume Control

Pressure-regulated volume control (PRVC) is a pressure-limited, time-cycled ventilation mode that adjusts inspiratory pressure to target a set tidal volume, based on the V_T of the previous breath. The main problem with the PRVC mode of the Maquet Servo 300 and to a lesser extent the Servo-i (Maquet, Inc., Bridgewater, New Jersey, formerly Siemens, Solna, Sweden) is the inaccuracy of V_T measurement performed at the ventilator end of the circuit, rather than at the airway opening.[24,25] This limitation can be overcome to some degree by the use of the circuit compliance feature and the use of a proximal flow sensor. More information on these ventilators can be found at www.maquet.com/criticalcare.

Volume-Assured Pressure Support

The volume-assured pressure support (VAPS) mode on the Bird VIP Gold (CareFusion, San Diego, California) is a hybrid mode, which works to ensure that the targeted V_T is reached. Each breath starts as a pressure-limited breath, but if the set tidal volume is not reached, the device converts to a flow (volume)-cycled mode. The resulting volume-controlled breath thus leads to prolongation of the inspiratory time and a passive increase in peak pressure. This rather prolonged inspiratory time may lead to expiratory asynchrony. Targeting tidal volume based on inspiratory V_T is susceptible to error in the presence of significant ETT leak. The focus is on ensuring a large enough V_T. There is no provision for automatically lowering inspiratory pressure as lung compliance improves, nor is provision made to avoid inadvertent hyperventilation and allow for automatic weaning.

The newer AVEA ventilator by CareFusion (San Diego, California) shares the basic features of VAPS, albeit with a more sophisticated microprocessor algorithm that avoids the excessively long inspiratory time, and adds a volume limit function that terminates inspiration if the upper V_T limit is exceeded. This added function should reduce the risk of volutrauma and hyperventilation, but it still does not lead to automatic weaning of inspiratory pressure and may lead to very short inspiratory times. More information on these ventilators can be found at www.carefusion.com. A new software modification that mimics the volume guarantee (VG) mode described below has recently been implemented in this device.

Volume Guarantee

The Dräger Babylog 8000 plus and the new Babylog VN500 offer a VG option that can be combined with any of the standard ventilator modes (A/C, SIMV, PSV). The VG mode is a volume-targeted, time-cycled, pressure-limited form of vetilation. The operator chooses a target V_T and selects a pressure limit up to which the ventilator operating pressure (the working pressure) can be adjusted. The microprocessor compares the V_T of the previous breath, using exhaled V_T to minimize possible artifact resulting from air leak, and adjusts the working pressure up or down to try to achieve the set V_T. The algorithm limits the amount of pressure increase from one breath to the next to avoid overcorrection that could lead to excessive V_T. This, and the fact that the exhaled V_T of the prior breath is used, means that, with very rapid changes in compliance or patient inspiratory effort, several breaths are needed to reach the target V_T. To minimize the risk of excessively large V_T, the microprocessor opens the expiratory valve, terminating any additional pressure delivery if the delivered V_T exceeds 130 percent of the previous breath. By design, the algorithm is geared toward slower adjustment for low V_T and more rapid adjustment for excessive, potentially dangerous volume delivery. The autoregulation of inspiratory pressure makes VG a self-weaning mode. Because weaning occurs in real time, rather than intermittently in response to blood gases, VG has the potential to achieve faster weaning from mechanical ventilation.

CLINICAL STUDIES OF VOLUME-TARGETED VENTILATION

Several early studies demonstrated the feasibility and efficacy of VG and showed that equivalent or lower peak pressures were needed to achieve similar gas exchange with a shift of the work of breathing from the ventilator to the infant.[26,27]

A short-term crossover study showed that VG combined with A/C, SIMV, or PSV led to significantly lower variability of V_T compared with A/C, PSV, or SIMV alone and that peak inspiratory pressures were similar.[28] The first randomized clinical trial of VG later demonstrated that, when combined with the A/C mode, VG maintained $PaCO_2$ and V_T within a target range more consistently than did A/C alone during the first 72 hours of life in preterm infants with uncomplicated RDS. The incidence of hypocapnia, defined as $PaCO_2$ <35 mmHg, was reduced by about 45 percent.[29] The crossover study documented that the VG device functions as intended in

the clinical setting, with the anticipated reduction of V_T variability.[28] The randomized trial demonstrated that excessively large V_T and hypocarbia could be reduced, although not eliminated, with the use of VG.[29] This suggested VG's potential to reduce many of the important adverse effects of mechanical ventilation.

A 2005 short-term crossover trial studied 12 extremely low birth weight (679 ± 138 g) infants to determine whether VG is more effective when combined with A/C or SIMV. As expected, V_T was more stable when VG was combined with A/C because the interval between supported breaths is longer during SIMV, leading to slower adjustment in working pressure. An unexpected finding was that, during SIMV, the infants had significantly lower and more variable SpO_2, and significantly more tachycardia and tachypnea. By design, the V_T was identical, but significantly higher peak inspiratory pressure (PIP) was required during SIMV to achieve the same V_T. The tachypnea, tachycardia, and lower, more variable oxygen saturation suggest that the infants were tiring during the SIMV period and contributing less spontaneous effort by the end of the two-hour period when the measurements were obtained.[30] This is because, during synchronized ventilation, the delivered V_T is the result of the combined inspiratory effort of the baby and the positive ventilator pressure. As the baby tires and contributes less, the ventilator needs to generate higher PIP to deliver the same V_T.

Finally, in a randomized trial of 53 infants with RDS, Lista and colleagues demonstrated decreased levels of pro-inflammatory cytokines and shorter durations of mechanical ventilation using VG combined with PSV rather than PSV alone. The duration of mechanical ventilation was 12.3 ± 3 days in the VG group compared to 8.8 ± 3 days in those on PSV alone.[31] By contrast, a subsequent similar study by the same authors, this time using a target tidal volume of 3 mL/kg, showed an *increase* in proinflammatory cytokines.[32] This was most likely a consequence of atelectasis that resulted from the combination of low V_T and low end-expiratory pressure of 3–4 cmH_2O that was used.[33]

A recent meta-analysis that included both VG studies, PRVC, and VCV studies reported that volume-targeted ventilation, compared to pressure-limited ventilation, reduced the combined outcome of death or BPD, reduced the risk of pneumothorax, and shortened the duration of mechanical ventilation. However, the included studies were quite small and, more important, many of the key outcomes reported in the meta-analysis were not prospectively collected or defined. In some of the studies, other variables beyond volume versus pressure targeting also differed. All the included studies focused on short-term physiologic outcomes, and none included BPD as a primary outcome.[34]

Importance of Open Lung Strategy

The findings of the second Lista study bring out the critical importance of distributing delivered tidal volume evenly into an optimally aerated lung. This key concept has not been widely appreciated and requires special emphasis. Lungs of preterm infants are very prone to atelectasis as a result of surfactant deficiency and an excessively compliant chest wall. Atelectasis is not uniform, but tends to occur in the dependent portion of the lung. Even a normal, physiologic V_T entering only the population of open alveoli will inevitably lead to overexpansion with subsequent lung injury. Thus, it is important to strive to optimize lung volume by using adequate distending airway pressure. In practical terms, this "open lung concept" is achieved by applying sufficient PEEP to improve oxygenation and wean FiO_2 to ≤ 0.35. *The benefits of volume-targeted ventilation cannot be realized without ensuring that this tidal volume is distributed evenly throughout the lungs.*

It remains to be seen whether the demonstrated short-term benefits of VG translate into significant reductions in the frequency of air leak, chronic lung disease, neuroimaging abnormalities, and length of hospitalization.

CLINICAL APPLICATION OF VENTILATION

Despite the lack of definitive evidence of synchronized ventilation's superiority to standard IMV, the benefits of synchronized ventilation are generally accepted. Very few if any NICUs have not adopted these techniques. The choice of SIMV or A/C is, to some extent, a matter of clinician preference and practice style. In reality, there is little difference between the two modalities in the acute phase of respiratory failure, especially in extremely premature or gravely ill infants who have little or no respiratory effort of their own or in infants who are heavily sedated or even paralyzed. Under these circumstances, we are really providing simple IMV, regardless of the ventilator mode selection. However, the differences between SIMV and AC/PSV become more pronounced during weaning and are especially important in the smallest infants with narrow ETTs. Prolonged ventilation with low SIMV rates should be avoided in these infants because it imposes an undesirably high work of breathing. Reyes and associates demonstrated that addition of PSV to support the spontaneous breathing during SIMV effectively compensates for the ineffective V_T during SIMV.[35]

STANDARD SYNCHRONIZED VENTILATION MODES

As with all pressure-limited, time-cycled ventilators, the operator must choose PIP, PEEP, T_I, ventilator rate (either directly or by separately adjusting inspiratory and expiratory time), and FiO_2. The initial steps are common to all forms of synchronized ventilation.

Initial Settings

PIP. Selection of the starting PIP is based on an estimation of the severity of disease and adequacy of chest rise. This setting is then adjusted to achieve an appropriate V_T, typically 4–7 mL/kg, measured at the airway opening. Contrary to popular opinion, the PIP requirement is not related to the baby's size, but to severity of illness. The misconception about PIP arose from the fact that larger babies cope with poorly compliant lungs more effectively than smaller ones because of their greater strength and endurance. Consequently, respiratory failure occurs at lesser degrees of illness severity in the smaller infant. However, even a small preterm infant may have very stiff lungs and may, at times, require fairly high pressures. On the other hand, the term infant with normal lungs who is ventilated for nonrespiratory reasons needs PIP only in the low teens to achieve a normal V_T. *Rapid improvement in compliance can take place following surfactant administration.*

PEEP. PEEP should be set in proportion to the current oxygen requirement because in virtually all neonatal lung diseases, hypoxemia is a reflection of ventilation-perfusion mismatch and intrapulmonary right-to-left shunting. This, in turn, reflects atelectasis and low lung volume. Thus, a high oxygen requirement can usually be attributed to low lung volume. It can be corrected by adequate PIP to open atelectatic alveoli and application of sufficient PEEP to maintain that recruitment. The exception to this rule is the infant with pulmonary hypertension with hypoxemia related to extrapulmonary shunting. A PEEP of 5 cmH_2O is usually adequate if the FiO_2 is 0.25–0.35, PEEP should be about 6 cmH_2O with an oxygen requirement between 0.35 and 0.5, and it should be 7–10 cmH_2O if the FiO_2 remains >0.6. Lung expansion on chest x-ray can also guide selection of the PEEP level.

Inspiratory Time. Selection of (T_I) should reflect the infant's time constants (a measure of how rapidly gas can get in and out of the lungs). Small preterm infants with RDS have very short time constants and should be ventilated with T_I of 0.3 second or less. Large infants or those with increased airway resistance (e.g., those with chronic lung disease or meconium aspiration) have longer time constants and require longer T_I, up to 0.5 second.

Ventilator Rate. The ventilator rate should reflect the severity of illness and whether the infant has much respiratory effort of his own. Infants with severe lung disease and little or no respiratory effort should generally be supported with a fairly rapid rate of 50–60 breaths per minute. Spontaneously breathing infants with less severe disease can be supported with a rate of around 40 breaths per minute, allowing them to trigger the ventilator. Because respiratory rate determines expiratory time (and vice versa), it is important to allow sufficient expiratory time to avoid air trapping resulting from incomplete exhalation. For this reason, it is important to avoid rates >60/minute in larger infants or those with increased airway resistance and >80/minute in small preterm infants. Adequacy of inspiratory and expiratory time can be verified by observing the ventilator flow waveform and making sure that flow returns to zero (baseline) before each expiration and inspiration begins.

Subsequent Adjustments

As the infant begins to improve and generate spontaneous respiratory effort, the ventilator rate should be lowered gradually to allow him to take over some of the work of breathing. This is important because a too rapid rate will override the infant's own effort and defeat the purpose of synchronized ventilation—namely, for the infant and the ventilator to work together. A low $PaCO_2$ is equally undesirable because it will suppress the infant's respiratory drive.

It is important to understand clearly how different ventilator variables affect gas exchange and how they interact with the underlying pathophysiology. A detailed discussion of these concepts is beyond the scope of this chapter, but the essentials are reviewed briefly.

Oxygenation is controlled by adjustments in FiO_2 and mean airway pressure, as discussed above. The goal should be to optimize lung volume and ventilation-perfusion matching and to lower FiO_2 to <0.35. PEEP is the most important determinant of mean airway pressure (Paw). PIP, inspiratory time, and rise time (how quickly plateau pressure is reached) are the other factors.

Ventilation (CO_2 elimination) is controlled by adjustments of ventilatory rate and V_T. In standard pressure-limited ventilation, V_T is determined by lung compliance and pressure amplitude (difference between PIP and PEEP). Thus, increasing PIP improves ventilation as well as oxygenation through its effect on V_T and Paw.

Increasing PEEP and/or lowering PIP decreases V_T if all other factors remain equal. However, if the increased PEEP results in recruitment (normalization) of lung volume, lung compliance will improve, which may improve ventilation, sometimes quite dramatically. This improvement in ventilation can lead to inadvertent hyperventilation—which the use of volume-targeted ventilation can avoid. Excessively high PEEP will cause overexpansion of the lungs, with resultant hemodynamic compromise and incomplete exhalation (lower V_T), resulting in hypercarbia. As the patient's lung disease evolves, significant changes in compliance and resistance will occur. Therefore, the appropriateness of all settings needs to be reevaluated regularly. For example, a PEEP of 6 or 7 cmH_2O, which would be quite appropriate early in the course of RDS when the lungs are stiff, becomes excessive as compliance and lung volume increase. Oxygen requirement is the best bedside tool to assess adequacy of lung volume.

Weaning

With SIMV, weaning is accomplished by reducing PIP as well as the ventilator rate. In general, the rate should not be reduced much until PIP has been reduced to relatively low values (<16–18 cmH_2O) that signify considerable improvement in lung compliance. Weaning the rate while the lungs are still quite stiff is likely to impose a high WOB. It may require excessively large V_T for the machine breaths to compensate for ineffective spontaneous breaths that may do little more than rebreathe the anatomic dead space. The rate should not be reduced to <10 breaths per minute, especially in small infants, because of the high work of breathing associated with small ETTs. Again, the addition of PSV to SIMV may compensate for these problems and is recommended if the ventilator has the capability. As a rule, infants who are able to generate adequate V_T and gas exchange with PIP of 15–18 cmH_2O and a rate of ten breaths per minute are ready for extubation.

With A/C and PSV, the infant controls the ventilator rate; therefore, lowering the set rate, which only acts as a backup in case of apnea, has little impact. Weaning is accomplished by lowering the PIP, which decreases the amount of support for each breath. This gradually transfers the WOB to the infant. When PIP has been reduced to 10–14 cmH_2O in small preterm infants and to 15–20 cmH_2O in larger infants, these infants are typically ready for extubation. In the small infants, these low pressures serve merely to overcome the added resistance of the ETT. In very premature infants, it is appropriate to lower the backup rate to 15–20 breaths per minute for a few hours prior to extubation to uncover inconsistent respiratory effort/periodic breathing that a higher backup rate might effectively mask.

VOLUME-TARGETED VENTILATION

Because VG is the most widely used and best studied modality of volume-targeted ventilation and because it is the technique with which I have extensive clinical experience, the clinical guidelines provided are specific for this modality. Though volume-targeted ventilation modes share certain characteristics, each device functions differently and may respond to perturbations in a different way. Consult the product literature of each manufacturer for specific clinical guidelines for their respective ventilators.

Initiation

- VG should be implemented as soon as possible after initiation of mechanical ventilation because this is the time when the most rapid changes in lung mechanics are likely to occur.
- The usual starting target V_T for most infants is 4–5 mL/kg during the acute phase of the illness. Infants with MAS may require slightly larger V_T (5–6 mL/kg) due to the larger alveolar dead space related to some degree of overinflation.
- The added dead space of the flow sensor becomes proportionally more significant in the smallest infants. For this reason, extremely low birth weight infants <700 g need V_T of 5.5–6 mL/kg. The effect is not large enough, however, to preclude the use of synchronized or volume-targeted ventilation.[36]
- Larger tidal volumes (as much as 6–8 mL/kg) are needed in older infants with chronic lung disease because of increased anatomic and physiologic dead space (dilated large airways and wasted ventilation resulting from poor ventilation-perfusion matching).
- The PIP should be set about 20 percent higher than the working pressure (the PIP currently needed to deliver the target V_T) to give the device adequate room to adjust PIP.
- Record not only the PIP limit, but also the working pressure, which is the true reflection of the level of support the infant is receiving.

Subsequent Adjustments

- Subsequent adjustment to the target V_T can be made based on $PaCO_2$, although adjustment is seldom necessary. The usual increment is 0.5 mL/kg.
- The PIP limit needs to be adjusted from time to time (the usual increment is 2–4 cmH_2O) to keep the PIP limit sufficiently close to the working pressure to avoid dangerously high V_T and at the same time high enough to avoid frequent alarms. In most infants, keeping the pressure limit 4–6 cmH_2O above average working pressure is appropriate.

  Note: The working pressure will default to the PIP limit if the flow sensor is temporarily removed (such as around the time of surfactant administration or delivery of nebulized medication), if its function is affected by reflux of secretions or surfactant, or if it malfunctions for any reason. The manual inspiration (activated by depressing a key on the front panel) also uses the set PIP limit. Ideally, when removing the flow sensor for significant periods, such as when nebulizing medications, adjust the PIP limit to roughly match the average or recent working pressures. To avoid volutrauma, keep the PIP limit sufficiently close to the actual PIP (~5–10 cmH_2O).
- If the infant appears agitated, with episodes of spontaneous hyperventilation, consider light sedation. (However, avoid oversedation, with complete suppression of respiratory effort.)
- If the infant is persistently tachypneic or is consistently breathing above the set V_T, his WOB is excessive. Consider increasing the V_T target even if the $PaCO_2$ and pH are normal. (However, if the $PaCO_2$ is low and the respiratory rate is high, sedation may be indicated.)
- If the low-V_T alarm sounds repeatedly, increase the pressure limit to allow the device to reach the desired V_T. Repeated alarms suggest that there has been a change in lung mechanics or patient respiratory effort (e.g., atelectasis, pneumothorax, pulmonary edema, entry of the ETT into the right mainstem bronchus). This early warning system is an important benefit of the VG mode and should not be ignored.
- If the pressure limit has to be increased substantially and/or repeatedly, verify that the V_T measurement is accurate (assess chest rise, obtain a blood gas). If it is, seek the cause of the change in lung mechanics (examine the patient, verify ETT position, obtain a chest x-ray).

Weaning

- When the target V_T is set at the low end of the normal range (usually 4 mL/kg in the acute phase, 1–2 mL/kg higher in BPD infants) and the $PaCO_2$ is allowed to rise to the low to mid-40s, weaning occurs automatically ("self-weaning").

- If the V_T is set too high and/or the $PaCO_2$ is too low, the baby will not have a respiratory drive and will not self-wean. Instead, lack of respiratory muscle training will cause him to become dependent on the ventilator.

- Avoid oversedation during the weaning phase.

- If an infant does not appear to be weaning as expected, despite apparently improving lung disease, try lowering V_T to 3.5 mL/kg, as long as the infant's blood gases are adequate and WOB does not appear excessive. However, remember that infants with chronic lung disease need relatively larger V_T. Lowering the V_T below the infant's physiologic need will result in excessive work of breathing because the infant will have to breathe through the ETT with little or no support from the ventilator.

- If a significant oxygen requirement persists, it may be necessary to increase the PEEP to maintain mean airway pressure as the PIP is automatically lowered.

- Most infants can be extubated when they consistently maintain V_T at or above the target value with delivered PIP <10–12 cmH$_2$O (<12–15 cmH$_2$O in infants >1 kg) with FiO$_2$ <0.35 and good sustained respiratory effort.

- Observing the graphic display of the working pressure is helpful in assessing for periodic breathing (variable respiratory effort) that may require methylxanthine administration to facilitate extubation.

SUMMARY

Many new modalities and techniques are available for the treatment of respiratory failure. Our understanding of how to use these devices to best effect, while improving constantly, remains somewhat behind the pace of technologic innovation. Improvements in outcomes, such as BPD, are becoming increasingly difficult to demonstrate because each incremental improvement leaves "the bar" that much higher. When combined with other lung protective strategies aimed at optimizing lung volume and ensuring even distribution of the delivered tidal volume, volume-targeted ventilation appears to offer the best hope of making a significant impact on ventilator-induced lung injury. However, avoiding mechanical ventilation through early use of continuous positive airway pressure with or without surfactant administration may still be the most effective way to reduce the risk of chronic lung disease.

REFERENCES

1. Keszler M, and Durand D. 2001. High-frequency ventilation. Past, present, and future. *Clinics in Perinatology* 28(3): 579–607.

2. Dimitriou G, Greenough A, and Cherian S. 2001. Comparison of airway pressure and airflow triggering systems using a single type of neonatal ventilator. *Acta Paediatrica* 90(4): 445–447.

3. Dimitriou G, et al. 1998. Comparison of airway pressure-triggered and airflow-triggered ventilation in very immature infants. *Acta Paediatrica* 87(12): 1256–1260.

4. Claure N, D'Ugard C, and Bancalari E. 2003. Elimination of ventilator dead space during synchronized ventilation in premature infants. *Journal of Pediatrics* 143(3): 315–320.

5. Chatburn RL, and Primiano FP Jr. 2001. A new system for understanding modes of mechanical ventilation. *Respiratory Care* 46(6): 604–621.

6. Schulze A, et al. 1999. Proportional assist ventilation in low birth weight infants with acute respiratory disease: A comparison to assist/control and conventional mechanical ventilation. *Journal of Pediatrics* 135(3): 339–344.

7. Mrozek JD, et al. 2000. Randomized controlled trial of volume-targeted synchronized ventilation and conventional intermittent mandatory ventilation following initial exogenous surfactant therapy. *Pediatric Pulmonology* 29(1): 11–18.

8. Chan V, and Greenough A. 1994. Comparison of weaning by patient triggered ventilation or synchronous intermittent mandatory ventilation in preterm infants. *Acta Paediatrica* 83(3): 335–337.

9. Dimitriou G, et al. 1995. Synchronous intermittent mandatory ventilation modes compared with patient triggered ventilation during weaning. *Archives of Disease in Childhood. Fetal and Neonatal Edition* 72(3): F188–F190.

10. Hummler H, et al. 1996. Influence of different methods of synchronized mechanical ventilation on ventilation, gas exchange, patient effort, and blood pressure fluctuations in premature neonates. *Pediatric Pulmonology* 22(5): 305–313.

11. Dreyfuss D, and Saumon G. 1993. Role of tidal volume, FRC, and end-inspiratory volume in the development of pulmonary edema following mechanical ventilation. *American Review of Respiratory Disease* 148(5): 1194–1203.

12. Dreyfuss D, and Saumon G. 1998. Ventilator-induced lung injury: Lessons from experimental studies. *American Journal of Respiratory and Critical Care Medicine* 157(1): 294–323.

13. Clark RH, Slutsky AS, and Gertsmann DR. 2000. Lung protective strategies of ventilation in the neonate: What are they? *Pediatrics* 105(1 part 1): 112–114.

14. Oxford Region Controlled Trial of Artificial Ventilation (OCTAVE) Study Group. 1991. Multicentre randomised controlled trial of high against low frequency positive pressure ventilation. *Archives of Disease in Childhood* 66(7 spec. no.): 770–775.

15. Greenough A, Milner A, and Dimitriou G. 2004. Synchronized mechanical ventilation for respiratory support in newborn infants. *Cochrane Database of Systematic Reviews* (4): CD000456.

16. Bernstein G, et al. 1996. Randomized multicenter trial comparing synchronized and conventional intermittent mandatory ventilation in neonates. *Journal of Pediatrics* 128(4): 453–463.

17. Chen JY, Ling UP, and Chen JH. 1997. Comparison of synchronized and conventional intermittent mandatory ventilation in neonates. *Acta Paediatrica Japonica* 39(5): 578–583.

18. Baumer JH. 2000. International randomised controlled trial of patient triggered ventilation in neonatal respiratory distress syndrome. *Archives of Disease in Childhood. Fetal and Neonatal Edition* 82(1): F5–F10.

19. Beresford MW, Shaw NJ, and Manning D. 2000. Randomised controlled trial of patient triggered and conventional fast rate ventilation in neonatal respiratory distress syndrome. *Archives of Disease in Childhood. Fetal and Neonatal Edition* 82(1): F14–F18.

20. Graziani LJ, et al. 1992. Mechanical ventilation in preterm infants: Neurosonographic and developmental studies. *Pediatrics* 90(4): 515–522.

21. Fujimoto S, et al. 1994. Hypocarbia and cystic periventricular leukomalacia in premature infants. *Archives of Disease in Childhood. Fetal and Neonatal Edition* 71(2): F107–F110.

22. Wiswell TE, et al. 1996. Effects of hypocarbia on the development of cystic periventricular leukomalacia in premature infants treated with high-frequency jet ventilation. *Pediatrics* 98(5): 918–924.

23. Singh J, et al. 2006. Mechanical ventilation of very low birth weight infants: Is volume or pressure a better target variable? *Journal of Pediatrics* 149(3): 308–313.

24. Cannon ML, et al. 2000. Tidal volumes for ventilated infants should be determined with a pneumotachometer placed at the endotracheal tube. *American Journal of Respiratory and Critical Care Medicine* 162(6): 2109–2112.

25. Chow LC, et al. 2002. Are tidal volume measurements in neonatal pressure-controlled ventilation accurate? *Pediatric Pulmonology* 34(3): 196–202.

26. Cheema IU, and Ahluwalia JS. 2001. Feasibility of tidal volume-guided ventilation in newborn infants: A randomized, crossover trial using the volume guarantee modality. *Pediatrics* 107(6): 1323–1328.

27. Herrera CM, et al. 2002. Effects of volume-guaranteed synchronized intermittent mandatory ventilation in preterm infants recovering from respiratory failure. *Pediatrics* 110(3): 529–533.

28. Abubakar KM, and Keszler M. 2001. Patient-ventilator interactions in new modes of patient-triggered ventilation. *Pediatric Pulmonology* 32(1): 71–75.

29. Keszler M, and Abubakar KM. 2004. Volume guarantee: Stability of tidal volume and incidence of hypocarbia. *Pediatric Pulmonology* 38(3): 240–245.

30. Abubakar K, and Keszler M. 2005. Effect of volume guarantee combined with assist/control vs synchronized intermittent mandatory ventilation. *Journal of Perinatology* 25(10): 638–642.

31. Lista G, et al. 2004. Impact of targeted-volume ventilation on lung inflammatory response in preterm infants with respiratory distress syndrome (RDS). *Pediatric Pulmonology* 37(6): 510–514.

32. Lista G, et al. 2006. Lung inflammation in preterm infants with respiratory distress syndrome: Effects of ventilation with different tidal volumes. *Pediatric Pulmonology* 41(4): 357–363.

33. Keszler M. 2006. Volume guarantee and ventilator-induced lung injury: Goldilock's rules apply. *Pediatric Pulmonology* 41(4): 364–366.

34. Wheeler K, et al. 2010. Volume-targeted versus pressure-limited ventilation in the neonate. *Cochrane Database of Systematic Reviews* (11): CD003666.

35. Reyes ZC, et al. 2006. Randomized, controlled trial comparing synchronized intermittent mandatory ventilation and synchronized intermittent mandatory ventilation plus pressure support in preterm infants. *Pediatrics* 118(4): 1409–1417.

36. Montazami S, Abubakar K, and Keszler M. 2006. Impact of instrumental dead space on volume guarantee mode of ventilation in extremely low birth weight infants. E-PAS 59: 468.

37. Bernstein G, Heldt GP, and Mannino FL. 1994. Increased and more consistent tidal volumes during synchronized intermittent mandatory ventilation in newborn infants. *American Journal of Respiratory and Critical Care Medicine* 150(5 part 1): 1444–1448.

38. Cleary JP, et al. 1995. Improved oxygenation during synchronized intermittent mandatory ventilation in neonates with respiratory distress syndrome: A randomized, crossover study. *Journal of Pediatrics* 126(3): 463–468.

39. Jarreau PH, et al. 1996. Patient triggered ventilation decreases the work of breathing in neonates. *American Journal of Respiratory and Critical Care Medicine* 153(3): 1176–1181.

40. Quinn MW, et al. 1998. Stress response and mode of ventilation in preterm infants. *Archives of Disease in Childhood. Fetal and Neonatal Edition* 78(3): F195–F198.

41. Smith KM, et al. 1997. Lower respiratory rates without decreases in oxygen consumption during neonatal synchronized intermittent mandatory ventilation. *Intensive Care Medicine* 23(4): 463–468.

NOTES

10 Complications of Positive Pressure Ventilation

Debbie Fraser, MN, RNC-NIC

The adaptation of mechanical ventilators for use in the neonatal population brought about a dramatic breakthrough in the care of premature infants. Further refinements and the development of technologies such as high-frequency ventilation combined with exogenous surfactant have further pushed back the boundaries of survival. Despite these advances, mechanical ventilation is not without risk. Barotrauma and volutrauma, resulting from the mechanical effects of positive pressure, and oxygen toxicity have harmful effects on many neonatal organs, including the lungs, heart, kidneys, eyes, and brain. Of special importance to all neonatal nurses is the risk for infection and airway trauma resulting from placement and use of the endotracheal tube. This chapter begins with a general discussion of lung trauma associated with volume, pressure, atelectasis, and oxygen. A review of some of the most common complications of mechanical ventilation—air leak syndromes, airway injury, pulmonary hemorrhage, and bronchopulmonary dysplasia (BPD)—follows. Patent ductus arteriosus (PDA) and retinopathy of prematurity (ROP) and their relationship to oxygen therapy are also discussed.

AIR LEAK SYNDROMES

Air leaks are produced by a rupture in the alveolus that allows air to escape into tissue where it is not normally found.[1] A review of the anatomy and physiology of the thorax and lungs will help the nurse understand why neonates are at especially high risk for developing air leak syndromes. The chest wall, or thoracic cage, consists of 12 thoracic vertebrae, 12 pairs of ribs, the sternum and diaphragm, and intercostal muscles. The

cone-shaped thoracic skeleton is quite flexible because of the presence of cartilage. The major respiratory muscle, the diaphragm, stretches across the bottom of the thorax, separating the thorax from the abdomen. Within the thorax are three subdivisions: the two lungs and the mediastinum. The mediastinum contains the thymus gland, the great vessels, the thoracic duct and small lymph nodes, the heart, a branch of the phrenic nerve, and parts of the trachea and esophagus.

The lungs and the thoracic cavity are lined by a double-layer membrane, or pleura: The parietal pleura lines the chest wall, diaphragm, and mediastinum; the visceral pleura covers each lung. These membranes lie in continuous contact with each other and form a potential space, called the pleural space, that contains a thin layer of serous fluid for lubrication and cohesion.

The elastic tissues of the lung and chest wall pull in opposite directions, creating a negative, or subatmospheric, pressure in the pleural space. These pressures are approximately -2.5 to -10 cmH$_2$O from base to apex during respiration.[2] In situations where air enters the pleural space, it interferes with the negative pressure, resulting in partial or total collapse of the lung.

Neonatal air leaks occur when large transpulmonary pressure swings, uneven alveolar ventilation, and air trapping result in alveolar overdistention and rupture. Uneven ventilation occurs, not only in neonates with immature lungs, but also in those with meconium, blood, or amniotic fluid aspiration or hypoplastic lungs. The air ruptures occur at the alveolar bases, and the air tracks along the perivascular sheaths of the pulmonary blood vessels or peribronchial tissues to the roots of the lung.

TABLE 10-1
Sites of Air Leak Syndromes

Site of Extraneous Air	Syndrome
Pulmonary interstitium (perivascular sheaths)	Interstitial emphysema
Alveoli trabeculae-visceral pleura	Pseudocysts
Pleural space	Pneumothorax
Mediastinum	Pneumomediastinum
Pericardial space	Pneumopericardium
Perivascular sheaths (peripheral vessels)	Perivascular emphysema
Vascular lumina (blood)	Air embolus
Subcutaneous tissue	Subcutaneous emphysema
Retroperitoneal connective tissue	Retroperitoneal emphysema
Peritoneal space	Pneumoperitoneum
Intestinal wall	Pneumatosis intestinalis
Scrotum	Pneumoscrotum

From: Korones SB. 2011. Complications. In *Assisted Ventilation of the Neonate,* 5th ed., Goldsmith JP, and Karotkin EM, eds. Philadelphia: Saunders, 407. Reprinted by permission.

Air may then rupture into the pleura, mediastinum, pericardium, or extrathoracic areas (Table 10-1).

Air leaks occur in 1–2 percent of all newborns; however, only a small percentage of these infants (0.05–0.07 percent) are thought to demonstrate symptoms.[3] Since the advent of surfactant therapy and improvements in neonatal ventilator technology, the incidence of air leaks has declined significantly. In a study done before surfactant use, Yu and associates reported that among 230 infants weighing 500–999 g, 35 percent had pulmonary interstitial emphysema (PIE), 20 percent had pneumothorax, 3 percent had pneumomediastinum, and 2 percent had pneumopericardium.[4] Post surfactant reports for infants 24–32 weeks gestation found that the incidence of pneumothoraces ranged from 3.7 to 10 percent.[5–7] The use of synchronized modes of ventilation has also been reported to result in lower rates of air leaks.[8]

In addition to decreased lung compliance resulting from inadequate surfactant production, several structural differences contribute to the premature infant's increased risk of developing an air leak. In a seminal work published in 1935, Macklin identified the presence of alveolar pores (pores of Kohn), which allow gases to move between ventilated and nonventilated alveoli. Because these pores increase in size and number with increasing lung maturity, premature infants may lack sufficient communication between adjacent lung units to prevent asymmetric ventilation.[9]

Risk factors for air leak syndromes include respiratory distress syndrome (RDS), meconium aspiration syndrome (MAS), hypoplastic lungs, congenital malformation, prematurity, endotracheal tube malposition, and overzealous resuscitation and suctioning.[10] Neonates on mechanical ventilation or continuous positive airway pressure (CPAP) are at much higher risk for air leaks, as are low birth weight (LBW) infants.[3] Sepsis and pneumonia caused by Pseudomonas or Candida have also been identified as potential risk factors.[11]

Mechanical ventilator factors that may increase the incidence of air leaks include positive end-expiratory pressure (PEEP), prolonged inspiratory time, high peak pressure, and breathing out of phase with the ventilator. An early study showed a 34 percent incidence of air leaks in infants receiving 3–8 cmH_2O of PEEP versus a 21 percent incidence in those not receiving PEEP.[12] One study reported a 50 percent incidence of air leaks when the inspiratory-to-expiratory (I:E) ratio was 1:1 or higher.[13] This finding was confirmed by a Cochrane review that identified a higher incidence of air leaks in infants ventilated with a long inspiratory time.[14] Prolonged inspiratory time can cause the infant to breathe against the ventilator, which can produce larger pressure and volume swings and lead to the rupture of alveoli. Studies have reported a higher incidence of air leaks with high peak inspiratory pressures (PIP) and mean airway pressures (Paw) >12 cmH_2O.[15,16] In a meta-analysis, patient-triggered ventilation was shown to decrease the risk of air leak compared with conventional ventilation.[17]

PULMONARY INTERSTITIAL EMPHYSEMA

PIE, a collection of gases in the connective tissue of the peribronchovascular sheaths, is a frequent complication in premature neonates with RDS who require mechanical ventilation.[10] Neonates with meconium or amniotic fluid aspiration or infection may also develop PIE, but premature infants are more prone to develop this condition because of their increased pulmonary connective tissue, which traps extra-alveolar air. Barotrauma, usually resulting from mechanical ventilation, combined with reduced lung compliance, causes rupture of small airways and alveoli, resulting in air in the interstitial spaces along the peribronchovascular, pleural, and interlobar passages.[10] This free air compromises lung ventilation

FIGURE 10-1
Pulmonary interstitial emphysema.

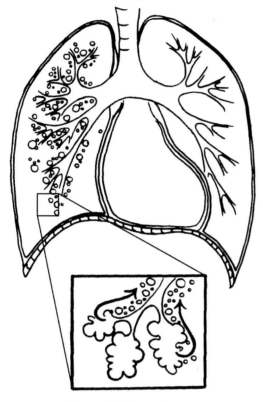

Interstitial emphysema

Adapted from: Korones S. 1986. Diseases of the lungs. In *High Risk Newborn Infants: The Basis for Intensive Nursing Care*, 4th ed. Philadelphia: Mosby, 252. Reprinted by permission.

FIGURE 10-2
Pulmonary interstitial emphysema.

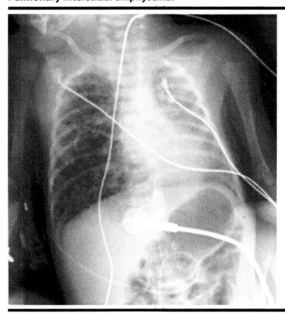

and pulmonary vascular circulation because it compresses alveoli and blood vessels (Figure 10-1). As a result, lung compliance decreases and pulmonary vascular resistance increases. There are case reports of PIE occurring in LBW infants receiving CPAP and in premature infants before CPAP or mechanical ventilation is initiated.[18–20] A study by Verma and colleagues also noted an independent relationship between antenatal magnesium sulfate exposure and PIE in extremely low birth weight (ELBW) infants.[21]

There are two varieties of PIE: a localized form and a diffuse form. The localized, unilateral form may involve one or more lobes of the lung and may be accompanied by mediastinal shift. Diffuse PIE occurs more often in premature infants on mechanical ventilation, because of barotrauma. Morbidity and mortality are highest in low birth weight and lower gestational age infants who develop PIE in the first 48 hours of life.[10] Premature infants with PIE are at great risk for developing BPD

and other air leak syndromes. In a study by Greenough and colleagues, 31 of 41 infants with PIE developed a pneumothorax, and 21 of these babies also developed an intraventricular hemorrhage (IVH).[22]

Clinically, neonates with PIE often exhibit deterioration in respiratory and cardiac status, necessitating additional ventilatory support. This can lead to a vicious cycle of increasing pressure causing more PIE.

The diagnosis of PIE is made radiographically. The classic picture is a "salt and pepper" pattern in which cyst-like radiolucent air pockets are visible against the dark background of lung parenchyma. Overinflation may be noted on the affected side (Figure 10-2). In some cases, the overinflated cysts characteristic of PIE can further enlarge to form pneumatoceles, which are visible on x-ray as cystic blebs.

When the diagnosis is in doubt, CT scanning has been shown to be of value in confirming the presence of PIE.[19]

Treatment

Several medical regimens—from conservative to surgical interventions—have been recommended for infants with PIE. In some infants, unilateral PIE can be managed by placing the neonate with the affected side down. This position improves oxygenation in the unaffected lung and may allow a reduction in PIP, which will help to resolve the PIE. If this approach is unsuccessful, selective mainstem bronchus intubation

FIGURE 10-3
Pneumomediastinum.

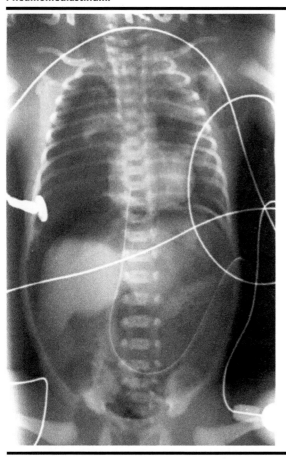

and bronchial occlusion are recommended.[23] The bronchus of the unaffected side is intubated for preferential ventilation while the affected lung resorbs interstitial air and becomes atelectatic. Improvement is generally seen in 3–72 hours.[24,25] Complications of this treatment include difficulty in left-side intubation, bronchial mucosal damage, infection, excessive secretions, hyperinflation of the intubated lung, and further air trapping.[10]

High-frequency ventilation—including high-frequency positive pressure, jet, and oscillatory ventilation—has been used effectively to treat diffuse PIE. In one study of 18 premature infants, high-frequency oscillatory ventilation was effective in improving oxygenation, CO_2 elimination, and circulation in infants with RDS and PIE.[26] High-frequency ventilation allows for adequate minute ventilation using lower airway pressures, which may reduce the amount of air leaking into the interstitial space.

A variety of other strategies, such as percutaneous evacuation of enlarged pneumatoceles, has been

described in case reports.[27,28] Surgical intervention—including pleurotomy, pneumonotomy, pneumonectomy, and lobectomy—has been utilized when the neonate does not respond to medical management.

Nursing Care

BPD is a frequent sequela in neonates surviving PIE. Nursing care of the neonate with PIE begins with close monitoring of all neonates who are intubated and mechanically ventilated. Initially, the nurse will note increasing oxygen and pressure requirements based on falling oxygen saturations and poor blood gas readings. Hypotension may also be noted.

Ventilatory management is crucial in preventing the development of further PIE. The endotracheal tube should be maintained in the proper position, above the level of the carina. Although the goal is to decrease Paw, thereby preventing further air leaks, neonates with lung disease often require higher levels of PIP and PEEP. Barotrauma can be reduced by using a synchronized mode of ventilation.[17]

The nurse should closely monitor oxygen saturations and blood gas levels so that ventilator changes can be made promptly. If the treatment of PIE necessitates the use of high-frequency ventilation, the nurse must be familiar with the equipment and maintain a high level of vigilance.

When treating PIE conservatively, the nurse should position the neonate on the affected side, using oxygen saturation levels and vital signs to monitor tolerance of the change in position. Follow-up x-ray examinations will determine if more aggressive therapy is needed.

Neonates who are treated with selective mainstem bronchus intubation should be monitored continuously. Adequate humidification and appropriate suctioning are vital to prevent plugging of the endotracheal tube and further development of PIE.

Pneumomediastinum

Pneumomediastinum occurs if the free air from a ruptured alveolus dissects along the perivascular and peribronchial tissue to the level of the hilum of the lung. At the hilum, air may accumulate in the mediastinum, causing a pneumomediastinum. If the pressure increases, air can dissect into the neck, producing subcutaneous emphysema, or into the thoracic cavity, causing a pneumothorax. Pneumomediastinum may also be an isolated air leak occurring in an otherwise healthy infant or following meconium aspiration.[1]

In healthy infants, a pneumomediastinum is usually asymptomatic. In more compromised infants, clinical signs include respiratory distress or mild cyanosis. The sternum may be thrust forward; muffled or distant heart sounds and a crunching noise may be heard over the pericardium. Blood gas readings and oxygen saturation levels indicate hypoxia and hypercarbia as a result of the pressure of free air on the lung and blood vessels.

The diagnosis of pneumomediastinum is made radiographically. The classic finding is the "sail sign": a windblown spinnaker sail appearance of the thymus (Figure 10-3). It may be necessary to do a lateral x-ray to clearly visualize air in the mediastinal space behind the sternum.

Medical management for pneumomediastinum involves conservative treatment. As with PIE, the goal is to maintain intrathoracic pressures as low as possible during mechanical ventilation. As with any mechanically ventilated neonate, the nurse must monitor the infant closely for respiratory deterioration. Pneumomediastinum may progress to a pneumothorax.

Pneumothorax

Spontaneous pneumothorax is estimated to occur in 1–2 percent of term and postterm infants, usually following the first few breaths after birth.[3] A pneumothorax can also result from aspiration of amniotic fluid and debris or meconium, the presence of congenital anomalies, or following bag and mask resuscitation. Tension pneumothorax can be a severe complication of mechanical ventilation, with free air quickly accumulating in the pleural cavity causing the lung to collapse, shifting the mediastinum, and severely impeding venous return and cardiac output (Figure 10-4).

A study comparing 44 infants with a pneumothorax in the first 24 hours of life to 88 control infants with no pneumothorax identified the following risk factors: male sex, low birth weight, low Apgar score at one minute, vacuum extraction, meconium-stained amniotic fluid, and the use of bag and mask ventilation.[29] The most significant risk factors are prematurity, respiratory distress, and high ventilatory pressures.[1] Neonates with MAS are at risk for air leaks because they often require mechanical ventilation, and ball-valve airway obstruction leads to further air trapping. One study reported that 12 percent of neonates with MAS develop pneumothorax.[30]

Infants with RDS are at risk for air leaks because of their stiff, noncompliant lungs. One study conducted

FIGURE 10-4
Tension pneumothorax.

Air fills the pleural space causing a shift of the trachea, heart, and mediastinum to the opposite side.

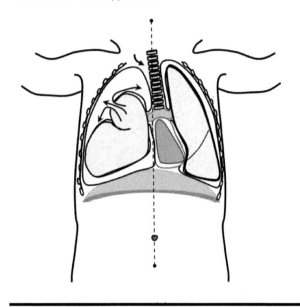

before the use of surfactant reported the incidence of pneumothorax to be 12 percent among infants with RDS not on mechanical ventilation, 11 percent in infants on CPAP, and 26 percent among those on mechanical ventilation.[31] Subsequently, a Cochrane review of surfactant administration in premature infants with RDS found that rates of pneumothorax and mortality were lower in infants receiving surfactant.[32] Walker and colleagues demonstrated that by instituting a clinical protocol of prophylactic administration of natural surfactant to infants <28 weeks gestation (N = 60), they were able to reduce the incidence of pneumothorax from 26.6 percent to 10 percent.[33] Development of a pneumothorax in infants with respiratory distress increases the risk of both chronic lung disease (CLD) and death.[34]

Premature neonates who have a pneumothorax are at high risk for developing a cerebral hemorrhage[35] because of intrathoracic pressure fluctuations in association with relative overperfusion of the periventricular circulation, lack of cerebral autoregulation, and inherent weakness of the periventricular capillary beds. Often these neonates on mechanical ventilation for RDS require high ventilatory pressures, which can increase intrathoracic pressure and reduce venous return. This can increase cerebral blood pressure, causing fragile capillaries to rupture. At the time of a pneumothorax, systemic

TABLE 10-2
Signs and Symptoms of Pneumothorax/Air Leaks

Profound generalized cyanosis
Bradycardia
Decrease in the height of the QRS complex on the monitor
Air hunger, including gasping and anxious facies
Diminished or shifted breath sounds
Chest asymmetry
Diminished, shifted, or muffled cardiac sound and point of maximal intensity
Severe hypotension and poor peripheral perfusion
Easily palpable liver and spleen
Subcutaneous emphysema
Cardiorespiratory arrest

Adapted from: Hagedorn MIE, et al. 2006. Respiratory diseases. In *Handbook of Neonatal Intensive Care*, 6th ed., Merenstein GB, and Gardner SL, eds. Philadelphia: Mosby, 625–626. Reprinted by permission.

TABLE 10-3
Factors that Interfere with Transillumination of a Pneumothorax

Chest wall edema
Darkly pigmented skin
Chest wall dressings or tape
Monitor probes or chest lead placement
Bright room lighting
Inadequate light from the transilluminator

hemodynamic changes markedly increase cerebral blood flow velocity and capillary pressure, which can lead to an IVH.[36,37] In some situations there is a loss of cerebral autoregulation. Systemic hypotension caused by the increased intrathoracic pressure can result in cerebral hypotension. As a consequence of altered cerebral perfusion, ischemia and IVH have been reported.[38] A similar relationship between pneumothorax and an increased risk for development of cerebral palsy has also been reported.[39]

Premature neonates on mechanical ventilation who have developed one pneumothorax should be monitored for bilateral pneumothoraces. Neonates at highest risk for bilateral pneumothoraces have PIE at the time of the initial pneumothorax.[40] Any infant who develops a spontaneous pneumothorax should be evaluated for cardiac and renal anomalies because of a noted correlation between these anomalies and pulmonary hypoplasia.[41]

Signs and Symptoms

The most common sign of a pneumothorax is respiratory distress, indicated by grunting, retractions, tachypnea, and cyanosis. In addition, there is a decrease in the pH, PaO_2, and oxygen saturations. Diagnosis cannot be made by these signs alone, however, because they also often accompany other causes of respiratory deterioration.

Because the incidence of pneumothorax has decreased, NICU staff may be less familiar than in the past with the often subtle clinical signs and symptoms of this disorder (Table 10-2). Lack of familiarity can delay diagnosis and increase the risk of hypoxia, elevated CO_2 levels, and blood pressure changes.[42] Unusual irritability or restlessness can be an early sign of pneumothorax. Transcutaneous CO_2 trends may provide an early indication of an impending air leak,[42] as can changes in the width of the QRS complex on the ECG monitor.[1]

Diminished breath sounds may be heard on the affected side, but this sign may be difficult to identify because of the small size of the chest and easily transmitted breath sounds in the neonate. It can be difficult to auscultate diminished breath sounds in the neonate with RDS because the lungs are stiff, noncompliant, and do not collapse in the same way as an adult's with a tension pneumothorax. If the pneumothorax is under tension, there may be a mediastinal shift and a shift in the cardiac point of maximal impulse (PMI).

Bradycardia, increased diastolic blood pressure followed by hypotension, increased central venous pressure, and distant heart sounds indicate very high intrathoracic pressures. Clinical findings of distended abdomen and palpable liver and spleen are useful signs of a tension pneumothorax causing displacement of the diaphragm. Other findings include unequal chest wall movement (especially decreased on the affected side), increased anteroposterior (AP) chest diameter, and hyper-resonance to percussion on the affected side.

Preliminary diagnosis of pneumothorax can be made by transillumination of the chest with a high-intensity fiberoptic light. This method has been successful in diagnosing a high percentage of pneumothoraces, with a false positive rate of 5 percent.[43] The nursery should be darkened as much as is safely possible and the probe placed directly on the infant's chest—initially superior to the nipple, then inferior to the nipple.[44] During transillumination of an infant with a pneumothorax, the examiner will note a larger area of illumination on the affected side than on the unaffected side. This corona of light will follow the shape of the chest

FIGURE 10-5
Pneumothorax.

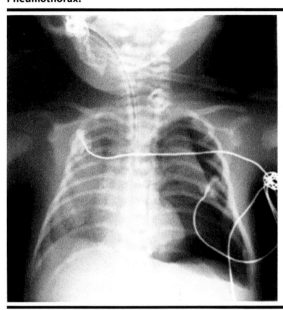

TABLE 10-4
X-ray Findings: Pneumothorax

1. Increased lucency on the affected side
2. Decreased or absent pulmonary vascular markings
3. Overall increase in the size of the affected hemithorax
4. Widened intercostal spaces
5. Flattened diaphragm on the affected side
6. Sharp edge sign (The cardiac border and the diaphragm are seen in sharp contrast.)
7. With tension pneumothorax, mediastinal shift with deviation of the trachea and heart to the opposite side, decreased volume and increased opacity of the opposite lung
8. With bilateral pneumothoraces, narrow cardiac silhouette

From: Carey BE. 1999. Neonatal air leaks: Pneumothorax, pneumomediastinum, pulmonary interstitial emphysema, pneumopericardium. *Neonatal Network* 18(8): 81. Reprinted by permission.

cavity and will vary with respiration and positioning. Table 10-3 lists factors that interfere with transillumination of a pneumothorax.

As with all forms of air leak, the diagnosis of a pneumothorax is confirmed radiographically (Figure 10-5). Anteroposterior and lateral films are necessary to document air that has risen to the anterior part of the thorax or for smaller pneumothoraces. A pneumothorax is identified as a pocket of air impinging on the lung. A mediastinal shift toward the opposite side indicates that the pneumothorax is under tension, and immediate intervention is indicated. Other radiographic findings of a pneumothorax include widened intercostal spaces and a depressed diaphragm (Table 10-4).

Treatment

In nonventilated infants, a pneumothorax can cause varying degrees of respiratory distress. Infants with mildly increased work of breathing may be given supplemental oxygen and monitored until the pneumothorax has resolved spontaneously. Treatments such as nasal CPAP that have the potential to increase the infant's end expiratory pressure should be avoided.

NEEDLE THORACENTESIS

The infant in severe respiratory distress with a tension pneumothorax requires immediate emergency treatment. Needle aspiration is necessary to decrease mortality and morbidity. Table 10-5 lists the equipment needed for needle aspiration. This equipment should be

kept in a clear plastic bag or container with the other emergency equipment in the nursery.

Following sterile preparation of the chest, the needle is inserted into the second or third intercostal space at the midclavicular line.[45] Air is aspirated out through the syringe, then vented out the stopcock (Figure 10-6). Following removal of the needle, the insertion site is covered with a clear occlusive dressing.

CHEST TUBE INSERTION

The insertion of a chest tube is performed using sterile technique. The neonate should be positioned with the affected side up. The chest wall is prepped with bacteriostatic solution and injected with 1 percent lidocaine to provide local anesthesia. Analgesia, such as fentanyl or morphine, should be given because chest tube placement is a painful procedure.

Using the traditional superior approach, the tube is inserted into the second intercostal space on or just lateral to the midclavicular line. The lateral approach uses the fifth to sixth intercostal space just lateral to the anterior axillary line. Care must be taken not to pierce

TABLE 10-5
Equipment for Needle Thoracentesis

Skin cleansing swabs
#18–20-gauge angiocatheter
T-connector
3-way stopcock
30–50 mL syringe
Transparent dressing

FIGURE 10-6
Insertion of a percutaneous catheter for drainage of a pneumothorax or pleural fluid.

Note that the needle has been removed and only the catheter remains in the pleural space.

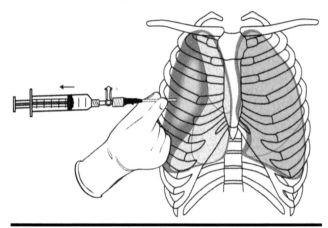

From: Kattwinkel J, ed. 2011. *Textbook of Neonatal Resuscitation*, 6th ed. Elk Grove Village, Illinois: American Academy of Pediatrics and American Heart Association, 244. Reprinted by permission.

the pectoralis muscle, lacerate the intercostal artery, or injure the nipple or breast tissue.

There are several techniques of chest tube placement: the blunt dissection, modified blunt dissection, and trocar methods. Once the chest tube enters the pleural space, the catheter "steams up." A purse-string suture is secured around the tube and the tube is immediately connected to a chest drainage system and tube placement verified radiographically. Complications following chest tube insertion involve improper placement of the tube causing injury to the heart, liver, spleen, and kidney. Significant breast deformities have also been reported as a result of chest tube placement.[46] The most serious complications include hemorrhage, lung perforation, infarction, phrenic nerve injury with eventration of the diaphragm, and cardiac tamponade.[47-50]

Nursing Care

The following nursing measures are important for neonates on mechanical ventilation who are at risk of developing pneumothorax:

1. Carefully monitor vital signs, including heart rate, respiratory rate, and blood pressure. Tachypnea and tachycardia followed by bradycardia and hypotension may indicate development of a pneumothorax.

2. Auscultate heart and breath sounds frequently. Diminished breath sounds may indicate inadequate functioning of the chest tube or development of a pneumothorax. A shift in the PMI may indicate a tension pneumothorax.

3. Closely evaluate arterial blood gas and oxygen saturation levels to determine appropriate oxygen and ventilator settings. The goal should be to use the minimum Paw necessary to obtain adequate ventilation.

4. Ensure the safety of the infant with chest tubes.
   - If chest tubes are inserted, ensure that the chest drainage system is set up correctly and evaluated hourly.
   - Immediately after chest tube insertion, check the water seal for oscillations and bubbling—indications of evacuation of air.
   - Set or fill the suction chamber to the prescribed level—usually between 5 and 25 cmH$_2$O, the average being 10–15 cmH$_2$O.
   - Check the collection chamber hourly and mark it every shift. If a chest tube has been inserted for a pneumothorax, there should be minimal drainage.
   - Observe the insertion site for drainage or signs of infection. An antibiotic ointment may be applied to the insertion site.

5. Tape all connector sites securely. Because of the weight of the connecting tubing, it is helpful to pin the first part of the tubing to the bed with a tab of tape to prevent accidental dislodgment. Measure the length of the chest tube from the insertion site to the connector every shift to assure that it has not slipped out.

6. Turn and position the neonate to facilitate the evacuation of air and fluid. Because air rises, positioning the neonate on the unaffected side will assist in air evacuation.

7. Monitor the neonate's tone and activity. Irritability and agitation can be early signs of pneumothorax.

8. Assess the neonate for signs of IVH. (Changes in cerebral blood flow can be caused by air leaks.) Clinical signs of a cerebral hemorrhage are similar to those of an air leak: respiratory distress, bradycardia, hypoxia, hypercarbia, and acidosis. Any premature neonate with pneumothorax should have serial cerebral sonograms.

9. Consider the use of medications to enhance cardiac output. Cardiac output may be compromised because of high intrathoracic pressure. Insertion of chest tubes may help, but volume expanders or vasopressor drugs may be necessary as well.

FIGURE 10-7
Pneumopericardium.

Air fills the pericardial sac causing a tamponade of the heart.

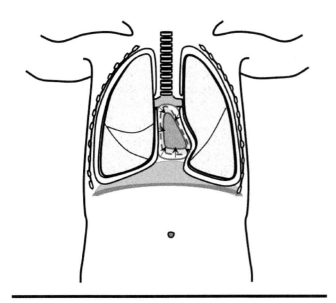

FIGURE 10-8
Pneumopericardium.

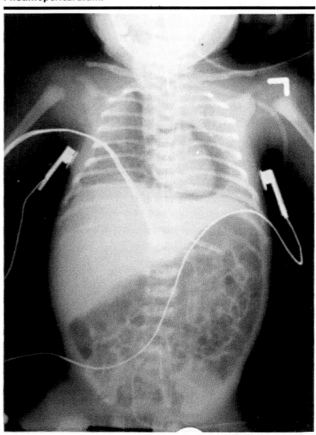

10. Evaluate the neonate's level of agitation and pain, and comfort or medicate as necessary. In the past, neonates were paralyzed if they were fighting mechanical ventilation. Sedation and analgesia are extremely important in caring for these critically ill neonates. Continuous fentanyl or morphine infusions may be helpful. Chest tube insertion and having the chest tube in place are quite painful.

11. Provide parents with accurate, honest, and understandable information regarding the complications of mechanical ventilation and treatment of the air leak. Reassure them that the chest tube will help their baby to breathe more comfortably.

PNEUMOPERICARDIUM

Pneumopericardium is a rare complication of mechanical ventilation seen particularly in preterm neonates. PIE and pneumomediastinum often precede the entry of air into the pericardial sac (Figure 10-7). Pneumopericardium usually occurs during the first few days of life and most often occurs when high ventilatory pressures are being used.

Cardiac tamponade as a result of pneumopericardium can develop very quickly. Death can occur if this condition is not diagnosed and treated promptly. Clinical signs of pneumopericardium include bradycardia, cyanosis, muffled heart sounds, and hypotension. Chest films using AP and lateral views reveal decreased heart size and air surrounding the heart (Figure 10-8).

A small pneumopericardium may be managed conservatively with close observation unless cardiac tamponade is evident.[51] Emergency treatment for tamponade includes needling the pericardial space. Starting under the xiphoid, the angiocath is advanced at a 30- to 40-degree angle aiming at the left shoulder. A thoracotomy tube may be connected to a closed drainage system usually for two to three days. Nursing care is similar to that for the infant with pneumothorax, with specific attention to cardiac output.

PNEUMOPERITONEUM

Another rare complication of mechanical ventilation is pneumoperitoneum. Air dissects through the diaphragm into the retroperitoneal space. Clinical signs of pneumoperitoneum include a firm, shiny, and distended abdomen. The cause of the pneumoperitoneum should be investigated because this complication is also associated with necrotizing enterocolitis (NEC), gastric rupture, and a perforated ulcer that may require surgery.

In the case of a pneumoperitoneum, the x-ray shows a dark layer of air over the abdomen that blurs the normal bowel pattern. A right lateral view demonstrates the liver clearly defined from the anterior abdominal wall.

Medical treatment is indicated if the neonate's respiratory status is severely compromised or if venous return to the heart is impeded. A soft catheter may be inserted into the peritoneum.

AIRWAY INJURY

Subglottic stenosis, tracheomalacia, bronchomalacia, tracheomegaly, necrotizing tracheobronchitis, and vocal cord injuries have been reported in infants requiring mechanical intubation and positive pressure ventilation.

Factors that appear to place intubated infants at risk for these complications include prolonged intubation, lack of an air leak around the endotracheal tube, repeated intubation, mechanical trauma from suctioning, gastroesophageal reflux, respiratory infection, hypoxia, hyperoxia, positive pressure ventilation, excessive movement of the endotracheal tube, and inadequate humidification of the endotracheal tube.[52,53] These complications are more common in infants with BPD but can develop in those who required only short-term intubation and ventilation.

At a minimum, any infant who is intubated will develop edema in the airway followed by acute inflammation if intubation continues for more than a few hours. Pressure from the endotracheal tube reduces mucosal capillary perfusion, which can lead to ischemia, irritation, congestion, edema, and eventually ulceration.[54,55] Progressive ulceration can lead to perichondritis, chondritis, and necrosis of the cricoid cartilage.[56] Granulation tissue grows at the margins of the injured area and can persist as thick tissue, leading to narrowing of the airways. These extensive changes can lead to fibrotic, firm scar tissue, which can cause subglottic stenosis and narrowing of the airways.[57] As a result, atelectasis and/or emphysema can develop. Many of these airway lesions contribute to the development of BPD.

Infants who have been intubated and ventilated for less than a week will have some edema, but their cries are normal within 24 hours after extubation. Infants who are extubated after one week to one month may have mild inspiratory and expiratory stridor lasting for a year or more.

Diagnosis of upper airway obstruction is often difficult to make in premature infants. Following extubation, the infant may have decreased bilateral breath sounds, mild retractions, and apnea. The premature infant may not always develop stridor. Infants who develop respiratory failure will require reintubation, and if the respiratory distress immediately disappears, upper airway injuries should be suspected.

Damage to the larynx can be caused by necrosis over the arytenoid cartilage and vocal cords. Necrosis occurs because the endotracheal tube is in contact with the area. As a result, there may be persistent ulceration and/or erosion of the vocal cords. Significant damage may affect vocalization and respirations.

SUBGLOTTIC STENOSIS

Subglottic stenosis ranges from mild to severe in the intubated infant. The overall incidence of this acquired condition in ventilated preterm infants weighing <1,500 g at birth is approximately 1 percent.[57] The lesion is usually associated with prolonged intubation and is diagnosed by bronchoscopy showing that the subglottic diameter (below the level of the glottic opening and above the level of the inferior margin of the cricoid cartilage) has become sufficiently narrow to cause symptoms of airway obstruction. The mildest form of subglottic stenosis is laryngeal edema.

Diagnosis of subglottic stenosis is made after physical examination, anteroposterior and lateral neck and chest x-ray films, and direct or fiberoptic laryngoscopy and bronchoscopy. In addition to respiratory distress, the infant may have mild to severe respiratory stridor that is not positional.

Treatment of mild respiratory difficulty includes elevating the head of the bed, providing humidified air, and administering racemic epinephrine. Treatment with steroids before extubation has been shown to be quite effective in premature infants.[58] No significant side effects have been noted with the short-term use of dexamethasone.

The more severe form of acquired subglottic stenosis is a "hard" scar of fibrotic tissue. To extubate infants with this condition, an anterior cricoid split with or without immediate cartilage graft interposition may be required to increase the airway diameter.[59] Some surgeons prefer a tracheostomy because it provides a long-term secure airway, but it too has its complications. If a tracheostomy is performed, decannulation occurs when the subglottic region has grown, usually in infants older than one year.[60]

TRACHEOMEGALY, TRACHEOMALACIA, AND BRONCHOMALACIA

Mechanical ventilation with positive pressure causing barotrauma can lead to dilation of the trachea and bronchi, resulting in tracheomegaly, tracheomalacia, or bronchomalacia. Tracheomegaly, diagnosed radiographically, results in an increase in the anatomic dead space, causing the infant to work harder at breathing to maintain normal carbon dioxide levels.[61] Tracheomalacia and bronchomalacia develop when the cartilaginous rings in the airway soften and fail to support the round shape of the trachea, resulting in widening of the posterior airway way leading to airway collapse.[62] The infant can develop expiratory stridor, wheezing, and atelectasis when the airway collapses or becomes obstructed on expiration. There are multiple factors for the pathogenesis of tracheomalacia and bronchomalacia, including barotrauma, immature airways, recurrent bacterial or viral infection, and pressure and irritation of the endotracheal tube.[63] Tracheo- and bronchomalacia has been successfully treated with PEEP and ventilation or CPAP. Such treatment may place the infant at higher risk for BPD.

NECROTIZING TRACHEOBRONCHITIS

Necrotizing tracheobronchitis, a necrotic inflammatory process involving the distal trachea and mainstem bronchi, is characterized by replacement of normal tracheal mucosa with acute inflammatory cells, mostly neutrophils. This process leads to sloughing of the mucosa, which can occlude the distal trachea. As a result of granulation, there may be impaired gas exchange, airway obstruction, and atelectasis. This lesion has been seen in neonates of all sizes and has been identified after just one day of ventilation.

Necrotizing tracheobronchitis has been associated with early work with high-frequency ventilation, but it has also been reported with conventional ventilation.[64] There are various theories for the pathogenesis of necrotizing tracheobronchitis, including lack of humidification. The presence of the endotracheal tube has been suggested as a factor that causes damage by (1) direct pressure, (2) barotrauma from the ventilator-transmitted piston effect, or (3) toxins from the plastic of the endotracheal tube. Bacterial or viral infection may play a role similar to that in infants with tracheo- and bronchomalacia or subglottic stenosis. Infants with severe birth asphyxia and/or shock may develop necrotizing tracheobronchitis because of the ischemia to the airway mucosa. A disturbance in hemodynamics or vascularization is postulated to play a role in the etiology of tracheobronchitis.[64]

Clinically, the infant with necrotizing tracheobronchitis may be asymptomatic, then suddenly deteriorate, with carbon dioxide retention that fails to respond to ventilator changes, suctioning, or reintubation. This is caused by the sloughing of the mucosa, which may occlude the distal trachea. Treatments have included excision or cauterization of the lesions, but this is difficult because of the relatively small airways of preterm infants. Obstruction can lead to lobar atelectasis or death.

Two types of lesions have been found on autopsy. Type I lesions show necrosis, mucosal hemorrhage, and ulcerations. Type II lesions, more chronic, show mucosal fibrosis and extensive squamous metaplasia.[65] The long-term outcome is unknown, but follow-up is important because Type II lesions are considered to be premalignant in the area of the larynx and glottis.

NURSING CARE AND AIRWAY INJURY PREVENTION

Prevention of airway injury should be a priority for nurses caring for any mechanically ventilated infant. An endotracheal tube of the correct size should be used, and only experienced clinicians should intubate the ELBW infant or the infant who is known to be difficult to intubate. Following intubation, the tube should be stabilized to prevent excessive movement and accidental extubation.

A chest x-ray should be taken to evaluate proper endotracheal tube placement. Once tube placement is confirmed, the length of the tube in relation to the infant's lip should be documented so that proper position can be checked every shift. When evaluating position by auscultating breath sounds, the caregiver should hear a slight air leak around the tube. Gas flow through the ventilator should be warmed and humidified sufficiently.

The nurse plays a major role in preventing airway damage from suctioning. Prior to suctioning, the nurse should select the appropriately sized suction catheter and know the exact measurement of the endotracheal tube. The suction catheter should not be passed beyond the length of the endotracheal tube. No more than $50-80$ cmH_2O pressure should be used when applying suction for five seconds. The frequency of suctioning should be individualized, based on the infant's breath sounds, respiratory status, and clinical condition. Oxygen saturation and clinical status should be closely monitored while weaning the infant to appropriate ventilator settings (see Chapter 7).

Mechanically ventilated infants require continuous monitoring to maintain the fine balance between hypoxia and hyperoxia. Assessment of changes in the infant's condition, oxygen saturation levels, and arterial blood gases is key to rapid initiation of appropriate ventilator changes to prevent complications.

Prevention of infection is a major challenge to the NICU team. The endotracheal tube prevents the cilia in the airway from clearing airway debris and potentially pathogenic bacteria or viruses. As a result, infection may develop, leading to the previously described airway lesions. Maintaining clean technique during intubation and endotracheal suctioning is important. If infection is suspected, antibiotics should be initiated and modified to specific organisms.

PULMONARY HEMORRHAGE

Pulmonary hemorrhage generally presents in the first week of life in neonates who require mechanical ventilation. Before the widespread use of exogenous surfactant, pulmonary hemorrhage occurred primarily in infants who were of low birth weight or small for gestational age, or in those with sepsis, asphyxia, or RDS.[66-69] Since the introduction of exogenous surfactant, pulmonary hemorrhage rates have increased. A meta-analysis done by Raju and Langenberg in 1993 demonstrated a 47 percent increase in the risk of pulmonary hemorrhage when surfactant is given.[70]

The risk of pulmonary hemorrhage in surfactant-treated infants increases with decreasing gestational age and birth weight and has also been noted to be higher following vaginal delivery, in male infants, and in the presence of a patent ductus arteriosus.[71,72]

The incidence of pulmonary hemorrhage depends on the definition used, and there is little consistency in the grading of the severity of bleeding.[73] Rates varying from 1 to 11 percent have been reported in the surfactant trials,[74-76] while an incidence of less than 5 percent in infants with RDS was reported in the meta-analysis done by Raju and Langenberg.[70]

More than 80 percent of infants with pulmonary hemorrhage have RDS, and the incidence of pulmonary hemorrhage is inversely proportional to gestational age. At autopsy, the incidence of hemorrhage in premature infants has been found to be 80 percent.[77] The extent of the hemorrhage may range from focal to massive (and fatal).

ETIOLOGY/PATHOPHYSIOLOGY

Pulmonary hemorrhage is speculated to be either the extreme result of pulmonary edema in the neonate or a consequence of increased transcapillary pore size, which allows red blood cells to enter the alveoli.[77] The most common causes of pulmonary edema are increased pulmonary microvascular pressure, reduced intravascular oncotic pressure, reduced lymphatic drainage, and increased microvascular permeability.[78] All result in increased fluid leakage into the pulmonary interstitium, increasing pulmonary lymphatic fluid. Pulmonary edema occurs as lung interstitial fluid increases; the fluid leaks into the alveoli after damage to the alveolar epithelium or distention caused by the interstitial fluid. Initially, only albumin leaks into the alveoli, but as the edema becomes more severe, capillary hemorrhage occurs. Pulmonary hemorrhage has been divided into three categories based on autopsy findings: (1) *interstitial hemorrhages* are characterized by hemorrhage in connective tissue spaces of the lung; (2) *lung hematomas* are accumulations of fresh blood in the interstitium of alveolar spaces; and (3) *intra-alveolar hemorrhages* are characterized by fresh blood filling alveoli in areas not directly adjacent to the interstitium, often extending into the bronchioles and bronchi to produce massive hemorrhage.

At-risk neonates also include those with asphyxia, shock, hypoxia, acidosis, and PDA, all of which can lead to left ventricular heart failure.

The premature infant with severe RDS who is on mechanical ventilation or a high oxygen concentration and who has heart failure secondary to increased pulmonary blood flow is at high risk for developing pulmonary edema and hemorrhage even before receiving surfactant therapy. And the pulmonary edema itself, is known to inhibit surfactant function.

Neonates with RDS who are treated with exogenous surfactant are at risk for pulmonary hemorrhage. The etiology of pulmonary hemorrhage following treatment with surfactant includes alterations in pulmonary hemodynamics because of a PDA, fragile capillaries resulting from extreme prematurity, barotrauma caused by mechanical ventilation, and a localized coagulopathy caused by the surfactant.[79,80] A review of 33 treatment trials using exogenous surfactant from 1980 to 1992 focused on the association between exogenous surfactant therapy and pulmonary hemorrhage. The natural surfactant trials reported a pulmonary hemorrhage incidence of 5.87 percent in treated infants versus

FIGURE 10-9
Pulmonary hemorrhage x-ray.

Infant with moderate respiratory distress.

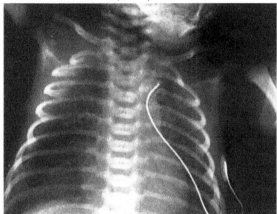

Three hours later, x-ray demonstrates a severe pulmonary hemorrhage.

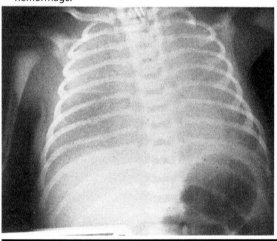

5.36 percent in controls; the synthetic trials reported an incidence of 2.51 percent in treated versus 1.04 percent in control infants. Analysis revealed that surfactant treatment and lower mean birth weight had a significant influence on the risk for a pulmonary hemorrhage. Interestingly, a PDA did not have an independent effect on the risk of a pulmonary hemorrhage.[70]

Factors associated with pulmonary hemorrhage include intrauterine growth retardation, massive aspiration, hypothermia, infection, oxygen therapy, severe Rh hemolytic disease, congenital heart disease, fluid overload, and coagulopathies. Although disseminated intravascular coagulation may precede pulmonary hemorrhage, most affected infants do not have a coagulopathy but may develop it after the hemorrhage occurs.[3]

Signs and Symptoms

Clinically, an infant with a pulmonary hemorrhage may initially present with blood-tinged fluid from the endotracheal tube. With a massive hemorrhage, there may then be a sudden deterioration and simultaneous appearance of bloody secretions in the endotracheal tube and/or the infant's mouth. The fluid has the appearance of fresh blood, but the hematocrit of the fluid is 15–20 points lower than that of the circulating blood.[3]

Usually, the infant becomes pale, cyanotic, hypotensive, and hypotonic, but term infants may become agitated secondary to the hypoxemia and begin to "fight" the ventilator. Signs of heart failure may be present, including tachycardia, murmur (related to the PDA), hepatosplenomegaly, and edema. Hypotension results from the blood and fluid loss, heart failure caused by hypoxemia, and acidosis. Auscultation of the chest reveals widespread crepitus and decreased air entry.

Diagnosis

A few infants may deteriorate clinically without apparent cause for an hour or two before the hemorrhage begins. Once the frank blood becomes evident, the diagnosis is made. Chest radiographic findings depend on whether the hemorrhage was focal or massive. It is often difficult to differentiate a focal hemorrhage from atelectasis or pneumonia. Massive hemorrhage reveals a "whiteout" reflecting atelectasis and opacifications with some air bronchograms (Figure 10-9).

Blood gases deteriorate rapidly following a massive hemorrhage, resulting in severe hypoxia, hypercarbia, and a marked metabolic acidosis. Although the hematocrit of the lung fluid is diluted, considerable amounts of blood may be lost. There are no specific white blood cell changes unless sepsis is present. Drawing of blood cultures is recommended following the hemorrhage. Development of disseminated intravascular coagulation is not uncommon after hemorrhage occurs.

Management

Control of pulmonary edema and heart failure in addition to positive pressure ventilation and oxygenation are critical in preventing pulmonary hemorrhage. Following administration of surfactant, the nurse should closely monitor the infant for signs of heart failure, hypotension, decreased air entry, and wet breath sounds.

Early detection and aggressive intervention are vital in the management of pulmonary hemorrhage. Infants experiencing pulmonary bleeding should be intubated and ventilated. They usually have severe lung diseases that require high PEEP and PIP. An increase in PEEP may be helpful in splinting the alveoli and reducing bleeding. This may help in redistributing lung fluid back into the interstitial space, improving ventilation and perfusion.[81]

Transfusion of blood products, including packed red blood cells, may be necessary because of acute blood loss. Infusions of fresh frozen plasma and administration of vitamin K may be successful in correcting clotting deficiencies. Antibiotic therapy should be started if not already instituted, because sepsis is a major risk factor for pulmonary hemorrhage. Inotropes and diuretics may be needed if heart failure develops.

Administration of surfactant following a pulmonary hemorrhage has been shown to improve oxygenation significantly.[82–84] It is postulated that the presence of hemoglobin in the alveoli may inhibit natural surfactant.[84]

Complications following pulmonary hemorrhage include air leaks and periventricular hemorrhage. The mortality rate after a pulmonary hemorrhage ranges from 30 to 90 percent, with 50–75 percent of the survivors developing CLD.[77]

Nursing Care

Care of the infant with a significant pulmonary hemorrhage includes all aspects of neonatal intensive care nursing. Maintaining an open airway is a major priority. During the first few hours after the hemorrhage, the endotracheal tube may require suctioning every 10–15 minutes. There is significant risk of bloody secretions blocking the tube. Breath sounds must be evaluated frequently.

The infant is often placed on maximum ventilator settings, requiring vigilant monitoring of arterial blood gases and vital signs. Monitoring for the development of air leaks is important because of high pressure settings. Based on evaluation of blood gases, ventilator settings may be changed, and sodium bicarbonate may be ordered. If hypotension occurs, fluids will be recalculated. Blood products and vasopressors may also be necessary.

Cardiovascular Complications

The respiratory and cardiovascular systems work in close harmony to provide the body with adequate oxygen and to remove waste products from the cells. The respiratory system affects cardiovascular function by altering venous return and pulmonary vascular resistance (PVR). Cardiac output depends on venous return to the heart, which is determined in part by differences between extrathoracic and intrathoracic pressures. Subatmospheric intrapleural pressure establishes a favorable pressure gradient for blood to flow back to the right atrium.

How Mechanical Ventilation Affects the Cardiovascular System

The use of CPAP or positive pressures from mechanical ventilation can affect the cardiovascular system by increasing intrathoracic pressure, which decreases venous return.[85] The diminished venous return along with compression of the ventricles caused by the increased intrathoracic pressure decreases cardiac output.

The impact of mechanical ventilation on cardiac output depends on the degree of pressure transmitted from the airway to the intrapleural space. This pressure is influenced by lung compliance. Neonates with RDS who have reduced lung compliance transmit significantly less pressure to the intrapleural space than do those with normal compliance, and so ventilation in these compromised neonates exerts little effect on venous return and cardiac output. The infants can generally tolerate high levels of PIP and PEEP without significant decreases in cardiac output. However, the premature infant who develops a tension pneumothorax has a sudden rise in intrathoracic pressure, which increases central venous pressure. These changes can result in IVH.

When neonates are recovering from RDS following surfactant therapy, compliance may increase rapidly along with increased intrapleural pressure. High ventilator pressures in these neonates can decrease cardiac output and increase venous pressure, leading to possible systemic hypotension, altered perfusion, and IVH.

Another potential complication of positive pressure ventilation and CPAP is a ventilation-to-perfusion mismatch ($\dot{V}_A/\dot{Q}_C$). This ratio describes the relationship between alveolar ventilation and capillary perfusion of the lung. In neonates with lung disease, even though CPAP or positive pressure is applied, areas that are atelectatic tend to remain so, while inflated regions tend to become further distended. The circulation responds by perfusing the areas of the lung that are distended and diminishing circulation in the atelectatic portions.[81] A maximum $\dot{V}_A/\dot{Q}_C$ mismatch occurs in an infant with a tension pneumothorax: Ventilation escapes into the pleural space, where no gas exchange occurs.

Mechanical ventilation increases airway pressure, which is also transmitted to the intraparenchymal pulmonary vessels. The effect is complex and depends on several factors, including the lung disease and compliance. In infants with RDS, there is a decrease in functional residual capacity (FRC), which can result in increased PVR. In infants with lung diseases treated with mechanical ventilation that overdistends the lung, the air spaces compress arterioles and capillaries, causing a $\dot{V}_A/\dot{Q}_C$ mismatch and leading to increased PVR.

Persistent pulmonary hypertension of the newborn (PPHN) is a well-known condition in which PVR remains elevated. During the transition to extrauterine life, PVR normally decreases. In the infant with PPHN, the PVR remains higher than the systemic blood pressure, resulting in a right-to-left shunt across the ductus arteriosus and/or foramen ovale, so blood bypasses the lungs. Clinically, neonates with this condition present with severe cyanosis, higher preductal and lower postductal oxygen saturations.

Hyperventilation with mechanical ventilation has been an important aspect of care because it has been shown to decrease PVR in infants with PPHN. Hyperventilation may not be necessary in treating milder cases and may result in complications, including air trapping. Moderate to severe PPHN may necessitate the use of high-frequency ventilation or ECMO (see Chapters 12 and 13).

Patent Ductus Arteriosus

Patent ductus arteriosus is a condition in which the cardiovascular system has a direct effect on ventilation and perfusion. Delayed ductal closure is inversely related to gestational age and presents a challenging problem for the team caring for the premature neonate on mechanical ventilation. The large left-to-right shunt and resulting cardiac failure aggravate preexisting pulmonary disease.

The ductus arteriosus (DA) arises from the distal dorsal sixth aortic arch and forms a bridge between the pulmonary artery and the dorsal aorta. During fetal life, it carries most of the right ventricular output and directs blood away from the fetal lungs and toward the descending aorta and placenta. Prostaglandin E_2, produced by tissue in the DA, plays an important role in maintaining patency of the ductus *in utero*.[86] The DA becomes more responsive to oxygen and less sensitive to the dilating effects of prostaglandin with increasing gestational age.

In the term neonate, the DA begins to constrict rapidly after delivery with the initiation of breathing and is usually functionally closed by 48 hours of age.[87] Muscle media indent into the lumen, and the intima increases in size to form intimal mounds or cushions that begin to occlude the ductus.[88] These intimal changes occur in conjunction with extensive constriction and shortening of the ductus as well as migration of smooth muscle cells from the media into the intima. Ductal constriction results from multiple factors, increased arterial oxygen tension being one of the most important.[86]

In preterm infants, closure of the DA is less predictable. A number of factors can delay closure, including lung disease that increases PVR, decreased ductal sensitivity to oxygen, increased circulating prostaglandins, and an increased ductal sensitivity to both prostaglandins and nitric oxide.[88,89] A study of 49 preterm infants found their serum levels of prostacyclin, a vasodilatory prostaglandin, to be higher than levels in adults, especially in those infants requiring higher ventilatory support. Higher prostacyclin levels were found in those infants in the study who developed a clinically significant PDA.[90]

Incidence

The incidence of PDA is 20 percent in infants born at >32 weeks gestation but increases to 60 percent in infants born at <28 weeks gestation; the incidence increases with decreasing gestational age and birth weight and the occurrence of RDS.[86] Among infants weighing <1,000 g, about 55–70 percent will have hemodynamic symptoms of a PDA.[87] An early study reported that surfactant therapy may increase the incidence of symptomatic PDA in mechanically-ventilated premature infants to as high as 90 percent.[91] Clinical and echocardiographic reports of these surfactant-treated infants showed that the PDA is of greater diameter, has more blood flow, and causes greater clinical deterioration.[92] A subsequent meta-analysis found that surfactant treatment had no effect on the incidence of PDA.[93]

Pathophysiology

Inflation and ventilation of the lungs at birth should decrease PVR and induce ductal constriction. The drop in PVR allows blood to flow from left to right (aorta to pulmonary artery), in the direction opposite of that fetal circulation. If PVR remains high, as it does during the acute phase of RDS, a bidirectional shunt may occur across the PDA.

The effects of the shunt through the PDA depend on several factors: diameter of the ductus, ductal tone, systemic vascular resistance and PVR, and left ventricular output. Quite often in premature neonates, especially those with RDS, the PVR remains elevated. In addition, persistent hypoxia may prevent the ductus from closing.

Before the use of surfactant, the development of a significant PDA usually corresponded to the diuresis phase of RDS. Following surfactant therapy, improved pulmonary compliance causes PVR to drop below systemic vascular resistance; a significant ductal shunt can develop rapidly as PVR drops.[88] Surfactant is thought to cause the release of circulating prostaglandins, which cause relaxation of smooth muscle, including that of the DA.

As respiratory distress resolves and PVR drops, left-to-right shunting predominates, placing stress on the heart and lung. In the premature infant, the ventricles are less distensible and generate less force; therefore, this can result in left ventricular enlargement from the PDA. Elevated left ventricular end-diastolic pressure results, which increases pulmonary venous pressure and causes pulmonary congestion. As a result, the infant develops right-sided heart failure and over time may develop pulmonary hypertension.[94]

In addition, the infant with RDS frequently has a low plasma oncotic pressure and increased capillary permeability, both of which respond to the increased microvascular perfusion by allowing leakage of plasma proteins into the alveolar space. This leads to pulmonary edema. This leakage may inhibit surfactant function and increase surface tension, thereby worsening the disease. Additionally, immature alveoli may be more sensitive to the presence of this fluid.[88] The pulmonary edema plus the continuous distention of pulmonary vessels during diastole may be factors in the development of pulmonary hemorrhage and BPD.[87,95]

In the presence of a left-to-right shunt such as a PDA, a term infant is capable of maintaining cardiac output by increasing left ventricular output. The premature infant's ventricles have less muscular organization and more water content, resulting in an inability to maintain cardiac output. This may cause a redistribution of systemic blood flow to the organs. Very low birth weight (VLBW) infants with PDA have been found to have increased blood flow in the ascending aorta and decreased flow in the descending aorta, findings that have been associated with IVH and NEC.[96–98]

Clinical Findings

Prior to the use of surfactant, clinical signs of a PDA did not usually appear until the third or fourth day of life, during the recovery phase of RDS. Although the ductus was patent, the elevated PVR secondary to lung disease diminished left-to-right shunting. As pulmonary functioning and oxygenation improved, PVR decreased. With the early administration of surfactant to infants with RDS, significant shunting through the ductus is seen much earlier. Infants born at less than 30 weeks gestation who have severe RDS also have a high incidence of persistent PDA.[99]

Moderate to large amounts of shunting through the PDA can result in congestive heart failure. Clinical signs include a hyperactive precordium, tachypnea, tachycardia, decreased urine output, increased pulse amplitude, and widened pulse pressure (difference between systolic and diastolic blood pressure is >30 mmHg). The increase in cardiac output and blood flow back to the left side of the heart cause the increased precordial activity and bounding pulses. The classic continuous murmur described in older infants is not always heard in premature infants.

Preterm infants may have a PDA that is clinically silent but hemodynamically significant. These infants can have a reduction in systolic and diastolic blood pressures severe enough to require inotropic drugs.[100] Research has demonstrated that the presence of a PDA for longer than six days is associated with a longer duration of oxygen therapy and mechanical ventilation.[101] Long-term effects of a PDA include poor weight gain, recurrent respiratory infections (because of increased lung fluid and left-sided heart failure), and the need for additional ventilator support.

Diagnosis

The diagnosis of PDA is based on clinical findings plus echocardiography. A poor correlation between clinical findings alone and a PDA diagnosis has been identified.[102] M-mode echocardiography provides measurement of the heart chambers and can be used to evaluate left ventricular function.[103] A color Doppler echocardiogram can determine the degree of shunting across the ductus, and two-dimensional echocardiography provides information about the size of the ductus. With M-mode, if the ratio of the size of the aortic root to the left atrium is greater than 1:1, the presence of a PDA is confirmed. Using echocardiography and Doppler diagnosis on day 3 of life, it is possible to predict PDAs that will later become symptomatic. In one study, a ductal diameter of >1.5 mm within the first 30 hours of life had a sensitivity of 83 percent in predicting the need for treatment of a PDA.[104] A chest x-ray of an infant with a PDA may be completely normal in the absence of significant left-to-right shunting, or it may demonstrate an enlarged left atrium and alveolar edema.[103]

Treatment

Definitive treatment of a PDA is closure. Conservative methods are implemented before pharmacologic therapy or surgical ligation. There has been some debate in the recent literature both about the need to treat the ductus and about when to initiate treatment. The lack of evidence showing any long-term benefit from treatment of a PDA has led some investigators to question the need for treatment.[89,105] Further, it has been suggested that although there is an *association* between a PDA and the morbidities discussed earlier in this section, there is little proof of causation.[94,106]

CONSERVATIVE APPROACHES

A study published in 2007, by Vanhaesebrouck and colleagues, demonstrated achievement of a 94 percent rate of ductal closure by employing a conservative approach of increased PEEP and fluid restriction.[107]

Prior to Vanhaesebrouck's study, it was generally accepted that fluid restriction, although recommended, was unlikely to close the PDA without other interventions,[86,106,108] but that it might confer some benefit by reducing the hemodynamic significance of the PDA.[109] A combination of fluid restriction and diuretics can lead to electrolyte imbalances, dehydration, and reduced caloric intake. According to one 1983 study, administration of furosemide was associated with an increased incidence of PDA.[110] It is speculated that this finding may have resulted from diuretic-induced release of renal prostaglandins.[86]

The use of PEEP has been shown to reduce the left-to-right shunt through the PDA.[100,107] Management of mechanical ventilation for the infant with a PDA is an important issue. Infants without RDS but with a large left-to-right shunt may have increased interstitial and peribronchiolar edema. Because lung compliance is relatively normal, high inflating pressures should be avoided. These high pressures may impair venous return and cardiac output, altering pulmonary perfusion and the $\dot{V}_A/\dot{Q}_C$ ratio.

PHARMACOLOGIC THERAPY: INDOMETHACIN AND IBUPROFEN

For a number of years, indomethacin has been the mainstay of pharmacologic therapy for a PDA. Debate continues regarding the criteria for initiating treatment (prophylactic vs symptomatic) and the length of treatment (short vs long course). More recently, ibuprofen has been approved for use in PDA treatment in the U.S. A number of trials comparing indomethacin and ibuprofen have been published, including three meta-analyses.[111–113] Indomethacin and ibuprofen are potent inhibitors of the cyclo-oxygenase pathway, which forms the various prostaglandins, and were originally developed as anti-inflammatory agents.

Indomethacin has been proven to be clinically effective in closing PDAs in premature infants within the first seven days of life, with successful closure in approximately 66–80 percent of cases.[114–116] More recent figures suggest that successful closure of a symptomatic PDA can be expected in 50 percent of 24- to 25-week-gestational-age infants receiving indomethacin and in 60 percent of infants >25 weeks gestational age.[117,118]

Administration of prophylactic indomethacin has been studied both in the prevention of PDA and also as a strategy to prevent IVH. Two studies have demonstrated the benefits of indomethacin prophylaxis on the incidences of PDA, PDA ligation, and severe intracranial hemorrhage (ICH).[119,120] A Cochrane review reached a similar conclusion.[101]

Evaluation of prophylactic treatment for PDA also found that indomethacin-treated infants required more oxygen, higher mean ventilatory pressures, and more doses of surfactant.[120–122] Because of the side effects of both indomethacin and ibuprofen and because prophylactic treatment has failed to demonstrate long-term benefits, this practice has been abandoned.

Use of indomethacin as a treatment for asymptomatic PDAs has also been examined. A meta-analysis done by Cooke and colleagues found a significant decrease in the incidence of symptomatic PDAs following treatment of asymptomatic PDAs with indomethacin.[123] Others argue that the use of indomethacin in asymptomatic infants unnecessarily puts them at risk of side effects without proven long-term benefit.[89,124]

Currently, intravenous indomethacin, 0.1–0.3 mg/kg/dose, is given every 12–24 hours for a total of three doses. In most cases, a single dose has not resulted in persistent constriction of the DA. Studies looking at the efficacy of a five- or six-day course of low-dose indomethacin (0.1 mg/kg/day) have found a lower incidence of fluid and electrolyte imbalances and also a lower rate of ductal reopening than with the traditional three-dose course.[125–127] However, a meta-analysis comparing the long-course (four doses or more) approach to a short (three-dose) course found only a borderline effect on the rate of PDA closure, with a greater risk of CLD in infants receiving the long course. The long course did result in a decreased risk of renal impairment, but an increased risk of NEC. The authors concluded that a prolonged course of indomethacin could not be recommended.[128]

Complications from indomethacin can be significant, so infants must be screened before therapy is initiated. Serum creatinine and electrolytes should be measured before treatment is started and before each subsequent dose is given.[87] Renal dysfunction can be a major complication. Indomethacin may be contraindicated if the serum creatinine is above 1.2–1.8 mg/dL or if urine output is less than 1 mL/kg/hour. If urine output decreases in an infant who has received indomethacin, the administration of low-dose dopamine has been suggested.

Platelet function may be impaired for at least a week after indomethacin administration. For this reason, indomethacin is contraindicated in infants with renal or gastrointestinal (GI) bleeding or with NEC. It is recommended that the neonate has a platelet count of at least 50,000/mm³ before initiation of indomethacin treatment.[87] Although the drug has been associated with occasional intestinal perforation, there has been no evidence of increased NEC. The increased incidence of GI perforation has been reported when indomethacin and postnatal steroids are administered concurrently.[129]

Indomethacin has been shown to decrease cerebral blood flow by 12–40 percent in premature infants.[116] There is concern that rapid infusion, which has been the standard practice, might reduce cerebral blood flow to excessively low levels, resulting in brain ischemia. Two studies have shown a significant decrease in cerebral blood flow velocities when the drug is given quickly over 5 minutes or slowly over 30 minutes. Therefore, further studies are necessary to determine the safest rate of administration.[130,131]

For a number of years ibuprofen has been used in Europe as an alternative to indomethacin. Studies have suggested that ibuprofen has an efficacy similar to that of indomethacin but without the significant reduction in renal function.[112,132,133] In a meta-analysis, indomethacin and ibuprofen had a similar rate of PDA closure with no differences in need for surgical ligation; mortality; or the incidence of IVH, NEC, or ROP. The

review found an increased rate of CLD in infants receiving ibuprofen.[134] Unlike indomethacin, ibuprofen has not been found to reduce the incidence of severe IVH.[135] Ibuprofen may be the drug of choice for closure of the ductus arteriosus because it has fewer short-term side effects.[117,136] No long-term follow-up data is available for ibuprofen as it was only approved for use in the United States in 2006.

Following administration of indomethacin or ibuprofen, the infant should be monitored for success of PDA closure. Significant improvements in lung compliance have been noted.[137] Mechanical ventilation pressures and rates can be lowered, thus exposing infants to lower Paw. Reopening of the ductus arteriosus is a common problem in infants weighing <1,000 g.

SURGICAL LIGATION

Surgical ligation of the PDA is usually reserved for infants for whom drug therapy is contraindicated or who fail to respond to conservative and/or drug therapy. Ligation through a left lateral thoracotomy can be done in a short time either in the operating room or at the bedside. Complications of ligation include laryngeal nerve paralysis, pneumothorax, infection, and chylothorax.[94,138] A significant number of postoperative infants experience hypotension, requiring inotropic support.[139] A recent study found an increased incidence of CLD, ROP, and neurodevelopmental abnormalities in ELBW infants requiring PDA ligation.[140] It is unclear from this study whether surgical ligation is causative or reflective of the degree of illness in this group.

A Cochrane review comparing surgical ligation with medical treatment with either ibuprofen or indomethacin found only one eligible trial to review.[113] This review does state that three observational studies noted that neonates undergoing surgical ligation for PDA had an increased risk for one or more of the following outcomes; chronic lung disease, retinopathy of prematurity, and neurosensory impairment.[113] That trial, from 1983, showed no difference in CLD, NEC, IVH, or mortality between the surgically and the pharmacologically treated groups.[116] Other surgical techniques, including video-assisted thoracoscopic clipping and catheter coil occlusion, have been explored, but limited neonatal experience has been reported.[141–143]

Nursing Care

Nursing care of the ventilated premature infant requires careful monitoring for signs of a PDA—especially after administration of surfactant. Changes in vital signs that suggest heart failure should be reported. A low mean arterial blood pressure may be an early sign of the patency of the ductus arteriosus in infants weighing <1,000 g. If possible, heart sounds should be auscultated while the infant is off the ventilator, and any murmurs or clicks should be noted. An increase in precordial activity is an extremely reliable sign of a significant PDA. Infants who require increasing ventilatory support or receive surfactant should be further evaluated for PDA.

Medical treatment is based on echocardiography, clinical signs, and unit standards. Before being given indomethacin or ibuprofen, the infant should be evaluated for signs of renal and platelet dysfunction, NEC, and recent IVH. Laboratory studies should include a complete blood count (CBC) with differential, platelet count, electrolytes, blood urea nitrogen (BUN), creatinine, and bilirubin levels.

Strict measurement of urine output before and during drug treatment will reflect renal dysfunction. Assessment for clinical bleeding includes heelstick sites, gastric drainage, and blood in the stool. Auscultation for the absence of a heart murmur during treatment is important. Even after the PDA has been determined to be closed, auscultation for recurrence of a murmur is important in VLBW infants. Retreatment may be considered.

If the infant is unresponsive to drug therapy and requires increased ventilatory support, surgical ligation is considered. Preoperative care includes stabilizing fluid and electrolyte levels, oxygenation, ventilation, and the infant's temperature. Packed red blood cells may be ordered and held for possible transfusion. The surgeon and neonatologist should discuss the benefits and risks of the surgery with the parents and obtain informed surgical consent.

Following surgical ligation, the nurse should assess the infant's vital signs and determine the need for pain medication. The thoracotomy site should be assessed for signs of bleeding or infection. The chest tube drainage system should be checked hourly for proper functioning and any drainage.

Bronchopulmonary Dysplasia

Bronchopulmonary dysplasia is a CLD that develops primarily in neonates who are born at 24–26 weeks gestation weighing <1,000 g and who receive prolonged oxygen therapy and/or positive pressure ventilation.[144] The increase in survival among very premature newborns has increased the number of infants with this disorder, challenging the health care system. In the literature the terms *BPD* and *CLD* are often used interchangeably, as they will be in this chapter.

Definitions: Old and New

In 1967, Northway, Rosan, and Porter described BPD as a type of CLD that developed in premature infants with severe RDS who were treated with positive pressure mechanical ventilation and oxygen.[145] These infants had severe respiratory failure at birth; required aggressive ventilatory support; and, as a result, developed severe lung injuries and remained dependent on oxygen for long periods of time. Originally, Northway's group postulated that oxygen toxicity caused BPD, but research has revealed that multiple complex mechanisms cause the disease. Northway and colleagues' description of BPD is now referred to as classic, or "old," BPD. This descriptor recognizes that in the postsurfactant, post–antenatal steroid era, the picture of BPD has changed and a "new" BPD has emerged. BPD is now known to occur in term and preterm neonates with a variety of neonatal conditions, including apnea, meconium aspiration, pneumonia, and congenital heart disease as well as primary lung disease. Today, infants with BPD may have only mild lung disease at birth and receive only brief periods of mechanical ventilation and oxygen therapy.

Northway and colleagues' original description of BPD outlined the radiologic, pathologic, and clinical criteria associated with four stages of the disease (Table 10-6).[145] Bancalari and associates, in 1979, further defined an infant with BPD as one who requires positive pressure ventilation for at least three days during the first week of life, has clinical signs of respiratory distress, requires supplemental oxygen to maintain an oxygen tension (PaO_2) of 50 torr for >28 days, and shows radiographic evidence of BPD.[146] Since its original description, the presentation and progression of BPD have changed, but the initial characteristics and definitions remain salient to an understanding of this disorder.

As smaller and sicker infants survive because of new technologies (including surfactant replacement therapy, high-frequency ventilation, and prenatal and postnatal steroids), new BPD has emerged. The severe form of BPD originally described was seen primarily in premature infants who were ventilated mechanically using high pressures and had prolonged exposure to high levels of inspired oxygen. New BPD is a milder form of CLD seen

TABLE 10-6
Stages of Bronchopulmonary Dysplasia (Classic)

Stage	Time	Pathologic Findings	Radiologic Findings	Clinical Features
I (mild)	2–3 days	Patchy loss of cilia; bronchial epithelium intact; profuse hyaline membranes	Air bronchograms; diffuse reticulogranularity (identical to RDS)	Identical to RDS
II (moderate)	4–10 days	Loss of cilia; fewer hyaline membranes; necrosis of alveolar epithelium; regeneration of bronchial epithelium; ulceration in bronchioles	Opacification; coarse, irregularly shaped densities containing small vacuolar radiolucencies	Increased O_2 requirements and increasing ventilatory support when recovery is expected; rales, retractions
III (severe)	10–20 days	Advanced alveolar epithelial regeneration; extensive alveolar collapse; bronchiolar metaplasia and interstitial fibrosis; bronchial muscle hypertrophy	Small radiolucent cysts in generalized pattern	Prolonged O_2 dependency; $PaCO_2$ retention; retractions; early barrel chest; severe acute episodes of bronchospasm
IV (advanced-chronic)	1 month	Obliterative bronchiolitis; active epithelial proliferation; peribronchial and some interstitial fibrosis; severe bronchiolar metaplasia	Dense fibrotic strands; generalized cystic areas; large or small heart; hyperinflated lungs; hyperlucency at bases	Increased chest anteroposterior diameter; cor pulmonale; frequent respiratory infection; prolonged O_2 dependency; failure to thrive

From Korones SB. 2011. In *Assisted Ventilation of the Neonate*, 5th ed., Goldsmith JP, and Karotkin EH, eds. Philadelphia: Saunders, 390. Reprinted by permission.

in smaller infants who do not necessarily have severe lung disease at birth.[147]

The newer descriptions of BPD reflect our understanding of the disorder as one of altered lung development with decreased numbers of alveoli and abnormal blood vessel development rather than lung damage.[144,148] However, a clear definition of BPD remains elusive. Some clinicians define BPD as a requirement for supplemental oxygen at day 28 of life; however, this definition may inaccurately label infants who have an acute illness at the end of the first month of life as having BPD or miss infants who subsequently develop the need for supplemental oxygen.[147] Others have proposed the need for oxygen at 36 weeks postmenstrual age as a better criterion for defining BPD.[149] In 2001, the National Institutes of Health (NIH) convened a consensus panel to address these inconsistencies. That panel agreed on the definition of BPD shown in Table 10-7. The NIH definition requires a minimum of 28 days of supplemental oxygen and defines the severity of the disease by the amount of oxygen required.[150] It is important to note that under this definition, infants being treated with supplemental oxygen for nonpulmonary problems—for example, for congenital anomalies such as diaphragmatic hernia—are not considered to have BPD unless they also have parenchymal lung disease. To further refine this definition, some clinicians have suggested that infants receiving supplemental oxygen at 28 days or 36 weeks corrected age, undergo an oxygen needs test. This test involves challenging the infant by gradually reducing the inspired oxygen to room air. Those infants with an oxygen saturation of <90 percent after 30 minutes on room air would be deemed to have BPD.[151]

INCIDENCE

The incidence of BPD is difficult to report because it depends both on the definition of BPD used and also on the accuracy of gestational age determination in the study population. A review by Bhandari and Panitch found the incidence of BPD, defined as oxygen need at 36 weeks postmenstrual age, to be about 30 percent among infants with birth weights <1,000 g.[152] This is similar to the rate of 35 percent found by Walsh and colleagues in a study of 1,598 inborn infants weighing <1,250 g who remained hospitalized at 36 weeks postmenstrual age.[151] Sahni and colleagues identified rates of BPD, defined as oxygen need at 28 and 36 weeks, to be 21.1 and 7.4 percent, respectively.[153] Ehrenkranz and colleagues applied the NIH definition of BPD in a retrospective review of 4,866 infants (birth weight ≤1,000 g, gestational age <32 weeks, alive at 36 weeks postmenstrual age) born between 1995 and 1999 and found that 77 percent of the infants met the criteria for BPD, with 30 percent having moderate disease and 16 percent severe BPD. Of those who met the NIH criteria and were seen in follow-up at 18–22 months corrected age, 35 percent had required rehospitalization for respiratory illnesses and 40 percent had received medications for a pulmonary condition.[154]

TABLE 10-7
Definition of Diagnostic Criteria for BPD

Gestational age	<32 weeks	≥32 weeks
Time point of assessment	36 week PCA or discharge to home, whichever comes first	>28 days, but <56 days postnatal age or discharge to home, whichever comes first
	Treatment with oxygen >21% for at least 28 days *plus*	
Mild BPD	Breathing room air at 36 weeks PCA or discharge, whichever comes first	Breathing room air by 56 days postnatal age or discharge, whichever comes first
Moderate BPD	Need* for <30% oxygen at 36 weeks PCA or discharge, whichever comes first	Need* for <30% oxygen at 56 days postnatal age or discharge, whichever comes first
Severe BPD	Need* for <30% oxygen and/or positive pressure, (PPV or NCPAP) at 36 weeks PCA or discharge, whichever comes first	Need* for ≥30% oxygen and/or positive pressure (PPV or NCPAP) at 56 days postnatal age or discharge, whichever comes first

Key: NCPAP = nasal continuous positive airway pressure; PCA = postconceptional age; PPV = positive-pressure ventilation.

*A physiologic test confirming that the oxygen requirement at the assessment time point remains to be defined. This assessment may include a pulse oximetry saturation range. BPD usually develops in neonates being treated with oxygen and PPV for respiratory failure, most commonly RDS. Persistence of clinical features of respiratory disease (tachypnea, retractions, rales) are considered common to the broad description of BPD and have not been included in the diagnostic criteria describing the severity of BPD. Infants treated with oxygen >21 percent and/or positive pressure for nonrespiratory disease (e.g., central apnea or diaphragmatic paralysis) do not have BPD unless they also develop parenchymal lung disease and exhibit clinical features of respiratory distress. A day of treatment with oxygen >21 percent means that the infant received oxygen >21 percent for more than 12 hours on that day. Treatment with oxygen >21 percent and/or positive pressure at 36 weeks PMA, or at 56 days postnatal age or discharge, should not reflect an "acute" event, but should rather reflect the infant's usual daily therapy for several days preceding and following 36 weeks PMA, 56 days postnatal age, or discharge.

From: Jobe AH, and Bancalari E. 2001. Bronchopulmonary dysplasia. *American Journal of Respiratory Critical Care Medicine* 163(7): 1726. Reprinted by permission.

PATHOGENESIS

Bronchopulmonary dysplasia has been attributed to oxygen toxicity, barotrauma, volutrauma, lung immaturity, inflammation, and infection (Figure 10-10). The causes are multifactorial and likely include acute lung injury, arrested lung development, as well as abnormal repair processes that occur in the lung. Normal lung growth and development are disrupted by a premature birth. The immature lung, already deficient in surfactant, is then exposed to adverse stimuli.

FIGURE 10-10
Factors contributing to the development of BPD.

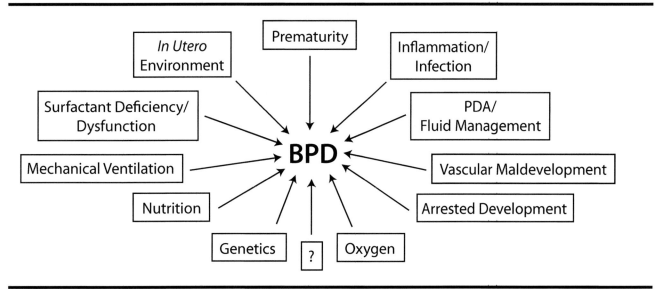

From: Chess PR, et al. 2006. Pathogenesis of bronchopulmonary dysplasia. *Seminars in Perinatology* 30(4): 172. Reprinted by permission.

FIGURE 10-11
Injury zones in the lung.

The upper graph shows a pressure-volume curve and indicates the low- and high-volume injury zones. Lung volumes for a normal adult, a term newborn, and a preterm infant with RDS are given in mL/kg in the lower graph. The low- and high-volume injury zones are indicated by arrows. The preterm lung is susceptible to injury with ventilation because of the small volume per kilogram between the two injury zones.

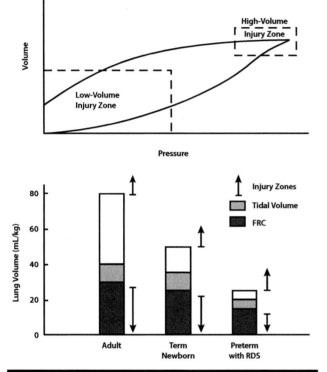

From: Jobe AH, and Ikegami M. 1998. Mechanisms initiating lung injury in the preterm. *Early Human Development* 53(1): 86. Reprinted by permission.

Oxygen

Oxygen has been implicated in the development of BPD since the disorder was first described in the 1960s.[145] Although the development of BPD in infants exposed to minimal or no supplemental oxygen supports the notion that oxygen is not essential for the development of BPD,[146,155] it continues to be implicated as a major factor.[156]

Two types of oxygen toxicity have been described in BPD. The first type results in damage from the toxic effects of oxygen on the lung tissue. The second type is indirect damage that results from maladaptive physiologic responses to hyperoxia. Ventilated infants are particularly at risk of injury as a result of the formation of toxic metabolites of oxygen, which damage the airway, the lining of the capillaries, and the

alveolar epithelium.[157] These by-products come in two forms: free radicals and reactive oxygen species (ROS). Free radicals include the superoxide radical ($O_2^-\cdot$)and the hydroxyl free radical (OH^-). Both reactive oxygen species have unpaired electrons in their outer orbital shells, a molecular conformation that makes it possible for both, but particularly the hydroxyl free radical, to damage DNA, proteins, and lipids. Essentially, free radicals destabilize organic molecules by either donating electrons to or accepting electrons from these species. In contrast, ROS include non-free radicals such as hydrogen peroxide (H_2O_2) and peroxynitrite ($ONOO^-$); ROS are nonradical by-products of oxygen metabolism that are injurious on their own and that may also be transformed into free radicals.

Free radicals and ROS are normal, physiologic by-products of a variety of cellular processes, including energy production, immune cell function, and drug metabolism. Under homeostatic conditions, the production of free radicals and ROS is balanced by endogenous antioxidants, which either act as scavengers or stimulate antioxidant enzymes such as superoxide dismutase (SOD), glutathione peroxidase (GPx), and catalase (CAT). Further antioxidant defenses are conferred by trace elements such as selenium and amino acids, including taurine.[158] Additionally, there is good evidence to suggest that exogenous molecules, such as antioxidant factors in breast milk (including lactoferrin and thioredoxin) and vitamins C and E, serve to reduce the toxicity of oxygen for the newborn infant.[159–161]

When hyperoxia, reperfusion, or inflammation cause increased free radical production that overwhelms the body's antioxidant defense mechanisms, these free radicals can damage cell membranes and unravel nucleic acids, a process referred to as oxidative stress.[162] Newborn infants in general, and premature infants in particular, are known to be at high risk for oxidative stress because of deficiencies in antioxidants.[162,163] Other causes of oxidative stress in this population include lung immaturity, which necessitates exposure to oxygen therapy; increased susceptibility to infections and inflammation; and the presence of free iron in the premature infant's system, which serves as a catalyst for ROS reactions.[164] There is mounting evidence that hyperoxia is a key injury stimulus in premature infants and that it is linked to the pathogenesis of a variety of disorders, including BPD and ROP.[157,165] Supporting this theory is the fact that, in animal models, prolonged exposure to oxygen is associated with markers of inflammation and the appearance of pro-inflammatory cytokines such as interleukin (IL)-1α.[166,167] Lung abnormalities such as decreased septation and decreased lung surface area have been found to persist even after recovery from hyperoxic exposure.[167] Furthermore, SOD and CAT decrease lung injuries associated with oxygen toxicity.[168] The appearance of the antioxidant SOD coincides with the onset of surfactant synthesis by Type II pneumocytes.[169]

Reactive oxygen species' injuries to epithelial and endothelial cells result in pulmonary edema and activation of inflammatory cells.[157] As pulmonary edema progresses, proteins leak into the alveoli, inhibiting the surface tension properties of surfactant, thereby exacerbating the surfactant deficiency of prematurity.[162] The resulting cycle of worsening atelectasis, decreased lung compliance, and increased $\dot{V}_A/\dot{Q}_C$ mismatch leads to the need for higher oxygen and ventilator settings, which increases oxidative stress.

In response to the direct damage to cells caused by oxygen free radicals, a second phase of damage occurs. This phase is characterized by the proliferation of alveolar Type II cells and, ultimately, tissue fibrosis.[157] A number of markers of peroxidation (oxidative damage) have been found in the tracheal fluid and urine of neonates who later develop BPD. These changes are often seen only a few hours or a day after birth, supporting the theory that prenatal inflammation is also important in the development of BPD.[170]

Lung Trauma

Positive pressure ventilation is known to be important in the pathogenesis of BPD because of the contribution of pressure (barotrauma) and volume (volutrauma) to initiation of the inflammatory cascade. Dreyfuss and Saumon report that mechanical ventilation in animals using volumes greater than lung capacity injures the alveoli, resulting in leukocyte migration into the lungs, increased tissue permeability, and leakage of fluid into the interstitial tissue and alveoli.[171] Equally damaging is ventilation using volumes below FRC, which results in cyclic collapse of the alveoli (atelectotrauma).[172] The lung injury zones are illustrated in Figure 10-11. Without adequate tools to measure FRC, it can be very difficult to avoid injury when mechanically ventilating a premature infant.

In some cases, it is likely that injury to the lungs begins during the initial resuscitation of the neonate as clinicians try to establish ventilation quickly. This finding was illustrated by Bjorklund and colleagues who found that as few as six breaths at high tidal volumes prior to surfactant administration resulted in significant lung injury in preterm lambs.[173]

Several studies have also demonstrated an inverse relationship between the development of BPD and PCO_2 levels.[174,175] In fact, Garland and colleagues reported that low PCO_2 before surfactant administration was a stronger predictor of BPD than was the severity of lung disease. This finding supports the theory that hyperventilation plays a significant role in lung injury and subsequent development of BPD.[172]

Inflammation and Infection

Inflammation is now recognized as playing a significant role in the development of BPD. Chorioamnionitis and the presence of elevated cytokine levels *in utero* initiate a pulmonary inflammatory response that is thought to alter wound healing, alveolarization, and vascular development in immature lungs.[176–178]

The pulmonary vasculature contains numerous neutrophils that can trigger an inflammatory response, resulting in the release of enzymes that ultimately disrupt the extracellular matrix of the lung.[179] This response can also be initiated after birth as a result of alveolar injury secondary to oxidative stress or mechanical injury.[176] Young and colleagues found a significant increase in BPD in infants weighing between 700 and 1,000 g with positive initial endotracheal cultures compared with those with cultures that did not grow bacteria.[180] The same association was not found for infants less than 700 g. Similarly, Watterberg and colleagues demonstrated that neonates born following chorioamnionitis experienced mild initial respiratory distress but needed more ventilatory support in the second week of life.[181]

Several infectious agents have been implicated in the development of BPD, among them Chlamydia and adenovirus.[182] *Ureaplasma urealyticum* has been identified as being associated with the development of BPD,[183] but it is unclear whether treating Ureaplasma with antibiotics reduces the incidence of BPD.[184] Studies have demonstrated that this organism may cause a chronic subclinical pneumonia, increasing ventilation and oxygen requirements. It has been suggested that infection may act as an additional stimulus in the inflammatory response, with recruitment of neutrophils and activation of the arachidonic acid cascade ultimately leading to BPD.

TABLE 10-8
Potentially Better Practices for Reducing CLD in LBW Infants

Practice	Level of Evidence*
Provide vitamin A supplementation	Level 1
Decrease fluid administration	Level 3
Administer postextubation CPAP	Level 1
Institute permissive hypercarbia	Level 2
Decrease supraphysiologic corticosteroid exposure in premature infants	Level 1
Provide prophylactic surfactant for infants with birth weights <1,000 g or delivery room CPAP for infants with birth weights >1,000 g	Level 1
Reduce ventilator days	Level 1–5
Use high-frequency ventilation or low tidal volume ventilation	Level 1–2
Provide gentle ventilation in the delivery room	Level 2–3

* Muir Gray Classification System 70:

Level 1—Strong evidence from at least one systematic review of multiple well-designed randomized controlled trials

Level 2—Strong evidence from at least one properly randomized controlled trial of appropriate size

Level 3—Evidence from well-designed trials without randomization including single group, prepost, cohort, time series, or matched case controls

Level 4—Evidence from well-designed nonexperimental studies preferably from more than one center or research group

Level 5—Opinion of respected authorities, based on clinical evidence, descriptive studies, or reports of expert committees

Adapted from: Sharek PF, et al. 2003. Evaluation and development of potentially better practices to prevent chronic lung disease and reduce lung injury in neonates. *Pediatrics* 111(4): e428. Reprinted by permission.

Nutrition

Compromised nutritional status may also exacerbate the development of BPD in the premature infant.[185] Adequate caloric and protein intake is required for cell growth and division. Copper, zinc, iron, manganese, and selenium are required cofactors for antioxidant enzymes and may be necessary for repair of elastin and collagen. Vitamin E may provide antioxidant protection, but research findings are inconclusive. Vitamin A deficiency may also play a significant role in the pathogenesis of BPD because this vitamin is essential for differentiation, integrity, and repair of respiratory epithelial cells.[185,186] Vitamin A supplementation in neonates has been shown to reduce the production of pro-inflammatory cytokines.[187] Malnutrition in the premature infant can impair macrophages and neutrophil and lymphocyte function, which protect the lung against infection.[188]

Other Risk Factors

Other factors that have been correlated with the pathogenesis of BPD include a genetic predisposition, excessive fluid intake, lipid infusion, and gas temperature and humidification in the ventilator circuit.[189] Research suggests that infants are more likely to develop BPD if there is a family history of airway reactivity (including asthma).[190,191] Fluid overload can cause pulmonary edema. Several studies have shown that a persistently patent ductus arteriosus increases the risk of developing BPD.[95,192]

Pathology

The pathologic features of BPD first described by Northway and colleagues are divided into four stages (see Table 10-6). This classic, or "old," BPD described by Northway and colleagues begins with an exudative and early repair stage. That stage is followed, in severe cases, by a chronic fibroproliferative phase marked by widespread fibrosis with atelectasis and emphysema, as well as capillary vascular damage resulting in reduced alveolar development.[145]

In the original descriptions of BPD, characteristics of mild disease included patchy loss of cilia accompanied by mucosal breakdown of the airway lining followed by edema of the bronchi, blood vessels, and alveolar septa. Infants with moderate BPD experienced extensive loss of cilia in the bronchial lining cells and had evidence of inflammatory cells. Areas of atelectasis and metaplasia of cells lining the conductive airways also occurred. Infants with severe BPD developed necrosis of the airway lining resulting in excessive amounts of debris containing necrotic epithelial cells, mucus, and inflammatory cells. Areas of atelectasis and hyperinflation caused a $\dot{V}_A/\dot{Q}_C$ mismatch.[193,194]

Upper airway damage in infants with traditional BPD included tracheal, subglottic, and bronchial stenosis; polyps; granulomas; and tracheo- and bronchomalacia. Airway hyperactivity was commonly found in infants with BPD and often persisted into childhood.

Lungs affected by BPD in the postsurfactant era are less likely to have significant fibrosis, airway or smooth muscle hypertrophy, or epithelial metaplasia.[195] Under the definition of BPD, lungs show uniform inflation with fewer but larger alveoli. Other findings include a disruption of the collagen network around the saccules and dysplastic Type II cells in the saccules.[196]

The proposed mechanism for these findings is a disruption in alveolarization occurring as a result of damage to the developing capillaries and the alveolar crest cells.[150] Before 36 weeks gestation, the functional respiratory units in the lung consist primarily of saccules. During the late saccular stage (after 20 weeks gestation), septal crest cells infiltrate these saccules, dividing each saccule into multiple alveoli. This septation process is accompanied by proliferation of alveolar capillaries that nourish the developing alveoli. Much of this development takes place in the relative hypoxemia found in the normal human fetus. Animal research suggests that inflammatory damage to the crest cells and the alveolar vasculature arrests septation, resulting in the findings of fewer, larger alveoli.[197]

Some researchers have proposed a three-stage model for the new definition of BPD, which might be useful in designing research studies.[198] The perinatal and early postnatal stage (Stage 1) represents opportunities to prevent BPD and is characterized by injury caused by inflammation. Evolving BPD (Stage 2) occurs at 7–14 days of age; interventions at this stage are aimed at diminishing the severity of the disease. In established BPD (Stage 3), which occurs at 21–35 days of age, characteristics include over-reactive airways, pulmonary edema, and oxygen dependency.

PREVENTION

Prevention of BPD begins with the elimination of preterm birth. If this is not possible, attempts should be made to accelerate lung maturity through administration of antenatal corticosteroids. The benefit of antenatal steroids in lessening the severity of RDS and, subsequently, BPD has been clearly shown.[199]

Numerous preventive strategies have been proposed, but few have been shown to significantly reduce the incidence of BPD in LBW infants. Using a research-to-practice translation process, representatives from nine member hospitals in the Neonatal Intensive Care Quality Collaborative developed a list of nine evidence-based potentially better practices (PBPs) aimed at reducing the incidence and severity of CLD in LBW infants.[200] Table 10-8 lists these practices. The levels of evidence supporting these PBPs varied. A report on the challenges and successes in implementing these PBPs was published.[201] The evidence supporting selected PBPs is presented in the following sections.

Avoid Ventilation

It was hoped that the introduction of surfactant therapy in the 1990s would reduce CLD. Although survival rates for LBW infants did increase following the introduction of this therapy, rates of BPD remained the same or increased.[202]

Assisted ventilation has come under intense scrutiny. Efforts have been made to reduce the impact of mechanical ventilation by avoiding intubation altogether, reducing the number of days on mechanical ventilation, and reducing the barotrauma and volutrauma linked to conventional mechanical ventilation. To this end, a variety of devices has been developed to support the LBW infant with respiratory disease. These include nasal CPAP (NCPAP) and nasal intermittent positive pressure ventilation (NIPPV), high-frequency ventilation (HFV), and synchronized mechanical ventilation (SIMV). None of these modes of ventilation have been shown to prevent BPD, but some results are promising.[202]

In a groundbreaking paper published in 1987, Avery and colleagues compared survival rates and rates of BPD in eight U.S. NICUs.[203] They found that, despite similar survival rates for LBW infants among the facilities, the incidence of BPD was significantly lower at Columbia Presbyterian Medical Center in New York. The most striking difference between Columbia and the other centers was the early use of nasal prong CPAP with less dependence on intubation and mechanical ventilation at Columbia. Similarly, Sahni and colleagues reported that in infants weighing <1,250 g managed primarily with bubble CPAP, the incidence of BPD was 7.4 percent.[153] In a study done in New Zealand, Meyer and colleagues examined the preferential use of bubble CPAP and noted an incidence of CLD of 19 percent compared with an average of 45 percent in 28 other centers. These investigators also noted a trend toward a decrease in late-onset sepsis.[204] Studies are now examining the early use of surfactant followed by rapid extubation to CPAP, an approach dubbed INSURE.[205] The use of the INSURE protocol at one institution in Sweden resulted in a 50 percent reduction in the number of infants requiring mechanical ventilation.[205]

A 2007 Cochrane review compared early surfactant replacement therapy followed by extubation to nasal CPAP with the use of rescue surfactant replacement and mechanical ventilation. The authors found that prophylactic surfactant and extubation to CPAP is associated with a reduction in the need for mechanical ventilation, fewer air leaks, and a lower incidence of BPD.[206]

In randomized controlled studies using NIPPV, a trend to lower rates of BPD among infants treated with NIPPV was noted, although the numbers did not reach statistical significance.[207,208] A more recent study published by Kugelman and colleagues found that in the 84 infants 28–33 weeks gestational age in their study, those randomized to NIPPV for the initial treatment of RDS were significantly less likely to require ventilation than were those in the CPAP group (25 percent vs 49 percent). Those infants also had significantly lower rates of BPD (5 percent vs 33 percent, *p*<.05, for infants <1,500 g).[209]

Permissive Hypercapnia

Permissive hypercapnia ($PaCO_2$ 45–55 mmHg) is another strategy that has been suggested to ensure a more gentle approach to ventilation aimed at reducing volutrauma and barotrauma. In addition to reduced barotrauma, animal data have demonstrated that lambs exposed to supplemental CO_2 to levels of 100 mmHg had fewer markers of pulmonary inflammation than did control lambs with normal levels of CO_2.[210] Clinical trials of permissive hypercapnia in human infants have been limited and have failed to demonstrate a consistent reduction in CLD.[211,212] The Cochrane review of this topic also failed to find a significant benefit to permissive hypercapnia.[213]

Fluid Restriction

Excessive lung water has been shown to be a risk factor for the development of BPD.[214] Lung injury and inflammation result in capillary leak, leading to pulmonary edema. Restricting fluid intake to the minimum necessary to provide adequate calories for growth has been recommended for infants at risk of developing BPD.[155,215] A meta-analysis examining fluid intake showed that restricted intake in preterm infants was associated with a lower risk of mortality and a trend toward a lower incidence of BPD.[109] Excessive sodium administration has also been shown to contribute to fluid retention and should be avoided.[216]

Antioxidant Therapy

Vitamin A is one of the only preventive strategies that has been clearly shown to reduce the incidence of BPD.[202] A randomized controlled trial of vitamin A supplementation in VLBW infants found that infants in the treatment group had significantly lower rates of oxygen dependency at 36 weeks than did control infants.[217] A Cochrane review of vitamin A in the prevention of BPD concurred with these findings.[218] Despite these conclusions, a survey of 207 Level III NICUs found that only 20 percent of training units and 13 percent of nontraining units routinely give vitamin A supplements to VLBW infants.[219]

Antioxidant agents other than vitamin A have been explored in the quest to reduce the incidence of BPD. These agents include intratracheal superoxide dismutase[220] and N-acetylcysteine.[221] Neither agent demonstrated a significant difference in BPD rates between study and control populations.

SIGNS AND SYMPTOMS

Early clinical signs of BPD may begin within the first week of life, when recovery from the initial disease (for example, RDS) is anticipated. Most LBW infants who develop "new" BPD have a relatively mild course of respiratory distress, but apnea or poor respiratory drive may delay extubation from mechanical ventilation.[95] These infants are weaned quickly to low ventilator settings and low concentrations of inspired oxygen. Following a honeymoon period with minimal or no supplemental oxygen, these infants progressively deteriorate, requiring increased ventilatory support. This deterioration may coincide with the onset of a symptomatic PDA or the diagnosis of a bacterial or viral infection.[155] Clinically, the infant may have retractions, diminished breath sounds, and fine crackles.

During the early phases of mild to moderate CLD, the changes on x-ray and in pulmonary function are usually mild. Persistent diffuse haziness may be the only change evident on x-ray.[155] As BPD progresses, a fine lacy pattern may develop in the parenchyma, and some hyperinflation with occasional large cysts may be seen on x-ray.[222]

A number of scoring systems have been developed to assist clinicians in predicting which infants with RDS will develop BPD.[223,224] The purpose of these scoring systems is, in part, to determine which infants to enroll in clinical trials investigating BPD treatments.[223] In these clinical trials, criteria found to be predictive of BPD development included the following two: a logistic regression analysis combining birth weight, five-minute Apgar scores, and PIP at 12 hours of age;[223] with FiO_2 >.30 and ventilation index <0.51 (10,000/peak pressure × rate × PCO_2) at 14 days.[224]

TREATMENT

The etiology and pathophysiology of BPD are multifactorial; the treatment is multifaceted. Management of the infant with BPD requires a multidisciplinary team in which all members are aware of the infant's response to various treatments. The goal is to promote growth and maintain homeostasis in all systems, while keeping the infant free from infection and gradually weaning the ventilator and oxygen. Prevention and early recognition of the many complications associated with BPD are essential.

Oxygen Therapy

The clinician, knowing that oxygen therapy is necessary but also causes further damage to the infant with BPD, must strive for a fine balance. As the Supplemental Therapeutic Oxygen for Prethreshold Retinopathy of Prematurity (STOP-ROP) study demonstrated, infants maintained at a higher oxygen saturation range had more severe BPD than did those in a lower range.[225] Although optimal oxygen levels for LBW infants are unknown, targeting an oxygen saturation of 88–92 should help to decrease the severity of BPD.[225] At the same time, adequate oxygen levels should be maintained to avoid pulmonary hypertension and promote tissue growth. Oxygen should be reduced gradually based on the infant's tolerance.

Using pulse oximetry and physical findings, the nurse should continuously assess the infant with BPD to determine oxygen requirements. During activities that may stress the infant—bathing; feeding; painful procedures, including laboratory work; and endotracheal tube suctioning—additional oxygen may be required. Following these activities, the infant should be given time to stabilize before the oxygen is reduced to baseline levels.

Parents should be taught to maintain adequate oxygen saturations at all times: while the infant is awake, feeding, and asleep. They also need to be taught to observe for respiratory distress, cyanosis, irritability, and early signs of respiratory infections.

Mechanical Ventilation

Like oxygen, mechanical ventilation is a known risk factor for infants with BPD. It is important to use the most modest settings possible to maintain appropriate levels of gas exchange. It is also important to set reasonable targets for PCO_2 and PO_2 and to work toward the shortest possible duration of mechanical ventilation. Few prospective randomized trials have been conducted to determine the combination of ventilator settings that either limits the severity or prevents the development of BPD; however, some general principles can be applied. To minimize both barotrauma and atelectotrauma, the lowest peak airway pressure that provides an adequate tidal volume should be used.[226] A PEEP adequate to avoid airway collapse is also important. Higher PEEP levels (6–8 cmH_2O) may be needed in infants with floppy airways secondary to prolonged ventilation.

Synchronized intermittent mandatory ventilation and pressure support ventilation (assist-control) are designed to improve interaction and reduce antagonism between infant-generated and mechanically generated breaths (see Chapter 9). The ability of SIMV to limit lung overdistention reduces the need for the neonate to fight the ventilator breaths. Intuitively, synchronized ventilation should be of benefit in reducing the incidence and severity of BPD; however, a large multicenter study failed to show any difference in the incidence of BPD.[227] A Cochrane review of synchronized ventilation did find a reduction of air leaks and a shorter duration of ventilation but did not find a reduction in the incidence of CLD with synchronized ventilators.[17] A Cochrane review of volume-targeted versus pressure limited ventilation did demonstrate a reduction in BPD, duration of ventilation, and airleaks for those infants receiving volume ventilation.[228] Studies that are more recent have demonstrated a positive effect of volume-targeted ventilation on lung inflammation in premature infants.[229,230] Longer-term follow-up is needed to assess for a reduction in BPD rates.

High-frequency ventilation (see Chapter 12) has been evaluated to determine its impact on BPD, again with mixed results. Thome and colleagues found that in infants 24–30 weeks, use of HFV with high lung volumes did not confer any benefit in preventing BPD compared with conventional ventilation.[231] A meta-analysis of two trials using high-frequency oscillatory ventilation (HFOV) concluded that the use of HFOV may reduce CLD rates somewhat, but the findings were inconsistent.[232] The Cochrane review of high-frequency jet ventilation (HFJV) found that the use of HFJV moderately reduces CLD rates but may increase the risk of IVH.[233]

Medications

Long-term management of infants with BPD often includes treatment with many drugs such as vitamins, diuretics, bronchodilators, and in some cases, steroids. The decision to use each drug should be individualized. The addition of each drug to the infant's management plan should be closely monitored to prevent the "polypharmacy" phenomenon associated with BPD care. For a detailed review of all medications used for the infant with BPD, see Chapter 11.

TABLE 10-9
Recommendations for Monitoring the Nutritional Status of Enterally Fed Hospitalized VLBW Infants

Intake/Output Monitoring	
Fluid intake (mL/kg/day)	Daily
Urine output (mL/kg/day)	Daily
Nutrient Intake	
Energy (kcal/kg/day)	Daily
Proteins (g/kg/day)	Daily if weight gain is poor
Anthropometric Monitoring	
Body weight (g)	Twice daily until stable, then daily
Length (cm)	Weekly
Head circumference	Weekly
Biochemical Monitoring	
Complete blood counts including platelet and reticulocyte count	Every 2 weeks
Serum electrolytes and blood urea nitrogen	Weekly if on diuretics or with fluid restriction; every 2 weeks when stable
Calcium, phosphorus, and alkaline phosphatase	Every 2 weeks
Total protein, albumin, prealbumin	Consider if weight gain is poor or blood urea nitrogen is low
Liver function tests	At 2 weeks, then every 2 weeks if there is evidence of cholestasis

Adapted from: Biniwale MA, and Ehrenkranz RA. 2006. The role of nutrition in the prevention and management of bronchopulmonary dysplasia. *Seminars in Perinatology* 30(4): 204. Reprinted by permission.

NUTRITION

Despite improvements in parenteral and enteral nutrition, postnatal growth failure is still seen in LBW infants, especially those with BPD.[234] For infants with BPD, the incidence of growth failure in the immediate postdischarge period is estimated to be between 30 and 67 percent.[235] Studies have shown that children with BPD have increased resting energy levels and that growth failure in this population may contribute to adverse pulmonary and developmental outcomes.[236,237] More specifically, infants with BPD have a metabolic rate approximately 25 percent higher than infants without BPD, leading to a caloric requirement 20–40 percent higher than age-matched infants without BPD.[188]

The increased work of breathing resulting from decreased lung compliance, increased airway resistance, and tachypnea is one of the factors interfering with normal growth. Another concern is the delay in initiating and advancing enteral feedings in the presence of respiratory disease, feeding intolerance, and other complications.[188]

Parenteral Nutrition

Providing adequate nutrition to the VLBW neonate at risk for BPD is often quite challenging. The overriding goal is to provide adequate calorie and protein intake to support a rate of growth similar to that seen *in utero*. It is important to address the neonate's nutritional needs beginning on the first day of life. Initially, nutrition is provided in parenteral form, with enteral feedings started as soon as the infant is medically stable, ideally within the first few days of life. Recommended parenteral intake on the first day of life is 80–100 mL/kg/day of fluid, 2–3 g/kg of protein, 0.5–1 g/kg of fat emulsion, and 4–6 mg/kg/minute of glucose.[188] Proteins, fats, and carbohydrates are gradually increased to 4 g/kg, 3 g/kg, and 10–12 mg/kg/minute, respectively. Some clinicians have been reluctant to provide protein in the first few days of life because of concerns regarding side effects such as metabolic acidosis; however, a study by Thureen and others demonstrated that a protein intake as high as 3 g/kg on day 1 of life was well tolerated by VLBW infants.[238]

Enteral Feedings

Breast milk or formula is introduced as soon as possible after delivery in the form of trophic feedings. Commonly, however, infants with respiratory distress have periods of feeding intolerance or medical complications such as a PDA or sepsis, that delay their progression to full enteral feedings. Feedings are started at small volumes and increased slowly to decrease the risk of NEC. Human breast milk, although the preferred source of nutrition, does not provide adequate calories, protein, or minerals to meet the increased metabolic needs of premature neonates. Fortification with human milk fortifier, liquid formula concentrate, or protein powder may be used to address the deficits.

Multivitamin supplementation, including vitamin D and iron, is indicated for infants receiving breast milk. Some support also exists for carnitine supplements as a mechanism for enhancing weight gain and catch-up growth.[239] Gastroesophageal reflux disease (GERD) often makes it difficult to provide adequate nutrition to infants with BPD. Reflux may alter lung function in these patients by causing aspiration of stomach contents and triggering bronchial reactivity. Neonates with suspected swallowing dysfunction should be evaluated by a feeding specialist. Conservative measures for managing reflux include thickening the feedings, decreasing the volume of the feeding by increasing the number of feedings, and elevating the head of the bed at a 30-degree angle. Nipple feeding the infant with BPD can be problematic because of the negative oral stimulation from the endotracheal tube, gastric feeding tubes, and frequent oral suctioning.

Electrolyte and mineral imbalances often accompany BPD as a result of fluid restriction, diuretics, dexamethasone, and other medications. Monitoring of serum electrolyte levels is important to determine appropriate amounts of supplementation. Table 10-9 displays a suggested schedule for nutritional monitoring.

Nursing Care

Caring for the infant with BPD can be a frustrating experience for even the most experienced nurse. Although infants with the newer form of BPD are less likely to develop profound bronchospasms, or BPD "snits," they may still have episodes of increased airway resistance or hypoxia in response to stress, handling, or discomfort. They may not respond as readily to the usual soothing techniques such as rocking, patting, holding, or talking.[240] Learning to interpret the infant's behavior is essential in supporting the infant and family. Major considerations in caring for infants with BPD include limiting environmental demands when the infant loses control and identifying early signs of loss of control. In addition, staff members understanding when intervention is needed, and knowing strategies to reduce stress is invaluable. Each infant should have an individualized developmental plan constructed by the neonatal team.

Infants with BPD are at increased risk of neuro-developmental delays beyond those associated with low birth weight alone. In a follow-up study done at eight years of age comparing term infants and VLBW infants with and without BPD, children from the BPD group demonstrated deficits in intelligence, reading, mathematics, and gross motor skills. Children in the BPD group were more likely to be enrolled in special education classes (54 percent) than were children in the VLBW-without-BPD group (37 percent) or term birth group (25 percent).[241] The risk for disabilities increases as birth weight decreases and more complications develop. Factors that appear to place infants with BPD at higher risk include moderate to severe IVH and low socioeconomic and parent education levels.[242]

Maximizing neurodevelopmental outcome in infants with BPD requires a multidisciplinary team approach. A team consisting of developmental specialists, physical therapists, speech therapists, neonatologists, and nurses should develop a plan of care to maximize neurologic growth and development. Goals include maximizing the environmental conditions in the NICU, reducing stress, and maintaining normal oxygen levels. Proper positioning in natural flexion using rolls and blankets is helpful. Minimizing stimulation and evaluating the infant's response to procedures using oxygen saturation monitoring as a guide are important. Evaluating and reporting the infant's responses to the various therapists help in developing an individualized plan of care.

Discharge planning should ensure that the family understands the plan of care, including handling, positioning, stimulation, and stress reactions. Teaching and supporting families who have an infant with BPD is a challenge for NICU nurses. The nurse is often coordinator of the various disciplines involved in the infant's care. Understanding their baby's treatment regimen and the importance of close medical follow-up may help with compliance and assist the parents in coping with the complexity of their infant's care. Parents need to be aware of the high risk of lower respiratory tract infections and rehospitalization despite optimal care and appropriate precautions. Preparing the infant and family for discharge is critical to a successful transition from the NICU environment to home. To assist NICUs in appropriate discharge planning, the American Academy of Pediatrics (AAP) has developed guidelines for the discharge of high-risk infants.[243] Before discharge, infants with BPD should be free from apnea, be taking all of their feedings by breast or bottle, and have oxygen requirements and medication regimens that are stable and manageable outside the hospital setting.[244] Care and attention must also be given to ensuring that the family is ready for discharge. Offering parents the opportunity to stay in the hospital overnight with their infant may help to ease the transition home.

Prognosis

Infants with BPD have an increased hospital readmission rate than their non-BPD counterparts, and respiratory abnormalities that persistent into adolescence.[245] The prognosis for infants with BPD is dependent on the severity of the disease and the infant's overall health status. A 1996 study reported that 50 percent of infants with severe BPD were readmitted to the hospital in the first year of life for lower respiratory tract infections.[246] This number has been reduced somewhat with the advent of respiratory syncytial virus prophylaxis, the main cause of respiratory infections requiring hospitalization in prematurely born infants.

Long-term follow-up of infants with BPD suggests that these children experience progressive normalization of lung mechanics and, to some extent, lung volumes; however, abnormalities of the small airways persist.[152] Other follow-up studies have found that children who had BPD as infants have no difference in exercise capacity and no difference in FRC but do have a decrease in forced expiratory volumes and forced vital capacity.[247] It has also been reported that at five years of age, BPD survivors have a higher incidence of asthma than the general population.[248]

RETINOPATHY OF PREMATURITY

One of the most common complications ascribed to the use of oxygen and mechanical ventilation in LBW infants is ROP. ROP is a disorder of retinal vascularization in the retina of a premature infant that causes a proliferation of abnormal vasculature, leading to visual loss from cicatrization (scarring) and retinal detachment. Immature retinal vessels are a prerequisite for the development of ROP. Initiated by an injury, ROP represents the healing process.

HISTORY

ROP was first described in 1942 by Terry, who called the disease *retrolental fibroplasia* because of the formation of scar tissue behind the lens of the eye in premature infants.[249] In the late 1940s and 1950s, the amount of blindness from this disorder was considered epidemic. Following a report of a controlled study by Patz and associates in the early 1950s showing that high concentrations of oxygen contributed to the development of retrolental fibroplasia, the use of oxygen was greatly curtailed.[250] Kinsey and Hemphill reported an ROP incidence of 71 percent with liberal use of oxygen and of 33 percent when oxygen use was curtailed.[251] Although the incidence of blindness in preterm infants decreased significantly with decreased use of oxygen, mortality and morbidity, including such conditions as cerebral palsy and lung disease, increased.[252]

The disorder was renamed retinopathy of prematurity in the 1980s because of its association with prematurity and its occurrence despite excellent oxygen monitoring and the absence of high oxygen blood levels. Cases of ROP have been reported in term infants and premature infants who did not receive oxygen, leading investigators to the current conclusion that ROP is multifactorial.[1]

INCIDENCE

The incidence of ROP is inversely related to birth weight and gestational age. There is a wide variation in the reported incidence of ROP, in part because of variations in screening criteria as well as differences in populations and the gestational ages of infants included in the studies. There is also a difference of opinion as to whether the incidence of ROP is increasing with greater survival rates among ELBW infants[253,254] or decreasing as a result of interventions such as the use of surfactant.[255]

In 1981, Phelps estimated that in the U.S. approximately 600 infants a year were at risk for blindness from ROP.[256] In 1990, the Cryotherapy for Retinopathy of Prematurity (CRYO-ROP) study, which involved 23 U.S. institutions and followed 4,009 infants, reported the incidence of ROP to be 47 percent in infants weighing 1,000–1,250 g, 78 percent in infants weighing 750–999 g, and 90 percent in infants weighing <750 g at birth. The overall rate of severe ROP—greater than threshold (Stage 3+ or greater)—was 22 percent. Multiple births and gender had no significant effect on the incidence. Caucasian infants had a higher chance of progressing to severe ROP than did African American infants.[257] In 2005, Good and colleagues from the Early Treatment for Retinopathy of Prematurity Cooperative Group compared then-current rates of ROP to those identified by the original CRYO-ROP study and found that, at 68 percent in 2005, rates of ROP had changed little since 1990.[257,258] A review of infants <1,250 g born between 1994 and 2000 found an increase in ROP over that time period from 40 to 54 percent, with a 2–5 percent rate of threshold ROP.[251] On the other hand, Hussain and colleagues reviewed 2,528 infants born between 1989 and 1997 at <37 weeks gestation and reported an overall incidence of ROP of 21 percent.[255] However, when the statistics were broken down by gestational age, the ROP rate for infants ≤28 weeks was 40.1 percent, with 9.8 percent of this group experiencing severe (Grade 3 or worse) ROP. Studies of ROP in infants born at >30 weeks gestation or ≥1,250 g demonstrated rates of ROP of 2–4.2 percent, with no infant >1,500 g developing ROP that needed to be treated.[255,259,260]

In the U.S., ROP is the second leading cause of childhood blindness, accounting for 6–20 percent of all cases.[261,262] In the United Kingdom, a follow-up study of infants with Stage 3 ROP found that 13 percent had a severe vision deficit.[263] Many middle-income areas such as South America and Eastern Europe are experiencing an exponential increase in the number of cases of severe ROP, with an estimated 50,000 cases of ROP-induced blindness being reported.[264] Infants of higher birth weights are at greater risk for ROP in these countries compared to those in high-income countries.[265]

PATHOPHYSIOLOGY

Knowledge of the development of retinal vasculature assists in understanding the disease, diagnosis, and treatment of ROP. Normal ocular development occurs in the hypoxic intrauterine environment. At 6 weeks gestation, the hyaloid artery enters the eye and begins to fill the vitreous cavity with blood vessels. The retina remains avascular until approximately 16 weeks gestation, when capillary precursor cells (spindle cells) start branching out from the tissue around the fetal optic nerve and slowly grow centrifugally toward the nasal edge of the optic disc. Spindle cells normally disappear by 21 weeks gestation. By 16–18 weeks, new blood vessels begin forming at the *ora serrata*, the central edge of the retina, reaching the temporal *ora serrata* at approximately 40–44 weeks gestation. The blood vessels behind the leading edge of capillaries gradually form arteries and veins.

In utero the fetus is exposed to a hypoxic environment with a PaO_2 of 30 mmHg.[266] This hypoxia is thought to be important in stimulating growth factors, which regulate normal vascular development *in utero*.[267] Two growth factors known to be important in both normal vessel growth and in the development of ROP are vascular endothelial growth factor (VEGF) and insulin-like growth factor (IGF-1). VEGF production occurs in response to hypoxia. Insulin-like growth factor is transported across the placenta and regulates neovascularization. Following premature delivery, IGF-1 levels fall quickly and remain low until endogenous production occurs. IGF-1 is postulated to be one of the factors not related to hypoxia that plays a role in ROP.[268,269] Studies have shown that IGF-1 levels are lowest in infants who later develop ROP.[270,271]

Phase 1 ROP

The first or acute phase of ROP occurs between birth and 30–32 weeks postmenstrual age and may progress slowly or rapidly.[266] Following premature birth, exposure to oxygen levels that are higher than those in the intrauterine environment suppresses VEGF, leading to a cessation of blood vessel development, vasoconstriction of existing immature retinal vessels, and ultimately to the destruction of some of the newly developed capillaries.[268,272] Falling levels of IGF-1 also play a role in the cessation of vascular growth. This cessation of vascular growth marks the beginning of Phase 1 ROP. In its early stages, this vasoconstriction may be reversible, but if it continues, there is tissue ischemia.

Phase 2 ROP

As the retina continues to grow, metabolic demands increase, and without adequate vascular development, local hypoxia occurs. This tissue hypoxia leads to the secretion of VGEF and new vessel growth (neovascularization). These vessels form at the junction of the avascular and vascularized retina in response to an increase in VEGF. If vascularization succeeds in reestablishing circulation to the central retina and to the peripheral avascular retina, ROP regresses, and any excess vessels are absorbed. In other cases, neovascularization erupts into the vitreous, and vessel growth is uncontrolled. These vessels may regress and heal, but the process can result in residual scarring that causes a neovascular ridge. As the scar tissue hardens and shrinks, it places traction on the retina, which can lead to detachment.[266] Phase 2 ROP occurs between 32 and 34 weeks postmenstrual age.[264]

Classification of ROP

An international classification system for ROP has been developed by ophthalmologists from six countries. First published in 1984 and updated in 1987 and 2005, this system describes ROP in terms of four characteristics or measures: the retinal location of the disease, the extent of involvement of the developing vasculature, the stage of the disease, and the presence or absence of dilated and tortuous vessels.[273]

LOCATION: ZONE I, II, OR III

Retinal vessel development occurs from the optic nerve in the posterior area of the eye toward the periphery. The location of the disease in one of three zones is a measure of how the progression of blood vessels has developed (Figure 10-12).

- **Zone I** is a small area extending from the optic nerve to twice the distance from the center of the optic nerve to the center of the macula.[273] Zone I disease is the most dangerous because progression to extensive scar tissue and total retinal detachment is most likely in this location.

FIGURE 10-12
Zones and clock hours of retinopathy of prematurity.

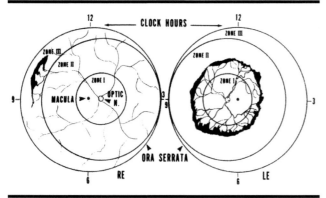

From: Phelps DL. 2006. Retinopathy of prematurity. In *Neonatal-Perinatal Medicine: Diseases of the Fetus and Infant*, 8th ed., Martin RJ, Fanaroff AA, and Walsh MC, eds. Philadelphia: Mosby, 1750. Reprinted by permission.

- **Zone II** extends from the edge of Zone I to the nasal ora serrata found at the 3-o'clock position in the right eye and the 9-o'clock position in the left eye.[273]
- **Zone III** is the remainder of the temporal retina, the last to be vascularized during fetal development.

EXTENT OF VASCULATURE INVOLVEMENT

The extent of the disease is defined by how many clock hours of the eye's circumference are diseased. Figure 10-12 illustrates both the zones and clock hours of ROP.

ROP STAGING

It is common for more than one stage of ROP to be present in the eye. However, staging of the eye as a whole is based on the most severe stage present.[273]

- **Stage 1** ROP is characterized by a sharp white line that lies within the plane of the retina and separates the vascular and avascular retina.
- **Stage 2** ROP displays a rolled ridge of scar tissue in the region of the white demarcation line. The ridge may be limited to a small area of the retina or may encircle the eye. Small tufts of new blood vessels, called *popcorn,* may be found behind the ridge.
- **Stage 3** ROP is characterized by neovascularization proliferating from the posterior aspect of the ridge out of the retina into the vitreous. Stage 3 is further subdivided into mild, moderate, or severe amounts of tissue reaching into the vitreous.
- **Stage 4** ROP is subtotal retinal detachment caused by the scar tissue formed in Stages 1–3. Stage 4a is a partial detachment in the periphery of the retina.

Stage 4b is a subtotal or total detachment involving the macula and fovea, usually with a fold extending through Zones I, II, and III.

- **Stage 5** ROP involves a complete retinal detachment, with the retina assuming a closed or partially closed funnel from the optic nerve to the front of the eye.
- **Plus disease** is a designation given to ROP when, at any of the stages, the posterior veins are enlarged and the arterioles are tortuous; it is expressed by adding a plus sign following the stage number (for example, Stage 3+). The plus sign indicates extensive ROP changes that may signify a rapidly progressive course. Other findings of plus disease include poor papillary dilation and vitreous haze.[273] In the CRYO-ROP study, the presence of plus disease significantly increased the chances of an unfavorable outcome.[274]
- **Pre-plus disease** is a category that was added during the 2005 revision of the ROP classification system. This identifier designates the presence of abnormal dilation and tortuosity of the posterior pole vessels that are not yet severe enough to be classified as plus disease. Over time, as dilation increases, pre-plus disease may progress to plus disease.[273]
- **Aggressive posterior ROP,** or **AP-ROP**, an unusually aggressive pattern of ROP development, has been reported in infants weighing <1,000 g.[273] Formerly termed *Rush disease*, AP-ROP develops earlier than usual (at three to five weeks after birth) and can progress rapidly to severe ROP with retinal detachment.[1]

THRESHOLD AND PRETHRESHOLD ROP

- **Threshold ROP** is a term used to designate Zone I or II changes found in a minimum of five uninterrupted clock hours or involvement of a total of eight clock hours.[1]
- **Prethreshold ROP** describes ROP changes that do not meet threshold ROP criteria in Zone I but that reach Stage 2+ or Stage 3 in Zone II. Infants with prethreshold disease require more frequent ROP examinations.[275]

Outcomes

The visual outcome for infants with ROP depends on the stage of the disease, whether the macula is involved, and the results of treatment. Because Stages 1–3 ROP generally occur in the peripheral retina, the macula is not affected. For most infants with Stage 1 or 2 ROP, the disease resolves spontaneously without scarring.[276] Although these infants do not require treatment, they are at greater risk for developing myopia, amblyopia, astigmatism, strabismus, and glaucoma.[272,277] In other studies, late peripheral retinal degeneration and late retinal detachment have been reported in teens and adults with ROP that regressed without treatment (regressive ROP).[278,279]

If they are not treated, infants with moderate to severe Stage 3 or Stage 4 ROP are at risk for reduced vision because scar tissue shrinks and then exerts traction on the retina. Moderate traction results in the distortion of the macula. In severe cases of ROP (Stages 4b and 5), the retina and macula may be totally detached, resulting in blindness. Untreated threshold disease leads to retinal detachment in about 50 percent of cases.[280]

Risk Factors

Since the 1950s, investigators have been looking at the many factors that may be associated with the development of ROP. Early studies identified prematurity and hyperoxia as the most important correlates with ROP.[264] During the resurgence of ROP that occurred in the 1970s and 1980s, the disorder occurred despite stringent oxygen controls, and gestational age was again noted to be the leading risk factor. Oxygen exposure continues to be a risk factor for the development of ROP but does not completely explain its occurrence.

In recognition of the complexity of ROP, many other risk factors have been studied, including blood transfusions, IVH, pneumothorax, mechanical ventilation, apnea, infection, hypercarbia, hypocarbia, PDA, administration of prostaglandin synthetase inhibitors (indomethacin), vitamin E deficiency, prenatal complications, and genetic factors. After controlling for immaturity, the sicker the infant, the more likely it is that serious ROP will develop. Because of the complexity and severity of illness in these infants who develop ROP, it remains difficult to determine precisely which factors increase the risk of ROP. For example, prenatal use of steroids appears to protect against ROP, but infants whose mothers received antenatal steroids are also less likely to be ill than are those who were not exposed to steroids.[281]

In most studies, birth weight and gestational age as well as the degree of serious illness, are among the primary risk factors for ROP.[282,283] Kim and colleagues also identified surfactant therapy and apnea as risk factors, noting that apnea not only increased the

risk of ROP but also worsened preexisting ROP.[283] In a study of 88 infants <34 weeks gestation at birth, Akkoyun and colleagues found that risk factors for severe ROP in their study population included birth weight, blood transfusions, and duration of mechanical ventilation.[284] Blood transfusions were also cited as a risk factor by Dutta and colleagues.[285] In another study of 159 infants with birth weights <1,600 g, significant risk factors for the development of ROP included birth weight ≤1,000 g, IVH, sepsis, and the use of dopamine or glucocorticoids.[286] Another review found that the primary risk factors for threshold ROP were maternal preeclampsia, birth weight, presence of pulmonary hemorrhage, and duration of ventilation.[287] In most cases, these risk factors are measures of the degree of illness experienced by LBW infants and may or may not play a direct role in the development of ROP.

Ethnic origin and country of birth have been found to correlate with the development of ROP. South Asian infants are more likely to develop severe ROP than are Caucasian infants,[288] and African American infants are less likely to develop ROP than are Caucasian infants.[289] Infants born in countries classified as middle income (for example, Latin America, Eastern Europe, and Thailand) were at increased risk of developing serious ROP and of becoming blind as a result.[262,290]

Prevention

Oxygen Levels

For many years, oxygen use has been the focus of attention as the primary cause of ROP. Early studies demonstrated a correlation between the duration of oxygen therapy and the development of ROP.[250,291,292] Other studies did not identify a clear correlation. An early multicenter study designed to assess the relationship between arterial oxygen levels and ROP failed to find any significant differences between study groups.[293] Another early study comparing transcutaneous oxygen ($TcPO_2$) levels demonstrated no difference in the incidence or severity of ROP at various $TcPO_2$ levels in infants weighing <1,000 g.[294] One 1992 study supports an association between the incidence and severity of ROP and the duration of exposure to transcutaneous oxygen levels of >80 mmHg.[295] This finding is supported by later work showing that lowering oxygen saturation alarm limits and implementing oxygen targeting guidelines and educational programs can reduce the incidence of severe ROP. In 2006, Vanderveen and colleagues reported that lowering oxygen alarm limits to the range of 85–93 percent in infants <1,250 g decreased prethreshold ROP from 17.5 percent to 5.6 percent.[296]

Ambient Light Levels

Exposure to high levels of ambient light has been suggested as a cause of progression of ROP. It is proposed that light can generate free radicals, which damage the developing retinal blood vessels. In 1985, Glass and colleagues reported a reduced incidence of ROP in neonates—especially those weighing <1,000 g—exposed to reduced (150 lux) compared with standard (600 lux) lighting in the nursery.[297] Two studies reported in 1988 and 1989 conflict with Glass and colleagues' findings, however.[298,299] A large multicenter, randomized clinical trial also failed to find a reduction in ROP as a result of reducing ambient light, a finding confirmed by a later Cochrane review.[300,301]

Dietary Supplements

A number of pharmacologic agents and dietary supplements have been examined to determine if they might play a role in the prevention of ROP. Several clinical and experimental studies have indicated that vitamin E (tocopherol) deficiency may cause ROP.[302–304] It has been theorized that premature infants have a deficiency of vitamin E, a naturally occurring antioxidant. Without sufficient amounts of vitamin E to protect the spindle cells in the retina, the free oxygen radicals destroy the cells.[305] Several infant trials using vitamin E reported mixed results in terms of lowering the incidence and severity of ROP.[302,304,306]

Even though vitamin E has been effective in some instances, there are concerns about the risks of sepsis, NEC, IVH, and retinal hemorrhage associated with its use.[304,307–309] Many of these problems were reported with use of intravenous pharmacologic megadoses or unapproved formulations of the vitamin. If vitamin E is administered, serum levels should be monitored to prevent overdose. More recently, a meta-analysis done by Brion and associates found that vitamin E supplementation did reduce the risk of both ROP and IVH in VLBW infants but increased the risk of sepsis.[310] These reviewers suggest that supplementation at high doses or producing levels >3.5 mg/dL is not supported by evidence.

Another supplement being studied is D-penicillamine, a potent antioxidant. Interest in this substance originated from work done by Lakatos and colleagues, who noted a low incidence of ROP among infants receiving D-penicillamine to prevent or treat hyperbilirubinemia.[311] A meta-analysis of this and one other study concluded that D-penicillamine may reduce the incidence of acute ROP and should be further investigated.[312,313] More recently, Christensen and colleagues compared 15 premature infants treated with D-penicillamine to 34 matched controls and found that a 14-day course of D-penicillamine decreased the odds of developing ROP from 60 percent to 21 percent with no short-term adverse effects noted.[314] The D-penicillamine treatment did not, however, reduce the need for ROP surgery in treated infants who did develop ROP.

A 1992 study reported beneficial effects of inositol, a dietary supplement.[315] A Cochrane review of two trials[315,316] using inositol to reduce morbidity in premature infants with respiratory distress reported a significant reduction in Stage 4 ROP and suggested the need for further randomized controlled trials.[317]

SCREENING

Screening guidelines for ROP have been published by the AAP, the American Academy of Ophthalmology, and the American Association for Pediatric Ophthalmology and Strabismus.[318] Recommendations from these guidelines identify the need for a skilled ophthalmologist to screen all infants with a gestational age of <32 weeks or a birth weight of <1,500 g, as well as selected infants with a birth weight of 1,500–2,000 g and an unstable clinical course. Examinations should be started when infants born at ≤27 weeks reach 31 weeks gestational age or at 4 weeks for infants born between 28 and 32 weeks gestational age.[319] The examining ophthalmologist determines the timing of subsequent examinations based on retinal findings. Generally, follow-up is required in one week or less for infants with Stage 1 or 2 ROP in Zone I or Stage 3 ROP in Zone II.

Some researchers have suggested that the AAP criteria be modified. Subhani and colleagues found that ELBW infants may develop significant ROP earlier than 31 or 32 weeks and that delays in screening in this population may miss prethreshold disease.[320] Others have suggested that the screening criteria could be safely modified to include only those infants born at <1,251 g and <30 weeks gestational age.[321,322] In a review of 205 LBW infants screened over an eight-year period, Mathew and colleagues identified ROP in five babies with birth weights >1,250 g and in eight babies born at >30 weeks gestation. In all of these babies, ROP was either Stage 1 or 2.[321]

Every NICU should have a program in place to identify infants who meet screening criteria and to schedule eye examinations for them. When an at-risk infant is discharged or transferred to another center, consideration must be given to the availability of appropriate follow-up.

To prepare the infant for a screening examination, the nurse administers mydriatic agents prescribed by the ophthalmologist. Drugs containing phenylephrine should be used cautiously if the infant has hypertension. Prior to and during the examination, a nurse should be at the bedside to monitor the infant's responses to the medication and examination. Resuscitative equipment should be available because neonates can react to the examination with apnea, bradycardia, increased blood pressure, and oxygen desaturation.

Using an indirect ophthalmoscope with a lid speculum and scleral depressors, the ophthalmologist examines each eye, evaluating all zones to determine retinal vascularization. If the infant does not tolerate the exam, it should be stopped and the infant treated appropriately. Administering atropine to an unstable infant has been recommended—especially if the examination is critical. Communication between members of the health care team and the family is particularly important in the screening and management of ROP. In addition to being aware of their infant's risk for developing ROP, parents should be counseled regarding the importance of ongoing follow-up with the ophthalmologist until retinal vascularization is complete.[318]

TREATMENT

The criteria for determining the need for intervention in ROP have been the subject of ongoing debate and much research.

Nonsurgical Treatment

Provision of supplemental oxygen to infants with prethreshold ROP has been studied as a method of preventing progression of the disease. The large multicenter STOP-ROP trial evaluated the safety and efficacy of maintaining oxygen saturations at between 96 and 99 percent in LBW infants with ROP. The investigators found that this therapy did not reduce the severity of ROP but did result in more adverse pulmonary complications. A small benefit was noted in infants with prethreshold ROP without plus disease compared with infants with plus disease, but this finding was not significant.[225] The systematic review conducted by Lloyd and colleagues in 2003 echoed this finding.[323]

FIGURE 10-13
Laser therapy.

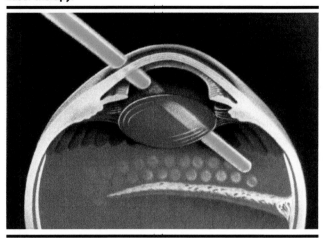

Courtesy of Coherent, Inc., Santa Clara, California.

Surgical Treatment

The AAP recommends surgical treatment for ROP when any of the following conditions exist: Zone I ROP at any stage when plus disease is present; Zone I ROP at Stage 3 in the absence of plus disease; and Stage 2 or 3 ROP in Zone II with plus disease.[318] Two effective treatments are available for infants with severe progressive ROP: cryotherapy and laser therapy.

Cryotherapy, which involves freezing the avascular area of the retina anterior to the area of disease, was originally the first-line treatment for ROP. It has largely been replaced by laser therapy and is today reserved for cases where blood or corneal haziness obscures the view of the retina.[324]

Despite the fact that its use is now limited, early evaluation of cryotherapy identified a significant benefit in infants with threshold ROP. In a multicenter trial of cryotherapy for ROP termed the CRYO-ROP study, 6 percent of infants weighing <1,250 g developed threshold ROP, 90 percent of whom were between 33 and 42 weeks gestation. Within 72 hours after threshold disease was detected, the infants were treated with cryotherapy. Cryotherapy was shown to improve visual outcome by 50 percent compared to those receiving no treatment.[276]

In the 10-year follow-up of the original CRYO-ROP study, similar results persisted, with 62 percent of the control eyes having unfavorable distance visual acuity compared with 44 percent of the treated eyes. Eyes that had disease in Zone I had a poor outcome at 10 years, whether treated or part of the control group, with 94 percent (15 of 16) having an unfavorable visual outcome.[325]

Laser photocoagulation (Figure 10-13), now the preferred treatment for ROP, acts in the same way as cryotherapy in destroying avascular tissue. The advantages of laser therapy include ease in treating more difficult locations such as Zone I, less trauma to the tissue, less discomfort for the infant, and fewer ocular and systemic complications such as intraocular hemorrhage and bradycardia.[326] A number of studies have evaluated laser therapy for ROP, and longer term follow-up data are now becoming available. Studies have shown that laser therapy is effective in preserving both distance and near vision in eyes with threshold ROP.[327] A ten-year follow-up of a randomized trial comparing laser treatment with cryotherapy found that eyes treated with laser therapy had better corrected visual acuity and less myopia than did cryotherapy-treated eyes.[328,329] A small risk of cataract development has been reported with laser therapy.[280]

If laser therapy is unsuccessful in preventing retinal detachment, scleral buckling may be indicated. Under general anesthesia, a silicone band is placed around the eye. This reduces the circumference of the eye enough that the retina can re-attach itself to the wall. However, if the scar continues to contract, the retina will again pull away from the posterior wall toward the center of the eye. Scleral buckling has been reported to have a 50–100 percent anatomic success rate for patients with Stage 4a or 4b ROP.[330] Favorable visual acuity of 20/60 to 18/400 has been reported with this technique, but if surgery is delayed, blindness may result.[331]

When retinal detachment progresses to Stage 5, a vitrectomy may be indicated. Two techniques, closed and open eye, have been reported, with comparable results. During this three- to four-hour procedure, the lens and vitreous humor are removed from the eye. The scar tissue is removed, and the retina is laid back against the eye wall. A study by Hartnett and colleagues demonstrated that after one procedure, anatomic attachment was more likely to be achieved in infants undergoing vitrectomy than in those receiving a scleral buckling procedure, but by the end of the follow-up period (six months) there was no difference in retinal attachment rates.[332]

In a follow-up analysis of infants in the Early Treatment for Retinopathy of Prematurity (ETROP) study[333] who developed retinal detachment, vitreoretinal surgery (vitrectomy and/or scleral buckling) resulted in macular attachment in 16 of 48 eyes. Macular attachment at the nine-month follow-up was achieved in 30 percent of the eyes treated with vitrectomy with or without buckling, in 60 percent of the eyes treated with scleral buckling alone, and in 17 percent of the 12 eyes followed with no surgery. The five eyes in which normal acuity was maintained after retinal surgery all had Stage 4a disease. In 11 eyes with Stage 5 ROP, vitreoretinal surgery resulted in some structural successes but poor functional outcomes, with 6 eyes having no light perception, 3 having light perception only, and the remaining 2 having low vision.[334]

Anti-VEGF Therapy

Following the recognition of the role that growth factors such as VEGF plays in the pathogenesis of ROP, work has been ongoing to develop more targeted treatments for ROP. One such treatment is the angiogenesis inhibitor, bevacizumab (Avastin, Genentech), which is given as an intraocular injection. Originally studied in oncology, bevacizumab has been successfully used to treat diabetic retinopathy in adults.[335] Bevacizumab is a monoclonal antibody that suppresses neovascularization of the retina by inhibiting vascular endothelial growth factor.[336,337] Bevacizumab has a large molecular weight and is therefore less likely to penetrate the retina and cause systemic effects; however, concerns remain regarding the safety and efficacy of anti-VEGF use in premature neonates.[337] In a systematic review of bevacizumab and ROP, Micieli and colleagues noted considerable variation in the dose and timing of treatment.[338] A large multicenter randomized controlled trial done by Mintz-Hittner and colleagues compared the use of bevacizumab to laser therapy in 150 neonates <1,500 g at birth with Stage 3+ ROP. The rate of recurrence of ROP was significantly higher with the conventional laser therapy group than with the intravitreal bevacizumab (42 percent vs 6 percent).[339] This study was not powered to establish the safety of the treatment. The follow-up phase of this study is ongoing until 2012.

Nursing Care

Caring for the mechanically ventilated infant who is at risk for ROP requires collaborative practice. Because of the multitude of current theories regarding the etiology of the disease, the NICU nurse needs to be aware of all the potential risk factors.

Until the role of oxygen in the development of ROP is clearly defined, current recommendations are that oxygen saturation levels for LBW infants be maintained between 85 and 93 percent.[296,340,341] Although a large randomized controlled trial has yet to be conducted, the studies by Chow and colleagues, Vanderveen and others, and Coe and associates demonstrate a clear reduction in ROP rates when lower oxygen saturation protocols are adopted.[296,340,331] When the infant's oxygen saturations reflect changes in oxygenation and ventilation, adjustments in the oxygen and ventilator settings should be made to keep oxygen saturations within acceptable levels while avoiding frequent changes in oxygen in response to brief variations in saturation levels.[340] Fluctuating PaO_2 levels have been found to increase the risk of threshold ROP in vulnerable infants.[342]

Each NICU should develop a screening and tracking program to ensure that at-risk infants are screened at appropriate intervals.[280] When infants are back-transported, appropriate arrangements for ROP screening should be in place, and the transfer documentation should communicate the infant's ROP status at transfer.

Nurses should educate and support parents of infants at risk for developing ROP. The neonatologist generally informs the parents of the possibility of ROP and the prognosis based on the infant's gestational age and early NICU course. Parents vary in their understanding of this complication. Following the initial ophthalmologic screening, parents are given information that may be difficult to understand. Their infant may have passed through the critical phase and may be off the ventilator, so they are not prepared for new problems. The nurse should assist the parents in understanding the diagnosis and possible treatment by giving them pamphlets and arranging meetings with the ophthalmologist and neonatologist. Parents need to be made aware of the critical importance of ongoing monitoring and follow-up, especially if discharge occurs before retinal vascularization is complete.[280]

Nursing care for the infant requiring ocular surgery is similar to that for any preoperative patient. All systems should be stabilized and baseline laboratory values and vital signs documented. The parents should understand the reason for the surgery, its potential risks, and its possible outcomes. Cryotherapy and laser therapy can be done in the NICU, but appropriate safety procedures, particularly for laser therapy, must be in place.

Following cryotherapy or laser therapy, all vital signs should be assessed as the infant is recovering. Respiratory status should be carefully monitored, especially in premature infants and infants with BPD. Eyelid edema and nasal stuffiness usually resolve in a few days. Eyedrops should be administered as ordered. The infant should be monitored for level of comfort and receive appropriate pain medication.

SUMMARY

As nurses, we are aware of the many benefits of mechanical ventilation, but we must be diligent in monitoring for the adverse effects. Nurses play a key role in recognizing early signs of potential complications and alerting the neonatal team. Support of the family through this stressful time is important.

REFERENCES

1. Korones SB. 2011. Complications. In *Assisted Ventilation of the Neonate*, 5th ed., Goldsmith JP, and Karotkin EH, eds. Philadelphia: Saunders, 389–425.

2. Wood BR. 2003. Physiologic principles. In *Assisted ventilation of the Neonate*, 4th ed., Goldsmith JP, and Karotkin EH, eds. Philadelphia: Saunders, 15–40

3. Whitsett JA, et al. 2005. Acute respiratory disorders. In *Avery's Neonatology: Pathophysiology and Management of the Newborn*, 6th ed., MacDonald MG, Mullett MD, and Seshia MMK, eds. Philadelphia: Lippincott Williams & Wilkins, 553–577.

4. Yu VY, et al. 1986. Pulmonary air leaks in extremely low birth weight infants. *Archives of Disease in Childhood* 61(3): 239–241.

5. Bloom BB, et al. 1997. Comparison of Infasurf (calf lung surfactant extract) to Survanta (beractant) in the treatment and prevention of respiratory distress syndrome. *Pediatrics* 100(1): 31–38.

6. Gortner L, et al. 1998. Early versus late surfactant treatment in preterm infants of 27 to 32 weeks' gestational age: A multicenter controlled clinical trial. *Pediatrics* 102(5): 1153–1160.

7. Kendig JW, et al. 1998. Comparison of two strategies for surfactant prophylaxis in very premature infants: A multicenter randomized trial. *Pediatrics* 101(6): 1006–1012.

8. Ozkan H, et al. 2004. Synchronized ventilation of very-low-birth-weight infants; report of 6 years' experience. *Journal of Maternal-Fetal and Neonatal Medicine* 15(4): 261–265.

9. Macklin CC. 1935. Pulmonic alveolar vents. *Journal of Anatomy* 69(part 2): 188–192.

10. Bhatt AJ, and Ryan RM. 2009. Pulmonary interstitial emphysema. *Emedicine*. Retrieved November 11, 2009, from http://emedicine.medscape.com/article/976801-overview.

11. Briassoulis GC, et al. 2000. Air leaks from the respiratory tract in mechanically ventilated children with severe respiratory disease. *Pediatric Pulmonology* 29(2): 127–134.

12. Berg TJ, et al. 1975. Bronchopulmonary dysplasia and lung rupture in hyaline membrane disease: Influence of continuous distending pressure. *Pediatrics* 55(1): 51–54.

13. Tarnow-Mordi WO, Narang A, and Wilkinson AR. 1985a. Lack of association between barotrauma and air leak in hyaline membrane disease. *Archives of Disease in Childhood* 60(6): 555–559.

14. Kamlin CO, and Davis PG. 2004. Long versus short inspiratory times in neonates receiving mechanical ventilation. *Cochrane Database of Systematic Reviews* (4): CD004503.

15. Greenough A, et al. 1984. Pancuronium prevents pneumothoraces in ventilated premature babies who actively expire against positive pressure inflation. *Lancet* 1(8367): 1–3.

16. Tarnow-Mordi WO, Sutton P, and Wilkinson AR. 1985b. Inspiratory:expiratory ratio and pulmonary interstitial emphysema. *Archives of Disease in Childhood* 60(5): 496–497.

17. Greenough A, et al. 2008. Synchronized mechanical ventilation for respiratory support in newborn infants. *Cochrane Database of Systematic Reviews* (1): CD000456.

18. Al-Abdi SY, and Singhal N. 2005. Pulmonary interstitial emphysema and continuous positive airway pressure in a premature infant. *Saudi Medical Journal* 26(10): 1627–1629.

19. Berk DR, and Varich LJ. 2005. Localized persistent pulmonary interstitial emphysema in a preterm infant in the absence of mechanical ventilation. *Pediatric Radiology* 35(12): 1243–1245.

20. Arioni C, et al. 2006. Pulmonary interstitial emphysema in preterm twins on continuous positive airway pressure. *Journal of Maternal-Fetal and Neonatal Medicine* 19(10): 671–673.

21. Verma RP, et al. 2006. Risk factors and clinical outcomes of pulmonary interstitial emphysema in extremely low birth weight infants. *Journal of Perinatology* 26(3): 197–200.

22. Greenough A, Dixon AK, and Robertson NR. 1984. Pulmonary interstitial emphysema. *Archives of Disease in Childhood* 59(11): 1046–1051.

23. Chalak LF, Kaiser JR, and Arrington RW. 2007. Resolution of pulmonary interstitial emphysema following selective left main stem intubation in a premature newborn: An old procedure revisited. *Paediatric Anaesthesia* 17(2): 183–186.

24. Weintraub Z, and Oliven A. 1988. Successful resolution of unilateral pulmonary interstitial emphysema in a premature infant by selective bronchial balloon catheterization. *Journal of Pediatric Surgery* 23(11): 1005–1006.

25. Weintraub Z, et al. 1990. A new method for selective left main bronchus intubation in premature infants. *Journal of Pediatric Surgery* 25(6): 604–606.

26. Nelle M, Zilow EP, and Linderkamp O. 1997. Effects of high-frequency oscillatory ventilation on circulation in neonates with pulmonary interstitial emphysema or RDS. *Intensive Care Medicine* 23(6): 671–676.

27. Arias-Camison JM, et al. 2001. Decompression of multiple pneumatoceles in a premature infant by percutaneous catheter placement. *Journal of Perinatology* 21(8): 553–555.

28. Fujii AM, and Moulton S. 2003. Percutaneous catheter evacuation of a pneumatocele in an extremely premature infant with respiratory failure. *Journal of Perinatology* 23(6): 516–518.

29. Ngerncham S, Kittiratsatcha P, and Pacharn P. 2005. Risk factors of pneumothorax during the first 24 hours of life. *Journal of the Medical Association of Thailand* 88(supplement 8): S135–S141.

30. Wiswell TE, Tuggle JM, and Turner BS. 1990. Meconium aspiration syndrome: Have we made a difference? *Pediatrics* 85(5): 715–721.

31. Madansky DL, et al. 1979. Pneumothorax and other forms of pulmonary air leaks in newborns. *American Review of Respiratory Disease* 120(4): 729–737.

32. Soll RF, and Blanco F. 2001. Natural surfactant extract versus synthetic surfactant for neonatal respiratory distress syndrome. *Cochrane Database of Systematic Reviews* (2): CD000144.

33. Walker MW, et al. 2002. Clinical process improvement: Reduction of pneumothorax and mortality in high-risk preterm infants. *Journal of Perinatology* 22(8): 641–645.

34. Powers WF, and Clemens JD. 1993. Prognostic implications of age at detection of air leak in very low birth weight infants requiring ventilatory support. *Journal of Pediatrics* 123(4): 611–617.

35. Linder N, et al. 2003. Risk factors for intraventricular hemorrhage in very low birth weight premature infants: A retrospective case-control study. *Pediatrics* 111(5 part 1): e590–e595.

36. Hill A, Perlman JM, and Volpe JJ. 1982. Relationship of pneumothorax to occurrence of intraventricular hemorrhage in the premature newborn. *Pediatrics* 69(2): 144–149.

37. Hillman K. 1987. Intrathoracic pressure fluctuation and periventricular haemorrhage in the newborn. *Australian Pediatrics Journal* 23(6): 343–346.

38. Mehrabani D, Gowen CW Jr, and Kopelman AE. 1991. Association of pneumothorax and hypotension with intraventricular hemorrhage. *Archives of Disease in Childhood* 66(1 spec. no.): 48–51.

39. Laptook AR, et al. 2005. Adverse neurodevelopmental outcomes among extremely low birth weight infants with a normal head ultrasound: Prevalence and antecedents. *Pediatrics* 115(3): 673–680.

40. Ryan CA, et al. 1987. Contralateral pneumothoraces in the newborn: Incidence and predisposing factors. *Pediatrics* 79(3): 417–421.

41. Katar S, et al. 2006. Symptomatic spontaneous pneumothorax in term newborns. *Pediatric Surgery International* 22(9): 755–758.

42. McIntosh N, et al. 2000. Clinical diagnosis of pneumothorax is late: Use of trend data and decision support might allow preclinical detection. *Pediatric Research* 48(3): 408–415.

43. Wyman ML, and Kuhns LR. 1977. Accuracy of transillumination in the recognition of pneumothorax and pneumomediastinum in the neonate. *Clinical Pediatrics* 16(4): 323–327.

44. Kuhns LR, et al. 1975. Diagnosis of pneumothorax pneumomediastinum in the neonate by transillumination. *Pediatrics* 56(3): 355–360.

45. Gardner SL, Enzman-Hines M, Dickey LA. 2011. Respiratory diseases. In Merenstein and Gardner's *Handbook of Neonatal Intensive Care*, 7th ed., Gardner SL, et al., eds. St. Louis: Mosby Elsevier, 581–677.

46. Rainer C, et al. 2003. Breast deformity in adolescence as a result of pneumothorax drainage during neonatal intensive care. *Pediatrics* 111(1): 80–86.

47. Marinelli PV, Ortiz A, and Alden ER. 1981. Acquired eventration of the diaphragm: A complication of chest tube placement in neonatal pneumothorax. *Pediatrics* 67(4): 552–554.

48. Stahly TL, and Tench WD. 1977. Lung entrapment and infarction by chest tube suction. *Radiology* 122(2): 307–309.

49. Quak JM, Szatmari A, and van den Anker JN. 1993. Cardiac tamponade in a preterm neonate secondary to a chest tube. *Acta Paediatrica* 82(5): 490–491.

50. Ary AH, et al. 1991. Neonatal paralysis caused by chest drains. *Archives of Disease in Childhood* 66(4 spec. no.): 441.

51. Pomerance JJ, et al. 1974. Pneumopericardium complicating respiratory distress syndrome: Role of conservative management. *Journal of Pediatrics* 84(6): 883–886.

52. Benjamin B. 1993. Prolonged intubation injuries of the larynx: Endoscopic diagnosis, classification and treatment. *Annals of Otology, Rhinology and Laryngology Supplement* 160: 1–15.

53. Sprecher RC, and Arnold JE. 2005. Upper airway lesions. In *Neonatal-Perinatal Medicine: Diseases of the Fetus and Infant*, 7th ed., Fanaroff AA, and Martin RJ, eds. Philadelphia: Mosby, 1146–1155.

54. McCulloch TM, and Bishop MJ. 1991. Complications of translaryngeal intubation. *Clinics in Chest Medicine* 12(3): 507–521.

55. Carlo WA, Martin RJ, Fanaroff AA. 2005. Assisted ventilation and complications of respiratory distress. In *Neonatal-Perinatal Medicine: Diseases of the Fetus and Infant*, 8th ed, Martin RJ, Fanaroff AA, and Walsh MC, eds. Philadelphia: Mosby, 1108–1122.

56. Donnelly WH. 1969. Histopathology of endotracheal intubation. An autopsy study of 99 cases. *Archives of Pathology* 88(5): 511–520.

57. Ratner I, and Whitfield J. 1983. Acquired subglottic stenosis in the very-low-birth-weight infant. *American Journal of Diseases of Children* 137(1): 40–43.

58. Davis PG, and Henderson-Smart DJ. 2001. Intravenous dexamethasone for extubation of newborn infants. *Cochrane Database of Systematic Reviews* (4): CD000308.

59. Richardson MA, and Inglis AF Jr. 1991. A comparison of anterior cricoid split with and without costal cartilage graft for acquired subglottic stenosis. *International Journal of Pediatric Otorhinolaryngology* 22(2): 187–193.

60. Sidman JD, Jaguan A, and Couser RJ. 2006. Tracheotomy and decannulation rates in a Level 3 neonatal intensive care unit: A 12-year study. *Laryngoscope* 116(1): 136–139.

61. Bhutani VK, Ritchie WG, and Shaffer TH. 1986. Acquired tracheomegaly in very preterm neonates. *American Journal of Diseases of Children* 140(5): 449–452.

62. Bye MR. 2009. Tracheomalacia. E Medicine. Accessed Nov 12 2009 from http://emedicine.medscape.com/article/1004463-overview

63. Sotomayor JL, et al. 1986. Large-airway collapse due to acquired tracheobronchomalacia in infancy. *American Journal of Diseases of Children* 140(4): 367–371.

64. Gaugler C, et al. 2004. Neonatal necrotizing tracheobronchitis: Three case reports. *Journal of Perinatology* 24(4): 259–260.

65. Hwang WS, et al. 1988. The histopathology of upper airway in the neonate following mechanical ventilation. *Journal of Pathology* 156(3): 189–195.

66. Rowe S, and Avery ME. 1966. Massive pulmonary hemorrhage in the newborn. Part 2: Clinical considerations. *Journal of Pediatrics* 69(1): 12–20.

67. Sly PD, and Drew JH. 1981. Massive pulmonary hemorrhage: A cause of sudden unexpected deaths in severely growth retarded infants. *Australian Paediatrics Journal* 17(1): 32–34.

68. Yeung CY. 1976. Massive pulmonary hemorrhage in neonatal infection. *Canadian Medical Association Journal* 114(2): 135–137.

69. Coffin CM, et al. 1993. Neonatal and infantile pulmonary hemorrhage: An autopsy study with clinical correlation. *Pediatric Pathology* 13(5): 583–589.

70. Raju TN, and Langenberg P. 1993. Pulmonary hemorrhage and exogenous surfactant therapy: A meta analysis. *Journal of Pediatrics* 123(4): 603–610.

71. Long W, et al. 1991c. Pulmonary hemorrhage after Exosurf Neonatal. In *Proceedings of the Exosurf Neonatal Treatment IND Investigators' Meeting*, Long WA, and Tilson HH, eds. Langhorn, Pennsylvania: Addis, 65–74.

72. Garland J, Buck R, and Weinberg M. 1994. Pulmonary hemorrhage risk in infants with a clinically diagnosed patent ductus arteriosus: A retrospective cohort study. *Pediatrics* 94(5): 719–723.

73. Pandit PB, et al. 1999. Outcome following pulmonary haemorrhage in very low birthweight neonates treated with surfactant. *Archives of Disease in Childhood. Fetal and Neonatal Edition* 81(1): F40–F44.

74. Long W, et al. 1991a. A controlled trial of synthetic surfactant in infants weighing 1250 g or more with respiratory distress syndrome. *New England Journal of Medicine* 325(24): 1696–1703.

75. Long W, et al. 1991b. Effects of two rescue doses of a synthetic surfactant on mortality rate and survival without bronchopulmonary dysplasia in 700- to 1350-gram infants with respiratory distress syndrome. *Journal of Pediatrics* 118(4 part 1): 595–605.

76. Leichty EA, et al. 1991. Reduction of neonatal mortality after multiple doses of bovine surfactant in low birth weight neonates with respiratory distress syndrome. *Pediatrics* 88(1): 19–28.

77. Raju TNK. 2006. Neonatal pulmonary hemorrhage. In *Manual of Neonatal Respiratory Care*, 2nd ed., Donn S, and Sinha SK, eds. Philadelphia: Mosby, 456–465.

78. Bland RD. 1982. Edema formation in the newborn lung. *Clinics in Perinatology* 9(3): 593–611.

79. Pramanik AK, Holtzman RB, and Merritt TA. 1993. Surfactant replacement therapy for pulmonary diseases. *Pediatric Clinics of North America* 40(5): 913–936.

80. Pappin A, et al. 1994. Extensive intraalveolar pulmonary hemorrhage in infants dying after surfactant therapy. *Journal of Pediatrics* 124(4): 621–626.

81. Malo J, Ali J, and Wood LD. 1984. How does positive end-expiratory pressure reduce intrapulmonary shunt in canine pulmonary edema? *Journal of Applied Physiology* 57(4): 1002–1010.

82. Greenough A. 2000. Expanded use of surfactant replacement therapy. *European Journal of Pediatrics* 159(9): 635–640.

83. Pandit PB, Dunn MS, and Colucci EA. 1995. Surfactant therapy in neonates with respiratory deterioration due to pulmonary hemorrhage. *Pediatrics* 95(1): 32–36.

84. Finer NN. 2004. Surfactant use for neonatal lung injury: Beyond respiratory distress syndrome. *Paediatric Respiratory Reviews* 5(supplement A): S289–S297.

85. Sherman TI, et al. 2003. Physiologic effects of CPAP: Application and monitoring. *Neonatal Network* 22(6): 7–16.

86. Wyllie J. 2003. Treatment of patent ductus arteriosus. *Seminars in Neonatology* 8(6): 425–432.

87. Hermes-DeSantis ER, and Clyman RI. 2006. Patent ductus arteriosus: Pathophysiology and management. *Journal of Perinatology* 26(supplement 1): S14–S18.

88. Clyman RI. 2004. Mechanisms regulating closure of the ductus arteriosus. In *Fetal and Neonatal Physiology*, 3rd ed, Polin RA, Fox WW, Abman SH, eds. Philadelphia: Saunders, 743–748.

89. Laughon MM, Simmons MA, and Bose CL. 2004. Patency of the ductus arteriosus in the premature infant: Is it pathologic? Should it be treated? *Current Opinion in Pediatrics* 16(2): 146–151.

90. Kluckow M, et al. 1999. Prostacyclin concentrations and transitional circulation in preterm infants requiring mechanical ventilation. *Archives of Disease in Childhood. Fetal and Neonatal Edition* 80(1): F34–F37.

91. Fujiwara T, et al. 1980. Artificial surfactant therapy in hyaline membrane disease. *Lancet* 1(8159): 55–59.

92. Heldt GP, et al. 1989. Closure of the ductus arteriosus and mechanics of breathing in preterm infants after surfactant replacement therapy. *Pediatric Research* 25(3): 305–310.

93. Soll RF, and McQueen MC. 1992. Respiratory distress syndrome. In *Effective Care of the Newborn Infant*, Sinclair JC, and Bracken MB, eds. Oxford: Oxford University Press, 325–368.

94. Clyman RI, and Chorne N. 2007. Patent ductus arteriosus: Evidence for and against treatment. *Journal of Pediatrics* 150(3): 216–219.

95. Rojas MA, et al. 1995. Changing trends in the epidemiology and pathogenesis of neonatal chronic lung disease. *Journal of Pediatrics* 126(4): 605–610.

96. Cotton RB, et al. 1981. Early prediction of symptomatic patent ductus arteriosus from perinatal risk factors: A discriminant analysis model. *Acta Paediatrica Scandinavica* 70(5): 723–727.

97. Martin CG, et al. 1982. Abnormal cerebral blood flow patterns in preterm infants with a large patent ductus arteriosus. *Journal of Pediatrics* 101(4): 587–593.

98. Fowlie PW, and Davis PG. 2003. Prophylactic indomethacin for preterm infants: A systematic review and meta-analysis. *Archives of Disease in Childhood. Fetal and Neonatal Edition* 88(6): F464–F466.

99. Clyman RI. 2005. Patent ductus arteriosus in the premature infant. In *Avery's Diseases of the Newborn*, 8th ed., Taeusch HW, Ballard RA, and Gleason CA, eds. Philadelphia: Saunders, 816–826.

100. Teixeira LS, and McNamara PJ. 2006. Enhanced intensive care for the neonatal ductus arteriosus. *Acta Paediatrica* 95(4): 394–403.

101. Fowlie PW, Davis PG, and McGuire W. 2010. Prophylactic intravenous indomethacin for preventing mortality and morbidity in preterm infants. *Cochrane Database of Systematic Reviews* (7): CD000174.

102. Alagarsamy S, et al. 2005. Comparison of clinical criteria with echocardiographic findings in diagnosing PDA in preterm infants. *Journal of Perinatal Medicine* 33(2): 161–164.

103. Schneider DJ, and Moore JW. 2006. Patent ductus arteriosus. *Circulation* 114(7): 1873–1882.

104. Kluckow M, and Evans N. 1995. Early electrocardiographic prediction of symptomatic patent ductus arteriosus in preterm infants undergoing mechanical ventilation. *Journal of Pediatrics* 127(5): 774–779.

105. Fowlie PW. 2005. Managing the baby with a patent ductus arteriosus. More questions than answers? *Archives of Disease in Childhood. Fetal and Neonatal Edition* 90(3): F190.

106. Knight DB. 2001. The treatment of patent ductus arteriosus in preterm infants. A review and overview of randomized trials. *Seminars in Neonatology* 6(1): 63–73.

107. Vanhaesebrouck S, et al. 2007. Conservative treatment for patent ductus arteriosus in the preterm. *Archives of Disease in Childhood. Fetal and Neonatal Edition* 92(4): F244–F247.

108. Bell EF, et al. 1980. Effect of fluid administration on the development of symptomatic patent ductus arteriosus and congestive heart failure in premature infants. *New England Journal of Medicine* 302(11): 598–604.

109. Bell EF, and Acarregui MJ. 2007. Restricted versus liberal water intake for preventing morbidity and mortality in preterm infants. *Cochrane Database of Systematic Reviews* (1): CD000503.

110. Green TP, et al. 1983. Furosemide promotes patent ductus arteriosus in premature infants with respiratory distress syndrome. *New England Journal of Medicine* 308(13): 743–748.

111. Ohlsson A, and Shah S. 2011. Ibuprofen for the prevention of patent ductus arteriosus in preterm and/or low birth weight infants. *Cochrane Database of Systematic Reviews* (7): CD000503.

112. Ohlsson A, and Shah S. 2011. Ibuprofen for the prevention of patent ductus arteriosus in preterm and/or low birth weight infants. *Cochrane Database of Systematic Reviews* (7): CD004213.

113. Malviya M, Ohlsson A, and Shah SS. 2008. Surgical versus medical treatment with cyclooxygenase inhibitors for symptomatic patent ductus arteriosus in preterm infants. *Cochrane Database of Systematic Reviews* (1): CD003951.

114. Merritt TA, et al. 1981. Early closure of the patent ductus arteriosus in very low-birth-weight infants: A controlled trial. *Journal of Pediatrics* 99(2): 281–286.

115. Yanagi RM, et al. 1981. Indomethacin treatment for symptomatic patent ductus arteriosus: A double-blind control study. *Pediatrics* 67(5): 647–652.

116. Gersony WM, et al. 1983. Effects of indomethacin in premature infants with patent ductus arteriosus: Results of a national collaborative study. *Journal of Pediatrics* 102(6): 895–906.

117. Koch J, et al. 2006. Prevalence of spontaneous closure of the ductus arteriosus in neonates at a birth weight of 1000 grams or less. *Pediatrics* 117(4): 1113–1121.

118. Cordero L, et al. 2007. Indomethacin prophylaxis or expectant treatment of patent ductus arteriosus in extremely low birth weight infants? *Journal of Perinatology* 27(3): 158–163.

119. Ment LR, et al. 1994. Low-dose indomethacin and prevention of intraventricular hemorrhage: A multicenter randomized trial. *Pediatrics* 93(4): 543–550.

120. Schmidt B, et al. 2006. Indomethacin prophylaxis, patent ductus arteriosus, and the risk of bronchopulmonary dysplasia: Further analyses from the Trial of Indomethacin Prophylaxis in Preterms (TIPP). *Journal of Pediatrics* 148(6): 730–734.

121. Van Overmeire B, et al. 2001. Early versus late indomethacin treatment for patent ductus arteriosus in premature infants with respiratory distess syndrome. *Journal of Pediatrics* 138(2): 205–211.

122. Yaseen H, et al. 1997. Effects of early indomethacin administration on oxygenation and surfactant requirement in low birth weight infants. *Journal of Tropical Pediatrics* 143(1): 42–46.

123. Cooke L, Steer P, and Woodgate P. 2003. Indomethacin for asymptomatic patent ductus arteriosus in preterm infants. *Cochrane Database of Systematic Reviews* (2): CD003745.

124. Benitz WE. 2011. Learning to live with patency of the ductus arteriosus in preterm infants. *Journal of Perinatology* 31(supplement 1): S42–S48.

125. Hammerman C, and Aramburo MJ. 1990. Prolonged indomethacin therapy for the prevention of recurrences of patent ductus arteriosus. *Journal of Pediatrics* 117(5): 771–776.

126. Rennie JM, and Cooke RW. 1991. Prolonged low dose indomethacin for persistent ductus arteriosus of prematurity. *Archives of Disease in Childhood* 66(1 spec. no.): 55–58.

127. Quinn D, Cooper B, and Clyman RI. 2000. Factors associated with permanent closure of the ductus arteriosus: A role for prolonged indomethacin therapy. *Pediatrics* 110(1 part 1): e10.

128. Herrera C, Holberton J, and Davis P. 2007. Prolonged versus short course of indomethacin for the treatment of patent ductus arteriosus in preterm infants. *Cochrane Database of Systematic Reviews* (2): CD003480.

129. Watterberg, KL, et al. 2004. Prophylaxis of early adrenal insufficiency to prevent bronchopulmonary dysplasia: A multicenter trial. *Pediatrics* 114(6): 1649–1657.

130. Mardoum R, et al. 1991. Controlled study of the effects of indomethacin on cerebral blood flow velocities in newborn infants. *Journal of Pediatrics* 118(1): 112–115.

131. Simko A, et al. 1994. Effects on cerebral blood flow velocities of slow and rapid infusion of indomethacin. *Journal of Perinatology* 14(1): 29–35.

132. Su PH, et al. 2003. Comparison of ibuprofen and indomethacin therapy for patent ductus arteriosus in preterm infants. *Pediatrics International* 45(6): 665–670.

133. Thomas RL, et al. 2005. A meta-analysis of ibuprofen versus indomethacin for closure of patent ductus arteriosus. *European Journal of Pediatrics* 164(3): 135–140.

134. Jones LJ, et al. 2011. Network meta-analysis of indomethacin versus ibuprofen versus placebo for PDA in preterm infants. *Archives of Disease in Childhood. Fetal and Neonatal Edition* 96(1): F45–F52.

135. Aranda JV, and Thomas R. 2006. Systematic review: Intravenous ibuprofen in preterm newborns. *Seminars in Perinatology* 30(3): 114–120.

136. Sekar KC, and Corff KE. 2008. Treatment of patent ductus arteriosus: Indomethacin or ibuprofen? *Journal of Perinatology* 28 (supplement 1): S60–S62.

137. Stefano J, et al. 1991. Closure of the ductus arteriosus with indomethacin in ventilated neonates with respiratory distress syndrome. Effects of pulmonary compliance and ventilation. *American Review of Respiratory Disease* 143(2): 236–239.

138. Mavroudis C, Backer CL, and Gevitz M. 1995. Forty-six years of patent ductus arteriosus division at Children's Memorial Hospital of Chicago. Standards for comparison. *Annals of Surgery* 220(3): 402–410.

139. Moin, F, Kennedy KA, and Moya FR. 2003. Risk factors predicting vasopressor use after patent ductus arteriosus ligation, *American Journal of Perinatology* 20(6): 313–320.

140. Kabra NS, et al. 2007. Neurosensory impairment after surgical closure of patent ductus arteriosus in extremely low birth weight infants: Results for the Trial of Indomethacin Prophylaxis in Preterms. *Journal of Pediatrics* 150(3): 229–234.

141. Mortier E, et al. 1996. Operative closure of patent ductus arteriosus in the neonatal intensive care unit. Acta Chirurgica Belgica 96(6): 266–268.

142. Hines MH, et al. 1998. Video-assisted thoracoscopic ligation of patent ductus arteriosus: Safe and outpatient. *Annals of Thoracic Surgery* 66(3): 853–858.

143. Forster R. 1993. Thoracoscopic clipping of patent ductus arteriosus in premature infants. *Annals of Thoracic Surgery* 56(6): 1418–1420.

144. Coalson JJ. 2006. Pathology of bronchopulmonary dysplasia. *Seminars in Perinatology* 30(4): 179–184.

145. Northway WH Jr, Rosan RC, and Porter DY. 1967. Pulmonary disease following respiratory therapy of hyaline-membrane disease. Bronchopulmonary dysplasia. *New England Journal of Medicine* 276(7): 357–368.

146. Bancalari E, et al. 1979. Bronchopulmonary dysplasia: Clinical presentation. *Journal of Pediatrics* 95(5 part 2): 819–823.

147. Bancalari E, and Claure N. 2006. Definitions and diagnostic criteria for bronchopulmonary dysplasia. *Seminars in Perinatology* 30(4): 164–170.

148. Jobe AJ. 1999. The new BPD: An arrest of lung development. *Pediatric Research* 46(6): 641–643.

149. Shennan AT, et al. 1988. Abnormal pulmonary outcomes in premature infants: Prediction from oxygen requirement in the neonatal period. *Pediatrics* 82(4): 527–532.

150. Jobe AH, and Bancalari E. 2001. Bronchopulmonary dysplasia. *American Journal of Respiratory and Critical Care Medicine* 163(7): 1723–1729.

151. Walsh MC, et al. 2004. Impact of a physiologic definition on bronchopulmonary dysplasia rates. *Pediatrics* 114(5): 1305–1311.

152. Bhandari A, and Panitch HB. 2006. Pulmonary outcomes in bronchopulmonary dysplasia. *Seminars in Perinatology* 30(4): 219–226.

153. Sahni R, et al. 2005. Is the new definition of bronchopulmonary dysplasia more useful? *Journal of Perinatology* 25(1): 41–46.

154. Ehrenkranz RA, et al. 2005. National Institutes of Child Health and Human Development Neonatal Research Network. Validation of the National Institutes of Health consensus definition of bronchopulmonary dysplasia. *Pediatrics.* 116(6): 1353–1360.

155. Bancalari E. 2001. Changes in the pathogenesis and prevention of chronic lung disease of prematurity. *American Journal of Perinatology* 18(1): 1–9.

156. Chess PR, et al. 2006. Pathogenesis of bronchopulmonary dysplasia. *Seminars in Perinatology* 30(4): 171–178.

157. Weinberger B, et al. 2002. Oxygen toxicity in premature infants. *Toxicology and Applied Pharmacology* 181(1): 60–67.

158. Tubman TR, Halliday HL, and McMaster D. 1990. Glutathione peroxidase and selenium levels in the preterm infant. *Biology of the Neonate* 58(6): 305–310.

159. Asikainen TM, and White CW. 2004. Pulmonary antioxidant defenses in the preterm newborn with respiratory distress and bronchopulmonary dysplasia in evolution: Implications for antioxidant therapy. *Antioxidants and Redox Signaling* 6(1): 155–167.

160. Todoroki Y, et al. 2005. Concentrations of thioredoxin, a redox-regulating protein, in umbilical cord blood and breast milk. *Free Radical Research* 39(3): 291–297.

161. Friel JK, et al. 2007. Impact of iron and vitamin C–containing supplements on preterm human milk: *In vitro. Free Radical Biology and Medicine* 42(10): 1591–1598.

162. Gitto E, et al. 2002. Causes of oxidative stress in the pre- and perinatal period. *Biology of the Neonate* 81(3): 146–157.

163. Higgins RD, et al. 2007. Executive summary of the workshop on oxygen in neonatal therapies: Controversies and opportunities for research. *Pediatrics* 119(4): 790–796.

164. Saugstad OD. 2003. Bronchopulmonary dysplasia-oxidative stress and antioxidants. *Seminars in Neonatology* 8(1): 39–49.

165. O'Donovan DJ, and Fernandes CJ. 2004. Free radicals and diseases in premature infants. *Antioxidants and Redox Signaling* 6(1): 169–176.

166. Deng H, Mason SN, and Auten RL Jr. 2000. Lung inflammation in hyperoxia can be prevented by antichemokine treatment in newborn rats. *American Journal of Respiratory and Critical Care Medicine* 162(6): 2316–2323.

167. Warner BB, et al. 1998. Functional and pathological effects of prolonged hyperoxia in neonatal mice. *American Journal of Physiology* 275(1 part 1): L110–L117.

168. Wilborn AM, Evers LB, and Canada AT. 1996. Oxygen toxicity to the developing lung of the mouse: Role of reactive oxygen species. *Pediatric Research* 40(2): 225–232.

169. Kotecha S. 2000. Lung growth: Implications for the newborn infant. *Archives of Disease in Childhood. Fetal and Neonatal Edition* 82(1): F69–F74.

170. Yoon BH, et al. 1999. A systemic fetal inflammatory response and the development of bronchopulmonary dysplasia. *American Journal of Obstetrics and Gynecology* 181(4): 773–779.

171. Dreyfuss D, and Saumon G. 1998. Ventilator-induced lung injury. *American Journal of Respiratory Diseases* 157(1): 294–323.

172. Jobe AH, and Ikegami M. 1998. Mechanisms initiating lung injury in the preterm. *Early Human Development* 53(1): 81–94.

173. Bjorklund LJ, et al. 1997. Manual ventilation with a few large breaths at birth compromises the therapeutic effect of subsequent surfactant replacement in immature lambs. *Pediatric Research* 42(3): 348–355.

174. Kraybill EN, et al. 1989. Risk factors for chronic lung disease in infants with birth weights of 751 to 1000 grams. *Journal of Pediatrics* 115(1): 115–120.

175. Garland JS, et al. 1995. Hypocarbia before surfactant therapy appears to increase bronchopulmonary dysplasia risk in infants with respiratory distress syndrome. *Archives of Pediatrics and Adolescent Medicine* 49(6): 617–622.

176. Van Marter LJ, et al. 2002. Chorioamnionitis, mechanical ventilation, and postnatal sepsis as modulators of chronic lung disease in preterm infants. *Journal of Pediatrics* 140(2): 171–176.

177. Jobe AH. 2003. Antenatal factors and the development of bronchopulmonary dysplasia. *Seminars in Neonatology* 8(1): 9–17.

178. Speer CP. 2006. Inflammation and bronchopulmonary dysplasia: A continuing story. *Seminars in Fetal and Neonatal Medicine* 11(5): 354–362.

179. Sweet DG, Halliday HL, and Warner JA. 2002. Airway remodelling in chronic lung disease of prematurity. *Paediatric Respiratory Reviews* 3(2): 140–146.

180. Young KC, et al. 2005. The association between early tracheal colonization and bronchopulmonary dysplasia. *Journal of Perinatology* 25(6): 403–407.

181. Watterberg KL, et al. 1996. Chorioamnionitis and early lung inflammation in infants in whom bronchopulmonary dysplasia develops. *Pediatrics* 97(2): 210–215.

182. Couroucli XI, et al. 2000. Detection of microorganisms in the tracheal aspirates of preterm infants by polymerase chain reaction: Association of adenovirus infection with bronchopulmonary dysplasia. *Pediatric Research* 47(2): 225–232.

183. Benstein BD, et al. 2003. Ureaplasma in lung. Part 2. Association with bronchopulmonary dysplasia in premature newborns. *Experimental and Molecular Pathology* 75(2): 171–177.

184. Schelonka RL, and Waites KB. 2007. Ureaplasma infection and neonatal lung disease. *Seminars in Perinatology* 31(1): 2–9.

185. Young TE. 2007. Nutritional support and bronchopulmonary dysplasia. *Journal of Perinatology* 27(supplement 1): S75–S78.

186. Van Marter LJ. 2006. Progress in discovery and evaluation of treatments to prevent bronchopulmonary dysplasia. *Biology of the Neonate* 89(4): 303–312.

187. Bessler H, et al. 2007. A comparison of the effect of vitamin A on cytokine secretion by mononuclear cells of preterm newborns and adults. *Neonatology* 91(3): 196–202.

188. Biniwale MA, and Ehrenkranz RA. 2006. The role of nutrition in the prevention and management of bronchopulmonary dysplasia. *Seminars in Perinatology* 30(4): 200–208.

189. Abman SH, and Groothius JS. 1994. Pathophysiology and treatment of bronchopulmonary dysplasia. *Pediatric Clinics of North America* 41(2): 277–315.

190. Smith J. 2003. An update on bronchopulmonary dysplasia: Is there a relationship to the development of childhood asthma? *Medical Hypotheses* 61(4): 495–502.

191. Evans M, et al. 1998. Associations between family history of asthma, bronchopulmonary dysplasia, and childhood asthma in very low birth weight children. *American Journal of Epidemiology* 148(5): 460–466.

192. Bancalari E, Claure N, and Gonzalez A. 2005. Patent ductus arteriosus and respiratory outcome in premature infants. *Biology of the Neonate* 88(3): 192–201.

193. Stocker JT. 1986. Pathologic features of long-standing "healed" bronchopulmonary dysplasia: A study of 28 3 to 40-month-old infants. *Human Pathology* 17(9): 943–961.

194. Bonikos DS, and Bensch KG. 1988. Pathogenesis of bronchopulmonary dysplasia. In *Bronchopulmonary Dysplasia*, Merritt TA, Northway WH, and Boynton BR, eds. Boston: Blackwell Scientific Publications, 33–58.

195. Coalson JJ, Winter V, and deLemos RA. 1995. Decreased alveolarization in baboon survivors with bronchopulmonary dysplasia. *American Journal of Respiratory and Critical Care Medicine* 152(2): 640–646.

196. Jobe AH. 2006. The new BPD. *NeoReviews* 7(10): e531–e545.

197. Coalson JJ, et al. 1999. Neonatal chronic lung disease in extremely immature baboons. *American Journal of Respiratory and Critical Care Medicine* 160(4): 1333–1346.

198. Walsh MC, et al. 2006. Summary Proceedings from the bronchopulmonary dysplasia group. *Pediatrics* 117(3 part 2): S52–S56.

199. Van Marter LJ, et al. 1990. Maternal glucocorticoid therapy and reduced risk of bronchopulmonary dysplasia. *Pediatrics* 86(3): 331–336.

200. Sharek PJ, et al. 2003. Evaluation and development of potentially better practices to prevent chronic lung disease and reduce lung injury in neonates. *Pediatrics* 111(4 part 2): e426–e431.

201. Burch K, et al. 2003. Implementing potentially better practices to reduce lung injury in neonates. *Pediatrics* 111(4 part 2): e432–e436.

202. Van Marter LJ. 2005. Strategies for preventing bronchopulmonary dysplasia. *Current Opinion in Pediatrics* 17(2): 174–180.

203. Avery ME, et al. 1987. Is chronic lung disease in low birth weight infants preventable? A survey of eight centers. *Pediatrics* 79(1): 26–30.

204. Meyer M, Mildenhall L, and Wong M. 2004. Outcomes for infants weighing less than 1000 grams cared for with a nasal continuous positive airway pressure-based strategy. *Journal of Paediatrics and Child Health* 40(1-2): 38–41.

205. Bohlin K, et al. 2007. Implementation of surfactant treatment during continuous positive airway pressure. *Journal of Perinatology* 27(7): 422–427.

206. Stevens TP, et al. 2007. Early surfactant administration with brief ventilation vs selective surfactant and continued mechanical ventilation for preterm infants with or at risk for respiratory distress syndrome. *Cochrane Database of Systematic Reviews* (4): CD003063.

207. Barrington KJ, Bull D, and Finer NN. 2001. Randomized trial of nasal synchronized intermittent mandatory ventilation compared with continuous positive airway pressure after extubation of very low birth weight infants. *Pediatrics* 107(4): 638–641.

208. Khalaf MN, et al. 2001. A prospective randomized, controlled trial comparing synchronized nasal intermittent positive pressure ventilation versus nasal continuous positive airway pressure as modes of extubation. *Pediatrics* 108(1): 13–17.

209. Kugelman A, et al. 2007. Nasal intermittent mandatory ventilation versus nasal continuous positive airway pressure for respiratory distress syndrome: a randomized, controlled, prospective study. *Journal of Pediatrics* 150(5): 521–526.

210. Strand M, Ikegami M, and Jobe AH. 2003. Effects of high PCO_2 on ventilated preterm lamb lungs. *Pediatric Research* 53(3): 468–472.

211. Mariani G, Cifuentes J, and Carlo WA. 1999. Randomized trial of permissive hypercapnia in preterm infants. *Pediatrics* 104(5 part 1): 1082–1088.

212. Carlo WA, et al. 2002. Minimal ventilation to prevent bronchopulmonary dysplasia in extremely-low-birth-weight infants. *Journal of Pediatrics* 141(3): 370–374.

213. Woodgate PG, and Davies MW. 2001. Permissive hypercapnia for the prevention of morbidity and mortality in mechanically ventilated newborn infants. *Cochrane Database of Systematic Reviews* (2): CD002061.

214. Adams EW, et al. 2004. Increased lung water and tissue damage in bronchopulmonary dysplasia. *Journal of Pediatrics* 145(4): 503–507.

215. Oh W, et al. 2005. Association between fluid intake and weight loss during the first ten days of life and risk of bronchopulmonary dysplasia in extremely low birth weight infants. *Journal of Pediatrics* 147(6): 786–790.

216. Hartnoll G, Betremieux P, and Modi N. 2001. Randomised controlled trial of postnatal sodium supplementation in infants of 25–30 weeks gestational age: Effects on cardiopulmonary adaptation. *Archives of Disease in Childhood. Fetal and Neonatal Edition* 85(1): F29–F32.

217. Tyson JE, et al.1999. Vitamin A supplementation for extremely-low-birth-weight infants. *New England Journal of Medicine* 340(25): 1962–1968.

218. Darlow BA, and Graham PJ. 2002. Vitamin A supplementation for preventing morbidity and mortality in very low birthweight infants. *Cochrane Database of Systematic Reviews* (4): CD000501.

219. Ambalavanan N, et al. 2003. A comparison of three vitamin A dosing regimens in extremely-low-birth-weight infants. *Journal of Pediatrics* 142(6): 656–661.

220. Davis JM, et al. 2003. Pulmonary outcome at 1 year corrected age in premature infants treated at birth with recombinant human CuZn superoxide dismutase. *Pediatrics* 111(3): 469–476.

221. Ahola T, et al. 2003. N-acetylcysteine does not prevent bronchopulmonary dysplasia in immature infants: A randomized controlled trial. *Journal of Pediatrics* 143(6): 713–719.

222. Toce SS, et al. 1984. Clinical and roentgenographic scoring systems for assessing bronchopulmonary dysplasia. *American Journal of Diseases of Children* 138(6): 581–585.

223. Sinkin RA, Cox C, and Phelps DL. 1990. Predicting risk for bronchopulmonary dysplasia: Selection criteria for clinical trials. *Pediatrics* 86(5): 728–736.

224. Rozycki HJ, and Narla L. 1996. Early versus late identification of infants at high risk of developing moderate to severe bronchopulmonary dysplasia. *Pediatric Pulmonology* 21(6): 345–352.

225. STOP-ROP Multicenter Study Group. 2000. Supplemental therapeutic oxygen for prethreshold retinopathy of prematurity (STOP-ROP), a randomized, controlled trial. Part 1: Primary outcomes. *Pediatrics* 105(2): 295–310.

226. Bancalari E, Wilson-Costello D, and Iben SC. 2005. Management of infants with bronchopulmonary dysplasia in North America. *Early Human Development* 81(2): 171–179.

227. Baumer JH. 2000. International randomised controlled trial of patient triggered ventilation in neonatal respiratory distress syndrome. *Archives of Disease in Childhood. Fetal and Neonatal Edition* 82(1): F5–F10.

228. Wheeler KI, et al. 2011. Volume-targeted versus pressure-limited ventilation for preterm infants. *Cochrane Database of Systematic Reviews* (11): CD003666.

229. Lista G, et al. 2004. Impact of targeted-volume ventilation on lung inflammatory response in preterm infants with respiratory distress syndrome (RDS). *Pediatric Pulmonology* 37(6): 510–514.

230. Lista G, et al. 2008. Volume guarantee versus high frequency ventilation: Lung inflammation in preterm infants. *Archives of Disease in Childhood. Fetal and Neonatal Edition* 93(4): F252–F256.

231. Thome U, et al. 1999. Randomized comparison of high-frequency ventilation with high-rate intermittent positive pressure ventilation in preterm infants with respiratory failure. *Journal of Pediatrics* 135(1): 39–46.

232. Cools F, et al. 2009. Elective high frequency oscillatory ventilation versus conventional ventilation for acute pulmonary dysfunction in preterm infants. *Cochrane Database of Systematic Reviews* (3): CD000104.

233. Bhuta T, and Henderson-Smart DJ. 2000. Elective high frequency jet ventilation versus conventional ventilation for respiratory distress syndrome in preterm infants. *Cochrane Database of Systematic Reviews* (2): CD000328.

234. Reynolds RM, and Thureen PJ. 2007. Special circumstances: Trophic feeds, necrotizing enterocolitis and bronchopulmonary dysplasia. *Seminars in Fetal and Neonatal Medicine* 12(1): 64–70.

235. Johnson DB, Cheney C, and Monsen ER. 1998. Nutrition and feeding in infants with bronchopulmonary dysplasia after initial hospital discharge: Risk factors for growth failure. *Journal of the American Dietetic Association* 98(6): 649–656.

236. Bott L, et al. 2006. Nutritional status at 2 years in former infants with bronchopulmonary dysplasia influences nutrition and pulmonary outcomes during childhood. *Pediatric Research* 60(3): 340–344.

237. Bhatia J, and Parish A. 2009. Nutrition and the lung. *Neonatology* 95(4): 362–367.

238. Thureen PJ, et al. 2003. Effect of low versus high intravenous amino acid intake on very low birth weight infants in the early neonatal period. *Pediatric Research* 53(1): 24–32.

239. Crill CM, et al. 2006. Carnitine supplementation in premature neonates: effect on plasma and red blood cell total carnitine concentrations, nutrition parameters and morbidity. *Clinical Nutrition* 25(6): 886–896.

240. Lund CL, and Collier SB. 1990. Nutrition and bronchopulmonary dysplasia. In *Bronchopulmonary Dysplasia: Strategies for Total Patient Care*, Lund CH, ed. Santa Rosa, California: NICU Ink, 75.

241. Short EJ, et al. 2003. Cognitive and academic consequences of bronchopulmonary dysplasia and very low birth weight: 8-year-old outcomes. *Pediatrics* 112(5): e359.

242. Bregman J, and Farrell EE. 1992. Neurodevelopmental outcome in infants with bronchopulmonary dysplasia. *Clinics in Perinatology* 19(3): 673–694.

243. American Academy of Pediatrics Committee on Fetus and Newborn. 1998. Hospital discharge of the high-risk neonate—Proposed guidelines. *Pediatrics* 102(2 part 1): 411–417.

244. Gracey K, et al. 2003. The changing face of bronchopulmonary dysplasia. Part 2: Discharging an infant home on oxygen. *Advances in Neonatal Care* 3(2): 88–98.

245. Kinsella JP, Greenough A, and Abman SH. 2006. Bronchopulmonary dysplasia. *Lancet* 367(9520): 1421–1431.

246. Furman L, et al. 1996. Hospitalization as a measure of morbidity among very low birth weight infants with chronic lung disease. *Journal of Pediatrics* 128(4): 447–452.

247. Allen JL, and Panitch HB. 2001. Lung function testing: Chronic lung disease of infancy. *Pediatric Pulmonology* 26 (supplement 23): 138–140.

248. Ng DK, Lau WY, and Lee SL. 2000 Pulmonary sequelae in long-term survivors of bronchopulmonary dysplasia. *Pediatrics International* 42(6): 603–607.

249. Terry TL. 1942. Extreme prematurity and fibroblastic overgrowth of persistent vascular sheath behind each crystalline lens. Part 1: Preliminary report. *American Journal of Ophthalmology* 25(2): 203–204.

250. Patz A, Hoeck LE, and DeLaCruz E. 1952. Studies on the effect of high oxygen administration in retrolental fibroplasia. I. Nursery observations. *American Journal of Ophthalmology* 35(9): 1248–1253.

251. Kinsey VE, and Hemphill FM. 1955. Etiology of retrolental fibroplasia and preliminary report of cooperative study of retrolental fibroplasia. *Transactions—American Academy of Ophthalmology and Otolaryngology* 59(1): 15–24.

252. Cross KW. 1973. Cost of preventing retrolental fibroplasia? *Lancet* 2(7835): 954–956.

253. Todd DA, Wright A, and Smith J. 2007. Severe retinopathy of prematurity in infants <30 weeks' gestation in New South Wales and the Australian Capital Territory from 1992 to 2002. *Archives of Disease in Childhood. Fetal and Neonatal Edition* 92(4): F251–F254.

254. O'Connor MT, et al. 2003. Is retinopathy of prematurity increasing among infants less than 1250 g birth weight? *Journal of Perinatology* 23(8): 673–678.

255. Hussain N, Clive J, and Bhandari V. 1999. Current incidence of retinopathy of prematurity, 1989–1997. *Pediatrics* 104(3): e26.

256. Phelps DL. 1981. Retinopathy of prematurity: An estimate of visual loss in the United States—1979. *Pediatrics* 67(6): 924–925.

257. Cryotherapy for Retinopathy of Prematurity Cooperative Group. 1990. Multicenter trial of cryotherapy for retinopathy of prematurity: One-year outcome—Structure and function. *Archives of Ophthalmology* 108(10): 1408–1416.

258. Good WV, et al. 2005. The incidence and course of retinopathy of prematurity: Findings from the early treatment for retinopathy of prematurity study. *Pediatrics* 116(1): 15–23.

259. Ahmed MA, Duncan M, and Kent A. 2006. Incidence of retinopathy of prematurity requiring treatment in infants born greater than 30 weeks' gestation and with a birthweight greater than 1250 g from 1998 to 2002: A regional study. *Journal of Paediatrics and Child Health* 42(6): 337–340.

260. Yanovitch TL, et al. 2006. Retinopathy of prematurity in infants with birth weight ≥1250 grams—Incidence, severity, and screening guideline cost-analysis. *Journal of the American Association for Pediatric Ophthalmology and Strabismus* 10(2): 128–134.

261. Steinkuller PG, et al. 1999. Childhood blindness. *Journal of the American Association for Pediatric Ophthalmology and Strabismus* 3(1): 26–32.

262. Gilbert C, et al. 1997. Retinopathy of prematurity in middle-income countries. *Lancet* 350(9070): 12–14.

263. Haines L, et al. 2005. UK population based study of severe retinopathy of prematurity: Screening, treatment, and outcome. *Archives of Disease in Childhood. Fetal and Neonatal Edition* 90(3): F240–F244.

264. Saugstad OD. 2006. Oxygen and retinopathy of prematurity. *Journal of Perinatology* 26(supplement 1): S46–S50.

265. Fleck BW, and McIntosh N. 2008. Pathogenesis of retinopathy of prematurity and possible preventative strategies. *Early Human Development* 84(2): 83–88.

266. Chen J, and Smith LE. 2007. Retinopathy of prematurity. *Angiogenesis* 10(2): 133–140.

267. Chan-Ling T, Gock B, and Stone J. 1995. The effect of oxygen on vasoformative cell division. Evidence that "physiological hypoxia" is the stimulus for normal retinal vasculogenesis. *Investigative Ophthalmology and Visual Science* 36(7): 1201–1214.

268. Smith LE. 2003. Pathogenesis of retinopathy of prematurity. *Seminars in Neonatology* 8(6): 469–473.

269. Smith LE. 2005. IGF-1 and retinopathy of prematurity in the preterm infant. *Biology of the Neonate* 88(3): 237–244.

270. Smith LE, et al. 1999. Regulation of vascular endothelial growth factor–dependent retinal neovascularization by insulin-like growth factor-1 receptor. *Nature Medicine* 5(12): 1390–1395.

271. Hellstrom A, et al. 2001. Low IGF-1 suppresses VEGF-a survival signaling in retinal endothelial cells: Direct correlation with clinical retinopathy of prematurity. *Proceedings of the National Academy of Sciences of the United States of America* 98(10): 5804–5808.

272. Stout AU, and Stout JT. 2003. Retinopathy of prematurity. *Pediatric Clinics of North America* 50(1): 77–87.

273. International Committee for the Classification of Retinopathy of Prematurity. 2005. The international classification of retinopathy of prematurity revisited. *Archives of Ophthalmology* 123(7): 991–999.

274. Schaffer DB, et al. 1993. Prognostic factors in the natural course of retinopathy of prematurity. *Ophthalmology* 100(2): 230–237.

275. Phelps DL. 2001. Retinopathy of prematurity: History, classifications and pathophysiology. *NeoReviews* 2(7): e153–e166.

276. Cryotherapy for Retinopathy of Prematurity Cooperative Group. 1996. Multicenter trial of cryotherapy for retinopathy of prematurity. Snellen visual acuity and structural outcome at 5½ years after randomisation. *Archives of Ophthalmology* 114(4): 417–442.

277. O'Connor AR, et al. 2002. Long-term ophthalmic outcome of low birth weight children with and without retinopathy of prematurity. *Pediatrics* 109(1): 12–18.

278. Tasman W, and Brown CC. 1988. Progressive visual loss in adults with retinopathy of prematurity. *Trans American Ophthalmologic Society* 86(1): 367–375.

279. Cats BP, and Tan K. 1989. Prematures with and without regressed retinopathy of prematurity: Comparison of long term (6–10 years) ophthalmological morbidity. *Journal of Pediatric Ophthalmology and Strabismus* 26(6): 271–275.

280. Phelps DL. 2001b. Retinopathy of prematurity: Practical clinical approach. *NeoReviews* 2(7): e174–e179.

281. Higgins RD, et al. 1998. Antenatal dexamethasone and decreased severity of retinopathy of prematurity. *Archives of Ophthalmology* 116(5): 601–605.

282. Quinn GE. 2005. The "ideal" management of retinopathy of prematurity. *Eye* 19(10): 1044–1049.

283. Kim TI, et al. 2004. Postnatal risk factors of retinopathy of prematurity. *Paediatric and Perinatal Epidemiology* 18(2): 130–134.

284. Akkoyun I, et al. 2006. Risk factors in the development of mild and severe retinopathy of prematurity. *Journal of the American Association for Pediatric Ophthalmology and Strabismus (AAPOS)* 10(5): 449–453.

285. Dutta S, et al. 2004. Risk factors of threshold retinopathy of prematurity. *Indian Pediatrics* 41(7): 665–671.

286. Liu PM, et al. 2005. Risk factors of retinopathy of prematurity in premature infants weighing less than 1600 g. *American Journal of Perinatology* 22(2): 115–120.

287. Shah VA, et al. 2005. Incidence, risk factors of retinopathy of prematurity among very low birth weight infants in Singapore. *Annals of the Academy of Medicine, Singapore* 34(2): 169–178.

288. Ng YK, et al. 1988. Epidemiology of retinopathy of prematurity. *Lancet* 2(8632): 1235–1238.

289. Saunders RA, et al, 1997. Racial variation in retinopathy of prematurity. *Archives of Ophthalmology* 115(5): 604–608.

290. Fielder AR, and Reynolds JD. 2001. Retinopathy of prematurity: Clinical aspects. *Seminars in Neonatology* 6(6): 461–475.

291. Campbell K. 1951. Intensive oxygen therapy as a possible cause of retrolental fibroplasia: A clinical approach. *Medical Journal of Australia* 2(2): 48–50.

292. Ashton N, and Cook C. 1954. Direct observation of the effect of oxygen on developing vessels: Preliminary report. *British Journal of Ophthalmology* 38(7): 433–440.

293. Kinsey VE, et al. 1977. PaO$_2$ levels and retrolental fibroplasia: A report of the cooperative study. *Pediatrics* 60(5): 655–668.

294. Bancalari E, et al. 1987. Influence of transcutaneous monitoring on the incidence of retinopathy of prematurity. *Pediatrics* 79(5): 663–669.

295. Flynn JT, et al. 1992. A cohort study of transcutaneous oxygen tension and the incidence and severity of retinopathy of prematurity. *New England Journal of Medicine* 326(16): 1050–1054.

296. Vanderveen DK, Mansfield TA, and Eichenwald EC. 2006. Lower oxygen saturation alarm limits decrease the severity of retinopathy of prematurity. *Journal of the American Association for Pediatric Ophthalmology and Strabismus* 10(5): 445–448.

297. Glass P, et al. 1985. Effect of bright light in the hospital nursery on the incidence of retinopathy of prematurity. *New England Journal of Medicine* 313(7): 401–404.

298. Hommura S, et al. 1988. Ophthalmic care of very low birthweight infants. Report 4. Clinical studies of the influence of light on the incidence of retinopathy of prematurity. *Nippon Ganka Gakkai Zasshi* 92(3): 456–461.

299. Ackerman B, Sherwonit E, and Williams J. 1989. Reduced incidental light exposure effect on the development of retinopathy of prematurity in low birth weight infants. *Pediatrics* 83(6): 958–962.

300. Reynolds JD, et al. 1998. Lack of efficacy of light reduction in preventing retinopathy of prematurity. *New England Journal of Medicine* 338(22): 1572–1576.

301. Phelps DL, and Watts JL. 2001. Early light reduction for preventing retinopathy of prematurity in very low birth weight infants. *Cochrane Database of Systematic Reviews* (1): CD000122. 302. Milner RA, et al. 1981. Vitamin E supplement in under 1,500 gram neonates. In *Retinopathy of Prematurity Conference.* Columbus, Ohio: Ross Laboratories, 703–716.

303. Finer NN, et al. 1982. Effect of intramuscular vitamin E on frequency and severity of retrolental fibroplasia. A controlled trial. *Lancet* 1(8281): 1087–1091.

304. Johnson L, et al. 1989. Effect of sustained pharmacologic vitamin E levels on incidence and severity of retinopathy of prematurity: A controlled clinical trial. *Journal of Pediatrics* 114(5): 827–838.

305. Kretzer FL, et al. 1983. Spindle cells as vasoformative elements in the developing human retina: Vitamin E modulation. In *Developing and Regenerating Vertebrate Nervous Systems*, Coates PW, Markwald RR, and Kenney AD, eds. New York: Alan R. Liss, 199–210.

306. Raju TN, et al. 1997. Vitamin E prophylaxis to reduce retinopathy of prematurity: A reappraisal of published trials. *Journal of Pediatrics* 131(6): 844–850.

307. Rosenbaum AL, et al. 1985. Retinal hemorrhage in retinopathy of prematurity associated with tocopherol treatment. *Ophthalmology* 92(8): 1012–1014.

308. Phelps DL, et al. 1987. Tocopherol efficacy and safety for preventing retinopathy of prematurity: A randomized, controlled, double-masked trial. *Pediatrics* 79(4): 489–500.

309. Ehrenkranz RA. 1989. Vitamin E and retinopathy of prematurity: Still controversial. *Journal of Pediatrics* 114(5): 801–803.

310. Brion LP, Bell EF, and Raghuveer TS. 2003. Vitamin E supplementation for prevention of morbidity and mortality in preterm infants. *Cochrane Database of Systematic Reviews* (4): CD003665.

311. Lakatos L, et al. 1986. Controlled trial of D-penicillamine to prevent retinopathy of prematurity. *Acta Paediatrica Hungary* 27(1): 47–56.

312. Lakatos L, et al. 1987. Controlled trial of use of D-penicillamine to prevent retinopathy of prematurity in very-low-birth-weight infants. In *Physiologic Foundations of Perinatal Care*, Stern L, Oh W, and Friis-Hansen B, eds. Philadelphia: Elsevier, 9–23.

313. Phelps DL, Lakatos L, and Watts JL. 2001. D-penicillamine for preventing retinopathy of prematurity in preterm infants. *Cochrane Database of Systematic Reviews* (1): CD001073.

314. Christensen RD, et al. 2007. D-penicillamine administration and the incidence of retinopathy of prematurity. *Journal of Perinatology* 27(2): 103–111.

315. Hallman M, et al. 1992. Inositol supplementation in premature infants with respiratory distress syndrome. *New England Journal of Medicine* 326(19): 1233–1239.

316. Hallman M, Jarvanpaa AL, and Pohjavuori M. 1986. Respiratory distress syndrome and inositol supplementation in preterm infants. *Archives of Disease in Childhood* 61(11): 1076–1083.

317. Howlett A, and Ohlsson A. 2003. Inositol for respiratory distress syndrome in preterm infants. *Cochrane Database of Systematic Reviews* (4): CD000366.

318. Section on Ophthalmology American Academy of Pediatrics, American Academy of Ophthalmology, American Association for Pediatric Ophthalmology and Strabismus. 2006. Screening examination of premature infants for retinopathy of prematurity. *Pediatrics* 117(2): 572–576.

319. Reynolds JD, et al. 2002. Evidence-based screening criteria for retinopathy of prematurity: Natural history data from the CRYO-ROP and LIGHT-ROP studies. *Archives of Ophthalmology* 120(11): 1470–1476.

320. Subhani M, et al. 2001. Screening guidelines for retinopathy of prematurity: the need for revision in extremely low birth weight infants. *Pediatrics* 107(4): 656–659.

321. Mathew MR, Fern AI, and Hill R. 2002. Retinopathy of prematurity: Are we screening too many babies? *Eye* 16(5): 538–542.

322. Ho SF, et al. 2005. Retinopathy of prematurity: An optimum screening strategy. *Journal of the American Association for Pediatric Ophthalmology and Strabismus* 9(6): 584–588.

323. Lloyd J, et al. 2003. Supplemental oxygen for the treatment of prethreshold retinopathy of prematurity. *Cochrane Database of Systematic Reviews* (2): CD003482.

324. Hutcheson KA. 2003. Retinopathy of prematurity. *Current Opinion in Ophthalmology* 14(5): 286–290.

325. Cryotherapy for Retinopathy of Prematurity Cooperative Group. 2001. Multicenter trial of cryotherapy for retinopathy of prematurity: Ophthalmological outcomes at 10 years. *Archives of Ophthalmology* 119(8): 1110–1118.

326. Subramanian KNS, Bahri M, Vincente G. 2009. Retinopathy of Prematurity. Emedicine. Accessed Nov 11 2009 from http://emedicine.medscape.com/article/976220-overview

327. McLoone E, et al. 2006. Long term functional and structural outcomes of laser therapy for retinopathy of prematurity. *British Journal of Ophthalmology* 90(6): 754–759.

328. Connolly BP, et al. 2002. A comparison of laser photocoagulation with cryotherapy for threshold retinopathy of prematurity at 10 years. Part 2: Refractive outcome. *Ophthalmology* 109(5): 936–941.

329. Ng EY, et al. 2002. A comparison of laser photocoagulation with cryotherapy for threshold retinopathy of prematurity at 10 years. Part 1: Visual function and structural outcome. *Ophthalmology* 109(5): 928–934.

330. Hunter DG, and Mukai S. 1992. Retinopathy of prematurity: Pathogenesis, diagnosis, and treatment. *International Ophthalmology Clinics* 32(1): 163–184.

331. Topilow HW, and Ackerman AL. 1989. Cryotherapy for Stage 3+ retinopathy of prematurity: Visual and anatomic results. *Ophthalmic Surgery* 20(12): 864–871.

332. Hartnett ME, et al. 2004. Comparison of retinal outcomes after scleral buckle or lens-sparing vitrectomy for Stage 4 retinopathy of prematurity. *Retina* 24(5): 753–757.

333. Early Treatment for Retinopathy of Prematurity Cooperative Group. 2003. Revised indications for the treatment of retinopathy of prematurity: Results of the early treatment for retinopathy of prematurity randomized trial. *Archives of Ophthalmology* 121(12): 1684–1694.

334. Repka MX, et al. 2006. Outcome of eyes developing retinal detachment during the Early Treatment for Retinopathy of Prematurity Study (ETROP). *Archives of Ophthalmology* 124(1): 24–30.

335. Arevalo JF, et al. 2011. Intravitreal bevacizumab (Avastin) for diabetic retinopathy: The 2010 GLADROF lecture. *Journal of Ophthalmology*. doi: 10.1155/2011/584238.

336. Hubbard GB. 2008. Surgical management of retinopathy of prematurity. *Current Opinion in Ophthalmology* 19(5): 384–390.

337. Salvin JH, et al. 2010. Update on retinopathy of prematurity: Treatment options and outcomes. *Current Opinion in Ophthalmology* 21(5): 329–334.

338. Micieli JA, Surkont M, and Smith AF. 2009. A systematic analysis of the off-label use of bevacizumab for severy retinopathy of prematurity. *American Journal of Ophthalmology* 148(4): 536–543.

339. Mintz-Hittner H, Kennedy K, and Chuang AZ. 2011. Efficacy of intravitreal bevacizumab for stage 3 retinopathy of prematurity. *New England Journal of Medicine* 364(7): 603–615.

340. Chow LC, Wright KW, and Sola A. 2003. Can changes in clinical practice decrease the incidence of severe retinopathy of prematurity in very low birth weight infants? *Pediatrics* 111(2): 339–345.

341. Coe K, et al. 2006. Special Premie Oxygen Targeting (SPOT): A program to decrease the incidence of blindness in infants with retinopathy of prematurity. *Journal of Nursing Care Quality* 21(3): 230–235.

342. York JR, et al. 2004. Arterial oxygen fluctuation and retinopathy of prematurity in very-low-birth-weight infants. *Journal of Perinatology* 24(2): 82–87.

NOTES

11 Neonatal Respiratory Pharmacotherapy

Susan Givens Bell, DNP, MABMH, RNC-NIC

A variety of drugs is used in the treatment of neonates with respiratory distress, including many that do not directly affect the lungs or pulmonary vasculature. This chapter focuses on only those medications that are administered for their direct effects on the pulmonary system. Those medications include exogenous surfactant, nitric oxide (NO) and related vasodilators, corticosteroids, and bronchodilators.

EXOGENOUS SURFACTANT

In his essay on the ten most significant areas of progress in neonatology, Nelson comments that "pulmonary surfactant...is unusual among biomedical advances in that it was not the product of serendipitous deductions, but rather was specifically sought out as the likely missing factor to account for the airless lungs of infants who died of RDS" (p. 734). The journey from discovery of endogenous pulmonary surfactant as the substance that lowers surface tension to approval of exogenous surfactant to prevent and treat neonatal respiratory distress syndrome (RDS) involved the cooperation of pediatricians, obstetricians, physiologists, and biochemists and took just over three decades.[1] In the mid- to late 1950s, researchers observed that low surface tension might be an important attribute of the lining of the alveoli in preventing collapse and atelectasis.[2–5] In 1959, Avery and Mead presented evidence that the substance responsible for this low surface tension was absent from the lungs of premature infants with hyaline membrane disease (HMD), later renamed RDS. Substances that accumulate spontaneously at the surface of a liquid, lowering its surface tension, are called surfactants.[6] Thus, it was postulated that the pathophysiology of HMD could be attributed to surfactant

deficiency.[7] This association of clinical illness with lack of surfactant brought clinical relevance to the field of surfactant research. The question remained, however: Could surfactant replacement ameliorate HMD? Clearly, further research was necessary. Surfactant had to be isolated, and its biochemical properties had to be characterized.[6] Chemical analysis of pulmonary surfactant revealed its essential components to be dipalmitoylphosphatidylcholine (DPPC) and phosphatidylglycerol along with four lung-specific apoproteins (surfactant-associated proteins [SP]).[6,8,9] Once it was discovered that DPPC is the principal component of surfactant, researchers attempted, albeit unsuccessfully, to treat RDS with aerosolized DPPC.[10] Clements explains that these trials failed, most likely because aerosol administration is not an efficient means of delivering substances to the alveoli, clinical management of sick neonates was relatively primitive in the late 1960s, and the adsorption and spread of the DPPC particles into the air-fluid interface of the alveoli was slow. Perhaps as a result of the failure of these early trials, systematic evaluation of surfactant therapy did not proceed for about a decade.[6]

In the 1970s researchers began to study the instillation of surfactant extract in premature animals.[11–13] Premature rabbits that received the surfactant extracts were noted to have improved pulmonary mechanics.[12] Furthermore, the surfactant appeared to protect the rabbits' immature lungs from injuries resulting from intermittent positive-pressure ventilation.[13] Encouraged by the success of the animal trials and after extensive studies establishing the safety of an artificial surfactant developed from cow lung, Fujiwara and colleagues tried the artificial surfactant on a group of ten infants with

TABLE 11-1
Comparison of Selected Natural Exogenous Pulmonary Surfactants

Surfactant (Brand Name)	Dose	Source	Contents	Comments
Beractant (Survanta)	4 mL/kg dose IT divided into 4 aliquots *Prophylaxis:* First dose as soon as possible after birth, preferably within 15 minutes, with up to 3 subsequent doses in the first 48 hours of life as indicated.* *Rescue treatment for RDS:* Up to 4 doses in the first 48 hours of life, no more frequently than every 6 hours.	Modified natural bovine lung extract	Phospholipids, neutral lipids, fatty acids, and SP-B and SP-C to which DPPC, palmitic acid, and tripalmitin have been added	▪ Allow to stand at room temperature for 20 minutes, or hold in the hand for at least 8 minutes to warm. ▪ Normal color is off-white to light-brown. ▪ If settling occurs, gently swirl vial. ▪ Do not shake. ▪ Do not filter. ▪ Discard unused portion of drug. ▪ Unopened vials that have been warmed to room temperature once may be refrigerated within 24 hours and stored for future use. ▪ Supplied in 4 mL and 8 mL vials.
Calfactant (Infasurf)	*Initial dose:* 3 mL/kg IT divided into 2 aliquots. Follow with up to 3 additional doses given at 12-hour intervals as indicated.*	Calf lung extract	Phospholipids, neutral lipids, fatty acids, and SP-B and SP-C	▪ Allow to warm to room temperature. ▪ Normal color is off-white. ▪ If settling occurs, gently turn vial upside down to uniformly suspend drug. ▪ Do not shake. ▪ Do not filter. ▪ Discard unused portion of drug. ▪ Unopened vials that have been warmed to room temperature once may be refrigerated within 24 hours and stored for future use. ▪ Supplied in 6 mL vials.
Poractant alfa (Curosurf)	*Initial dose:* 2.5 mL/kg IT divided into 2 aliquots. Follow with up to 2 additional doses of 1.25 mL/kg at 12-hour intervals as indicated.*	Modified porcine-derived minced lung extract	Phospholipids, neutral lipids, fatty acids, and SP-B and SP-C	▪ Allow to warm to room temperature. ▪ Normal color is creamy white. ▪ If settling occurs, gently turn vial upside down to uniformly suspend drug. ▪ Do not shake. ▪ Do not filter. ▪ Discard unused portion of drug. ▪ Unopened vials that have been warmed to room temperature once may be refrigerated within 24 hours and stored for future use. ▪ Supplied in 1.5 mL and 3 mL vials.

* Based on clinical assessment and condition and radiologic evidence.

Key: SP-B = surfactant-associated protein B; SP-C = surfactant-associated protein C; IT = intratracheally.

Compiled from: Taketomo CK, Hodding JH, and Kraus DM. 2009. *Pediatric Dosage Handbook,* 16th ed. Hudson, Ohio: Lexi-Comp, 166–167, 218–219, 1013; and Zenk KE, Sills JH, and Koeppel RM. 2003. *Neonatal Medications & Nutrition: A Comprehensive Guide,* 3rd ed. Petaluma, California: NICU Ink, 85–86, 107–110.

severe RDS, reporting the results of this first successful trial of an artificial surfactant in humans in 1980.[14] During the 1980s, research on exogenous pulmonary surfactant, including multiphase clinical trials, continued. In 1990, the U.S. Food and Drug Administration (FDA) approved the first exogenous surfactant for the prevention and treatment of RDS in premature neonates, the artificial surfactant colfosceril palmitate with cetyl alcohol and tyloxapol (Exosurf Neonatal).[15] Since the approval of natural, animal-derived surfactants, artificial surfactants have fallen out of favor. Exosurf is no longer available in North America. The discussion that follows covers three widely used natural surfactants, reviews meta-analyses of clinical surfactant studies, and reflects on some unanswered questions regarding surfactant therapy. Recent research on use of surfactant therapy for other neonatal respiratory disease processes is also reported.

NATURAL SURFACTANTS

In July 1991, the FDA approved the first natural, animal-derived surfactant, beractant, for the treatment of neonates at risk for or with RDS. In the late 1990s, two other natural, animal-derived surfactants received FDA approval: calfactant in 1998 and poractant alfa in 1999.[15]

Beractant (Survanta, Ross Products Division, Abbott Laboratories, Columbus, Ohio) is a modified natural bovine lung extract containing phospholipids, neutral lipids, fatty acids, and the surfactant-associated proteins B and C (SP-B and SP-C). Colfosceril palmitate, palmitic acid, and tripalmitin are added to the natural components to mimic the surface tension–lowering characteristics of naturally occurring human surfactant.[16–18] The lipophilic SP-B and SP-C facilitate the adsorption and spread of phospholipids at the alveolar air-fluid interface. The presence of naturally occurring SP-B in the lung is necessary for the packaging of surfactant into the lamellar bodies, where it is stored before it is secreted into the air spaces.[16] Surfactant-associated protein B is essential for lung function. Calfactant (Infasurf, Forest Pharmaceuticals, St. Louis, Missouri) is an organic-solvent extract of alveolar lavage fluid from calf lungs. Calfactant contains phospholipids, primarily phosphatidylcholine; neutral lipids; fatty acids; and SP-B and SP-C and does not require further modification.[16,17] The SP-B concentration in calfactant approximates that in human surfactant.[18]

Poractant alfa (Dey Pharma LP, Napa, California) is a modified extract of minced porcine lungs. It contains phospholipids, including DPPC; neutral lipids; fatty acids; and SP-B and SP-C.[16]

Doses and frequency of repeat dosing for the three natural surfactants can be found in Table 11-1. Several techniques are described for administration. The trachea should be suctioned to clear secretions before administration. The surfactant should be allowed to warm to room temperature before instillation. Warming may be accomplished by allowing the vial to stand for 20 minutes, or the suspension may be warmed in the hand for 8 minutes. The first administration technique uses a 5-French, end-hole catheter that has been shortened so

FIGURE 11-1
Schematic representation of a side-port endotracheal tube adapter.

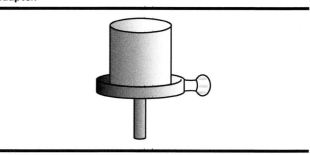

that its tip protrudes just beyond the end of the endotracheal tube above the carina. The entire content of the surfactant vial is drawn into a plastic syringe using a larger than 20 gauge needle. Surfactant should not be filtered or shaken. The syringe is attached to the shortened catheter, and the catheter is filled with surfactant. Excess surfactant is flushed through the catheter so that only the prescribed dose remains in the syringe. Ideally, the catheter is then inserted into the endotracheal tube via a neonatal suction valve so that the surfactant can be given without interrupting mechanical ventilation. Alternatively, the surfactant can be instilled through the catheter by briefly disconnecting the infant from the ventilator, inserting the catheter into the endotracheal tube, administering an aliquot of the medication, removing the dosing catheter, and then reconnecting the ventilator and ventilating the infant for at least 30 seconds or until stable.

The Survanta dose is divided into four 1 mL/kg aliquots. Each quarter-dose is given over 2–3 seconds, repositioning the infant with each aliquot. Manufacturer-recommended positions are[19]

- Head and body inclined 5–10 degrees down, with head turned to the right
- Head and body inclined 5–10 degrees down, with head turned to the left
- Head and body inclined 5–10 degrees up, with head turned to the right
- Head and body inclined 5–10 degrees up, with head turned to the left

The infant is ventilated for a minimum of 30 seconds following each quarter-dose to allow time for him to stabilize.[18] After administration, avoid suctioning for one hour, unless clinically indicated.[20]

The Infasurf dose is divided into two equal aliquots. Each is given in small bursts over 20–30 breaths during the inspiratory phase, with the infant's head in a neutral position. Following administration of each aliquot, the infant is positioned with either the left or the right side dependent, to facilitate distribution of the surfactant. An alternative method for instilling Infasurf is to use a Luer-Lock side-port endotracheal tube adapter (Figure 11-1). The procedure otherwise remains the same. A specific waiting period for suctioning following administration has not been established for Infasurf.[21]

The Curosurf dose is also divided into two equal aliquots. Supplemental oxygen is provided to maintain the oxygen saturation within the prescribed range. With the infant's head in a midline position, the first aliquot is instilled. The infant is then positioned with either the right or the left side down. The procedure is repeated for the second aliquot, positioning the infant with the opposite side down following administration. Ventilator settings are adjusted to maintain blood gases within prescribed limits. Alternatively, Curosurf may be administered through the proximal end of the secondary lumen of a double-lumen endotracheal tube (Figure 11-2). The entire volume of the Curosurf dose is given over one minute without interruption in ventilation. The airway should not be suctioned for one hour following administration, unless clinically indicated.[22]

All three natural, animal-derived surfactants are well tolerated. Reflux of the medication into the endotracheal tube or deterioration of the infant's condition requires either slowing or temporarily halting the procedure. Oxygen concentration and ventilator settings are adjusted as needed. As with artificial surfactant, there is a risk for pulmonary hemorrhage.[17] The neonate requires close monitoring following surfactant administration. Rapid improvement in lung function with improved oxygenation and lung compliance necessitates changes in FiO_2 and ventilator settings.

COMPARISON OF SURFACTANTS

Surfactant administration for the prevention and treatment of RDS is one of the most widely studied neonatal therapies. Moya and Maturana provide an excellent review of U.S. and U.K. studies comparing animal-derived surfactants and past and current synthetic surfactants. Those surfactants included in the review were Exosurf (GalxoSmithKline, Brentford, U.K.), Pumactant (Britannia Pharmaceutical, Redhill, Surrey, U.K.), the animal-derived surfactants, Survanta, Infasurf, Curosurf, and Alveofact (Boehringer Ingelheim, Ingelheim, Germany), and a novel synthetic surfactant lucinactant (Surfaxin) (Discovery Laboratories, Warrington, Pennsylvania). Lucinactant is

an experimental surfactant containing a peptide mimic of human SP-B.[23] A summary of their findings are discussed here.[24]

In comparisons of Exosurf and animal-derived surfactants, the authors note that the use of animal-derived surfactant does not result in a reduced risk of mortality or bronchopulmonary dysplasia (BPD). The advantage of animal-derived surfactants appears to be related to faster weaning and decreased risk of pneumothorax when used for the treatment of RDS.[24]

No important differences in major outcomes were noted in comparison studies of particular animal-derived surfactants. Curosurf may provide a survival advantage over the other animal-derived surfactants; however, the authors note that their data were derived from studies of lesser quality and with smaller sample sizes and therefore must be interpreted with caution.[24]

Studies comparing Surfaxin with either synthetic surfactants containing only phospholipids or animal-derived surfactant show promising results suggesting that Sufaxin functions better clinically than phospholipid-only surfactants and at least as well as the animal-derived surfactants.[24] Other potential advantages of a synthetic surfactant that mimics the action of SP-B over the animal-derived surfactants are absence of immunogenicity, absence of risk of disease transmission, and the ability to mass-produce the product with a high degree of consistency.[25] Finally, the authors found no differences when side effects of the various surfactants were evaluated prospectively in comparison studies. The authors note the paucity of follow-up studies and suggest that follow-up should be a component of future surfactant studies.[24]

ALTERNATIVE METHODS FOR SURFACTANT ADMINISTRATION

There is a trend toward managing premature infants using the INSURE (INtubation-SURfactant-Extubation) described by Dani and colleagues.[26] Premature infants in whom RDS is initially managed with nasal continuous positive airway pressure (CPAP) are intubated to administer surfactant, then immediately extubated and nasal CPAP is reinstituted. Infants are weaned from CPAP as tolerated.[26,27] In a recent study, Dani and colleagues found that birth weight <750 g and RDS severity, evaluated as PaO_2/FiO_2 <218 and a/ApO_2 <44, are independent risk factors for INSURE failure.[27]

Dargaville and associates investigated the feasibility of a method of minimally invasive surfactant therapy (MIST) in 11 spontaneously breathing neonates on

CPAP. The CPAP mask or nasal prongs were removed. A 16 gauge, 130 mm long vascular catheter was inserted, to a predetermined depth, through the vocal cords under direct laryngoscopy. A syringe of Curosurf (Chiesi Farmceutici, Parma, Italy), 1.25 mL/kg, was then attached to the catheter. The surfactant was administered in a single bolus for infants who were 25–28 weeks gestational age and in two boluses, 10 seconds apart, for infants who were 29–34 weeks gestational age. Following surfactant administration, the catheter was immediately removed and CPAP was reinstituted. The researchers determined that this technique is feasible and that safety and efficacy studies of this technique are needed.[28]

Finer and colleagues examined the feasibility and safety of prophylactic aerosolized surfactant delivery in 17 premature infants on nasal CPAP. The researchers used Aerosurf ([lucinactant for inhalation] Discovery Laboratories, Warrington, Pennsylvania), a peptide-containing synthetic surfactant. The infants tolerated the aerosolized surfactant well. Further studies are needed to determine the efficacy of this technique.[29]

SURFACTANT-RELATED CONTROVERSIES AND ETHICAL CONCERNS

Surfactants are considered a safe and effective treatment and are the standard of care for infants at risk for or with established RDS.[30] As Jobe points out, however, strategies regarding which neonates to treat and when and how to initiate treatment remain controversial topics in neonatology. Specific variables in surfactant therapy include timing (at delivery or after initial stabilization), ventilatory support before and after therapy (CPAP or mechanical ventilation and type of mechanical ventilation), techniques for treatment (pharyngeal at delivery, number and volume of boluses for each treatment), and management after treatment. Each of these variables is complicated further by each infant's gestational age, birth weight, and clinical condition at delivery.[30] Two recent studies explored some of these variables.[31,32]

In a multicenter, randomized clinical trial, Escobedo and associates studied the efficacy and safety of elective surfactant therapy for preterm infants with mild to moderate RDS who did not require mechanical ventilation. The trial was performed on 132 neonates with birth weights ≥1,250 g, gestational ages of ≤36 weeks, and postnatal ages of 4–24 hours. Oxygen requirement was ≥40 percent for at least 1 hour, and the infants had no immediate need for intubation. Infants were randomly

FIGURE 11-2
Schematic representation of a double-lumen endotracheal tube.

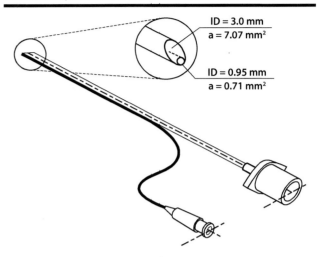

ID = 3.0 mm
a = 7.07 mm²

ID = 0.95 mm
a = 0.71 mm²

Key: ID = inside diameter; a = area (internal cross-sectional).

From: Valls-i-Soler A, et al. 1998. A randomized comparison of surfactant dosing via a dual-lumen endotracheal tube in respiratory distress syndrome. *Pediatrics* 101(4): e4. Reprinted by permission.

assigned to intubation and surfactant therapy (beractant) with expedited extubation or to expectant management with subsequent intubation and surfactant therapy if clinically indicated. The primary outcome measure was duration of mechanical ventilation. The researchers found that the infants in the intervention group had a small but statistically significant increase in the median duration of mechanical ventilation: 2.2 hours (0.6, 41) versus 0 hours (0, 38.5) for the control group. They found no significant differences between the two groups in median duration of CPAP, duration of oxygen therapy, or length of stay. Additionally, there were no significant differences in complications, including pulmonary air leaks, pulmonary hemorrhage, intraventricular hemorrhage (IVH), death, or airway complications (e.g., stridor). The researchers noted, however, that because there was a low incidence of complications in this population, a much larger study would be necessary to exclude any clinically important differences in these adverse outcomes. Based on their findings, the researchers do not recommend elective intubation for administration of surfactant in larger preterm neonates with mild to moderate respiratory distress.[31] There is a need for further large clinical trials and meta-analysis to support these results.

Kaiser and coworkers sought to determine whether surfactant administration affects cerebral and systemic hemodynamics and gas exchange in very low birth weight (VLBW) infants and to determine which of three factors—PaCO$_2$, mean arterial blood pressure (MABP), and PaO$_2$—has the greatest influence on changes in mean cerebral blood flow velocity (mCBFv) after surfactant administration. Fourteen neonates with birth weights of 832 ± 162 g and gestational ages of 25.7 ± 1.5 weeks were enrolled in the study. The researchers found a consistent rise in middle cerebral artery mCBFv. Peak velocity occurred approximately 10–20 minutes after surfactant administration and persisted for approximately 45 minutes. Changes in mCBFv during surfactant instillation were highly associated with changes in PaCO$_2$. Changes in MABP during surfactant administration had much less impact on mCBFv than did changes in PaCO$_2$. No apparent relationship was noted between PaO$_2$ and changes in mCBFv after surfactant administration.[32]

Even though the study by Kaiser and colleagues was small, the implications for clinical practice are significant. The researchers assert that their results support the notion that techniques for surfactant treatment could be improved to minimize potential harm related to changes in cerebral blood flow.[32] Citing other studies in which fluctuations in arterial blood gases and hemodynamics were prevented using alternative techniques for surfactant administration, the authors raise some interesting points. Saliba and associates found that infusing surfactant slowly, rather than as a bolus, prevented changes in mCBFv, most likely by preventing increases in PaCO$_2$. In their study, infants received Exosurf rapidly over 5 minutes or by slow infusion over 15 minutes.[33] However, fast bolus instillation versus slow infusion again raises the issue addressed by Wang and coworkers of distribution of surfactant throughout the lungs.[34] Saliba and colleagues reported that the rapid-instillation and slow-infusion methods were equally effective in improving acute clinical outcome based on alveolar-arterial gradients in the two groups 72 hours after the initial dose of surfactant.[33] In a separate study, reducing the number of aliquots from six to two decreased both the duration and amplitude of PaCO$_2$ increases.[35] Using either an endotracheal tube adapter with a side-port or a dual-lumen endotracheal tube may eliminate the changes in cerebral blood flow velocity that result from loss of functional residual capacity related to disconnection from mechanical ventilation during surfactant instillation.[36,37]

In the side-port study, Valls-i-Soler and associates compared the instillation of the entire dose of poractant over 1 minute via the side port of the endotracheal tube adapter with the standard delivery technique. There was no significant difference in PaCO$_2$ before and after surfactant instillation, nor was there a significant difference in PaCO$_2$ between the two groups.[36] Similar results were found when administration of the entire dose of poractant over 1 minute via a dual-lumen endotracheal tube was compared with the standard delivery method. Again, there was no significant difference in PaCO$_2$ before and after surfactant instillation, nor was there a significant difference in PaCO$_2$ between the two groups.[37] Cerebral blood flow velocity was not measured in either of these studies.

Although Kaiser and coworkers demonstrated that mCBFv was highly associated with PaCO$_2$, one must be careful when generalizing results of multiple studies. Additionally, nebulized surfactant has been noted to have a minimal effect on cerebral blood flow in an animal model.[38] Dijk and colleagues note, however, that improvement in the nebulization efficiency of neonatal ventilators is necessary before this mode of surfactant delivery can be used as an alternative for human neonates. Using a surfactant product that requires smaller dosing volumes than beractant (4 mL/kg/dose) may decrease large-airway clogging and minimize or prevent changes in PaCO$_2$.[38] Initially, Kaiser and associates suggest that the use of a continuous blood gas system would allow active ventilatory management to maintain the necessary ventilation and oxygenation levels and thus diminish hemodynamic and blood gas changes associated with surfactant administration.[32] Clearly, more research is necessary before questions regarding the best technique for surfactant administration are definitively answered.

The presence of bovine or porcine products in natural, animal-derived surfactants raises ethical concerns of consent and issues of cultural sensitivity.[39] Adappa and coworkers address the question of consent, noting that two families declined to participate in a clinical trial of a new artificial surfactant. A Hindu family did not want their infant to receive beractant because it is a bovine-derived product and cows are sacred in the Hindu religion. A Muslim family wished to avoid the use of a porcine product. Other religions have dietary restrictions that may preclude infants whose parents practice them from receiving surfactant products derived from specific animals.[40] Seventh Day Adventists and Jews are prohibited or strongly discouraged from consuming pork, and the most devout among Hindus avoid pork as well. The most devout Buddhists avoid consumption of both beef and pork.[41] With these dietary restrictions in mind, Adappa and colleagues ask if consent for treatment with surfactant should be presumed. This also highlights the importance of having an artificial surfactant available as an alternative for families who prefer to avoid the use of animal-derived pharmaceutical products.

SURFACTANT THERAPY IN OTHER ACUTE NEONATAL RESPIRATORY DISEASES

There are several reports in the literature of surfactant treatment for acute neonatal respiratory diseases other than RDS. These include meconium aspiration syndrome (MAS),[42–50] pneumonia,[51] and bronchiolitis secondary to respiratory syncytial virus (RSV).[52]

MAS and Surfactant Therapy

The premise of surfactant therapy in MAS is evidence of disturbances of the surfactant system in infants with this disorder. Dargaville and associates found that, compared with normal controls, infants with MAS receiving mechanical ventilation had normal levels of surfactant phospholipid and surfactant-associated protein A, but high concentrations of potential surfactant inhibitors (including total protein, albumin, and phosphatidylserine) associated with hemorrhagic pulmonary edema.[53] Four randomized clinical trials of surfactant for meconium aspiration in term and near term infants met inclusion criteria for a systematic review by El Shahed and colleagues.[43,48–50] Analysis of these four trials revealed that in infants with MAS, surfactant may decrease the severity of respiratory illness. Additonally, surfactant therapy may decrease the number of infants with progressive respiratory failure who required extracorporeal membrane oxygenation. The relative efficacy of surfactant administration for MAS compared to or in conjunction with inhaled nitric oxide (iNO), liquid ventilation, surfactant lavage, and high-frequency ventilation remains to be examined.[54]

Another potential surfactant therapy under investigation for treatment of MAS is surfactant lavage. Large-volume lung lavage with dilute surfactant has been effective in removing particulate meconium from the lung in an animal model of MAS.[55] Wiswell and coworkers reported a small randomized clinical trial of surfactant lavage in term neonates with MAS. Twenty-two neonates were enrolled in a study to compare broncho-alveolar lavage (BAL) using a dilute surfactant (lucinactant [Surfaxin]) with standard care for MAS. Infants in the treatment group received a total of 48 mL/kg of dilute surfactant divided into a series of three lavages (16 mL/kg each), a specific protocol of surfactant instillation, and suctioning with an in-line suction device.

The procedure had to be stopped in 20 percent of the infants because of hypoxemia or hypotension. One-third of the subjects reached failure criteria (oxygen index* [OI] >25 or an increase in OI to >50 percent above baseline) despite being lavaged. Even though the lavaged infants had a more rapid decline in OI than those who received standard care, the difference was not statistically significant. In fact, none of the differences between the groups—including mean days to extubation, mean days until discontinuation of oxygen, and mean days to discharge from the NICU—were significant.[23]

Kinsella suggests that it may be reasonable to consider the early use of exogenous surfactant as a small-volume bolus for neonates with MAS and evidence of parenchymal lung disease but without echocardigraphic evidence of significant pulmonary hypertension.[56] It remains to be seen whether surfactant lavage is an appropriate regimen in the treatment of MAS. The U.S. FDA has approved a large phase III trial to evaluate the safety and efficacy of this approach to MAS.[23]

A protocol has been developed for the systematic review of therapeutic lung lavage for MAS in neonates. The primary objective of this review is to evaluate the safety and efficacy of pulmonary lavage with saline, surfactant, or perfluorocarbon in infants with MAS, with particular focus on the impact of lavage on mortality and morbidity. The reviewers will also evaluate, by subgroup analysis of controlled lavage therapy, which lavage fluid, at what volume, and at what time has the greatest effect on mortality and morbidity in this population.[57]

Pneumonia, RSV-related Bronchiolitis, and Surfactant Therapy

Other potential targets for surfactant therapy are pneumonia and RSV-related bronchiolitis. Numerous investigators have reported alterations in surfactant function in both animal models and humans with acute respiratory illness and inflammation. Acute lung injury in the mouse model results in decreased expression of SP-B.[58] The release of phospholipase C by *Pseudomonas aeruginosa* in patients with cystic fibrosis may affect surfactant function by catalyzing surfactant phospholipid hydrolysis.[59] The fatty acid composition of various pulmonary surfactant phospholipids is altered in acute RDS (ARDS) and in severe pneumonia in mechanically ventilated adult patients.[60] Kerr and Paton noted a reduction in surfactant proteins A, B, and D in the BAL fluid in children with RSV infection. Viral invasion of type II pneumocytes and other pulmonary cells may reduce

---

* OI = (FiO$_2$ × Paw [mean airway pressure] × 100)/PaO$_2$

surfactant protein synthesis.[61] Surfactant proteins A and D play a role in the lung's defense against pathogens.[62] It is not clear if SP-A and SP-D bind to RSV and are subsequently phagocytized, thus reducing the concentration of these surfactant proteins in the BAL fluid, or if a primary reduction in SP-A or SP-D causes reduced immunity to RSV or increased susceptibility to respiratory failure from RSV.[61]

Herting and colleagues found that surfactant administration improved gas exchange in preterm and term infants with Group B streptococcal (GBS) pneumonia. However, this improvement was notably slower than in the control group of premature infants with RDS without infection. The researchers suggest that the slower response in the GBS group may be related to larger quantities of surfactant inhibitors in the bronchoalveolar space in this group. In addition, the complication rate was higher in the GBS group. Thirty percent of the infants in the GBS group died, compared with 19 percent in the RDS group. Pneumothorax and intracranial hemorrhage (ICH) occurred, respectively, in 19 percent and 43 percent of the GBS group. Thirteen percent of the control group experienced pneumothorax; 35 percent had an ICH.[51]

In a small study of 19 infants with RSV, Tibby and associates noted that the infants who received two 4 mL/kg doses of surfactant (beractant) within 24 and 48 hours of initiation of mechanical ventilation for respiratory failure did not demonstrate the deterioration in lung compliance and resistance that was observed in the placebo group. The treatment group had a more rapid improvement over the first 60 hours following enrollment in the study, but they did not show improvement in lung mechanics or indices of gas exchange (OI, ventilation index [VI], or alveolar-arterial gradient*) during the first 30 hours following enrollment. In fact, surfactant administration caused a transient worsening of these indices, but they resolved within 2 hours. Based on their findings, the researchers asked whether surfactant therapy for RSV bronchiolitis has the potential to reduce number of ventilator days and length of hospital stay. Although this small study lacked statistical power, there was a trend toward reduction in mean duration of ventilation, hospital stay, and hospital stay in the surfactant-treated group.[52] Clearly, there is a need for further study to assess the efficacy of surfactant therapy in NICU patients with pneumonia and RSV-related bronchiolitis.

* VI = respiratory rate × peak-inspiratory pressure × $PaCO_2/1,000$.
   Alveolar-arterial gradient $(AaDO_2) = (FiO_2 \times [760 \text{ mmHg} - 47 \text{ mmHg}] - [PaCO_2/0.8]) - PaO_2$. *Note:* 760 mmHg is atmospheric pressure; 47 mmHg is the partial pressure of water vapor.

Congenital Diaphragmatic Hernia and Surfactant Therapy

There are conflicting data on surfactant deficiency in infants with congenital diaphragmatic hernia (CDH). A study using a lamb model demonstrated that all components that contribute to surfactant function are deficient in CDH. There was both a quantitative and a qualitative reduction in the phospholipid component. Not only were total phospholipids significantly decreased, even with normalization per gram of lung weight in the hypoplastic lung, but the percentage of phospholipids that was phosphatidylcholine was also decreased. Both SP-A and SP-B were significantly reduced as well. The researchers suggest that a possible mechanism for these abnormalities is dysfunction of the type II pneumocytes.[63]

Moya and coworkers found that both SP-A and saturated phosphatidylcholine levels in the amniotic fluid were lower in fetuses with CDH than in gestational age–matched controls. The researchers assert that it is unclear whether these deficiencies are a result of delayed lung maturation or if the degree of lung dysplasia is the cause.[64]

IJsselstijn and colleagues evaluated concentrations of different surfactant phospholipids and the fatty acid composition of phosphatidylcholine in BAL fluid in 18 infants with CDH (13 on conventional ventilation, 5 on ECMO) and 19 controls (13 on conventional ventilation, 6 on extracorporeal membrane oxygenation [ECMO]). The control subjects were ventilated postoperatively for nonpulmonary-related problems; those on ECMO were being treated for primary pulmonary disease. The researchers found that this series of infants with CDH did not have phosphatidylcholine and phosphatidylglycerol concentrations or lethicin:sphingomyelin ratios that were significantly different from those of the control group. However, there was a trend toward decreased values in all three measurements in the CDH group.[65]

Cogo and associates developed a technique to measure surfactant synthesis and turnover in vivo in human neonates with CDH. The results of the study revealed moderately but significantly reduced amounts of surfactant disaturated phosphatidylcholine (DSPC) and SP-A from tracheal aspirates of 14 infants with CDH. However, the rate of endogenous surfactant synthesis was not statistically different between infants with CDH and those with normal lungs. The authors hypothesize that the alteration in surfactant among infants with CDH may be related to enhanced catabolism or perhaps impairment of surfactant secretion.[66]

Despite limited and conflicting evidence, some centers have incorporated surfactant therapy into their treatment protocols for infants with CDH.[67,68] A protocol for a systematic review of surfactant use in CDH has been developed. The objectives of this systematic review will be to determine whether surfactant administration decreases morbidity and mortality and reduces the need for assisted ventilation and ECMO in neonates with CDH. The reviewers will conduct a separate subgroup analysis to evaluate and compare prophylactic and rescue surfactant therapy strategies.[69] In animal studies, it appears that prophylactic delivery-room administration of surfactant is more beneficial than rescue administration.[70] However, prophylactic administration requires antenatal diagnosis of CDH.[71] Lally asserts that until surfactant therapy in infants with CDH has demonstrable efficacy in controlled clinical trials, exogenous surfactant should be used with caution in neonates with CDH.[72]

Chronic Lung Disease and Surfactant Therapy

The etiology of neonatal chronic lung disease (CLD) is multifactorial. Among the factors that contribute to the development of CLD are barotrauma or volutrauma induced by mechanical ventilation, oxygen toxicity, nosocomial infection, increased pulmonary blood flow secondary to patent ductus arteriosus, and inflammation.[73,74] SP-D may have a protective role in these processes. SP-D's activities include promoting clearance of invading pathogens from the airway and down-regulating the pro-inflammatory response to pathogens. SP-D also has antioxidant properties, which may play a role in promoting normal alveolar repair after injury by diminishing chronic inflammation. SP-D may further promote alveolar repair by promoting clearance of apoptotic cells from the airway.[75] Interestingly, infants who develop CLD by day 28 of age have been shown to have significantly lower levels of SP-D on days 2 and 3 of life than those who do not develop CLD.[76] It is now possible to produce biologically active fragments of SP-D that could potentially be used therapeutically. This area of surfactant therapy requires further study to evaluate the potential benefits in neonates at risk for or with CLD.[75]

NITRIC OXIDE AND RELATED VASODILATORS

The discovery by vascular biology researchers that endothelium-derived relaxation factor is NO generated both skepticism and excitement in the scientific community. Hailed as molecule of the year by Science in 1992,[77] NO has become an important therapeutic agent in the

FIGURE 11-3
Endothelium-dependent relaxation: The action of NO.

In response to a hormone or neurotransmitter (e.g., acetylcholine, substance P, histamine, bradykinin, or adenosine triphosphate) and in the presence of NOS, NO is produced from the amino acid L-arginine in the vascular endothelium. Subsequently, NO stimulates sGC to convert GTP to cGMP. Accumulation of cGMP causes relaxation of the vascular smooth muscle, resulting in vascular dilation.

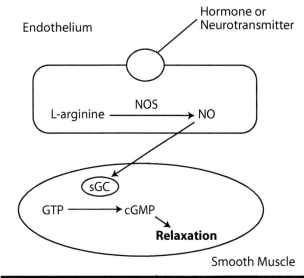

Adapted from: Bell SG. 2004. The story of nitric oxide: From rascally radical to miracle molecule. *Neonatal Network* 23(4): 49. Reprinted by permission.

management of severe respiratory failure in term and near-term neonates. This discussion of NO addresses the use of iNO in term and near-term neonates, reviews the literature on iNO use in other neonatal populations, and explores the use of NO-related vasodilators in neonates with severe respiratory failure.

Severe hypoxic respiratory failure in term and near-term (>34 weeks gestation) neonates has several causes. They include MAS, pneumonia with or without sepsis, RDS, pulmonary hypoplasia associated with CDH or oligohydramnios, and persistent pulmonary hypertension of the newborn (PPHN). All of the diagnoses are frequently associated with reversible increased pulmonary vascular resistance (PVR). Increased PVR leads to right-to-left shunting at the foramen ovale or ductus arteriosus level or both and to ventilation-perfusion mismatching.[78]

Endogenous NO is produced from the amino acid L-arginine in the vascular endothelium under hormonal or neurotransmitter (e.g., acetylcholine, substance P, histamine, bradykinin, or adenosine triphosphate) influence and in the presence of nitric oxide synthase (NOS). Subsequently, NO stimulates soluble guanylate cyclase

TABLE 11-2
PPHN Treatment Modalities before Widespread iNO Therapy

Treatment Modality	Mean Percentage (Percentage range) of Neonates Receiving Treatment
Hyperventilation*	66 (33–92)
Continuous alkali infusion (sodium bicarbonate, tris(hydroxymethyl)aminomethane [tromethamine or THAM])	75 (27–93)
Sedation	94 (77–100)
Paralysis	73 (33–98)
Inotropes (dopamine, dobutamine, isoproterenol, epinephrine, others)	84 (46–100)
Vasodilators (tolazoline, sodium nitroprusside, adenosine, prostaglandin E$_1$, others)	39 (13–81)
Surfactant administration	36 (12–71)
High-frequency ventilation	39 (0–63)
Inhaled nitric oxide[†]	8 (no range given)
Extracorporeal membrane oxygenation[‡]	34 (0–85)

* Hyperventilation = PaCO$_2$ <35 mmHg for >12 hours, maximum peak inspiratory pressure, maximum mean airway pressure; maximum ventilatory rate.

[†] Available at six centers in the study.

[‡] Available at nine centers and by transport from the remaining three units.

Adapted from: Walsh-Sukys MC, et al. 2000. Persistent pulmonary hypertension of the newborn in the era before nitric oxide: Practice variation and outcomes. *Pediatrics* 105(1 part 1): 14–20.

(sGC) to convert guanosine triphosphate (GTP) to cyclic guanosine monophosphate (cGMP). The accumulation of cGMP causes relaxation of the vascular smooth muscle, resulting in vasodilation (Figure 11-3).[79]

Although not solely responsible for the decrease in pulmonary vascular resistance during transition at birth, endogenous NO clearly plays a role.[80–82] Furthermore, research in an animal model has demonstrated that intrauterine events that result in endothelial disruption and NO inhibition may produce the pathophysiology seen in neonates with PPHN.[81] This research provides a link between nitric oxide and PPHN.

In 1992, reports of uncontrolled clinical trials of iNO appeared promising.[83,84] From October 1993 to December 1994, before use of iNO to treat PPHN became widespread, Walsh-Sukys and coworkers prospectively evaluated the variety of therapies used to treat PPHN in 12 NICUs participating in the National Institute of Child Health and Human Development Neonatal Research Network. Table 11-2 identifies the therapies and the percentage of neonates managed with each therapy. Death, use of oxygen at 28 days of age, duration of intubation, and duration of oxygen administration were the primary end points of the study. The researchers found no significant difference in mortality among the centers in the study. Overall mortality was 11 percent (range: 4–33

percent). None of the therapies was clearly associated with a reduction in mortality.[85]

Finer and Barrington completed a systematic review of 12 randomized, controlled studies of iNO in term and near-term neonates.[86–97] The entry criteria for all of the studies were fairly consistent, except for one trial that studied only infants with CDH[95] and one that enrolled both preterm and term neonates.[92] However, most of the results for the term and preterm groups in the latter study were reported separately.[92]

The objectives of Finer and Barrington's review were to determine whether treatment of hypoxemic term and near-term neonates with NO improves oxygenation and reduces the rate of death and the requirement for ECMO. Effects on long-term neurodevelopmental outcome were also reviewed, using information from a follow-up study,[98] to the two 1997 Neonatal Inhaled Nitric Oxide Study Group (NINOS) studies.[94,95] Finer and Barrington have added two additional studies.[99,100] Based on the evidence, including neurodevelopmental and medical outcomes, Finer and Barrington concluded that near-term and term neonates with hypoxic respiratory failure who are unresponsive to other therapy, excluding those with CDH, should have a trial of iNO. It is very effective in reducing the need for ECMO.[101] The authors note that early initiation of iNO does not appear to reduce the need for ECMO or decrease mortality. Starting iNO when OI is

TABLE 11-3
Nitric Oxide for Neonates with Hypoxic Respiratory Failure: Therapeutic Information

Dose

Infants >34 weeks gestation: Initially, 20 ppm.[264] Wean dose as tolerated to maintain PaO_2 within prescribed respiratory care plan. Doses >20 ppm may be effective in a limited number of patients.[94] However, doses >20 ppm increase the risk for methemoglobinemia and elevated nitrogen dioxide (NO_2) levels. NO therapy may be maintained for up to 14 days.[264]

Administration

NO is administered as a gas via inhalation in constant concentration ranges in parts per million throughout the entire respiratory cycle using devices approved by the U.S. FDA.[265]

Cautions and Contraindications

- Echocardiogram is recommended to rule out congenital heart disease.[265] Inhaled NO therapy is contraindicated in neonates who are dependent on right-to-left shunting of blood.[264]

- Inhaled NO therapy should be directed by a physician and administered by staff qualified by education and experience in its use. Centers offering iNO must be able to provide multisystem support, generally including ECMO. If iNO is administered in centers without ECMO capabilities, criteria and mechanisms for timely transfer to an ECMO center should be established. Inhaled NO therapy must continue without interruption during the transfer process.[265]

- Off-label or experimental use of iNO in other neonatal populations requires a formal protocol, with approval by the institutional review board and informed parental consent.[265]

- Administration of 100% oxygen is not possible during iNO therapy because the iNO dilutes the oxygen in the inspiratory circuit.[18]

    Occupational Exposure: Exposure limits for NO and NO_2 are 25 ppm and 5 ppm, respectively.[18]

Adverse Effects

- Hematologic

    - Methemoglobinemia may decrease the oxygen delivery capacity of the red blood cells. The risk for methemoglobinemia rises with increased iNO concentrations. Methemoglobin levels peak between 8 and 40 hours after initiation of therapy. NO concentration should be reduced or therapy discontinued for methemoglobin.[18] Methemoglobinemia that does not respond when iNO therapy is decreased or discontinued can be treated with intravenous methylene blue.[264] If treatment with 2 doses of methylene blue, 1–1.5 mg/kg/dose given 1 hour apart, is unsuccessful in reducing the methemoglobin level, exchange transfusion may be necessary.[18]

    - One mechanism of action of iNO is prevention of platelet clumping, resulting in anticoagulant action.[264] The neonate should be observed for signs of prolonged bleeding.

- Pulmonary: Elevated NO_2 levels may cause acute lung injury. An NO_2 level >3 ppm is an indication to reduce iNO concentration or discontinue therapy.[264]

Pharmacokinetics/Pharmacodynamics

Absorption: Inhaled NO diffuses from the alveoli to pulmonary vascular smooth muscle.[18]

Metabolism and Elimination: Inhaled NO is inactivated by hemoglobin, producing methemoglobin, and is subsequently metabolized to nitrate and nitrite in the urine and plasma. The exact amounts of metabolites produced and the precise steps involved in the metabolism of NO remain unclear.[266]

Weaning

- Weaning from iNO can begin when the patient is clinically stable and the PaO_2 is >50 torr.[94]

- Increasing FiO_2 by 0.1–0.2 is reasonable. (A mean decline in PaO_2 of 19 torr is associated with weaning of iNO.)[267]

- Infants with higher PaO_2 before weaning can be expected to have a greater decline in PaO_2 during weaning than those infants with lower PaO_2.[267]

- Previous treatment with surfactant appears to enhance the oxygenation reserve when weaning from iNO.[267]

- For infants on ≤20 ppm iNO, wean by 50% every 12 hours as tolerated until a dose of 5 ppm is reached.[94]

- Avoid attempting to wean directly from 5 ppm to 0 ppm.[267] Infants can be weaned by 1 ppm at least daily and possibly more frequently if OI is <10.[94]

- Infants who have echocardiographic evidence of pulmonary hypertension may show greater declines in PaO_2 during weaning of iNO.[267]

- A 30 torr decline in PaO_2 has been associated with discontinuing iNO from 1 ppm. Some infants may experience repeated weaning failures. In these cases, iNO should be weaned to ≤0.5 ppm before it is stopped.[267]

Nursing Implications

- Monitor according to institutional protocols. These protocols are designed to prevent toxicity associated with iNO administration.[265]

- Obtain a baseline methemoglobin level before beginning therapy, and every 12–24 hours thereafter. Ideally, levels should be maintained <2.5%.[18] However, if the infant is improving on iNO, perhaps a slightly higher methemoglobin level can be tolerated. Once the level is >2.5 percent, more frequent monitoring should be done.

- Monitor continuous inline iNO, NO_2, and O_2 levels.

Withdrawal of iNO in Nonresponders

- If after a 30-minute trial of iNO there is no response, iNO can be safely withdrawn without a significant increase in OI from baseline.[268]

Adapted from: Bell SG. 2004. The story of nitric oxide: From rascally radical to miracle molecule. *Neonatal Network* 23(4): 48. Reprinted by permission.

>25 or the PaO_2 is <100 mmHg while receiving 1.0 FiO_2 is consistant with the current literature.[95]

ECMO is a therapy of proven value; however, it is invasive, expensive, and associated with important complications (see Chapter 13). Reducing the need for ECMO by using a less invasive and safer therapy does suggest a therapeutic advance.[101] Table 11-3 provides therapeutic information on the use of NO for neonates with hypoxic respiratory failure.

EARLY VERSUS STANDARD iNO THERAPY

Based on clinical trials, the recommended threshold for initiating iNO in neonatal respiratory failure is an OI ≥25.[88,90,94,96] Konduri and and colleagues noted that subgroup analysis in an earlier trial of iNO in neonates with severe respiratory failure suggested greater reductions in both the need for ECMO and the mortality rate among infants who were enrolled at the lowest severity of illness—that is, at an OI of 25–30—than among those whose illness was more severe when treatment was started.[99]

A subsequent study evaluated the hypothesis that early initiation (OI ≥15 and <25) of iNO in neonatal respiratory distress would further reduce both the need for ECMO and mortality compared with standard iNO therapy. The researchers also evaluated the effectiveness of an initial low dose (5 parts per million [ppm]) of iNO in improving oxygenation compared with the standard initial dose of 20 ppm of iNO.[99] Two hundred ninety-nine infants were randomized to early iNO therapy (n = 150) or standard therapy (n = 149). Early iNO therapy did increase oxygenation without increasing short-term iNO toxicity. However, the early improvement in oxygenation did not translate into reductions in the need for ECMO or the mortality rate.[99]

Konduri and associates found that an initial iNO dose of 5 ppm was effective in improving oxygenation at an OI of 15–25. Many of the infants who did not respond at 5 ppm had an increase in PaO_2 of >20 mmHg at a dose of 20 ppm. This indicates that exposure to low-dose iNO does not compromise response to higher doses if they are necessary.[99] This finding is consistent with previously reported findings of dose-dependent response.[102,103]

Of the 299 infants enrolled in the study by Konduri and coworkers, 266 survived to 18 to 24 months (130 in the early iNO group and 136 in the control group. Two hundred thirty-four (121 from the early iNO group and 113 from the control group) were seen for neurodevelopment follow-up. The researchers found that there was no difference between groups in the incidence of neurodevelopmental impairment (27 percent of the early iNO group and 25 percent of the controls) or hearing loss (early iNO 23 percent, control 24 percent). Although the mental development index was similar in the two groups, psychomotor development scores were slightly higher in the control group. Konduri and colleagues concluded that early use of iNO in term and near-term neonates is not associated with increased neurodevelopmental impairment or early hearing loss at 18 to 24 months.[104]

Sadiq and associates also evaluated earlier initiation of iNO in infants with PPHN. Severe PPHN is generally defined as an alveolar-arterial gradient ($AaDO_2$) of >600 torr or an OI >25. The researchers enrolled infants with $AaDO_2$ values between 500 and 599—neonates with moderate PPHN—in a study to assess the effectiveness of iNO in improving their oxygenation and preventing progression to severe PPHN. Forty infants were randomized to the early iNO group and 40 to the control group. Those in the treatment group received iNO beginning at 10 ppm and progressing in steps of 10–20 ppm every 30 minutes until no further improvement in PaO_2 was noted or until a maximum of 80 ppm iNO was reached. In infants who responded, the iNO concentration was titrated to achieve maximum improvement in PaO_2. The iNO concentration was weaned once the FiO_2 had been weaned to 0.3–0.5 or if the methemoglobin level exceeded 5 percent.[105]

Nonresponse was defined as ≤20 percent improvement in $AaDO_2$ or OI. Nonresponders were weaned from iNO over several minutes. Treatment failure was defined as $AaDO_2$ ≥600 torr for more than two hours. Infants in either the treatment group or the control group who met this exit criterion were eligible for other therapies (e.g., ECMO, prostacyclin, iNO) at the discretion of the attending neonatologist. Only 6 of the 40 infants in the iNO group, compared with 27 of the 40 infants in the control group, progressed to severe PPHN. The outcome variables of ECMO and oxygen requirement at 28 days were the same for both groups. Use of iNO rescue in control group infants who went on to develop severe PPHN may account for the lack of difference in these outcome variables. The researchers concluded that treatment of moderate PPHN with iNO improves PaO_2 and prevents progression to severe PPHN. Furthermore, they noted that infants in the iNO group had a significant decrease in the need for ventilatory support, especially in the first 36 hours after initiation of iNO therapy. This trend in decreased support continued for up to 120 hours.[105]

iNO and CDH

As mentioned earlier, iNO did not improve the outcomes of need for ECMO or the mortality rate of infants with CDH.[101] Three studies reported in 2002, 2003, and 2004 provide further evaluation of this CHD population.[106–108] Okuyama and colleagues evaluated outcomes in 30 infants who were treated with iNO and early surgical repair (n = 17) compared with delayed surgical repair (n = 13) during two time periods. From 1988 to 1995 (period 1), delayed surgical repair after a prolonged stabilization period of >48 hours was used to manage infants with CDH. From 1996 to 2000 (period 2), early surgical repair following a brief (up to 48 hours) stabilization period in combination with iNO was used for infants with CDH. During both study periods, high-frequency ventilation was used regardless of clinical status. ECMO was considered for patients with postductal OI >40 for several hours and postductal $AaDO_2$ >610 torr for more than 8 hours. From 1994 on, patients with arterial oxygen saturations of <90 percent received iNO. In study period 1, 31 percent of the infants were treated with iNO; in study period 2, 59 percent received iNO. Only 6 percent of the infants in period 2 required ECMO, compared with 62 percent in period 1. Only 50 percent of the infants studied were treated with iNO. The researchers conclude that use of iNO may have contributed to the more favorable outcome in study period 2. They also note that the use of high-frequency ventilation may have contributed to the improved response to iNO and decreased need for ECMO in study period 2.[106]

Sebald and associates completed a retrospective study of 27 neonates with isolated left-sided CDH sent to their facility for evaluation for ECMO. Fifteen of the infants met ECMO criteria, OI >40 for more than 4 hours despite optimized medical management on iNO, PaO_2 <40 for 2 hours, and/or development of cardiovascular failure unresponsive to aggressive volume and vasopressor/inotropic therapy. The remaining 12 could be managed medically. Clinically relevant variables selected for univariate logistic regression analysis were birth weight <3.3 kg, Apgar <5, transfer age >12 hours, FiO_2 >0.95, pH <7.35, HCO_3 <23 mEq/liter, and air leak. The researchers found that the only variable significantly associated with the need for ECMO was the presence of an air leak. In fact, infants with isolated left-sided CDH who developed pulmonary air leak before admission and who were treated with iNO for 6 hours after admission were 22 times more likely to require ECMO than those who did not experience pulmonary air leak. Ten of the

12 infants (83.3 percent) in the non-ECMO group survived to discharge or transfer back to the referring hospital, compared with 8 of 15 (53.3 percent) in the ECMO group. Based on their findings, the researchers assert the importance of immediate referral to an ECMO center for infants with CDH and hypoxic respiratory failure who develop pulmonary air leak.[107]

The third study evaluated the use of iNO in infants with CDH who developed late pulmonary hypertension (PH). Early iNO was initiated at 20 ppm for infants with CDH who had echocardiographic evidence of extrapulmonary bidirectional or right-to-left shunting or evidence of severe left ventricular dysfunction. The concentration of iNO was reduced to 6 ppm in the first 24 hours of therapy. After 96 hours of therapy, the iNO concentration was decreased to 2–5 ppm. Attempts to withdraw iNO were made during echocardiogram to evaluate for changes in pulmonary artery pressure. Inhaled NO was immediately restarted for any patient who had hypoxemia requiring an increase in FiO_2 to >0.6 and/or a marked elevation of pulmonary hypertension to systemic or suprasystemic levels of pulmonary artery pressure. If the pulmonary arterial pressure remained less than two-thirds of the systemic pressure, iNO was not restarted.[108] Some of the infants who met criteria for extubation, defined as FiO_2 <0.4 and ventilator rate <15 breaths per minute (bpm), still showed evidence of PH when iNO was discontinued. These patients were extubated and placed in an oxygen hood at 40 percent oxygen with NO blended in to provide 5 ppm. After 12–24 hours of treatment with hood O_2 and NO, the delivery system was changed to provide iNO via nasal cannula (NC). The delivery system was configured to mix low-flow NO blended with oxygen at a flow rate of 1 liter/minute to achieve an iNO concentration of 5–10 ppm. Measured nasopharyngeal concentrations of iNO were 2.4 ± 0.4 ppm at 5 ppm and 5.4 ± 0.5 ppm at 10 ppm.[108]

Ten (21 percent) of the infants in the study were successfully treated with NC iNO for late or sustained PH associated with CDH. NC-iNO was discontinued when pulmonary artery pressure was subsystemic as evidenced by echocardiogram during weekly trials off iNO. Median duration of NC-iNO therapy was 17 days (range: 5–60 days). The researchers concluded that iNO can be successfully delivered via nasal cannula to newborns with CDH with prolonged PH. This mode of iNO delivery potentially decreases the duration of mechanical ventilation.[108]

iNO and Ventilation Management

In patients with PPHN complicated by significant parenchymal lung disease, clinical trials and case studies indicate that there is greater improvement in oxygenation if iNO is used in combination with high-frequency ventilation than if either therapy is used independently.[93,109] Because suboptimal lung volume has a negative impact on the efficacy of iNO, high-frequency ventilation is used to recruit and sustain lung volume, allowing the iNO to reach resistant vessels within the lung.[110]

In a review of a single center's five years of experience using iNO and gentle ventilation (GV) to treat neonates with PH of varying etiologies, researchers found that iNO was effective and well tolerated in combination with GV. The principles of GV employed by the authors included low ventilator settings and maintenance of spontaneous respirations to maintain PaO_2 between 50 and 70 mmHg and $PaCO_2$ between 40 and 60 mmHg. If sedation was required, low-dose phenobarbital or, rarely, midazolam (Versed) was used. Paralysis, opiate infusions, and deliberate respiratory or metabolic alkalosis were avoided. The initial iNO dose was 25 ppm. Inhaled NO concentrations were maintained and ventilator settings weaned as oxygenation improved. When the difference between preductal and postductal oxygen saturations was insignificant on FiO_2 >0.6, weaning of iNO by 5 ppm every two to four hours was attempted until a concentration of 5 ppm was reached. If the infant remained stable on 5 ppm, iNO was discontinued and FiO_2 was kept constant. A decrease in oxygen saturation by 10 percent or below 85 percent was considered a weaning failure, and iNO was restarted at 5 ppm. After the infant stabilized, FiO_2 was increased by 0.4, and weaning was again attempted. Once the infant was stable off iNO, FiO_2 was weaned as tolerated.[111]

A total of 229 infants was included in the study. The overall survival rate was 72 percent. Forty-five infants (19.7 percent) failed iNO therapy and required ECMO. The average duration of iNO therapy was 90 ± 166 hours, and the mean number of ventilator days was 9.9 ± 14 days. Infants with MAS or PPHN had the most favorable response to iNO and GV. Infants with CDH or sepsis were more likely to require ECMO than were those with MAS or PPHN.[111]

Neurodevelopmental Outcome after iNO Treatment

Five published studies address neurodevelopmental follow-up for term and near-term infants treated with iNO.[98,112–115] Outcomes in the study by Ellington and coworkers were assessed strictly via telephone interviews and included parental reports of specific conditions (e.g., cerebral palsy [CP], hearing deficit, visual deficits, hyperactivity, mental retardation) and hospital use, along with parental ratings of general health, cognitive and motor development, behavior problems, temperament, and satisfaction with hospital stay.[113] For patients who presented for follow-up in the other four studies, assessment included a history and physical, neurologic examination, and testing using the Bayley Scales of Infant Development when possible.[98,112,114,115] These studies report a number of neurodevelopmental sequelae, including CP, visual and hearing deficits, and developmental delays. Predisposing factors likely include therapies used to treat PPHN, such as respiratory alkalosis and systemic vasodilators. In addition, central nervous system damage may be related to the underlying disease process. Many of the infants treated for PPHN with severe handicaps had significant perinatal or postnatal hypoxic-ischemic events.[112]

Results of all five studies showed that neurodevelopmental outcomes for patients in the iNO groups were similar to those for infants treated conventionally or with ECMO.[98,112–115] Between 77.6 and 90.1 percent of iNO-treated infants showed normal neurologic outcomes.[98,112–115] These overall results are promising. To assess the long-term success of iNO therapy, follow-up of survivors ideally should continue through school age.[112]

iNO and Premature Neonates

Over the years, several studies have shown evidence of PH in premature newborns with RDS.[116–118] In a study by Golan and colleagues, 6 of 24 premature neonates with RDS who did not respond to surfactant therapy were noted to have clinical or echocardiographic evidence of PPHN. The mean gestational age of the infants in this study was 27 ± 2 weeks (range: 25–30 weeks) with a mean birth weight of 1,092 ± 212 g.[118] Lack of response in premature neonates to conventional therapies with hypoxic respiratory failure and the long-term impact of CLD have prompted researchers to assess the efficacy of iNO in this population.

In a systematic review, Barrington and Finer sought to determine if premature neonates <35 weeks gestation with hypoxic respiratory failure benefit from iNO therapy. Outcome criteria included mortality rate, rate of BPD, incidence of IVH, and neurodevelopmental outcome. The review revealed that, as a rescue therapy, iNO does not appear to be effective in premature infants.

Early use of iNO does not affect serious brain injury or improved survival without BPD. However, later use of iNO, between 7 and 21 days of age, may be effective.[119] This conclusion is based in part on the work of Ballard and colleagues, who found that iNO improved pulmonary outcome in premature infants at risk for CLD when iNO is initiated between 7 and 21 days of age. There also was no apparent short-term adverse effects.[120]

One study included in the review did demonstrate a decrease in the number of days of assisted ventilation.[121] At the time of the last substantive addition to the review in November 2005, the reviewers note two studies that presented data on long-term developmental follow-up of premature infants who received iNO therapy.[122,123]

In the study by Mestan and associates, 82 percent of the survivors were evaluated for neurodevelopmental outcome at two years corrected age. Abnormal developmental outcome was defined as disability (CP, bilateral blindness, or bilateral hearing loss) or delay (no disability, but one score of 70 or less on the Bayley Scales of Infant Development II). Twenty-four percent of the children in the iNO group had abnormal developmental outcome, compared to 46 percent of those in the placebo group. A 47 percent decrease in the risk for cognitive impairment was the primary factor in the improved neurodevelopmental outcome in the iNO group.[122]

Field and coworkers looked at neurodevelopmental outcome at one year of age and found no difference between groups. The earlier follow-up and lack of formal testing in this study makes any comparison with the Mestan study difficult.[123] Therefore, no meta-analysis is available.[116] In an earlier study of neurodevelopmental outcome in preterm infants treated with iNO in a controlled clinical trial, 42 infants <32 weeks gestational age were enrolled in the original trial at 96 hours of age if they were at high risk for death or development of CLD.[124] The infants were randomly assigned to one of four treatment groups: (1) 5–20 ppm iNO for 72 hours, (2) 0.5–1 mg/kg/day dexamethasone for six days, (3) both drugs together, (4) continued conventional management. Ten infants received iNO alone, and ten received both iNO and dexamethasone.[125]

Of the 42 infants in the original study, 25 survived until discharge from the hospital. Three of the surviving infants subsequently died of complications related to CLD before study follow-up. At the time of assessment, the infants were 30 months of age, corrected for prematurity. Four out of 7 (57 percent) of the iNO group showed neurodevelopmental delays, compared with 64 percent of the control group. None of those in the iNO group

were assessed as having severe neurodisability or CP. The researchers concluded that there was no evidence of a significant effect on neurodevelopmental outcome in preterm neonates treated with iNO.[124]

There is limited research on the safety and efficacy of iNO in the treatment of neonatal CLD, but as noted earlier, CLD is associated with PH.[126] One study evaluated whether iNO improved oxygenation without adverse effects in VLBW infants with developing CLD.[127] Thirty-three infants with a mean birth weight of 736 g (range: 509–1,250 g), mean gestational age of 25.3 weeks, and mean age of 19 days were enrolled in the study. The infants initially received 20 ppm iNO. After 3 hours, researchers decided whether to continue iNO therapy based on evidence of efficacy (a decrease in FiO_2 ≥0.10, an increase in oxygen saturation ≥10 percent, or transcutaneous partial pressure of oxygen improved by 1.3 kilopascals. If there was evidence of improvement, iNO was continued at 20 ppm. After 36 hours, iNO was decreased to 15 ppm, followed by a decrease of 2–3 ppm every 12 hours to a dose of 2 ppm as tolerated, based on no worsening of oxygenation. Treatment was discontinued after seven days provided there was no evidence of dependency. If an infant showed signs of iNO dependency, iNO therapy was continued, with attempts to discontinue it every 24–48 hours.[127]

Neonatal CLD is defined as the continuing need for supplemental oxygen at 36 weeks postconceptional age (PCA). All 33 infants showed improvement during the initial 3-hour trial. After 48 hours, 2 infants showed no further decrease in FiO_2, and iNO was discontinued. The remaining 31 infants continued on iNO and showed improvement at 3 hours and at 72 hours. Four of the 33 infants enrolled in the study died before discharge from the hospital. Of the remaining 29 infants, 1 remained on mechanical ventilation, 2 were on CPAP, and 22 were on supplemental oxygen via NC at 36 weeks PCA. At 44 weeks PCA, 3 of the infants remained hospitalized, 2 were on supplemental oxygen via NC, and 1 was breathing room air. Of 26 infants who had been discharged, 9 were breathing room air, and 17 continued on supplemental oxygen at home. When the infants reached six months of age, 25 charts were available for review. Ten infants continued on supplemental oxygen by NC, and 15 were on room air. The researchers concluded that their results did not provide sufficient support for widespread use of iNO in premature infants with evidence of developing CLD.[127]

In 2011, the conclusions of the National Institutes of Health Development Conference on iNO therapy in premature infants were published in *Pediatrics*. The panel concluded that: (1) The available evidence does not support the use of iNO as early-routine, early-rescue, or late-rescue for premature infants <34 weeks gestational age. (2) There are rare clinical situations, such as pulmonary hypertension, in which iNO may benefit the premature infant of <34 weeks gestation. These situations have not been adequately studied and therefore the clinician should discuss the potential risks, benefits, and uncertainties of iNO therapy with the family. (3) Future research should focus on the the gap between lung development and function in infants at risk for CLD. (4) Previous research showing potential benefit of iNO has generated hypotheses. Unless new evidence emerges, strategies that have been shown to be ineffective are discouraged. Research should focus on timing of initiation of therapy, dose, and duration of therapy, ideally randomizing these elements separately. (5) Based on currently available evidence, hospitals, clinicians, and the pharmaceutical industry should not market iNO for premature infants of <34 weeks gestational age.[128]

OTHER PULMONARY VASODILATORS

Inhaled NO has become the gold standard for treating near-term and term infants with severe hypoxic respiratory failure. Currently, iNO is the only drug approved specifically for treating hypoxic respiratory failure in this population. However, because of the technology required for iNO administration, the importance of immediate access to an ECMO center should the patient fail to respond to iNO, and the cost (approximately $3,000 per day in the U.S.), iNO is not universally available.[129] Some infants do not respond to iNO and go on to require ECMO. Others respond to iNO, but experience rebound hypoxemia and pulmonary hypertension when weaning of iNO is begun. Thus, the search for other selective pulmonary vasodilators continues. L-arginine, nitroprusside, adenosine, and phosphodiesterase inhibitors are NO-related medications that have been described in the literature as potential therapeutic agents for PPHN.[130–135] Prostacyclin, which plays a role in normal transition following delivery, is another option discussed in the literature.[135–138]

L-arginine

Recall from Figure 11-3 (p. 247) that the amino acid L-arginine is a precursor for NO. Additionally, research has shown that infants with PPHN have low plasma concentrations of both arginine and NO metabolites. The concurrent low presence of precursors of NO and

NO breakdown products suggests that inadequate production of NO plays a significant role in the pathogenesis of PPHN.[139] Provision of exogenous arginine would be expected to increase endogenous NO production. Clinically, this increase in NO production would be manifested as a rise in PaO_2 and a reduction in the OI.

In a case report of five neonates with PPHN, a one-time infusion of 500 mg/kg of L-arginine over 30 minutes resulted in a mean increase in PaO_2 from 37 mmHg to 84 mmHg 90 minutes after the infusion in four of the five infants. Over the five hours following the infusion, a 33–50 percent reduction in OI was also noted. No adverse effects were observed.[130]

In a more recent case study, a neonate with PPHN who responded positively to treatment with high-frequency ventilation and iNO failed three attempts to discontinue iNO therapy. The infant was noted to have severe desaturation related to right-to-left extrapulmonary shunting through the ductus arteriosus and foramen ovale. Dipyridamole (a phosphodiesterase inhibitor, see discussion later in this section) alone was ineffective in achieving successful discontinuation of iNO. However, a combination of dipyridamole and L-arginine allowed iNO to be discontinued successfully.[131]

Increased PVR is associated with pulmonary endothelial dysfunction following cardiovascular surgery. Ten infants with a mean age of 0.62 year (no neonates) had elevated PVR following surgery for repair of a ventricular septal defect or atrial septal defect. As a condition of the study protocol, these infants received an L-arginine infusion at 15 mg/kg/minute for 35 minutes, beginning 25 minutes into the protocol and ending at the conclusion of the protocol (60 minutes). The L-arginine infusion resulted in a significant fall of the PVR index ($PVRI = PVR \times m^2$). There were no negative effects on mean arterial pressure. These infants also received Substance P at 1 picomole (pmol)/kg/minute for 20 minutes, beginning 40 minutes into the study protocol. An immediate, transient fall in systemic blood pressure was noted with the Substance P infusion. Systemic blood pressure reached steady state in 2–3 minutes, and none of the infants required an increase in blood pressure support. A further significant fall in PVRI was noted. Finally, the infants received 20 ppm of iNO for the final 10 minutes of the protocol. There was no further significant decline in PVRI with the addition of iNO. The researchers concluded that endogenous NO release (which is maximally stimulated by intravenous administration of L-arginine and Substance P) reversed postoperative elevations in PVR. Inhaled NO produced little additional effect.[140]

Sodium Nitroprusside

Sodium nitroprusside (SNP) is an antihypertensive agent and an NO donor that reduces preload via venous dilation and decreased venous return to the heart. This decreases left ventricular end-diastolic pressure and afterload via arteriolar relaxation, resulting in reductions in systemic vascular resistance, systolic arterial pressure, and mean arterial pressure.[18] The action of nitrovasodilators such as SNP is the result of their ability to release NO.[141] Sodium nitroprusside is a direct NO donor—that is, at physiologic pH, NO is released directly from the parent compound.[142]

Continuous intravenous administration of SNP causes nonselective vasodilation, with the potential for systemic hypotension.[132] Research has shown that nebulized SNP produces prompt, significant, selective reduction of pulmonary artery pressure (PAP) in a porcine model of pulmonary hypertension.[143] In a later study comparing iNO and nebulized SNP in the porcine model, researchers found an equivalent response with the two drugs: Both caused a rapid, significant, selective reduction of PAP.[132]

Palhares and colleagues assessed the effectiveness of inhaled SNP in ten neonates with severe hypoxemia. They observed increases in PaO_2, SaO_2, and the PaO_2:FiO_2 ratio at one hour and at six to eight hours of treatment. Significant changes in systemic blood pressure were not observed. There was no evidence of cyanide toxicity or methemoglobinemia in any of the neonates.[144]

Mestan and associates evaluated the effect of nebulized SNP in 22 term neonates with hypoxic respiratory failure. On entry into the study, infants received 5 mg aqueous SNP dissolved in 2 mL of 0.9 percent sodium chloride and nebulized into the inspiratory arm of the ventilator circuit at a flow rate of 2 liters/minute over a period of 20 minutes. This was followed by a 25 mg dose of SNP administered in the same manner. Ventilator settings remained constant during nebulized SNP treatment, and changes in other medical interventions were not allowed. Following the nebulized SNP, all of the infants were started on iNO at 20–40 ppm. Pre- and postductal oxygen saturations, systemic arterial blood pressure, and heart rate were monitored continuously and recorded at 5-minute intervals before and during each 20-minute period of nebulized SNP treatment. Arterial blood gas values and methemoglobin levels were obtained before treatment and after each 20-minute treatment period.[122]

Fourteen of the 22 infants had a positive response, defined as a >20 percent increase in PaO_2, to the nebulized SNP. Mean PaO_2 increased from a baseline of 64.6 ± 5.6 mmHg to 90.1 ± 15.3 mmHg with the 5 mg dose and to 113.2 ± 20.4 mmHg with the 25 mg dose. Neither mean systemic arterial pressure nor heart rate significantly changed during the treatments. The mean percentage change in OI with nebulized SNP was identical to that seen with iNO.[122]

The researchers assert that administration of nebulized SNP results in significant and dose-dependent improvement in oxygenation in term neonates with clinical or echocardiographic evidence of PPHN. The duration of treatment in this study was brief, however; further investigation is needed to determine the potential for toxicity with sustained doses. The researchers conclude that nebulized SNP may be beneficial in treating infants with hypoxic respiratory failure when iNO is not readily available. However, large randomized, placebo-controlled trials are needed to determine the true benefit of nebulized SNP in the treatment of hypoxic respiratory failure in neonates.[122]

Adenosine

Neonatal nurses are familiar with adenosine for the treatment of supraventricular tachycardia. Adenosine is a short-acting purine nucleoside that potentially slows conduction through the atrioventricular node and suppresses automaticity of both atrial and Purkinje tissues.[145] Because of its vasoactive properties and short half-life (approximately ten seconds), adenosine also has potential as a selective pulmonary vasodilator.[146] The action of endogenous adenosine in the pulmonary vasculature is mediated through A_2 receptors located in the vascular smooth muscle and is partially dependent on endothelium-derived NO.[147,148] Three studies in the neonatal population have evaluated the effectiveness of adenosine infusion for the management of PPHN.[133,149,150]

Konduri and coworkers studied the effect of continuous intravenous infusion of adenosine 25–50 mcg/kg/minute versus a placebo infusion of 0.9 percent sodium chloride on oxygenation, ventilator support, blood pressure, and heart rate in 18 infants with PPHN. Nine infants were randomized into each group. A positive response to the adenosine infusion was defined as an increase of ≥20 torr in the postductal PaO_2. Secondary outcomes for the study were IVH, BPD, need for ECMO, and death. The adenosine infusion was started at 25 mcg/kg/minute. If there was no response at that dose after 30 minutes, the infusion was increased to

50 mcg/kg/minute. If the increased dose did not produce a response after 30 minutes, the study was terminated, and the infant was provided with standard care for PPHN, including ECMO if criteria were met. A drop in PaO_2 below 60 torr was also a condition for halting the study. If the infant showed a positive response to adenosine, the infusion was continued for a maximum of 24 hours. The 24-hour limit was imposed in this study because of concern over the potential for prolonged bleeding time and bradycardia. Postductal arterial blood gases, blood pressure, heart rate, and ventilator settings were noted just before the start of the infusion, 30 minutes after the infusion was started, and 30 minutes after the infusion increase if it was required. All of the infants were managed on conventional ventilation while in the study.[133]

None of the infants in the control group had a response to the placebo. Four of the nine infants in the adenosine group showed a significant improvement in PaO_2 at an infusion rate of 50 mcg/kg/minute. All four of those infants had MAS complicated by PPHN. Two of the four infants who demonstrated a positive response required ECMO for poor oxygenation after the infusion was stopped. There were no adverse effects on heart rate or blood pressure.[133]

Adenosine infusion caused short-term improvement in oxygenation in infants with severe respiratory failure compared with a placebo. Konduri and colleagues offer several explanations for the lack of response in the remaining five infants in the adenosine group: (1) The presence of a large right-to-left shunt made delivery of adenosine to the pulmonary circulation difficult. (2) There was a ventilation/profusion mismatch. (3) The patient was unable to release NO in response to adenosine stimulation, related to endothelial cell dysfunction and limited ability to synthesize NO. Adenosine infusion did not decrease ventilator requirements or the need for ECMO. There were no differences in the incidence of BPD and mortality between the two groups. Two infants in the control group had Grade I IVH, compared with none in the adenosine group. Further studies are needed to determine the optimum effective dose of adenosine for infants with PPHN. Additionally, large clinical trials are required to determine the impact of adenosine on mortality and on the need for ECMO.[133]

Patole and associates studied the effect of adenosine infusion in six infants—three term, three preterm—with PPHN following failure of conventional therapy including iNO. Gestational age of the infants in this case report was 26–42 weeks. Birth weight ranged from 805 to 3,870 g.

Infants received 0.03 mg/kg/minute, 0.06 mg/kg/minute, and a maximum of 0.09 mg/kg/minute adenosine infusion via a right arterial catheter. A positive response was defined is an increase in PaO_2 of >20 mmHg. If no response was observed at a starting dose of 0.03 mg/kg/minute, the infusion was stopped for 20 minutes and then resumed at a higher dose of 0.06 mg/kg/minute. If no response was observed at this rate, the infusion was stopped again for 20 minutes and then resumed at a maximum dose of 0.09 mg/kg/minute. The authors do not identify the time frame for a positive response at each infusion rate. Three of the infants survived; three died. Of those who died, support for one preterm infant was withdrawn because of diagnoses of arthrogyposis and lung hypoplasia. The other two infants, a preterm infant who died from renal failure and a term newborn with MAS who died as the result of a pulmonary hemorrhage followed by bleeding from multiple sites (suggestive of disseminated intravascular coagulation), showed persistent improvement in oxygenation until their deaths. The three infants who survived had a positive response to adenosine at an infusion rate of 0.03 mg/kg/minute. The authors assert that adenosine may be an important option for the treatment of PPHN.[149]

In a later study, Ng and coworkers looked at the effects of concurrent administration of iNO and adenosine in nine neonates with PPHN. The infants were all term, with a mean birth weight of 3,600 g. They were receiving 15–25 ppm iNO and dopamine at 5–15 mcg/kg/minute and yet remained hypoxic, with echocardiographic evidence of increased pulmonary artery pressure. All infants were on high-frequency ventilation. Adenosine was infused via a central vein at 50 mcg/kg/minute. In an attempt to further improve oxygenation in one neonate, the researchers increased the infusion rate to 80 mcg/kg/minute for five minutes. Mild systemic hypotension was noted at the increased infusion rate; it resolved when the infusion was decreased to 50 mcg/kg/minute. Oxygenation index, PaO_2, systemic mean arterial blood pressure, estimated PAP by echocardiography, and SpO_2 were monitored, and pulmonary-to-systemic arterial pressure ratios were calculated.[150]

Six infants who had minimal improvement in oxygenation in response to 3–23 hours of iNO therapy responded positively to adenosine infusion. Inhaled NO was discontinued in these infants between 0.5 and 8 hours of initiation of adenosine. These six infants showed a significant increase in PaO_2, fall in PAP, and fall in pulmonary-to-systemic arterial pressure ratios. The remaining three infants, with diagnoses of CDH, capillary alveolar dysplasia, and MAS, did not show significant improvement in oxygenation, PAP, or other variables. Two of the infants with MAS, one responder and one nonresponder, received ECMO. The majority of infants had an increase in systemic mean blood pressure associated with improved blood flow through the pulmonary vasculature. There were no episodes of bradycardia.[150]

Ng and colleagues assert that adenosine may be a viable alternative to iNO in situations where iNO therapy may not be practical. Such situations might include transport, stabilization in smaller NICUs where iNO therapy is not available, and developing countries. Further study is needed to determine the impact of concurrent adenosine and iNO administration on the need for ECMO and on mortality.[150]

Phosphodiesterases and Phosphodiesterase Inhibitors

Phosphodiesterases (PDEs) are enzymes responsible for controlling the intracellular levels of the cyclic neucleotides guanosine monophosphate and adenosine monophosphate (cAMP) by degradation.[151] It follows that degradation—and thus lower intracellular levels of cGMP and cAMP—would impact pulmonary vascular dilation. Pharmacologic regulation of these pathways with PDE inhibitors has been the focus of research in a variety of populations, including neonates. The PDE5 family has been implicated in the control of pulmonary vascular resistance.[152] Drugs that inhibit the action of PDE5 are of interest in the treatment of PPHN. Four PDE inhibitors—dipyridamole, sildenafil, pentoxifylline, and zaprinast—are described here.

Researchers evaluated the pulmonary and systemic effects of the specific PDE5 inhibitor dipyridamole in an animal model of persistent pulmonary hypertension. There were three experimental conditions in that study: (1) iNO alone for 15 minutes following 30 minutes of observation, (2) a 45-minute dipyridamole infusion alone, and (3) a 45-minute dipyridamole infusion with the addition of iNO for the final 15 minutes. Inhaled NO at a concentration of 5 ppm significantly decreased PAP, increased pulmonary blood flow, and decreased PVR. There was no change in aortic pressure. The 45-minute dipyridamole infusion at 0.02 mg/kg/minute resulted in a significant decrease in PAP, PVR, and aortic pressure measured at 30 minutes and 45 minutes. There was a significant increase in pulmonary blood flow at 20 minutes and 45 minutes as well. In the third group, the 30-minute infusion of dipyridamole alone increased

pulmonary blood flow and decreased PVR and aortic pressure. There was a trend toward decreased PAP, but it was not statistically significant. The addition of iNO for the final 15 minutes significantly increased pulmonary blood flow and significantly decreased PAP and PVR. There was no further decrease in aortic pressure with the addition of iNO. The changes in pulmonary hemodynamics observed during the 15-minute combined iNO and dipyridamole therapy were not significantly greater than those observed with iNO therapy alone. The observed decreases in aortic pressure in both groups receiving dipyridamole translated into significant systemic hypotension. The researchers concluded that the clinical application of dipyridamole, alone or in combination with iNO, will be limited by its effect on systemic arterial pressure.[153]

In another animal model of pulmonary hypertension, researchers showed that low-dose dipyridamole, 10 mcg/kg/minute, reduced mean PAP and PVR. There was also a significant reduction in systemic vascular resistance (SVR), but the concomitant decrease in mean arterial pressure was reported to be clinically acceptable. The combination of iNO and dipyridamole was more effective in decreasing PVR than was iNO alone, but it did not have a significant effect on mean PAP.[154]

Dipyridamole appears to attenuate rebound pulmonary hypertension on discontinuation of iNO. Intravenous dipyridamole increases serum cGMP concentrations. The researchers hypothesized that the serum cGMP levels reflect, at least to some degree, the cGMP levels in the pulmonary vascular smooth muscle and therefore may protect against rebound pulmonary hypertension. They concluded that low-dose intravenous dipyridamole enhances the effects of iNO with moderate but clinically acceptable changes in systemic hemodynamics and can prevent rebound pulmonary hypertension when iNO is discontinued.[154]

There are several case reports of dipyridamole use in neonates, three of which involve its use in neonates with CDH.[155–157] Kinsella and associates assert that response to iNO may be limited by an inability to sustain adequate levels of cGMP in the vascular smooth muscle. They examined the clinical effects of dipyridamole on the response to iNO in an infant with CDH requiring ECMO. The infant had developed bleeding complications, and iNO was initiated to expedite decannulation. Inhaled NO was effective in decreasing PAP, but PVR and right-to-left shunting via the ductus arteriosus persisted. The addition of 0.6 mg/kg dipyridamole enhanced the effects of the iNO, ductal shunting was reversed to left-to-right, and the infant was weaned from ECMO.[155]

Thebaud and coworkers report transient enhancement of iNO with dipyridamole in two infants with CDH who ultimately died. The researchers comment that dipyridamole was employed as a rescue therapy in response to secondary deterioration. Whether earlier initiation of dipyridamole would have resulted in improved oxygenation for a longer period of time is open to supposition.[156]

Dipyridamole has also been used to successfully wean a term neonate with CDH from iNO. Initially treated with high-frequency ventilation and iNO, the infant required ECMO on day 3 of life. ECMO was discontinued after two days because of clots in the circuit. The infant tolerated removal from ECMO well. Surgical repair of the CDH was performed on day 7 of life. Following surgery, iNO was reinstituted at 20 ppm for exacerbation of PH. Over a three-week period, ventilator settings and iNO had been weaned. However, once the infant was on 2 ppm iNO, several daily attempts to wean from 2 ppm to 0 ppm were unsuccessful. After eight attempts, a dose of dipyridamole 0.4 mg/kg/minute was given over 10 minutes and repeated every 12 hours for a total of three doses. After the second dose, the infant was successfully weaned from iNO. There was a transient decrease in systemic blood pressure in the 30 minutes following infusion of the first dose of dipyridamole, but systemic blood pressure remained unchanged with the subsequent two doses.[157]

Sildenafil, a specific PDE5 inhibitor, has perhaps generated the most interest as a therapy for PPHN. To date, there is only one published randomized clinical trial of sildenafil in infants.[158] Following cardiovascular surgery for the repair of ventricular septal defect or atrial septal defect with a large amount of left–to-right shunting, 15 infants were entered in the clinical study. They were randomized to receive 20 ppm iNO with the addition at 20 minutes of intravenous sildenafil 0.35 mg/kg infused over 20 minutes or intravenous sildenafil 0.35 mg/kg with the addition of 20 ppm iNO at 20 minutes. None of the infants in the study was a neonate. Average age in the iNO-first group was 139 days; the average in the sildenafil-first group was 123 days. By 20 minutes, infants in the iNO-first group had a 7.8 ± 2.1 percent reduction in PAP. Mean systemic arterial pressure (SAP), left atrial pressure (LAP), central venous pressure (CVP), and cardiac index remained unchanged. The PVRI fell by 17 ± 5 percent. The SVR index (SVRI) was unchanged. The addition of sildenafil did not have any further influence on PAP. However, SAP fell by 13.4 ± 2.7 percent.

LAP, CVP, and cardiac index remained unchanged. Sildenafil produced an additional 16 ± 5.2 percent drop in PVRI; however, SVRI was reduced significantly, by 22 ± 5.4 percent. There was an initial improvement in oxygenation along with a significant decline in OI and $AaDO_2$. The addition of sildenafil reduced PaO_2 and increased both the OI and the $AaDO_2$.[158]

In the sildenafil-first group, PAP showed a tendency to fall by 10.4 ± 4.1 percent, along with a 17 ± 1.8 percent reduction in SAP. The addition of iNO resulted in a further reduction in PAP below baseline (preoperative). There was a 12.8 ± 5.7 percent decline in PVRI and a 23 ± 2.1 percent drop in SVRI. The addition of iNO resulted in a further reduction of PVRI by 7.8 ± 2 percent without any effect on the SVRI. Sildenafil decreased PaO_2 and increased the OI and $AaDO_2$. Administration of iNO did not result in any changes in these variables.[158]

The four main findings described by Stocker and colleagues were that intravenous sildenafil (1) reduces PVR, (2) enhances the vasodilator effects of iNO, (3) results in a significant decrease in systemic blood pressure with systemic vasodilation, and (4) causes a deterioration in oxygenation that does not respond to iNO therapy. The study was halted early because of the last two findings. The researchers felt that the side effects of sildenafil outweighed any potential benefit in this group of infants.[158]

Azt and Wessel provide three case reports, one of a neonate, in which oral sildenafil was used to ameliorate the effects of iNO withdrawal. The first infant was a six-week-old who underwent surgical resection of an obstructive membrane within the left atrium. Postoperative management included a trial of iNO at 20 ppm that selectively reduced mean PAP from 57 mmHg to 33 mmHg. Inhaled NO increased plasma cGMP from 12 pmol/mL at baseline to 28 pmol/mL. After three unsuccessful attempts at weaning the iNO, a 1 mg dose of oral sildenafil was given via a nasogastric tube. Ninety minutes after sildenafil administration, the infant was successfully weaned from the iNO.[159]

A term newborn underwent surgical correction of total anomalous pulmonary venous return (TAPVR) on day 1 of life. Inhaled NO at 20 ppm was used to manage postoperative PH. On postoperative day 3, an attempt at withdrawal of iNO failed. Inhaled NO therapy was reinstituted at 20 ppm, and sildenafil 1 mg was given via a nasogastric tube. Before NO was withdrawn, cGMP levels were 19 pmol/mL; one hour after iNO was restarted at 20 ppm and sildenafil was administered, the cGMP level was 30 pmol/mL. Seventy minutes after the sildenafil dose, the infant was successfully weaned from iNO.[159]

The third infant was a four-month-old who underwent surgical repair of pulmonary vein stenosis after neonatal repair of TAPVR. Inhaled NO at 80 ppm resulted in a modest decrease in PAP from 27 mmHg to 19 mmHg. Levels of cGMP increased from 27 pmol/mL at baseline to 135 pmol/mL on iNO therapy. After three failed attempts at withdrawal of iNO, sildenafil 1.1 mg was given via nasogastric tube. Seventy minutes after sildenafil administration, iNO was withdrawn. There was an immediate increase in PAP, requiring reinstitution of iNO. There was a minimum increase in cGMP levels following sildenafil administration in this infant, who was known to have problems with gastrointestinal absorption.[159] This third case study illustrates an important aspect of medication administration in sick neonates and infants. Although this infant's absorption problem was apparently an ongoing issue, critically ill infants may have questionable gastrointestinal absorption and may be at increased risk for ischemic insult to the gut.[160]

Sildenafil appeared more promising in two animal models of neonatal pulmonary hypertension. In an animal model of hypoxic PH, researchers sought to determine whether nebulized sildenafil with or without iNO would produce selective pulmonary vasodilation. The major findings of this study were that nebulized sildenafil (1) produced selective pulmonary vasodilation without systemic vasodilation, (2) potentiated the pulmonary vasodilating effects of iNO, and (3) did not increase the venous admixture via intrapulmonary right-to-left shunting.[160,161]

In an animal model of neonatal pulmonary hypertension related to MAS, researchers evaluated the effects of intravenous sildenafil on pulmonary hemodynamics and oxygenation and compared the effects with those of iNO. The control group received only mechanical ventilation, the NO group received iNO at 20 ppm, and the sildenafil group received 2 mg/kg over two hours. The intravenous sildenafil completely reversed the changes in pulmonary vascular resistance in this model of MAS. Sildenafil lowered mean aortic pressure by 5 ± 11 percent, but this was not statistically significant. SVR was unchanged. Sildenafil produced changes in pulmonary hemodynamics comparable to those observed with iNO therapy. Neither sildenafil nor iNO had a significant effect on oxygenation.[160]

Based on these animal studies, it appears that sildenafil may be useful as an adjunct to iNO therapy. The case studies illustrate sildenafil's potential for preventing rebound hypertension after iNO withdrawal. The side effects reported by Stocker and associates are concerning, however.[158] In addition, there is a case report in the literature of severe ROP in a preterm neonate treated with sildenafil for PH.[162] Pharmacokinetic studies are needed to determine optimal dosing, and further clinical studies, to determine efficacy and safety as well as optimal mode of administration to maximize benefits and minimize potential side effects.

There are two case reports of use of the nonspecific PDE inhibitor pentoxifylline (PTXF) for neonatal respiratory illness: one in a premature infant with PPHN and the other in infants with BPD.[163,164] Pentoxifylline is a methylxanthine derivative with bronchodilator, diuretic, and respiratory muscle stimulant effects.[164]

Lauterbach reported the use of intravenous PTXF infusion in an infant born at 34 weeks gestational age with radiographic evidence of pneumonia and confirmation of PPHN by echocardiography. After three hours of age, PTXF infusion was begun at an unspecified dose for six hours. The infant received identical doses on two subsequent days. There was significant improvement in oxygenation and ventilation, allowing for reduction in FiO_2 and ventilator rate. Lauterbach suggests that the influence of PTXF on PPHN can be attributed to its action on the pulmonary vasculature via stimulation of endogenous NO.[163]

Lauterbach and Szymura-Oleksiak reported the use of nebulized PTXF in five spontaneously breathing infants who developed BPD despite treatment with surfactant, corticosteroids, and furosemide. The infants received nebulized PTXF 10 mg/kg/dose four times a day (every six hours) for six consecutive days. During the first three days of therapy, the researchers identified a tendency toward a decreased oxygen requirement; the oxygen requirement was significantly reduced by day 6 of PTXF therapy. One infant had continuing oxygen needs, but the requirement had decreased from 70 percent to 25 percent. Within the subsequent five days, this infant no longer required supplemental oxygen. None of the infants had further need for supplemental oxygen.[164]

Zaprinast is an experimental, specific PDE5 inhibitor that has not been approved for clinical use.[134] Researchers have come to the following conclusion based on their studies in animal models. In a lamb model of pulmonary hypertension, the animals received iNO at 5 ppm, 10 ppm, and 20 ppm followed by a continuous intravenous infusion of zaprinast at 0.1 mg/kg/minute. The lambs had a dose-dependent reduction in mean PAP in response to the iNO; the greatest response was at a dose of 20 ppm. Zaprinast did not change the magnitude of mean PAP reduction, but it did cause a statistically significant reduction in PVR. Zaprinast also prolonged the duration of action of the iNO at all three concentrations. For example, at 20 ppm iNO alone, the half-time of vasodilator response was 2.1 ± 0.2 minutes; with the addition of the zaprinast infusion, the half-time of vasodilator response was 12.3 ± 2 minutes. Zaprinast did not cause systemic vascular dilation. It potentiated and prolonged the action of iNO without changing its pulmonary vascular selectivity in this animal model of PH.[165]

Thusu and coworkers found that the combination of iNO at 6 ppm and a continuous zaprinast infusion at 0.05 mg/kg/minute was more effective in reducing PAP than was either drug alone. Additionally, the combined therapy did not have a negative effect on systemic blood pressure. The researchers concluded that zaprinast significantly enhances the effect of iNO in newborn lambs with persistent pulmonary hypertension. They further speculated that PDE inhibition may increase the response rate to iNO or may possibly permit use of lower concentrations of iNO.[166]

In a model of sepsis-induced PH, Steinhorn and colleagues had similar results using a 0.25 mg/kg bolus dose of zaprinast followed by continuous infusion over 20 minutes to provide a total dose of 1.3 ± 0.07 mg/kg and concomitant administration of iNO at a concentration of 45 ppm. Zaprinast was noted to have no effect when administered alone, but it did enhance pulmonary vasodilation in response to iNO. The researchers concluded that pharmacologic inhibition of PDE5 may be a useful adjuvant to iNO in the treatment of PPHN.[167]

In a rat model of hypoxic PH, both iNO alone at 20 ppm and zaprinast alone at 0.3 mg/kg/minute decreased the pulmonary hypertensive response to hypoxia. The combination of iNO and zaprinast totally eliminated the hypertensive response. The researchers caution against extrapolating their results to human subjects.[168]

Finally, in a lamb model of acute PH, Ichinose and associates evaluated the effect of iNO alone at 5 ppm and 20 ppm; nebulized zaprinast generated from solutions of 10 mg/mL, 20 mg/mL, 30 mg/mL, and 50 mg/mL; and two combinations of iNO and zaprinast: the first of 5 ppm iNO and zaprinast 10 mg/mL nebulized solution; the second of 20 ppm iNO and zaprinast 10 mg/mL nebulized solution. Both doses of iNO alone resulted in prompt pulmonary vasodilation without any effect on mean SAP or SVR. Nebulized zaprinast solutions of 20 mg/mL and 30 mg/mL produced selective reductions in PAP and PVR without decreasing SAP or SVR.

However, in addition to further decreases in PAP and PVR, the 50 mg/mL zaprinast solution also caused a significant decrease in SAP. The duration of action of zaprinast was significantly longer than that of iNO. The combination of iNO, at either concentration, and zaprinast 10 mg/mL nebulized solution reduced PAP and PVR more than did either agent alone. The duration of action of the combined agents was longer than that of iNO alone. The researchers concluded that the use of a cGMP-selective phosphodiesterase inhibitor alone or in combination with iNO may be a useful noninvasive therapy for acute PH.[169]

Prostacyclin

Prostaglandin I_2 (PGI_2), or prostacyclin, is an endogenous vasodilator synthesized in the vascular endothelium in three steps: (1) Arachidonic acid is mobilized from the endothelial-cell-membrane phospholipids as a result of the activation of the enzyme phospholipase A_2. (2) Cyclooxygenase catalyzes the conversion of arachidonic acid to prostaglandin H_2 (PGH_2). (3) PGI_2 synthase isomerizes PGH_2 to PGI_2.[170] PGI_2-induced elevation in cAMP causes vascular relaxation.[171] PGI_2 plays an important role in the transition of the pulmonary circulation at birth. Inhibition of prostaglandin synthesis dramatically attenuates the normal decline in PVR.[172] In the postnatal period, a function of PGI_2 is lessening pulmonary vasoconstriction in response to hypoxia.[170] However, alterations in PGI_2 synthesis may be implicated in the pathogenesis of neonatal PH.[173]

PGI_2 is now the primary therapy for PH, except PPHN. It can be delivered by a variety of routes including intravenously (epoprostenol [Flolan] GlaxoSmithKline, Brentford, Middlesex, UK), subcutaneously (treprostinil sodium [Remodulin—previously UT-15 or Uniprost, United Therapeutics Corp., Silver Spring, Maryland), aerosolized (iloprost, [Ventavis] CoTherix, South San Francisco), and orally (beraprost, United Therapeutics). There is evidence of intravenous prostacyclin's efficacy in patients of all ages with primary PH and in patients with PH related to congenital heart disease.

There are several disadvantages to epoprostenol therapy. Epoprostenol has a half-life of only three to five minutes, necessitating a continuous intravenous infusion. The infusion must be remixed daily in an alkali buffer. Tolerance to epoprostenol results in a need to escalate the dose to maintain therapeutic response. Rapid withdrawal can result in fatal pulmonary hypertension.[174] In addition, because intravenous prostacyclin is not a specific pulmonary vasodilator, significant systemic hypotension may occur during intravenous administration. Management with the more stable analogs Remodulin, iloprost, and beraprost is more attractive in the pediatric population.[174] Discussion of PGI_2 administration for PPHN in the literature has focused on the use of the aerosolized or endotracheal PGI_2.[137,175,176] Suzuki and coworkers reported on the use of oral beraprost sodium in a six-month-old infant and a four-month-old infant both with congenital heart disease.[177] Four neonates with PPHN, three with MAS, and one with a postmortem diagnosis of alveolar capillary dysplasia (ACD) who did not respond to iNO received aerosolized intravenous prostaglandin. The intravenous form was dissolved in 20 mL of the alkaline diluent provided by the manufacturer to deliver PGI_2 50 ng/kg/minute continuous via the ventilator circuit. Fresh solution was added every four hours. Within one hour, there was a significant improvement in PaO_2, and within two hours, there was a significant decline in OI. The infant (who was later diagnosed with ACD) had only a transient improvement in oxygenation. The three surviving infants received iNO for 5–8 days and PGI_2 for 7–18 days. They were extubated within three weeks of starting PGI_2 therapy and had normal oxygen saturations without tachypnea in room air at the time of discharge from the NICU. Administration of aerosolized prostacyclin was not associated with changes in systemic blood pressure, heart rate, or temperature in this case report.[137]

Ehlen and Wiebe provide a case report of a term infant with Down syndrome who presented with respiratory distress at 90 minutes of age followed by rapid deterioration following pulmonary hemorrhage by 9 hours of age. An echocardiogram revealed a right-to-left shunt at the level of the ductus arteriosus. Management included high-frequency ventilation, iNO (initially at 40 ppm, then at 20 ppm), repeat surfactant lavages, vasopressors (dopamine, norepinephrine, and epinephrine), dexamethasone (for blood pressure management), and alkalization. Cranial ultrasound at 24 hours of age demonstrated bilateral Grade II–III IVH. Transfer to an ECMO center was not an option because of the infant's status. Furthermore, ECMO was contraindicated because of the IVH. At 30 hours of age, with parental consent, iloprost administration began.[175]

The infant initially received 2 mcg of iloprost via a nasogastric tube placed at the tip of the endotracheal tube, without interrupting ventilation. Up to the age of 39 hours, the infant received three more endotracheal doses of iloprost every 90–120 minutes. Endotracheal administration of iloprost resulted in a 10–20 percent

decrease in mean systemic arterial blood pressure. After 39 hours of age, adequate oxygenation was achieved (PaO_2 of at least 60–80 mmHg). An echocardiogram revealed a complete conversion of the right-to-left ductal shunting, along with decreased right ventricular pressure. Over the following days, the infant developed multiorgan system failure and died at four days of age. The authors concluded that further investigation is needed to determine the efficacy of aerosolized iloprost alone or in combination with endotracheal administration in infants with PPHN.[175]

Four premature neonates, 26.7–33.7 weeks gestational age and birth weights of 745–2,300 g, with persistent pulmonary hypertension related to RDS in three infants and to septicemia in the fourth, received endotracheal prostacyclin. They received a bolus through a catheter at the distal end of the endotracheal tube 1–2 hours after extrapulmonary shunting was established by echocardiography. Two of the infants received three subsequent endotracheal instillations of prostacyclin. A third infant received continuous endotracheal instillation of the prostacyclin solution at 1 mL/kg/hour for 12 hours. The fourth received only the initial endotracheal instillation.[176]

Following the initial bolus administration, there was a significant decrease in OI and a significant increase in the PaO_2:FiO_2 ratio. There was no change in mean systemic arterial pressure associated with endotracheal instillation of prostacyclin. The authors assert that improved oxygenation was most likely the result of decreased PVR and reversal of extrapulmonary shunting via the ductus arteriosus and the foramen ovale. The positive effects of the prostacyclin on oxygenation were reversed when the drug was withdrawn. The procedure was reported to be well tolerated, and no side effects were observed. The authors suggest that surfactant might serve as a potential carrier for endotracheal prostaglandin administration. Long-term outcomes were not described in this group of premature infants.[176]

Both infants reported by Suzuki and colleagues had Down syndrome and atrial septal defect (ASD) with pulmonary hypertension. Both showed noted improvement in their PH on long-term beraprost therapy. One infant was started on beraprost 1.5 mcg/kg/day at the age of 6 months. By 9 months of age, an echocardiogram revealed spontaneous closure of the ASD and regression of the PH. A further decline in pulmonary artery pressure was noted at cardiac catheterization at 15 months of age. Home oxygen therapy and beraprost were discontinued at 20 months of age. The second infant was

TABLE 11-4
Relative Potency of Corticosteroids

Corticosteroid	Equivalent Dose (mg)	Biological Half-life (hours)	Anti-inflammatory Potency Multiples (when compared to hydrocortisone)
Dexamethasone (Decadron)	0.75	36–54	20–30
Hydrocortisone (Solu-Cortef)	20	8–12	1
Methylprednisolone (Solu-Medrol)	4	18–36	5

Adapted from: Zenk KE, Sills JH, and Koeppel RM. 2003. *Neonatal Medications & Nutrition: A Comprehensive Guide*, 3rd ed. Petaluma, California: NICU INK, 182. Reprinted by permission.

started on beraprost 1.5 mcg/kg/day at 4 months of age. This infant also demonstrated improvement over time; the beraprost was discontinued at 29 months of age. The authors assert that beraprost along with conventional treatment for PH (oxygen, digoxin, and diuretics) contributed to the regression of PH in these infants.[177]

The pulmonary vasodilator drugs discussed in this section present intriguing possibilities for the management of PPHN. Clearly, there is a need for randomized clinical trials, including pharmacokinetic studies, before any of these medications become a part of mainstream therapy for neonates with acute hypoxic respiratory failure.

CORTICOSTEROIDS

The role of corticosteroids in the treatment of premature infants remains both controversial and poorly defined.[178] This discussion of corticosteroids describes the impact of antenatal corticosteroids on the neonate. It also addresses the use of postnatal corticosteroids to prevent and treat CLD, to facilitate extubation, and in other neonatal respiratory illnesses.

ANTENATAL CORTICOSTEROID THERAPY

Antenatal corticosteroid therapy has been heralded as one of the two greatest advances in the prevention of RDS (surfactant is the other).[179] Corticosteroids have been used in pregnant women at risk for preterm (before 34 weeks gestation) delivery since Liggins and Howie reported in 1972 that antenatal betamethasone decreased the incidence of RDS and increased survival in preterm infants.[180]

A systematic review of 21 clinical trials of antenatal corticosteroids that included 3,885 women and 4,269 infants [180–200] confirmed this report. However, the use of this therapy was not widespread until the National

Institutes of Health held a consensus development conference in 1994.[201]

The reviews found that use of antenatal steroids is associated with an overall reduction in neonatal death, RDS, cerebroventricular hemorrhage, necrotizing enterocolitis, respiratory support, NICU admissions, and systemic infections in the first 48 hours of life. The authors concluded that the evidence supports the use of a single dose of antenatal corticosteroids for fetal lung maturation in women at risk for preterm delivery. There continues to be a need for further study regarding optimal dose to delivery interval, effects in multiple gestations, and long-term effects into adulthood.[202]

There is evidence to suggest that betamethasone is preferable to dexamethasone for antenatal corticosteroid therapy. Both of these steroids cross the placenta and have similar biologic activity.[203] But, the significant decrease in neonatal mortality following administration of corticosteroids has been demonstrated for betamethasone, not for dexamethasone.[204,205] In an animal model, betamethasone was more potent than dexamethasone in accelerating lung maturity.[206] Furthermore, researchers have found that antenatal betamethasone, not antenatal dexamethasone, is associated with a decreased risk for cystic periventricular leukomalacia among preterm infants with gestational ages from 24 to 31 weeks.[207] Finally, sulfites used as preservatives in various forms of injectable dexamethasone on the market in Europe and the U.S. may have neurotoxic effects, so dexamethasone should be used with caution during the perinatal period.[208]

Researchers have compared the effectiveness of a single course of antenatal steroids with multiple weekly courses when the risk of preterm delivery continues into the weeks following the initial corticosteroid course. They found that weekly antenatal steroids do not improve neonatal morbidity.[209] In fact, another source states that three or more weekly courses of antenatal corticosteroids are associated with increased mortality. This increase in mortality could not be explained by confounding maternal risk factors, increased infection, or other morbidities associated with prematurity; rather, it was associated with increased incidence of severe lung disease. The researchers speculate that excessive exposure to antenatal corticosteroids may have a detrimental effect on alveolarization.[210] Baud suggests that if the risk of preterm delivery persists following an initial course of antenatal corticosteroids, a second course should be administered two weeks after the first course and no more than two courses should be given.[203]

Researchers have also assessed the effect of antenatal corticosteroid therapy on birth weight and head circumference, weight gain and head circumference growth in the NICU, and mortality and long-term morbidity in growth-restricted infants.[211–223] Antenatal corticosteroids may be associated with decreases in birth weight and head circumference independent of other antenatal factors such as preeclampsia, race, maternal smoking, nulliparity, prolonged premature rupture of membranes, and multiple gestation. The reduction in head circumference persists even after controlling for decreased birth weight. The researchers assert that the clinical significance of the findings is not known.[211] Interestingly, antenatal corticosteroids were not found to affect postnatal weight gain or head circumference growth.[212]

In their study of growth-restricted infants, Schaap and associates compared infants whose mothers received steroids >24 hours but <7 days before delivery with infants whose mothers did not receive steroids. The primary outcome measure was survival without disability or handicap at two years of age. Results revealed that survival without disability or handicap at two years of age was more frequent in the steroid group. Long-term follow-up at school age showed a significant negative effect on physical growth in the steroid group; however, no differences in behavior, based on the *Diagnostic and Statistical Manual of Mental Disorders* criteria for attention-deficit hyperactivity disorder, were observed. The researchers concluded that the follow-up data demonstrating significantly higher survival without disability in the antenatal steroid group far outweighed the negative effects of steroids on physical growth.[213]

In summary, a single course of antenatal corticosteroids decreases the incidence of RDS and mortality. Current research does not support the use of multiple courses when the risk of preterm delivery persists. In fact, three or more courses of antenatal corticosteroids may be detrimental. Because of the potential for neurotoxicity related to dexamethasone administration, betamethasone appears to be the corticosteroid of choice. Although antenatal steroids do impact birth weight and head circumference, the significance of these findings is not known at present. Antenatal steroids do not affect weight gain and head circumference growth in the NICU. The benefits of antenatal steroids for growth-restricted infants outweigh the negative effects on physical growth in this population.

POSTNATAL CORTICOSTEROIDS

Although the benefits of antenatal corticosteroid administration have been clearly established, there is considerable debate about the benefits and risks of steroids administered to the neonate postnatally. Three systematic reviews of postnatal steroid administration looked at 39 studies.[214–216] Twenty of the studies evaluated early preventive corticosteroid treatment (within 96 hours of birth).[216] Seven trials evaluated moderately early preventive corticosteroid therapy (at 7–14 days of age).[215] Twelve studies evaluated delayed corticosteroid therapy for infants more than three weeks of age with CLD.[214]

The reviewers found that early administration of postnatal corticosteroids in preterm infants resulted in the short-term benefits of (1) earlier extubation and, decreased risk of CLD and (2) decreased risk of either death or CLD at 28 days of age and 36 weeks postconception. However, there were significant short- and long-term side effects. There was a short-term risk of gastrointestinal bleeding, intestinal perforation, hyperglycemia, and hypertension. Long-term risks were abnormal neurologic examination and CP. The reviewers assert that none of the studies in the review had the power to identify important adverse long-term neurosensory outcomes. Because of the risks of potential short-term and long-term adverse effects versus the potential short-term benefits, the reviewers suggest that it is appropriate to curtail early postnatal corticosteroid therapy for prevention of CLD. The majority (85 percent) of the studies in this review evaluated dexamethasone; the remaining three used hydrocortisone. The researchers further recommend that future studies should include the use of potentially safer steroids such as hydrocortisone and perhaps methylprednisone. (Table 11-4 compares three corticosteroids.) The importance of long-term neurodevelopment follow-up is strongly emphasized.[216]

The review of moderately early steroid therapy did not reveal greater benefit than risk. There was a reduction in failure to extubate, a decreased incidence of CLD, and a decrease in mortality. However, increases in infection, hyperglycemia, hypertension, gastrointestinal bleeding, and hypertrophic cardiomyopathy were seen in infants treated with steroids. The same methodologic issues regarding assessment of long-term outcomes exist in the studies evaluated in this review as in the studies of early steroid treatment. The reviewers recommend reserving moderately early steroid therapy for those infants who cannot be weaned from mechanical ventilation.

TABLE 11-5
Dexamethasone Tapering Doses

Days	Dose
1–7	0.25 mg/kg every 12 hours
8–14	0.12 mg/kg every 12 hours
15–21	0.05 mg/kg every 12 hours
22–28	0.02 mg/kg every 12 hours

Adapted from: Yeh TF, et al. 2004. Outcomes at school age after postnatal dexamethasone therapy for lung disease of prematurity. *New England Journal of Medicine* 350(13): 1304–1313.

Furthermore, they suggest minimizing both dose and duration of therapy, but no specific recommendations are made in this regard.[215]

Infants who are ventilator dependent with CLD after three weeks of age were noted to improve, at least briefly, following a course of dexamethasone. Steroid therapy facilitated extubation and reduced the need for subsequent steroid therapy and for home oxygen therapy. Short-term effects of hyperglycemia and hypertension were noted in this review as well, but more notable were the long-term adverse effects of severe ROP and abnormal neurologic examination. Once more, however, there were methodologic limitations regarding long-term follow-up in the studies in this review. Again, the reviewers recommend limited use of delayed corticosteroid therapy in infants who cannot be weaned from mechanical ventilation.[214]

In an attempt to answer concerns regarding neurodevelopmental outcome in infants treated postnatally with corticosteroids, Barrington performed a meta-analysis of those studies with adequate neurodevelopmental follow-up, defined as follow-up to at least one year of age. The primary outcome measures in this review were CP rate and neurodevelopmental impairment, which was defined as a developmental score less than two standard deviations below the mean or CP or blindness. Eight studies met the criterion of having follow-up to at least one year of age for this review. Steroids were given either early or moderately early. There was "contamination" of the control groups in at least three of these studies because up to 43 percent of the controls received steroids as rescue therapy. The meta-analysis revealed that infants who are treated with postnatal steroids are more likely to have CP and neurodevelopmental impairment. The studies with less contamination showed a clearer difference between treatment and control groups. The author asserts that "the single most effective intervention which could currently be introduced for improving

neurodevelopmental outcome of extremely low birth weight infants would be to immediately abandon the use of postnatal steroids for chronic lung disease" (p. 7). The short-term benefits of postnatal steroids are accompanied by the variety of short-term adverse consequences described earlier. The long-term adverse effects do not seem to be associated with any proven long-term benefit.[217]

Yeh and coworkers studied the outcomes at school age in children who had participated in a double-blind trial of early (initiated within 12 hours of delivery) postnatal dexamethasone administration for prevention of CLD. Of the 262 infants in the initial study, 159 survived. Of the survivors, 146 children, 72 in the dexamethasone group and 74 in the control group, were included in the follow-up study.[218] As neonates, the children in the dexamethasone group had received 0.25 mg/kg intravenous dexamethasone every 12 hours for one week, followed by a taper dose over the following three weeks (Table 11-5). The results of the initial study revealed that early dexamethasone significantly decreased the incidence of CLD at either 28 days (16 percent in the treatment group versus 31 percent in the control group) or 36 weeks gestational age (20 percent in the treatment group versus 37 percent in the control group). Infants treated with dexamethasone required oxygen concentrations ≥40 percent for a shorter duration than did the controls. The frequency of IVH and the mortality were similar in both groups.[219]

At the time of follow-up, the mean age of the children in the dexamethasone group was 8.3 ± 0.9 years and in the control group, 8.1 ± 0.8 years. The researchers found that children who received early dexamethasone therapy were more likely to have delays in somatic growth, impaired neuromotor and cognitive functions, and disability at school age.[218] This study provides further support for the recommendation to avoid routine systemic dexamethasone to prevent or treat CLD of prematurity.

Inhaled corticosteroids have also been evaluated for prevention of CLD in premature neonates. A systematic review comparing inhaled corticosteroids with systemic corticosteroids revealed that inhaled corticosteroids administered within the first two weeks of life resulted in a slight increase in the incidence of CLD at 36 weeks compared with early administration of systemic steroids. There was no evidence that inhaled steroids decreased either the incidence of CLD at 28 days or 36 weeks or the combined outcome of either CLD or mortality at 28 days or 36 weeks compared with systemic steroids. An increased incidence of patent ductus arteriosus (PDA), a longer duration of mechanical ventilation, and a longer duration of supplemental oxygen were associated with inhaled corticosteroids. The reviewers concluded that the use of inhaled corticosteroids cannot be recommended for the prevention of CLD in ventilated preterm infants.[220]

In a separate systematic review, the same researchers compared inhaled corticosteroids with systemic corticosteroids for the treatment of CLD in preterm infants. They found no distinct advantage of inhaled steroids over systemic steroids in the treatment of ventilator-dependent preterm infants. Additionally, there was no difference in the side-effect profiles for inhaled or systemic corticosteroids. The reviewers concluded that they could not recommend the use of inhaled steroids for the treatment of ventilator-dependent preterm infants.[221]

In a joint statement, the American Academy of Pediatrics (AAP) and the Canadian Paediatric Society (CPS) presented the following conclusions regarding the use of postnatal corticosteroids to treat or prevent CLD in preterm infants:[222]

- Systemic dexamethasone decreases the incidence of CLD and extubation failure in preterm infants who are mechanically ventilated, but it does not decrease overall mortality.
- Systemic dexamethasone administration in VLBW infants is associated with an increased risk of short- and long-term complications, including impaired growth and neurodevelopmental impairment.
- There are no short- or long-term benefits of inhaled corticosteroids in the prevention or treatment of CLD.

Based on those findings, the AAP and CPS make the following recommendations:[222]

- The routine use of systemic dexamethasone for the prevention or treatment of CLD in VLBW infants is not recommended.
- Use of systemic dexamethasone should be limited to randomized, double-blind, controlled trials. The primary outcome measure of these studies should be survival without long-term developmental impairment. Contamination and crossover should be avoided.
- Long-term developmental follow-up of participants in clinical trials of dexamethasone is strongly encouraged.
- Clinical trials of alternative inhaled or systemic anti-inflammatory corticosteroids are needed before further recommendations can be made about the forms.
- Outside of randomized, controlled trials, the use

of corticosteroids should be limited to exceptional clinical situations, such as an infant on maximum ventilatory and oxygen support. In such cases, the parents should be fully informed about the short- and long-term risks of corticosteroids and agree to the treatment.

CORTICOSTEROIDS TO FACILITATE EXTUBATION

Endotracheal tubes may injure the upper airway, resulting in laryngeal edema. Laryngeal edema, in turn, may cause extubation failure. Can corticosteroids play a role in facilitating extubation? A systematic review attempted to address this question. The reviewers assessed the effects of intravenous dexamethasone on the incidence of endotracheal reintubation, stridor, atelectasis, and adverse side effects in neonates having their endotracheal tubes removed following a period of intermittent positive-pressure ventilation.[223]

Dexamethasone was effective in reducing stridor using a higher and multiple-dose strategy of 0.25 mg/kg intravenously four hours before planned extubation, then every eight hours for a total of three doses.[223,224] A trend toward decreased atelectasis was also noted, but once again, this result was heavily influenced by the high-risk population.[223] Because dexamethasone is not without potential adverse effects (including glucosuria and hyperglycemia reported in this review), it would be desirable to define the group in which intravenous dexamethasone would be more effective. The reviewers concluded that use of intravenous dexamethasone to facilitate extubation should be restricted to those infants who are at particularly high risk for reintubation.[223]

It is important to note that the studies included in this review[224–226] were published before use of exogenous surfactant, antenatal steroids, and a trend toward early extubation to nasal continuous positive airway pressure became common aspects of neonatal intensive care.[223] A Medline search did not identify any recent randomized controlled trials of corticosteroids to facilitate extubation. Thus, the relevance of this therapy is questionable.

CORTICOSTEROIDS IN OTHER NEONATAL RESPIRATORY ILLNESSES

MAS and Corticosteroid Therapy

Several studies have demonstrated that inflammation plays a key role in meconium-induced lung dysfunction.[227–232] Thus, it has been suggested that anti-inflammatory glucocorticoids may limit the pulmonary damage after meconium aspiration.[233,234]

TABLE 11-6
Inhaled Bronchodilators

Bronchodilator	Category	Dose	Mechanism of Action	Pharmacodynamics	Side Effects/Comments
Isoproterenol (Isuprel)	β-adrenergic agonist (nonspecific)	**Intermittent nebulization:** *Preterm:* 1% 0.05 mL/dose every 1–2 hours *Term:* 1% 0.1 mL/dose every 1–2 hours • 1% solution = 10 mg/mL. Dilute to 3 mL with normal saline or other compatible medications for nebulization.	Acts on both β_1 and β_2 receptors. Relaxes smooth muscle of bronchial tree.	*Onset of action:* 2–5 minutes *Duration of action:* 0.5–1 hour	Increase interval of nebulization if heart rate is >180 bpm (if baseline heart rate is <150 bpm) or >200 bpm (if baseline heart rate is >150 bpm). Expect a moderate increase in heart rate following inhalation treatment; this may indicate absorption and therapeutic response. Saliva may be pink or red because isoproterenol turns these colors when exposed to air.
Albuterol, salbutamol (Proventil, Ventolin)	β-adrenergic agonist (specific)	**Intermittent nebulization:** 0.083% 0.6–1.2 mL every 2–6 hours* • 0.083% = 0.83 mg/mL. Dilute to 3 mL with normal saline. **MDI:** 1–2 puffs every 6 hours • 90 mcg/puff	β_2-adrenergic stimulation, resulting in bronchodilation and vasodilation. Possible enhancement of mucociliary transport and redistribution of pulmonary blood flow. Inhibition of histamine release from mast cells, resulting in vasodilation.	*Onset of action:* Within 5 minutes *Duration of action:* 4–6 hours	Expect increased myocardial contractility and conduction as a result of minor β_1 effects. May cause tachycardia, arrhythmias, hypokalemia, and irritability.
Metaproterenol (Alupent)	β-adrenergic agonist (specific)	**Intermittent nebulization:** 0.4% 0.13 mL/kg/dose every 3–6 hours • 0.4% = 4 mg/mL. Dilute to 3 mL with normal saline or other compatible medications for nebulization.	β_2-adrenergic stimulation, resulting in bronchodilation and vasodilation. Inhibition of histamine release from mast cells, resulting in vasodilation. Increased ciliary motility.	*Onset of action:* 5–30 minutes *Duration of action:* 2–6 hours	Expect increased myocardial contractility and conduction as a result of minor β_1 effects. May cause tachycardia, arrhythmias, blood pressure increases, and hyperglycemia. Tolerance may develop with prolonged use. Decrease dose or increase interval of nebulization if heart rate is >180 bpm (if baseline heart rate is <150 bpm) or >200 bpm (if baseline heart is >150 bpm). Expect a moderate increase in heart rate following inhalation treatment; this may indicate absorption and therapeutic response. When respiratory status improves, try to lengthen the interval between doses. If respiratory distress continues after 1–3 doses, consider increasing the dose or decreasing the interval between dosing. Do not increase dose if the infant is experiencing side effects at the present dose.

(continued on next page)

TABLE 11-6
Inhaled Bronchodilators *(continued)*

Bronchodilator	Category	Dose	Mechanism of Action	Pharmacodynamics	Side Effects/Comments
Terbutaline (Brethine, Brethaire)	β-adrenergic agonist (specific)	**Intermittent nebulization:** 0.01–0.03 mg/kg/dose every 2–6 hours • Use intravenous form (1 mg/mL) for nebulization. • Dilute to 3 mL with normal saline or other compatible medications for nebulization. **MDI:** 2 puffs every 4–12 hours • 0.2 mg/puff	Bronchodilation by relaxation of bronchial musculature and vasodilation. Inhibition of histamine release from mast cells, resulting in vasodilation. Increased ciliary motility.	*Onset of action:* 5–30 minutes *Duration of action:* 3–6 hours	Decrease dose or increase interval of nebulization if heart rate is >180 bpm (if baseline heart rate is <150 bpm) or >200 bpm (if baseline heart rate is >150 bpm). Expect a moderate increase in heart rate following inhalation treatment; this may indicate absorption and therapeutic response. When respiratory status improves, try to lengthen the interval between doses. If respiratory distress continues after 1–3 doses, consider increasing the dose or decreasing the interval between dosing. Do not increase dose if the infant is experiencing side effects at the present dose.
Atropine	Anticholinergic agent	**Intermittent nebulization:** 0.03–0.05 mg/kg/dose every 6–8 hours • Maximum dose 2.5 mg/dose • Dilute to 3 mL with normal saline or other compatible medications for nebulization.	Competitive inhibition of acetylcholine on bronchial smooth muscle, resulting in dilation.	*Onset of action:* 15 minutes *Peak effect:* 15–90 minutes *Duration of action:* Not reported specifically for inhalation; up to 4 hours following oral dosing	Causes greater dilation of larger than of smaller airways. Usually well tolerated as a respiratory treatment. Tachycardia: Monitor heart rate before, during, and after dose. Taper to lowest effective dose. Decrease dose or increase interval of nebulization if heart rate is >180 bpm (if baseline heart rate is <150 bpm) or >200 bpm (if baseline heart rate is >150 bpm). If respiratory distress continues after 1–3 doses, consider increasing the dose or decreasing the interval between dosing. Do not increase dose if the infant is experiencing side effects at the present dose.
Ipratropium (Atrovent)	Anticholinergic agent	**Intermittent nebulization:** **Neonates** 25 mcg/kg/dose every 8 hours **Infants** 125–250 mcg every 8 hours • Supplied in 2.5 mL vial (200 mcg/mL) **MDI:** 1–2 puffs every 6 hours • 17 mcg/puff	Competitive inhibition of acetylcholine on bronchial smooth muscle, resulting in dilation. Some additive effect when given with β-adrenergic agonists.	*Onset of action:* Slow. Maximum bronchodilation occurs 1–2 hours after dose. *Duration of action:* 6–8 hours	Benzalkonium chloride and edetic acid in the solution may cause bronchospasms. Rebound hyper-responsiveness may occur when drug is discontinued. Systemic absorption is poor. If respiratory distress continues after 1–3 doses, consider increasing the dose or decreasing the interval between dosing. Do not increase dose if the infant is experiencing side effects at the present dose.

* Other dosing recommendations can be found in the literature.
Key: bpm = beats per minute; MDI = metered-dose inhaler.

Compiled from: Zenk KE, Sills JH, and Koeppel RM. 2003. *Neonatal Medications & Nutrition: A Comprehensive Guide,* 3rd ed. Petaluma, California: NICU Ink, 17–21, 78–81, 332–333, 339–342, 380–381, 545–547; and Taketomo CK, Hodding JH, and Kraus DM, eds. 2009. *Pediatric Dosage Handbook,* 16th ed. Hudson, Ohio: Lexi-Comp, 141–142, 683–684.

A systematic review of steroid therapy for MAS[235] included only two studies, which were published 22 years apart.[236,237] A total of 85 neonates was included in the two studies. Infants in the earlier study received either an initial dose of 20 mg/kg intravenous hydrocortisone followed by the same dose every 12 hours for four doses (n = 17) or a placebo (n = 18).[236] In the more recent study, infants received either intravenous dexamethasone (n = 27) or a placebo (n = 23). The dosing schedule for the dexamethasone was an initial dose of 1 mg/kg/dose, followed by 0.5 mg/kg/dose every 12 hours on days 1–3, and then 0.25 mg/kg/dose every 12 hours on days 4–7, for a total of 15 doses.[237] Based on these two studies, the reviewers concluded that the evidence for assessing the efficacy of steroid therapy in the treatment of MAS is inadequate.[235]

A 2004 nonrandomized study compared three different strategies for the treatment of MAS: standard therapy, BAL with dilute surfactant, and BAL plus a single dose of intravenous dexamethasone 0.5 mg/kg. There were significant differences between the group that was treated with BAL plus dexamethasone and the group treated with BAL alone. The infants in the BAL-plus-steroids group demonstrated a greater and more sustained improvement in OI; greater reductions in oxygen requirement, days on iNO, and duration of mechanical ventilation; and a shorter length of hospitalization than the infants in the other two groups. The researchers concluded that BAL within the first hour of life combined with a single dose of intravenous dexamethasone may be an effective treatment for MAS. The authors note that there have not been any reports of iatrogenic complications of steroid therapy in term neonates after a single dose of steroids; however, follow-up should include neurologic evaluation.[238] As noted earlier, the safety and efficacy of BAL with dilute surfactant are as yet unproven; randomized, controlled clinical trials are necessary to evaluate the safety and efficacy of steroids alone or in combination with BAL.

RSV Bronchiolitis and Corticosteroid Therapy

Corticosteroids have also been suggested as a treatment for RSV bronchiolitis.[239] The premise for this suggestion is that the anti-inflammatory action of these drugs will reduce bronchiolar swelling and therefore relieve airway obstruction.[240] Two meta-analyses have reported on the use of corticosteroids for acute viral bronchiolitis in infants and young children.[241,242] Neither of these reviews is specific to patients cared for in the NICU. The findings of these meta-analyses conflict.

Garrison and colleagues reported a statistically significant improvement in clinical symptoms, length of hospital stay, and duration of symptoms.[241] Patel and associates reported no difference in length of hospitalization or clinical score in infants and young children treated with corticosteroids compared with a placebo. They also found no difference between groups in respiratory rate, oxygen saturation, and hospital revisit or readmission rates. The reviewers concluded that the evidence does not support the use of corticosteroids to treat bronchiolitis in infants and young children.[242] The AAP does not recommend the use of corticosteroids to treat RSV in hospitalized infants.[243]

Corticosteroids appear to be therapeutic agents in search of a respiratory illness. Their efficacy has not been demonstrated consistently in the treatment of MAS or RSV. The use to facilitate extubation in those infants at highest risk for reintubation may prove efficacious, but it is essential to define this population to avoid unnecessary exposure to corticosteroids. Despite the call for additional randomized trials of postnatal steroids in premature infants, Barrington asserts that it is doubtful that a major benefit of corticosteroids will be discovered, especially a benefit that will significantly outweigh the increased risk of neurodevelopmental impairment.[244] This sentiment is echoed by others, who stress that the continued prescription of postnatal steroids in the absence of sufficient evidence of a decisive benefit could undermine the progress that has been made in the care of our most vulnerable neonates.[245]

BRONCHODILATORS

The bronchodilators used in neonates are divided into three therapeutic categories: adrenergic agonists, anticholinergic agents, and xanthines. Methylxanthines are described in Chapter 3. The focus of this section is inhaled (nebulized or metered-dose inhaler [MDI]) adrenergic and anticholinergic agents.

Bronchodilators have been used to prevent and treat CLD in premature infants. In CLD, the muscles of the small airways become hypertrophic. Potentially, bronchodilators can dilate the hypertrophic airways, improving compliance and tidal volume and decreasing pulmonary resistance.[246]

ADRENERGIC AGONISTS

A variety of inhaled β-adrenergic agonists is available. Those that have been described in the treatment of neonates include the nonspecific adrenergic agonist isoproterenol and the specific adrenergic agonists albuterol, metaproterenol, and terbutaline (Table 11-6).[247–251] Albuterol has been the β-adrenergic agonist most widely studied in neonates and is preferred over isoproterenol. Metaproterenol has fewer side effects than isoproterenol but may cause greater cardiac stimulation than albuterol because of its lower β_2-selectivity. Albuterol and terbutaline are equipotent and produce similar bronchodilator response.[18]

Few recent studies of the use of inhaled adrenergic agents have been published. In fact, in a systematic review, Ng and coworkers found only one study[247] of bronchodilators that met the inclusion criteria for the review, primarily because the only outcome measure in the excluded studies was pulmonary mechanics. The reviewers were interested in a broader range of outcomes, including the primary outcomes of mortality within the study period and CLD (that is, oxygen dependency at 28 days of life or 36 weeks corrected gestational age with compatible radiographic sign) and the secondary outcomes of number of days on oxygen, number of ventilator days, PDA, pulmonary interstitial emphysema, pneumothorax, grade of IVH, necrotizing enterocolitis, sepsis, and adverse effects for bronchodilators administered prophylactically. For treatment of CLD, the primary outcome measure was mortality within the study period. Secondary outcome measures were the same as just described.[246]

Denjean and colleagues studied the efficacy of inhaled albuterol and beclomethasone (an inhaled steroid) for prevention of BPD in 173 preterm infants with gestational ages less than 31 weeks. The infants were 9.8–10.1 days of age on entry into the study. They were randomized into four groups and received a placebo plus placebo, placebo plus albuterol, placebo plus beclomethasone, or albuterol plus beclomethasone. The medications and placebos were delivered via MDIs using a spacer device during 30 seconds of manual administration. The major criteria for the efficacy of albuterol or beclomethasone were diagnosis of BPD, mortality during mechanical ventilation, and oxygen therapy. The researchers found that inhaled albuterol and beclomethasone did not prevent BPD. In addition, these treatments failed to modify the need for ventilator support or oxygen supplementation.[247] The researchers concluded that there is not enough evidence to support the use of albuterol or beclomethasone or the combination of both for the prevention of CLD in premature infants. Further studies are needed to assess the efficacy of this and other bronchodilators in the prevention and treatment of CLD.[246]

FIGURE 11-4
Schematic representation of an MDI adapted to a spacer device for use in the intubated neonate.

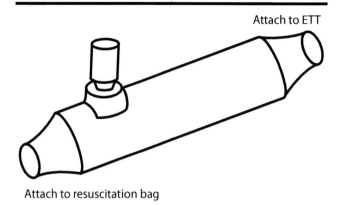

Attach to ETT

Attach to resuscitation bag

Anticholinergic Agents

The inhaled anticholinergic agents used in neonates are atropine and ipratropium (see Table 11-6). A literature search revealed even fewer recent studies on the use of anticholinergic agents in neonates than on the use of β-adrenergic agonists. Inhaled nebulized atropine can cause relaxation of bronchial smooth muscle tone and bronchodilation of the airways by inhibiting vagal activity. Ipratropium is chemically related to atropine but has fewer systemic side effects. Ipratropium is used to treat nonacute bronchospasms associated with CLD. Because albuterol has a faster onset of action than ipratropium, it is the preferred drug for acute bronchospasms.[18]

Everard and associates performed a systematic review of anticholinergic drugs for wheeze in children less than two years of age. None of the included studies were specific to infants in the NICU.[252–257] The review concluded that there was not enough evidence to support the use of anticholinergic agents in infants and young children under the age of two with wheeze. The reviewers did note, however, that parents who use these agents at home report benefits.[258]

AEROSOL DELIVERY SYSTEMS

Several factors are considered in the delivery of inhaled medications to the neonate. The particle size produced by the therapeutic aerosol is ideally in an optimal range for deposition in the lung. Reduced airway diameter resulting from disease, edema, and secretions is a major influence on the deposition of these drugs. Small-particle aerosols are best delivered to the distal airways by some nebulizers and MDIs with a spacer device (Figure 11-4).[259]

TABLE 11-7
Comparison of Inhalation Delivery Systems for Bronchodilators

Delivery System	Advantages	Disadvantages
Nebulizer (jet, ultrasonic)	No specific inhalation technique required Aerosolizes most drug solutions Delivers large doses Suitable for infants	Time-consuming Bulky Not portable Contents easily contaminated Relatively expensive Poor delivery efficiency Drug waste Wide performance variations among models and in various operating conditions
Pressured metered-dose inhaler (pMDI)	Compact Portable Multidose Inexpensive Sealed environment (prevents drug degradation) Consistent dosing	Inhalation technique requires coordination (dose delivered with inspiration) High oral deposition Maximum dose of 5 mg Limited range of available drugs

Adapted from: Labiris NR, and Dolovich MB. 2003. Pulmonary drug delivery. Part II: The role of inhalant delivery devices and drug formulations in therapeutic effectiveness of aerosolized medications. *British Journal of Clinical Pharmacology* 56(6): 600–612.

Nebulizers

There are two types of nebulizers: the jet nebulizer and the ultrasonic nebulizer. The jet nebulizer uses compressed air or oxygen, which is passed through a narrow orifice, creating an area of low pressure at the outlet of the adjacent liquid feed tube. This causes the drug solution to be drawn up from the reservoir and shattered into droplets in the gas stream. An ultrasonic nebulizer uses a piezoelectric crystal that vibrates at 1–3 megahertz to generate a fountain of liquid in the nebulizer chamber. Higher-frequency vibrations produce smaller droplets of medication.[260]

Nebulized medications can be delivered into the ventilator and CPAP circuit or given by face mask or blow-by for extubated infants. Ultrasonic nebulizers are more expensive than jet nebulizers. Additionally, they cannot be used for more viscous medications such as antibiotics.[261] Researchers have demonstrated that MDIs with spacers result in more efficient delivery of inhaled medications than do jet nebulizers in a mechanically ventilated neonatal lung model.[262] Because of the relative inefficiency of nebulization and these devices' need for more processing and maintenance, there has been a trend toward the use of MDIs with spacers.[261] Table 11-7

compares the advantages and disadvantages of nebulizers and MDIs.

MDIs with Spacers

The use of an MDI without the use of a spacer is not appropriate or practical in neonates. With a spacer, metered-dose inhaled medications can be delivered to ventilated and nonventilated infants. For the ventilated infant, the spacer is attached at the proximal end to the endotracheal tube adapter and to the resuscitation bag at the distal end. For the extubated neonate, a face mask is attached to the proximal end of the spacer. In either case, the delivery of the medication is coordinated with inspiration. Drugs delivered by MDI are propelled with either chlorofluorocarbons or hydrofluorokanes.[260]

Summary

Four general therapeutic categories of drugs—surfactant, iNO and other pulmonary vasodilators, corticosteroids, and bronchodilators—for management of neonatal respiratory disorders have been presented. Both surfactant and iNO are effective in management of the neonatal respiratory diseases for which they are approved by the U.S. FDA. In light of negative neurodevelopmental outcomes, the use of corticosteroids should be limited to those infants in whom all other therapies have failed. Informed parental consent is recommended before steroid administration. Clearly, other medications (e.g., NO-related vasodilators) need further study in controlled, randomized clinical trials before their widespread use can be supported. Because of limited clinical pharmaceutical studies, children in general—and neonates in particular—have become therapeutic orphans.[263] This situation appears to be changing. It is essential that we focus on randomized trials and not on anecdotal reports when making therapeutic decisions for our vulnerable patients. Nurses have an important role to play in these trials in administering medications and documenting clinical findings.

References

1. Nelson NM. 2000. A decimillennium in neonatology. *Journal of Pediatrics* 137(5): 731–735.
2. Pattle RE. 1955. Properties, function, and origin of the alveolar lining layer. *Nature* 175(4469): 1125–1126.
3. Clements JA. 1957. Surface tension of lung extracts. *Proceedings of the Society of Experimental Biology and Medicine* 95(1): 170–172.
4. Brown ES. 1957. Lung area from surface tension effects. *Proceedings of the Society of Experimental Biology and Medicine* 95(1): 168–170.
5. Pattle RE. 1958. Properties, function, and origin of the alveolar lining layer. *Proceedings of the Royal Society of London. Series B: Biological Sciences* 148(931): 217–240.
6. Clements JA. 1997. Lung surfactant: A personal perspective. *Annual Review of Physiology* 59: 1–21.

7. Avery ME, and Mead J. 1959. Surface properties in relation to atelectasis and hyaline membrane disease. *AMA Journal of Diseases of Children* 97(5 part 1): 517–523.

8. Klaus MH, Clements JA, and Havel RJ. 1961. Composition of surface-active material isolated from beef lung. *Proceedings of the National Academy of Science of the United States of America* 47: 1858–1859.

9. Pattle RE, and Thomas LC. 1961. Lipoprotein composition of the film lining the lung. *Nature* 189: 844.

10. Chu J, et al. 1967. Neonatal pulmonary ischemia. Part I: Clinical and physiological studies. *Pediatrics* 40 (4 supplement): S709–S782.

11. Enhorning G, and Robertson B. 1972. Lung expansion in the premature rabbit fetus after tracheal disposition of surfactant. *Pediatrics* 50(1): 58–66.

12. Fujiwara T, et al. 1979. Improved pulmonary pressure volume characteristics in premature newborn rabbits after tracheal instillation of artificial surfactant. *IRCS Journal of Medical Science* 7: 312.

13. Fujiwara T, et al.. 1979. Improved lung-thorax compliance and prevention of neonatal pulmonary lesion in prematurely delivered rabbit neonates subjective to IPPV after tracheal instillation of artificial surfactant. *IRCS Journal of Medical Science* 7: 313.

14. Fujiwara T, et al. 1980. Artificial surfactant therapy in hyaline-membrane disease. *Lancet* 1(8159): 55–59.

15. U.S. Food and Drug Administration. 2004. Label and approval history, Exosurf Neonatal. Drugs@FDA. Retrieved July 21, 2004, from www.accessdata.fda.gov/scripts/cder/drugsatfda.

16. Merrill JD, and Ballard RA. 2003. Pulmonary surfactant for neonatal respiratory disorders. *Current Opinion in Pediatrics* 15(2): 149–154.

17. Taketomo CK, Hodding JH, and Kraus DM, eds. 2009. Beractant. *Pediatric Dosage Handbook*, 16th ed. Hudson, Ohio: Lexi-Comp, 166-167, 218–219, 1013.

18. Zenk KE, Sills JH, and Koeppel RM. 2003. *Neonatal Medications & Nutrition: A Comprehensive Guide*, 3rd ed. Petaluma, California: NICU Ink, 85–86, 107–110, 436–438, 17–21, 339–342, 380–381, 545–547, 78–81, 332–333, 429–432, 387–395.

19. Abbott Nutrition, Abbott Laboratories. Survanta dosing video. Retrieved November 25, 2011, from http://abbottnutrition.com/Products/Survanta.aspx?CMS=Survanta-Dosing-Video.

20. Abbott Nutrition, Abbott Laboratories. 2009. Survanta (beractant) intratracheal suspension. Manufacturer's product literature. Columbus, Ohio.

21. Ony, Inc. 2011. Infasurf (calfactant) intratracheal suspension. Manufacturer's product literature. Amhearst, New York.

22. Cornerstone Therapeutics, Inc. 2010. Curosurf user guide. Manufacturer's product literature. Cary, North Carolina.

23. Wiswell TE, et al. 2002. A multicenter, randomized, controlled trial comparing Surfaxin (lucinactant) lavage with standard care for treatment of meconium aspiration syndrome. *Pediatrics* 109(6): 1081–1087.

24. Moya F, and Maturana, A. 2007. Animal-derived surfactants versus past and current synthetic surfactants: Current status. *Clinics in Perinatology* 34(1): 145–177.

25. Sinha SK, et al. 2005. A multicenter, randomized, controlled trial of lucinactant versus poractant alfa among very premature infants at high risk for respiratory distress syndrome. *Pediatrics* 115(4): 1030–1038.

26. Dani C, et al. 2004. Early extubation and nasal continuous positive airway pressure after surfactant treatment for respiratory distress syndrome among preterm infants <30 weeks' geatation. *Pediatrics* 113(6): e560–e563.

27. Dani C, et al. 2010. The INSURE method in preterm infants of less than 30 weeks' gestation. *Journal of Maternal-Fetal and Neonatal Medicine*, 23(9): 1024–1029.

28. Dargaville PA, et al. 2011. Preliminary evaluation of a new technique of minimally invasive surfactant therapy, *Archives of Disease in Childhood. Fetal and Neonatal Edition* 96(4): F243–F248.

29. Finer NN, et al. 2010. An open label, pilot study of Aerosurf combined with nCPAP to prevent RDS in preterm neonates. *Journal of Aerosol Medicine and Pulmonary Drug Delivery* 23(5): 303–309.

30. Jobe AH. 2004. Surfactant for RDS: When and how? *Journal of Pediatrics* 144(6): 2A.

31. Escobedo MB, et al. 2004. Early surfactant for neonates with mild to moderate respiratory distress syndrome: A multicenter, randomized trial. *Journal of Pediatrics* 144(6): 804–808.

32. Kaiser JR, Gauss CH, and Williams DK. 2004. Surfactant administration acutely affects cerebral and systemic hemodynamics and gas exchange in very-low-birth-weight infants. *Journal of Pediatrics* 144(6): 809–814.

33. Saliba E, et al. 1994. Instillation rate effects of Exosurf on cerebral and cardiovascular haemodynamics in preterm neonates. *Archives of Disease in Childhood. Fetal and Neonatal Edition* 71(3): F174–F178.

34. Wang Z, et al. 1996. Differential activity and lack of synergy of lung surfactant protein SP-B and SP-C in interactions with phospholipids. *Journal of Lipid Research* 37(8): 1749–1760.

35. Lundstrom KE, and Greisen G. 1996. Changes in EEG, systemic circulation and blood gas parameters following two or six aliquots of porcine surfactant. *Acta Paediatrica* 85(6): 708–712.

36. Valls-i-Soler A, et al. 1997. A simplified surfactant dosing procedure in respiratory distress syndrome: The ìside-holeî randomized study. *Acta Paediatrica* 86(7): 747–751.

37. Valls-i-Soler A, et al. 1998. A randomized comparison of surfactant dosing via a dual-lumen endotracheal tube in respiratory distress syndrome. *Pediatrics* 101(4): e4.

38. Dijk PH, Heikamp A, and Bambang Oetomo S. 1997. Surfactant nebulisation prevents the adverse effects of surfactant therapy on blood pressure and cerebral blood flow in rabbits with severe respiratory failure. *Intensive Care Medicine* 23(10): 1077–1081.

39. Sattar SP, et al. 2004. Inert medication ingredients causing nonadherence due to religious beliefs. *Annals of Pharmacotherapy* 38(4): 621–624.

40. Adappa R, et al. 2003. Use of animal surfactant: Should we seek consent? *Archives of Disease in Childhood. Fetal and Neonatal Edition* 88(4): F351.

41. Kittler PG, Sucher KP, and Four Winds Food Specialists. 2000. *Religious Food Practices*. Retrieved July 23, 2004, from https://asiarecipe.com/religion.html.

42. Auten RL, et al. 1991. Surfactant treatment of full-term newborns with respiratory failure. *Pediatrics* 87(1): 101–107.

43. Findlay RD, Taeusch HW, and Walther FJ. 1996. Surfactant replacement therapy for meconium aspiration syndrome. *Pediatrics* 97(1): 48–52.

44. Halliday HL, Speer CP, and Robertson B. 1996. Treatment of severe meconium aspiration syndrome with porcine surfactant. *European Journal of Pediatrics* 155(12): 1047–1451.

45. Ibara S, et al. 1995. Management of meconium aspiration syndrome by tracheobronchial lavage and replacement of surfactant-TA. *Acta Paediatrica Japonica* 37(1): 64–67.

46. Khammash H, et al. 1993. Surfactant therapy in full-term neonates with severe respiratory failure. *Pediatrics* 92(1): 135–139.

47. Lam BC, and Yeung CY. 1999. Surfactant lavage for meconium aspiration syndrome: A pilot study. *Pediatrics* 103(5 part 1): 1014–1018.

48. Lotze A, et al. 1998. Multicenter study of surfactant (beractant) use in the treatment of term infants with severe respiratory failure. *Journal of Pediatrics* 132(1): 40–47.

49. Chinese Collaborative Study Group for Neonatal Respiratory Diseases. 2005. Treatment of severe meconium aspiration with porcine sufactant: A multicenter, randomized, controlled trial. *Acta Paediatrica* 94(7): 896–902.

50. Maturana A, et al. 2005. A randomized trial of natural surfactant for moderate to severe meconium aspiration syndrome. *Pediatric Academic Societies Meeting Abstract* 57: 1545.

51. Herting E, et al. 2000. Surfactant treatment of neonates with respiratory failure and Group B streptococcal infection. *Pediatrics* 106(5): 957–964.

52. Tibby SM, et al. 2000. Exogenous surfactant supplementation in infants with respiratory syncytial virus bronchiolitis. *American Journal of Respiratory and Critical Care Medicine* 162(4 part 1): 1251–1256.

53. Dargaville PA, South M, and McDougall PN. 2001. Surfactant and surfactant inhibitors in meconium aspiration syndrome. *Journal of Pediatrics* 138(1): 113–115.

54. El Shahed AI, et al. 2007. Surfactant for meconium aspiration syndrome in full term/near term infants. *Cochrane Database of Systematic Reviews* (3): CD002054.

55. Dargaville PA, et al. 2003. Therapeutic lung lavage in the piglet model of meconium aspiration. *American Journal of Respiratory and Critical Care Medicine* 168(4): 456–463.

56. Kinsella JP. 2003. Meconium aspiration syndrome: Is surfactant lavage the answer? *American Journal of Respiratory and Critical Care Medicine* 168(4): 413–414.

57. Dargaville PA, Mills JF, and Soll RF. 2002. Therapeutic lung lavage for meconium aspiration syndrome in newborn infants. *Cochrane Database of Systematic Reviews* (1): CD003486.

58. Ingenito EP, et al. 2001. Decreased surfactant protein-B expression and surfactant dysfunction in a murine model of acute lung injury. *American Journal of Respiratory Cell and Molecular Biology* 25(1): 35–44.

59. Lema G, et al. 2000. Pseudomonas aeruginosa from patients with cystic fibrosis affects function of pulmonary surfactant. *Pediatric Research* 47(1): 121–126.

60. Schmidt R, et al. 2001. Alteration of fatty acid profiles in different pulmonary surfactant phospholipids in acute respiratory distress syndrome and severe pneumonia. *American Journal of Respiratory and Critical Care Medicine* 163(1): 95–100.

61. Kerr MH, and Paton JY. 1999. Surfactant protein levels in severe respiratory syncytial virus infection. *American Journal of Critical Care Medicine* 159(4 part 1): 1115–1118.

62. van Golde LMG. 1995. Potential role of surfactant proteins A and D in innate lung defense against pathogens. *Biology of the Neonate* 67(supplement 1): 2–17.

63. Wilcox DT, et al. 1997. Contributions by individual lungs to the surfactant status in congenital diaphragmatic hernia. *Pediatric Research* 41(5): 686–691.

64. Moya FR, et al. 1995. Fetal lung maturation in congenital diaphragmatic hernia. *American Journal of Obstetrics and Gynecology* 173(5): 1401–1405.

65. IJsselstijn H, et al. 1998. Prospective evaluation of surfactant composition in bronchoalveolar lavage fluid of infants with congenital diaphragmatic hernia and of age-matched controls. *Critical Care Medicine* 26(3): 573–580.

66. Cogo PE, et al. 2002. Surfactant synthesis and kinetics in infants with congenital diaphragmatic hernia. *American Journal of Respiratory and Critical Care Medicine* 166(2): 154–158.

67. Somaschini M, et al. 1999. Impact of new treatments of respiratory failure on outcome of infants with congenital diaphragmatic hernia. *European Journal of Pediatrics* 158(10): 780–784.

68. Finer NN, et al. 1998. Congenital diaphragmatic hernia: Developing a protocolized approach. *Journal of Pediatric Surgery* 33(9): 1331–1337.

69. Moya F, et al. 2003. Surfactant for newborn infants with congenital diaphragmatic hernia. *Cochrane Database of Systematic Reviews* (2): CD004209.

70. O'Toole SJ, et al. 1996. Surfactant decreases pulmonary vascular resistance and increases pulmonary blood flow in the fetal lamb model of congenital diaphragmatic hernia. *Journal of Pediatric Surgery* 31(4): 507–511.

71. O'Toole SJ, et al. 1996. Surfactant rescue in the fetal lamb model of congenital diaphragmatic hernia. *Journal of Pediatric Surgery* 31(8): 1105–1109.

72. Lally KP. 2002. Congenital diaphragmatic hernia. *Current Opinion in Pediatrics* 14(4): 486–490.

73. Bancalari E. 1998. Corticosteroids and neonatal chronic lung disease. *European Journal of Pediatrics* 157(supplement 1): S31–S37.

74. Speer CP. 1999. Inflammatory mechanisms in neonatal chronic lung disease. *European Journal of Pediatrics* 158(supplement 1): S18–S22.

75. Clark H, and Reid K. 2003. The potential of recombinant surfactant protein D therapy to reduce inflammation in neonatal chronic lung disease, cystic fibrosis, and emphysema. *Archives of Disease in Childhood* 88(11): 981–984.

76. Beresford MW, and Shaw NJ. 2002. The role of pulmonary surfactant proteins A, B, and D in the preterm infants ventilated for respiratory distress receiving different surfactant therapies. *Early Human Development* 66(1): 47–49.

77. Koshland DE. 1992. The molecule of the year. *Science* 258(5090): 1861.

78. Finer NN, and Barrington KJ. 2000. Nitric oxide therapy for the newborn infant. *Seminars in Perinatology* 24(1): 59–65.

79. Gianetti J, Bevilacqua S, and De Caterina R. 2002. Inhaled nitric oxide: More than a selective pulmonary vasodilator. *European Journal of Clinical Investigation* 32(8): 628–635.

80. Abman SH, et al. 1990. Role of endothelium-derived relaxing factor during transition of pulmonary circulation at birth. *American Journal of Physiology–Heart and Circulatory Physiology* 259(6 part 2): H1921–H1927.

81. Fineman JR, et al. 1994. Chronic nitric oxide inhibition in utero produces persistent pulmonary hypertension in newborn lambs. *Journal of Clinical Investigation* 93(6): 2675–2683.

82. Colnaghi M, et al. 2003. Endogenous nitric oxide production in the airways of preterm and term infants. *Biology of the Neonate* 83(2): 113–116.

83. Kinsella JP, et al. 1992. Low-dose inhalation nitric oxide in persistent pulmonary hypertension of the newborn. *Lancet* 340(8823): 819–820.

84. Roberts JD, et al. 1992. Inhaled nitric oxide in persistent pulmonary hypertension of the newborn. *Lancet* 340(8823): 818–819.

85. Walsh-Sukys MC, et al. 2000. Persistent pulmonary hypertension of the newborn in the era before nitric oxide: Practice variation and outcomes. *Pediatrics* 105(1 part 1): 14–20.

86. Barefield ES, et al. 1996. Inhaled nitric oxide in term infants with hypoxemic respiratory failure. *Journal of Pediatrics* 129(2): 279–286.

87. Christou H, et al. 2000. Inhaled nitric oxide reduces the need for extracorporeal membrane oxygenation in infants with persistent pulmonary hypertension of the newborn. *Critical Care Medicine* 28(11): 3722–3727.

88. Clark RH, et al. 2000. Low-dose nitric oxide therapy for persistent pulmonary hypertension of the newborn. *New England Journal of Medicine* 342(7): 469–474.

89. Cornfield DN, et al. 1999. Randomized, controlled trial of low-dose inhaled nitric oxide in the treatment of term and near-term infants with respiratory failure and pulmonary hypertension. *Pediatrics* 104(5 part 1): 1089–1094.

90. Davidson D, et al. 1998. Inhaled nitric oxide for the early treatment of persistent pulmonary hypertension of the term newborn: A randomized, double-masked, placebo-controlled, dose-response, multicenter study. *Pediatrics* 101(3 part 1): 325–334.

91. Day RW, et al. 1996. Acute response to inhaled nitric oxide in newborns with respiratory failure and pulmonary hypertension. *Pediatrics* 98(4 part 1): 698–705.

92. Franco-Belgium Collaborative NO Trial Group. 1999. Early compared with delayed inhaled nitric oxide in moderately hypoxaemic neonates with respiratory failure: A randomised controlled trial. *Lancet* 354(9184): 1066–1071. (Published erratum in *Lancet*, 1999, 354[9192]: 1826.)

93. Kinsella JP, et al. 1997. Randomized, multicenter trial of inhaled nitric oxide and high-frequency oscillatory ventilation in severe, persistent pulmonary hypertension of the newborn. *Journal of Pediatrics* 131(1 part 1): 55–62.

94. Neonatal Inhaled Nitric Oxide Study Group. 1997. Inhaled nitric oxide in full-term and nearly full-term infants with hypoxic respiratory failure. *New England Journal of Medicine* 336(9): 597–604. (Published erratum in *New England Journal of Medicine*, 1997, 337[6]: 434.)

95. Neonatal Inhaled Nitric Oxide Study Group. 1997. Inhaled nitric oxide and hypoxic respiratory failure in infants with congenital diaphragmatic hernia. *Pediatrics* 99(6): 838–845.

96. Roberts JD, et al. 1997. Inhaled nitric oxide and persistent pulmonary hypertension of the newborn. *New England Journal of Medicine* 336(9): 605–610.

97. Wessel DL, et al. 1997. Improved oxygenation in a randomized trial of inhaled nitric oxide for persistent pulmonary hypertension of the newborn. *Pediatrics* 100(5): e7.

98. Neonatal Inhaled Nitric Oxide Study Group. 2000. Inhaled nitric oxide in term and near-term infants: Neurodevelopmental follow-up of the Neonatal Inhaled Nitric Oxide Study Group (NINOS). *Journal of Pediatrics* 136(5): 611–617.

99. Konduri GG, et al. 2004. A randomized trial of early versus standard inhaled nitric oxide therapy in term and near-term newborn infants with hypoxic respiratory failure. *Pediatrics* 113(3 part 1): 559–564.

100. Sadiq HF. 1998. Treatment of persistent pulmonary hypertension of the newborn with nitric oxide: A randomized trial. *Pediatric Research* 43: 192A.

101. Finer NN, and Barrington KJ. 2006. Nitric oxide for respiratory failure in infants born at or near term. *Cochrane Database of Systematic Reviews* (2): CD000399.

102. Tworetzky W, et al. 2001. Inhaled nitric oxide in neonates with persistent pulmonary hypertension. *Lancet* 357(9250): 118–120.

103. Finer NN, et al. 2001. Randomized, prospective study of low-dose versus high-dose inhaled nitric oxide in the neonate with hypoxic respiratory failure. *Pediatrics* 108(4): 949–955.

104. Konduri GG, et al. 2007. Inhaled nitric oxide for term and near term newborn infants with hypoxic respiratory failure: Neurodevelopmental follow-up. *Journal of Pediatrics* 150(3): 235–240.

105. Sadiq HF, et al. 2003. Inhaled nitric oxide in the treatment of moderate persistent pulmonary hypertension of the newborn: A randomized controlled, multicenter trial. *Journal of Perinatology* 23(2): 98–103.

106. Okuyama H, et al. 2002. Inhaled nitric oxide with early surgery improves the outcome of antenatally diagnosed congenital diaphragmatic hernia. *Journal of Pediatric Surgery* 37(8): 1188–1190.

107. Sebald M, et al. 2004. Risk of need for extracorporeal membrane oxygenation support in neonates with congenital diaphragmatic hernia treated with inhaled nitric oxide. *Journal of Perinatology* 24(3): 143–146.

108. Kinsella JP, et al. 2003. Noninvasive delivery of inhaled nitric oxide therapy for late pulmonary hypertension in newborn infants with congenital diaphragmatic hernia. *Journal of Pediatrics* 142(4): 397–401.

109. Hoehn T, Krause M, and Hentschel R. 1998. High-frequency ventilation augments the effect of inhaled nitric oxide in persistent pulmonary hypertension of the newborn. *European Respiratory Journal* 11(1): 234–238.

110. Kinsella JP, and Abman SH. 1998. Inhaled nitric oxide and high frequency oscillatory ventilation in persistent pulmonary hypertension of the newborn. *European Journal of Pediatrics* 157(supplement 1): S28–S30.

111. Gupta A, et al. 2002. Inhaled nitric oxide and gentle ventilation in the treatment of pulmonary hypertension of the newborn—A single-center, 5-year experience. *Journal of Perinatology* 22(6): 435–441.

112. Rosenberg AA, et al. 1997. Longitudinal follow-up of a cohort of newborn infants treated with inhaled nitric oxide for persistent pulmonary hypertension. *Journal of Pediatrics* 131(1 part 1): 70–75.

113. Ellington, M, et al. 2001. Child health status, neurodevelopmental outcome, and parental satisfaction in a randomized, controlled trial of nitric oxide for persistent pulmonary hypertension of the newborn. *Pediatrics.* 107(6): 1351–1356.

114. Lipkin, PH, et al. 2002. Neurodevelopmental and medical outcomes of persistent pulmonary hypertension in term newborns treated with nitric oxide. *Journal of Pediatrics* 140(3): 306–310.

115. Clark RH, et al. 2003. Low-dose nitric oxide therapy for persistent pulmonary hypertension: 1-year follow-up. *Journal of Perinatology* 23(4): 300–303.

116. Halliday H, et al. 1977. Respiratory distress syndrome: Echocardiographic assessment of cardiovascular function and pulmonary vascular resistence. *Pediatrics* 60(4): 444–449.

117. Walther FJ, Benders MJ, and Leighton JO. 1992. Persistent pulmonary hypertension in premature neonates with severe respiratory distress syndrome. *Pediatrics* 90(6): 899–904.

118. Golan A, et al. 1995. Pulmonary hypertension in respiratory distress syndrome. *Pediatric Pulmonology* 19(4): 221–225.

119. Barrington KJ, and Finer NN. 2010. Inhaled nitric oxide for respiratory failure in preterm infants. *Cochrane Database of Systematic Reviews* (1): CD000509.

120. Ballard RA, et al. 2006. Inhaled nitric oxide in preterm infants undergoing mechanical ventilation. *New England Journal of Medicine* 355(4): 343–353.

121. Kinsella JP, et al. 1999. Inhaled nitric oxide in premature neonates with severe hypoxaemic respiratory failure: A randomised controlled trial. *Lancet* 354(9184): 1061–1065.

122. Mestan KKL, et al. 2005. Neurodevelopmental outcomes of premature infants treated with inhaled nitric oxide. *New England Journal of Medicine*, 353(1): 23–32.

123. Field D, et al. 2005. Neonatal ventilation with inhaled nitric oxide versus ventilator support without inhaled nitric oxide for preterm infants with severe respiratory failure: The INNOVO multicentre randomized controlled trial (ISRCTN 17821339). *Pediatrics* 115(4): 926–936.

124. Bennett AJ, et al. 2001. Neurodevelopmental outcome in high-risk preterm infants treated with inhaled nitric oxide. *Acta Paediatrica* 90(5): 573–576.

125. Subhedar NV, Ryan SW, and Shaw NJ. 1997. Open randomised controlled trial of inhaled nitric oxide and early dexamethasone in high risk preterm infants. *Archives of Disease in Childhood. Fetal and Neonatal Edition* 77(3): F185–F190.

126. Jobe AH, and Bancalari E. 2001. Bronchopulmonary dysplasia. *American Journal of Respiratory and Critical Care Medicine* 163(7): 1723–1729.

127. Clark PL, et al. 2002. Safety and efficacy of nitric oxide in chronic lung disease. *Archives of Disease in Childhood. Fetal and Neonatal Edition* 86(1): F41–F45.

128. Sessons F. 2011. NIH Consensus Development Conference statement: Inhaled nitric oxide therapy for premature infants. *Pediatrics* 127(2): 363–369.

129. Mestan KK, et al. 2003. Cardiopulmonary effects of nebulized sodium nitroprusside in term infants with hypoxic respiratory failure. *Journal of Pediatrics* 143(5): 640–643.

130. McCaffrey MJ, et al. 1995. Effects of L-arginine infusion on infants with persistent pulmonary hypertension of the newborn. *Biology of the Neonate* 67(4): 240–243.

131. Saidy K, and al-Alaiyan S. 2001. The use of L-arginine [correction of F-arginine] and phosphodiesterase inhibitor (dipyridamole) to wean from inhaled nitric oxide. *Indian Journal of Pediatrics* 68(2): 175–177.

132. Schreiber MD, et al. 2002. Direct comparison of the effects of nebulized nitroprusside versus inhaled nitric oxide on pulmonary and systemic hemodynamics during hypoxia-induced pulmonary hypertension in piglets. *Critical Care Medicine* 30(11): 2560–2565.

133. Konduri GG, et al. 1996. Adenosine infusion improves oxygenation in term infants with respiratory failure. *Pediatrics* 97(3): 295–300.

134. Travadi JN, and Patole SK. 2003. Phosphodiesterase inhibitors for persistent pulmonary hypertension of the newborn: A review. *Pediatric Pulmonology* 36(6): 529–535.

135. Weinberger B, et al. 2001. Pharmacologic therapy of persistent pulmonary hypertension of the newborn. *Pharmacology & Therapeutics* 89(1): 67–79.

136. Abman SH, and Stenmark KR. 1992. Changes in lung eicosanoid content during normal and abnormal transition in perinatal lambs. *American Journal of Physiology* 262(2 part 1): L214–L222.

137. Kelly LK, et al. 2002. Inhaled prostacyclin for term infants with persistent pulmonary hypertension refractory to inhaled nitric oxide. *Journal of Pediatrics* 141(6): 830–832.

138. Rose F, et al. 1999. Prostacyclin enhances stretch-induced surfactant secretion in alveolar epithelial type II cells. *American Journal of Respiratory and Critical Care Medicine* 160(3): 846–851.

139. Pearson DL, et al. 2001. Neonatal pulmonary hypertension—Urea-cycle intermediates, nitric oxide production, and carbamoyl-phosphate synthetase function. *New England Journal of Medicine* 344(24): 1832–1838.

140. Schulze-Neick I, et al. 1999. L-arginine and substance P reverse the pulmonary endothelial dysfunction caused by congenital heart surgery. *Circulation* 100(7): 749–755.

141. Feelisch M. 1991. The biochemical pathways of nitric oxide formation from nitrovasodilators: Appropriate choice of exogenous NO donors and aspects of preparation and handling of aqueous NO solutions. *Journal of Cardiovascular Pharmacology* 17(supplement 3): S25–S33.

142. Ignarro LJ, Napoli C, and Loscalzo J. 2002. Nitric oxide donors and cardiovascular agents modulating the bioactivity of nitric oxide: An overview. *Circulation Research* 90(1): 21–28.

143. Meadow W, et al. 1998. Effects of nebulized nitroprusside on pulmonary and systemic hemodynamics during pulmonary hypertension in piglets. *Pediatric Research* 44(2): 181–186.

144. Palhares DB, Figueiredo CS, and Moura AJ. 1998. Endotracheal inhalatory sodium nitroprusside in severely hypoxic newborns. *Journal of Perinatal Medicine* 26(3): 219–224.

145. Bakshi F, Barzilay Z, and Paret G. 1998. Adenosine in the diagnosis and treatment of narrow complex tachycardia in the pediatric intensive care unit. *Heart and Lung* 27(1): 47–50.

146. Utterback DB, et al. 1994. Basis for the selective reduction of pulmonary vascular resistance in humans during infusion of adenosine. *Journal of Applied Physiology* 76(2): 724–730.

147. McCormack DG, Clarke B, and Barnes PJ. 1989. Characterization of adenosine receptors in human pulmonary arteries. *American Journal of Physiology* 256(1 part 2): H41–H46.

148. Steinhorn RH, et al. 1994. Endothelium-dependent relaxations to adenosine in juvenile rabbit pulmonary arteries and veins. *American Journal of Physiology* 266(5 part 2): H2001–H2006.

149. Patole S, et al 1998. Improved oxygenation following adenosine infusion in persistent pulmonary hypertension of the newborn. *Biology of the Neonate* 74(5): 345–350.

150. Ng C, et al. 2004. Adenosine infusion for the management of persistent pulmonary hypertension of the newborn. *Pediatric Critical Care Medicine* 5(1): 10–13.

151. Essayan DM. 2001. Cyclic nucleotide phosphodiesterases. *Journal of Allergy and Clinical Immunology* 108(5): 671–680.

152. Beavo JA. 1995. Cyclic nucleotide phosphodiesterases: Functional implications of multiple isoforms. *Physiological Reviews* 75(4): 725–748.

153. Dukarm RC, et al. 1998. Pulmonary and systemic effects of the phosphodiesterase inhibitor dipyridamole in newborn lambs with persistent pulmonary hypertension. *Pediatric Research* 44(6): 831–837.

154. Foubert L, et al. 2002. Intravenous dipyridamole enhances the effects of inhaled nitric oxide and prevents rebound pulmonary hypertension in piglets. *Pediatric Research* 52(5): 730–736.

155. Kinsella JP, et al. 1995. Dipyridamole augmentation of response to nitric oxide. *Lancet* 346(8975): 647–648.

156. Thebaud B, et al. 1999. Dipyridamole, a cGMP phosphodiesterase inhibitor, transiently improves the response to inhaled nitric oxide in two newborns with congenital diaphragmatic hernia. *Intensive Care Medicine* 25(3): 300–303.

157. Buysee C, et al. 2001. The use of dipyridamole to wean from inhaled nitric oxide in congenital diaphragmatic hernia. *Journal of Pediatric Surgery* 36(12): 1864–1865.

158. Stocker C, et al. 2003. Intravenous sildenafil and inhaled nitric oxide: A randomised trial in infants after cardiac surgery. *Intensive Care Medicine* 29(11): 1996–2003.

159. Azt AM, and Wessel DL. 1999. Sildenafil ameliorates effects of inhaled nitric oxide withdrawal. *Anesthesiology* 90(1): 307–310.

160. Shekerdemian LS, Ravn HB, and Penny DJ. 2002. Intravenous sildenafil lowers pulmonary vascular resistance in a model of neonatal pulmonary hypertension. *American Journal of Respiratory and Critical Care Medicine* 165(8): 1098–1102.

161. Ichinose F, et al. 2001. Nebulized sildenafil is a selective pulmonary vasodilator in lambs with acute pulmonary hypertension. *Critical Care Medicine* 29(5): 1000–1005.

162. Marsh CS, Marden B, and Newsom R. 2004. Severe retinopathy of prematurity (ROP) in a premature baby treated with sildenafil acetate (Viagra) for pulmonary hypertension. *British Journal of Ophthalmology* 88(2): 306–307.

163. Lauterbach R. 1993. Pentoxifylline treatment of persistent pulmonary hypertension of the newborn. *European Journal of Pediatrics* 152(5): 460.

164. Lauterbach R, and Szymura-Oleksiak J. 1999. Nebulized pentoxifylline in successful treatment of five premature neonates with bronchopulmonary dysplasia. *European Journal of Pediatrics* 158(7): 607.

165. Ichinose F, et al. 1995. Prolonged pulmonary vasodilator action of inhaled nitric oxide by zaprinast in awake lambs. *Journal of Applied Physiology* 78(4): 1288–1295.

166. Thusu KG, et al. 1995. The cGMP phosphodiesterase inhibitor zaprinast enhances the effect of nitric oxide. *American Journal of Respiratory and Critical Care Medicine* 152(5 part 1): 1605–1610.

167. Steinhorn RH, Gordon JB, and Tod ML. 2000. Site-specific effect of guanosine 3',5'-cyclic monophosphate phosphodiesterase inhibition in isolated lamb lungs. *Critical Care Medicine* 28(2): 490–495.

168. Nagamine J, Hill LL, and Pearl RG. 2000. Combined therapy with zaprinast and inhaled nitric oxide abolishes hypoxic pulmonary hypertension. *Critical Care Medicine* 28(7): 2420–2424.

169. Ichinose F, Adrie C, Hurford WE, Bloch KD, and Zapol WM. 1998. Selective pulmonary vasodilation induced by aerosolized zaprinast. *Anesthesiology* 88(2): 410–416.

170. Shaul PW. 1999. Regulation of vasodilator synthesis during lung development. *Early Human Development* 54(3): 271–294.

171. Vane JR. 1983. Nobel lecture. Adventures and excursions in bioassay— The stepping stones to prostacyclin. *Postgraduate Medical Journal* 59(698): 743–758.

172. Leffler CW, Tyler TL, and Cassin S. 1978. Effect of indomethacin on pulmonary vascular response to ventilation of fetal goats. *American Journal of Physiology* 234(4): H346–H351.

173. Badesch DB, et al. 1989. Decreased arterial wall prostaglandin production in neonatal calves with severe chronic pulmonary hypertension. *American Journal of Respiratory Cell and Molecular Biology* 1(6): 489–498.

174. Aschner JL. 2004. New therapies for pulmonary hypertension in neonates and children. *Pediatric Pulmonology* 37(supplement 26): S132–S135.

175. Ehlen M, and Wiebe B. 2003. Iloprost in persistent pulmonary hypertension of the newborn. *Cardiology in the Young* 13(4): 361–363.

176. De Jaegere AP, and van den Anker JN. 1998. Endotracheal instillation of prostacyclin in preterm infants with persistent pulmonary hypertension. *European Respiratory Journal* 12(4): 932–934.

177. Suzuki H, et al. 2002. Beraprost sodium for pulmonary hypertension with congenital heart disease. *Pediatrics International* 44(5): 528–529.

178. Jobe AH. 2004. Postnatal corticosteroids for preterm infants—Do what we say, not what we do. *New England Journal of Medicine* 350(13): 1349–1351.

179. St. John EB, and Carlo WA. 2003. Respiratory distress syndrome in VLBW infants: Changes in management and outcomes observed by the NICHD Neonatal Research Network. *Seminars in Perinatology* 27(4): 288–292.

180. Liggins GC, and Howie RN. 1972. A controlled trial of antepartum glucocorticoid treatment for prevention of the respiratory distress syndrome in premature infants. *Pediatrics* 50(4): 515–525.

181. Block MF, Kling OR, and Crosby WM. 1977. Antenatal glucocorticoid therapy for the prevention of respiratory distress syndrome in the premature infant. *Obstetrics & Gynecology* 50(2): 186–190.

182. Taeusch HW Jr, et al. 1979. Risk of respiratory distress syndrome after prenatal dexamethasone treatment. *Pediatrics* 63(1): 64–72.

183. Doran TA, et al. 1980. Results of a double-blind controlled study on the use of betamethasone in the prevention of respiratory distress syndrome. *American Journal of Obstetrics and Gynecology* 136(3): 313–320.

184. Schutte MF, et al. 1980. The influence of betamethasone and orciprenaline on the incidence of respiratory distress syndrome in the newborn after preterm labour. *British Journal of Obstetrics and Gynaecology* 87(2): 127–131.

185. Teramo K, Hallman M, and Raivio KO. 1980. Maternal glucocorticoid in unplanned premature labor. Controlled study on the effects of betamethasone phosphate on the phospholipids of the gastric aspirate and on the adrenal cortical function of the newborn infant. *Pediatric Research* 14(4 part 1): 326–329.

186. Collaborative Group on Antenatal Steroid Therapy. 1984. Effects of antenatal dexamethasone administration in the infant: Long-term follow-up. *Journal of Pediatrics* 104(2): 259–267.

187. Nelson LH, et al. 1985. Premature rupture of membranes: A prospective, randomized evaluation of steroids, latent phase, and expectant management. *Obstetrics & Gynecology* 66(1): 55–58.

188. Parsons MT, et al. 1988. Steroid, antibiotic and tocolytic versus no steroids, antibiotic and tocolytic management in patients with preterm PROM at 25–32 weeks. Proceedings of the 8th Annual Meeting of the Society of Perinatal Obstetricians, Las Vegas 44: 4432.

189. Gamsu HR, et al. 1989. Antenatal administration of betamethasone to prevent respiratory distress syndrome in preterm infants: Report of a UK multicentre trial. *British Journal of Obstetrics and Gynaecology* 96(4): 401–410.

190. Morales WJ, et al. 1989. Use of ampicillin and corticosteroids in premature rupture of membranes: a randomized study. *Obstetrics & Gynecology* 73(5 part 1): 721–726.

191. Cararach V, et al. 1990. A multicentric prospective randomized study in premature rupture of membranes (PROM). Respiratory and infectious complications in the newborn. Proceedings of 12th European Congress of Perinatal Medicine, September 11–14, Lyon, France, 216.

192. Carlan SJ, et al. 1991. Pharmacologic pulmonary maturation study in preterm premature rupture of membranes. *American Journal of Obstetrics and Gynecology* 164(1 part 2): 371A.

193. Garite TJ, et al. 1992. A randomized, placebo-controlled trial of betamethasone for the prevention of respiratory distress syndrome at 24 to 28 weeks gestation. *American Journal of Obstetrics and Gynecology* 166(2): 646–651.

194. Kari MA, et al. 1994. Prenatal dexamethasone treatment in conjunction with rescue therapy of human surfactant: A randomized placebo-controlled multicenter study. *Pediatrics* 93(5): 730–736.

195. Lewis DF, et al. 1996. Preterm premature ruptured membranes: A randomized trial of steroids after treatment with antibiotics. *Obstetrics & Gynecology* 88(5): 801–805.

196. Silver RK, et al. 1996. Randomized trial of antenatal dexamethasone in surfactant-treated infants delivered before 30 weeks' gestation. *Obstetrics & Gynecology* 87(5 part 1): 683–691.

197. Amorian MM, Santos LC, and Faundes A. 1999. Corticosteroid therapy for prevention of respiratory distress syndrome in severe preeclampsia. *American Journal of Obstetrics and Gynecology* 180(5): 1283–1288.

198. Pattinson RC, et al. 1999. The use of dexamethasone in women with preterm premature rupture of membranes—a multicentre, double-blind, placebo-controlled, randomised trial. Dexiprom Study Group. *South African Medical Journal* 89(8): 865–870.

199. Qublan HS, et al. 2001. The effect of antenatal corticosteroid therapy on pregnancies complicated by premature rupture of membranes. *Clinical & Experimental Obstetrics & Gynecology* 28(3): 183–186.

200. Fekih M, et al. 2002. Value of prenatal corticotherapy in the prevention of hyaline membrane disease in premature infants. *Tunisie Medicale* 80(5): 260–265.

201. National Institutes of Health. 1994. Report of the Consensus Development Conference on the effect of corticosteroids for fetal maturation on perinatal outcomes. *NIH Consensus Statement* 12(2): 1–24.

202. Roberts D, and Dalziel S. 2006. Antenatal corticosteroids for accelerating fetal lung maturation for women at risk of preterm birth. *Cochrane Database of Systematic Reviews* (3): CD004454.

203. Baud O. 2004. Antenatal corticosteroid therapy: Benefits and risks. *Acta Paediatrica* 93(444 Supplement): 6–10.

204. Crowley PA. 1995. Antenatal corticosteroid therapy: A meta-analysis of the randomized trials, 1972 to 1994. *American Journal of Obstetrics and Gynecology* 173(1): 322–335.

205. Ballard PL, and Ballard RA. 1995. Scientific basis and therapeutic regimens for use of antenatal glucocorticoids. *American Journal of Obstetrics and Gynecology* 173(1): 254–262.

206. Christensen HD, Sienko AE, Rayburn WF, Gonzalez CL, and Coleman FH. 1997. A placebo-controlled, blinded comparison between betamethasone and dexamethasone to enhance lung maturation in the fetal mouse. *Journal of the Society for Gynecologic Investigation* 4(3): 130–134.

207. Baud O, et al. 1999. Antenatal glucocorticoid treatment and cystic periventricular leukomalacia in very premature infants. *New England Journal of Medicine* 341(16): 1190–1196.

208. Baud O, et al. 2001. Neurotoxic effects of fluorinated glucocorticoid preparations on the developing mouse brain: Role of preservatives. *Pediatric Research* 50(6): 706–711.

209. Jazayeri A, Gevrila B, and Sincich T. 2001. Repeated antenatal corticosteroid treatments: Do they reduce neonatal morbidity? *Journal of Reproductive Medicine* 46(9): 788–790.

210. Banks BA, et al. 1999. Multiple courses of antenatal corticosteroids (ANCS): Association with increased mortality and early severe lung disease (ESLD) in preterm neonates. *Pediatrics* 104(3 part 3): 739A.

211. Thorp JA, et al. 2002. Does antenatal corticosteroid therapy affect birth weight and head circumference? *Obstetrics & Gynecology* 99(1): 101–108.

212. Thorp JA, et al. 2002. Effect of antenatal and postnatal corticosteroid therapy on weight gain and head circumference growth in the nursery. *Obstetrics & Gynecology* 99(1): 109–115.

213. Schaap AH, et al. 2001. Effects of antenatal corticosteroid administration on mortality and long-term morbidity in early preterm, growth restricted infants. *Obstetrics & Gynecology* 97(6): 954–960.

214. Halliday HL, Ehrenkranz RA, and Doyle LW. 2009. Delayed (>7 days) postnatal corticosteroids for chronic lung disease in preterm infants. *Cochrane Database of Systematic Reviews* (1): CD001145.

215. Halliday HL, Ehrenkranz RA, and Doyle LW. 2008. Moderately early (7–14 days) postnatal corticosteroids for preventing chronic lung disease in preterm infants. *Cochrane Database of Systematic Reviews* (4): CD001144.

216. Halliday HL, Ehrenkranz RA, and Doyle LW. 2010. Early (<8 days) postnatal corticosteroids for preventing chronic lung disease in preterm infants. *Cochrane Database of Systematic Reviews* (1): CD001146.

217. Barrington KJ. 2001. The adverse neuro-developmental effects of postnatal steroids in the preterm infant: A systematic review of RCTs. *BioMed Central Pediatrics* 1(1): 1. Retrieved August 14, 2004, from www.biomedcentral.com/1471-2431/1/1.

218. Yeh TF, Lin YJ, Lin HC, et al. 2004. Outcomes at school age after postnatal dexamethasone therapy for lung disease of prematurity. *New England Journal of Medicine* 350(13): 1304–1313.

219. Yeh TF, et al. 1997. Early postnatal dexamethasone therapy for the prevention of chronic lung disease in preterm infants with respiratory distress syndrome: A multicenter clinical trial. *Pediatrics* 100(4): e3.

220. Shah SS, et al. 2007. Inhaled versus systemic corticosteroids for preventing chronic lung disease in ventilated very low birth weight preterm neonates. *Cochrane Database of Systematic Reviews* (2): CD002058.

221. Shah SS, et al. 2007. Inhaled versus systemic corticosteroids for the treatment of chronic lung disease in ventilated very low birth weight preterm infants. *Cochrane Database of Systematic Reviews* (3): CD00002057.

222. American Academy of Pediatrics, Committee on Fetus and Newborn and Canadian Paediatric Society, Fetus and Newborn Committee. 2002. Postnatal corticosteroids to treat or prevent chronic lung disease in preterm infants. *Pediatrics* 109(2): 330–338.

223. Davis PG, and Henderson-Smart DJ. 2007. Intravenous dexamethasone for extubation of newborn infants. *Cochrane Database of Systematic Reviews* (4): CD000308.

224. Couser RJ, et al. 1992. Effectiveness of dexamethasone in preventing extubation failure in preterm infants at increased risk for airway edema. *Journal of Pediatrics* 121(4): 591–596.

225. Courtney SE, et al. 1992. Effects of dexamethasone on pulmonary function following extubation. *Journal of Perinatology* 12(3): 246–251.

226. Ferrara TB, et al. 1989. Routine use of dexamethasone for the prevention of postextubation respiratory distress. *Journal of Perinatology* 9(3): 287–290.

227. Cleary GM, and Wiswell TE. 1998. Meconium-stained amniotic fluid and the meconium aspiration syndrome: An update. *Pediatric Clinics of North America* 45(3): 511–529.

228. Davey AM, Becker JD, and Davis JM. 1993. Meconium aspiration syndrome: Physiological and inflammatory changes in a newborn piglet model. *Pediatric Pulmonology* 16(2): 101–108.

229. Holopainen R, et al. 1999. Human meconium has high phospholipase A_2 activity and induces cellular injury and apoptosis in piglet lungs. *Pediatric Research* 46(5): 626–632.

230. de Beaufort AJ, et al. 1998. Effect of interleukin 8 in meconium on in-vitro neutrophil chemotaxis. *Lancet* 352(9122): 102–105.

231. Zagariya A, et al. 2000. Cell death and lung cell histology in meconium aspirated newborn rabbit lung. *European Journal of Pediatrics* 159(11): 819–826.

232. Jones CA, et al. 1996. Undetectable interleukin (IL)-10 and persistent IL-8 expression early in hyaline membrane disease: A possible developmental basis for the predisposition to chronic lung inflammation in preterm newborns. *Pediatric Research* 39(6): 966–975.

233. Wiswell TE. 2001. Advances in the treatment of the meconium aspiration syndrome. *Acta Paediatrica* 90(436 supplement): S28–S30.

234. Kääpä P. 2004. Corticosteroid treatment in meconium aspiration syndrome: A solution for better outcome? *Acta Paediatrica* 93(1): 5–7.

235. Ward M, and Sinn J. 2003. Steroid therapy for meconium aspiration syndrome in newborn infants. *Cochrane Database of Systematic Reviews* (4): CD003485.

236. Yeh TF, et al. 1977. Hydrocortisone therapy in meconium aspiration syndrome: A controlled study. *Journal of Pediatrics* 90(1): 140–143.

237. Wu JM, et al. 1999. The role of pulmonary inflammation in the development of pulmonary hypertension in newborn with meconium aspiration syndrome (MAS). *Pediatric Pulmonology* 19(supplement): 205–208.

238. Salvia-Roigés MD, et al. 2004. Efficacy of three treatment schedules in severe meconium aspiration syndrome. *Acta Paediatrica* 93(1): 60–65.

239. Panitch HB. 2003. Respiratory syncytial virus bronchiolitis: Supportive care and therapies designed to overcome airway obstruction. *Pediatric Infectious Disease Journal* 22(2 supplement): S83–S88.

240. Buckingham SC, et al. 2002. A randomized, double-blind, placebo-controlled trial of dexamethasone in severe respiratory syncytial virus (RSV) infection: Effects on RSV quantity and clinical outcome. *Journal of Infectious Disease* 185(9): 1222–1228.

241. Garrison MM, et al. 2000. Systemic corticosteroids in infant bronchiolitis: A meta-analysis. *Pediatrics* 105(4): e44.

242. Patel H, Platt R, and Lozono JM. 2004. Glucocorticoids for acute viral bronchiolitis in infants and young children. *Cochrane Database of Systematic Reviews* (1): CD004878.

243. American Academy of Pediatrics, Committee on Infectious Diseases. 2003. Respiratory syncytial virus. In *Red Book: The 2003 Report of the Committee on Infectious Disease*, 26th ed., Pickering LK, ed. Elk Grove Village, Illinois: American Academy of Pediatrics, 523–528.

244. Barrington KJ. 2001. Postnatal steroids and neurodevelopmental outcomes: A problem in the making. *Pediatrics* 107(6): 1425–1426.

245. Finer NN, et al. 2000. Postnatal steroids: Short-term gain, long-term pain? *Journal of Pediatrics* 137(1): 9–13.

246. Ng GYT, da Silva O, and Ohlsson A. 2006. Bronchodilators for the prevention and treatment of chronic lung disease in preterm infants. *Cochrane Database of Systematic Reviews* (2): CD003214.

247. Denjean A, et al. 1998. Inhaled salbutamol and beclomethasone for preventing broncho-pulmonary dysplasia: A randomised double-blind study. *European Journal of Pediatrics* 157(11): 926–931.

248. Fok TF, et al. 1998. Randomised crossover trial of salbutamol aerosol delivered by metered dose inhaler, jet nebuliser, and ultrasonic nebuliser in chronic lung disease. *Archives of Disease in Childhood. Fetal and Neonatal Edition* 79(2): F100–F104.

249. Kao LC, et al. 1984. Effect of isoproterenol inhalation on airway resistance in chronic bronchopulmonary dysplasia. *Pediatrics* 73(4): 509–514.

250. Kao LC, Durand DJ, and Nickerson BG. 1989. Effects of inhaled metaproterenol and atropine on the pulmonary mechanics of infants with bronchopulmonary dysplasia. *Pediatric Pulmonology* 6(2): 74–80.

251. Sosulski R, et al. 1986. Physiologic effects of terbutaline on pulmonary function of infants with bronchopulmonary dysplasia. *Pediatric Pulmonology* 2(5): 269–273.

252. Henry RL, et al. 1984. Nebulised ipratropium bromide and sodium cromoglycate in the first two years of life. *Archives of Disease in Childhood* 59(1): 54–57.

253. Mallol J, et al. 1987. Use of nebulized brochodilators in infants under 1 year of age: Analysis of four forms of therapy. *Pediatric Pulmonology* 3(5): 298–303.

254. Mallol J, et al. 1987. Bronchodilator effect of fenoterol and ipratropium bromide in infants with acute wheezing: Use of MDI with a spacer device. *Pediatric Pulmonology* 3(5): 352–356.

255. Wang EE, et al. 1992. Bronchodilators for treatment of mild bronchiolitis: A factorial randomised trial. *Archives of Disease in Childhood* 67(3): 289–293.

256. Naspitz CK, and Sole D. 1992. Treatment of acute wheezing and dyspnea attacks in children under 2 years old: Inhalation of fenoterol plus ipratropium bromide versus fenoterol. *Journal of Asthma* 29(4): 253–258.

257. Schuh S, et al. 1992. Efficacy of adding nebulized ipratropium bromide to nebulized albuterol therapy in acute bronchiolitis. *Pediatrics* 90(6): 920–923.

258. Everard ML, et al. 2008. Anticholinergic drugs for wheeze in children under the age of two years. *Cochrane Database of Systematic Reviews* (2): CD001279.

259. Dolovich M. 1999. Aerosol delivery to children: What to use, how to choose. *Pediatric Pulmonology* 18(supplement): 79–82.

260. Labiris NR, and Dolovich MB. 2003. Pulmonary drug delivery. Part II: The role of inhalant delivery devices and drug formulations in therapeutic effectiveness of aerosolized medications. *British Journal of Clinical Pharmacology* 56(6): 600–612.

261. Cole CH. 2000. Special problems in aerosol delivery: Neonatal and pediatric considerations. *Respiratory Care* 45(6): 646–651.

262. Lugo RA, et al. 2001. Albuterol delivery in a neonatal ventilated lung model: Nebulization versus chlorofluorocarbon- and hydrofluoroalkane-pressurized metered dose inhalers. *Pediatric Pulmonology* 31(3): 247–254.

263. Shirkey H. 1999. Therapeutic orphans. *Pediatrics* 104(3 part 2): 583–584.

264. INO Therapeutics. 2001. INOmax (nitric oxide) for inhalation. Manufacturer's product literature. Clinton, New Jersey. Retrieved February 13, 2004, from www.inotherapeutics.com/assets/package_insert/package_insert_1.htm.

265. American Academy of Pediatrics, Committee on Fetus and Newborn. 2000. Use of inhaled nitric oxide. *Pediatrics* 106(2 part 1): 344–345.

266. Moncada S, and Higgs A. 1993. The L-arginine–nitric oxide pathway. *New England Journal of Medicine* 329(27): 2002–2012.

267. Sokol GM, et al. 2001. Changes in arterial oxygen tension when weaning neonates from inhaled nitric oxide. *Pediatric Pulmonology* 32(1): 14–19.

268. Carriedo H, and Rhine W. 2003. Withdrawal of inhaled nitric oxide from nonresponders after short exposure. *Journal of Perinatology* 23(7): 556–558.

NOTES

12 High-Frequency Ventilation: The Current Challenge to Neonatal Nursing

Debbie Fraser, MN, RNC-NIC

Since the late 1970s, conventional mechanical ventilation (CMV) has been used with increasing success to treat infants suffering from a variety of cardiorespiratory diseases.[1] The addition of surfactant therapy has further increased survival rates and lessened morbidity.[2] Although death occurs in fewer and fewer patients, complications such as bronchopulmonary dysplasia (BPD, defined as oxygen need at 36 weeks postmenstrual age) and pulmonary air leak syndrome may occur in some survivors. BPD is estimated to occur in 30 percent of infants with birth weights <1,000 g.[3] These complications have been attributed to oxygen toxicity, barotrauma, volutrauma, lung immaturity, inflammation, and infection.[4]

In an attempt to avoid damaging the newborn infant's fragile alveoli, researchers and clinicians have sought a method of ventilation that uses smaller tidal volumes and lower pressures than traditional time-cycled, pressure-limited conventional ventilation. High-frequency ventilation (HFV) is such a method.[5] This chapter presents an overview of HFV and the nursing management and care of infants receiving this therapy.

High-frequency ventilation is a type of mechanical ventilation that uses small tidal volumes at rates of at least 150 breaths per minute.[5] The respiratory frequencies (breaths or cycles) generally range from 300 breaths per minute or 5 Hertz (Hz) to 900 breaths per minute or 15 Hz.[6]

Since the late 1980s, HFV has become an increasingly popular method of providing respiratory support to infants with severe lung disease.[7] Data from neonates enrolled in the Vermont Oxford database reveal that, since 1996, more than 25 percent of infants born weighing <1,500 g have been treated with HFV.[8] Use of HFV has expanded from experimental therapy in a few nurseries to a common means of respiratory support in a number of countries.

With HFV, respiratory gas flow and support of oxygenation and ventilation can be provided by various systems, including jet impulse and bias flow oscillations by piston or diaphragm drivers.[9,10] Currently, the U.S. Food and Drug Administration (FDA) has approved two devices for providing HFV to neonates in the U.S.[11] These are the Bunnell Life Pulse high-frequency jet ventilator (HFJV) (Bunnell Inc., Salt Lake City, Utah) and the SensorMedics 3100A high-frequency oscillatory ventilator (HFOV) (SensorMedics, Inc., Yorba Linda, California). In Canada and the United Kingdom, the Dräger Babylog HFOV (Dräger Medical, Lübeck, Germany) is also used. HFV has influenced neonatal nursing care since its introduction and continues to do so.[12–14]

A Physiologic Framework

Despite having been studied for decades, HFV is a phenomenon that is still being described and explored. A framework for understanding this modality is established first by addressing how conventional ventilation works and what concepts from CMV are also used to support respiratory gas exchange during HFV. Then the unique concepts that make HFV work for the infant with lung disease are discussed.

Conventional Mechanical Ventilation

The CMV device supports gas exchange by mimicking many normal physiologic processes. Fresh gas is

FIGURE 12-1
CO$_2$ elimination equation.

CO$_2$ Elimination:

- CMV: $\dot{V}CO_2 = V_T \times f$
- HFV: $\dot{V}CO_2 = (V_T)^a \times f^b$
  a = 1.5–2.2
  b = 0.5–1

f = frequency, V$_T$ = Tidal volume
$\dot{V}CO_2$ = volume of CO$_2$ per unit of time

Adapted from: Clark R. 1994. High frequency ventilation. *Journal of Pediatrics* 124(5): 661–670; and Fredberg JJ. 1989. Summary: Pulmonary mechanics during high frequency ventilation. *Acta Anesthesiology Scandinavica* (90 supplement): 170–171. Reprinted by permission.

FIGURE 12-2
Pendelluft.

Representation of interregional gas mixing caused by different time constants in two lung units. The fast (1) time constant unit can be seen to be filling at end expiration. The slow (2) time constant unit fills at the end of inspiration. Tracheal flow is zero at this time, and this effect thus augments alveolar tidal volume.

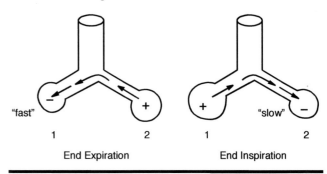

"fast"   +   +   "slow" –
  1   2   1   2

End Expiration   End Inspiration

From: Wetzel RC, and Gioia FR. 1987. High frequency ventilation. *Pediatric Clinics of North America* 34(1): 20. Reprinted by permission.

delivered to the lungs as bulk flow in tidal volumes much greater (>6–8 mL/kg) than anatomic dead space (ADS). During inspiration, positive pressure is used to force bulk gas flow through the larger airways. Gas moves through the smaller airways and to the alveolar region mostly by passive diffusion. Varying amounts of positive end-expiratory pressure (PEEP) are used to prevent airway and alveolar collapse (see Chapter 7).

Oxygenation during CMV depends mostly on the amount of ambient oxygen (FiO$_2$) and the mean airway pressure (Paw) used to deliver the gas.[15,16] The effect of Paw on oxygenation may be related to enhanced alveolar recruitment and stabilization, creating an optimal lung volume.[9,17] Carbon dioxide (CO$_2$) elimination during CMV is dependent upon alveolar ventilation, which is the product of tidal volume (minus dead space) and respiratory frequency.[17]

Exhalation during CMV is a passive event occurring by the natural recoil of the chest. The time necessary to deflate (or inflate) the lung is known as the *time constant*. It takes three to five time constants for the lung to empty to its functional residual capacity (FRC). If the time allowed for exhalation is shorter than the time constant, gas trapping will occur, leading to alveolar distention and impaired carbon dioxide elimination.[18,19]

HIGH-FREQUENCY VENTILATION

During HFV, respiratory gas exchange can be explained by a combination of traditional gas exchange concepts (bulk flow) described previously and unique concepts (mixing) described below.[6,20] As in CMV, oxygenation during HFV depends on Paw and ambient FiO$_2$.[21] The Paw used to support the lung volume may be higher or lower than that required during CMV,

depending upon the device and where the pressure is measured. Raising the Paw with HFV may lead to an increase in lung volumes.[6] The key is having optimal lung volumes for the disease state being treated.[22]

By using a combination of bulk flow and mixing, HFV can be very effective in eliminating carbon dioxide. Tidal volume and respiratory frequency influence the rate of carbon dioxide elimination. This relationship is illustrated in Figure 12-1. Small changes in the volume of gas delivered during HFV can produce large changes in carbon dioxide removal.[6] This makes careful monitoring of CO$_2$ during HFV imperative.

As with CMV, tidal volume delivery for all HFV devices is sensitive to lung compliance and resistance. For HFJV devices (such as the Bunnell Life Pulse), tidal volume change is generally related to amplitude or ΔP (peak inspiratory pressure [PIP] – PEEP) as long as the inspiratory time does not vary. For HFV devices, effective oxygenation requires an adequate FRC and an optimal lung volume.[23–26]

Another important factor affecting CO$_2$ elimination is gas trapping in the lung. To reduce the risk of gas trapping, there must be sufficient time for exhalation, and lung overinflation must be avoided.[19] All HFV devices can cause gas trapping if used inappropriately. Avoiding lung overinflation, using the shortest inspiratory time possible, ensuring sufficient exhalation time, and eliminating obstructions reduce the risk of gas trapping.[18,19,27,28]

FIGURE 12-3
The quicker the puff, the sharper the spike.

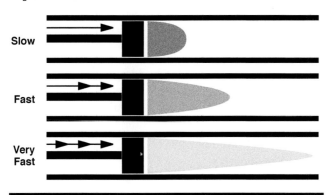

Forward movement of gas in the center and backward movement of gas at the walls.

Adapted from: Henderson Y, Chillingworth FP, and Whitney JL. 1915. The respiratory dead space. *Journal of Physiology* 38(1): 5. Reprinted by permission.

GAS EXCHANGE MECHANISMS

During HFV, gas exchange occurs even when tidal volume approaches or is less than ADS. Numerous physiologic mechanisms are responsible. The most important of these are convection and diffusion.

Convection

During HFV, high kinetic/potential energy breaths are given. Although the individual volumes of each breath may be less than ADS, gas movement can still occur in a bulk fashion.[6] Direct aeration of proximal airways and central alveolar units can occur because of short transit times from the main airways.[20] These alveolar units may provide a significant portion of the total gas exchange because of local hyperventilation.[29] That is, the PCO_2 in these central units may be much lower than in the surrounding or more peripheral alveolar units.

Convective mixing and recirculation of gas can occur between neighboring respiratory units during the whole respiratory cycle. This interregional mixing, or "pendelluft," occurs because of the different time constants of the respiratory units. This mixing results in out-of-phase gas movements and facilitates convective exchange (Figure 12-2).[6]

Convective flow streaming is another means of gas transport. Henderson and colleagues showed that the more energy or speed that generates a puff of smoke, the greater the forward movement of the center of the puff (Figure 12-3).[30] A parabolic-shaped puff or breath is formed from the development of asymmetric velocity profiles. During exhalation, there are blunt flow profiles

FIGURE 12-4
Asymmetric velocity profiles.

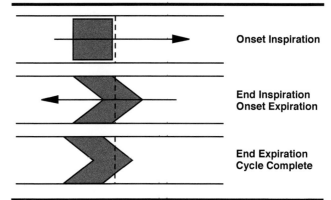

From: Wetzel RC, and Gioia FR. 1987. High frequency ventilation. *Pediatric Clinics of North America* 34(1): 22. Reprinted by permission.

in the opposite direction, but the elongated center portion does not return to the starting point. At the end of a breath, there is a small net forward movement (Figure 12-4). During HFV (especially jet ventilation), gas tends to flow down the center or inner core of the tube (or airway) and out along the outer walls (Figure 12-5).[31]

Diffusion and Taylor Dispersion

Diffusion describes gas exchange by random (Brownian) motion. This exchange occurs in any part of the lung where there is a gradient, not just in the terminal respiratory units.

In 1954, Taylor described the augmented movement and radial diffusion of gas in situations of parabolic gas

FIGURE 12-5
Helical pattern of convective streaming during HFJV.

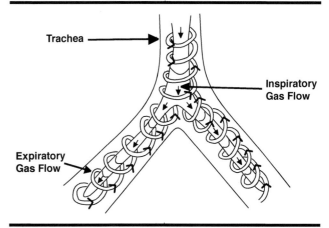

Adapted by Solon JF, from: Rausch K via Ellis R, unpublished data, Milpitas, California. Reprinted by permission.

FIGURE 12-6
Taylor dispersion.

The inspiratory gas front is parabolic, and this provides a greatly
increased area over which radial molecular diffusion can occur, as
represented by the arrows.

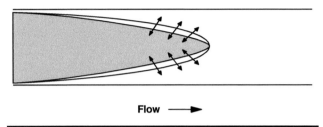

Flow ⟶

From: Wetzel RC, and Gioia FR. 1987. High frequency ventilation.
Pediatric Clinics of North America 34(1): 21. Reprinted by permission.

FIGURE 12-7
**Mechanisms of gas transport predominating in given lung
regions.**

1 Convection
2 Taylor Type
3 Velocity Profiles
4 Interregional (Pendelluft)
5 Molecular Diffusion

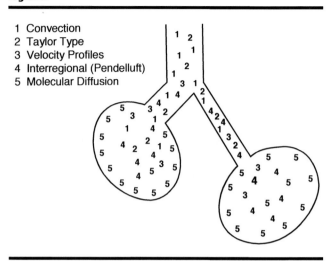

From: Wetzel RC, and Gioia FR. 1987. High frequency ventilation.
Pediatric Clinics of North America 34(1): 23. Reprinted by permission.

flow (HFV breath) (Figure 12-6).[32] In a parabolic gas flow
situation, fresh gas moves down the center of the airway
and is surrounded by expired gases at the periphery of
the airway. This sets up a concentration gradient of CO_2
and oxygen (O_2) causing O_2 to diffuse from the higher
concentration in the center of the airway to the lower
concentration at the periphery.[6]

During HFV, this diffusion process is facilitated by
the increased surface area between two gases because
of increased viscous drag.[33] Actual gas exchange can be
hampered by Taylor dispersion because of the diffusion
of carbon dioxide from the expiring gas into the fresh
gas; however, the high-energy HFV cycles probably
result in the delivery of more fresh gas to the respiratory
units before significant contamination can occur. This
preserves the diffusion gradient needed to move CO_2 out
of the blood.

Various aspects of direct ventilation and convective
and diffusive mechanisms of gas transport are probably
responsible for the majority of gas exchange during
HFV. These mechanisms are not restricted to any one
anatomic area. Convective forces, however, are probably
more dominant in areas where bulk flow occurs and
diffusion forces in areas where it stops. There must also
be areas of overlap and simultaneous operation (Figure
12-7).

CLINICAL DEVICES

Anecdotal and experimental evidence has
accumulated to support the use of HFV therapy in
various disease states and clinical situations, which
are presented in Table 12-1. When considering the
indications for HFV, the clinician must individualize
them to each NICU. The type of device, experience

with the device, and alternate therapies must all be
considered.

HFV therapy must be used early enough to improve
outcome and decrease complications, rather than
being used as a last resort. Yet use should not begin so
early as to expose the infant to unnecessary risks and
complications. Whenever possible, HFV should be used
in the context of a research study, to build the knowledge
and experience base. Finally, based on current data, HFV
should not be used in situations where CMV has a track
record of success.

GENERAL CONCEPTS

HFV is provided to the patient by specialized devices,
which are classified and compared based on the method
of HFV employed and their operating characteristics.
The HFV devices currently in clinical use deliver gas
during inspiration under positive pressure.

Table 12-2 lists some general operating characteristics
of HFJV and HFOV devices. An understanding of key
concepts will be useful in managing the patient on HFV:

- **Frequency** (or rate) refers to the breaths or cycles
  the machine can deliver.
- **Waveform** refers to the "shape" of the breath
  delivered. Waveform may influence how gas travels
  in and out of the lung.
- **Exhalation** refers to how the gas gets out of the lung.
  Passive exhalation relies on the natural recoil of the
  chest (as in CMV). Active exhalation refers to pulling

TABLE 12-1
Clinical Indications for Use of High-Frequency Ventilation

Severe respiratory failure
Extraventilatory air leak syndromes
Failing CMV
Persistent pulmonary hypertension
Before and after other therapies
ECMO
Cardiac surgery
Congenital diaphragmatic hernia surgery
Airway surgery

Adapted from: Karp T. 1993. High frequency ventilation: Life in the fast lane? Presented at Neonatal Nurses National Conference, Nottingham, England, September 25; and Clark RH. 1994. High-frequency ventilation. *Journal of Pediatrics* 124(5): 661–670. Reprinted by permission.

TABLE 12-2
General Operating Characteristics of HFJV and HFOV Devices

Characteristic	HFJV	HFOV
Frequency in cycles/minute (Hz/minute)	150–660 (2.5–12)	300–3,000 (5–50)
Inspiratory waveform	Triangular/spike	Sine wave
Exhalation	Passive	Active
Tidal volume (usually)	<CMV >Anatomic dead space	<CMV < or >anatomic dead space

or assisting the gas out of the chest by generating a type of pull or "negative" pressure during exhalation.

- The **inspiratory-to-expiratory (I:E)** ratio refers to the time allotted to inspiration compared with expiration for each breath. The I:E ratio is affected by rate. When the time for inspiration is the same as that for expiration, the I:E ratio is 1:1. For most devices, especially those with passive exhalation, more time is needed for expiration than for inspiration.

- **Tidal volume** (in Table 12-2) refers to the size of the breath in relation to ADS. The amount of pressure used, gas flow, endotracheal tube size (or change in size), and time allowed for inspiration all contribute to determining tidal volume. In general, the more pressure, gas flow, and time allowed for inspiration, as well as the larger the endotracheal tube, the larger the delivered tidal volume.

HFV may be provided as a single therapy or in combination with traditional mechanical ventilation. The device may be a stand-alone machine (SensorMedics 3100A HFOV), a stand-alone machine that works in tandem with a conventional ventilator (Bunnell Life Pulse HFJV), or a machine that combines both capabilities (Dräger Babylog). Manufacturers constantly change device configurations, so users must keep up to date on manufacturer recommendations.

Monitoring Issues

Currently, most neonatal ventilation is provided by positive pressure. The caregiver monitors the pressure signal produced by various pressure transducers, with results displayed either on the ventilator or on an attached monitor. The pressure readings during CMV are most often sampled at the patient connector and measured by a transducer located in the ventilator.

The pressure values displayed usually represent the pressure transmitted through the endotracheal tube to the lung.[9] As the ventilator rate increases, the endotracheal tube acts as a resistor, decreasing the amplitude of the signal. Thus, at high rates, the pressure in the lung can be less than that measured at the endotracheal tube connector. The exception is when gas trapping occurs, in which case the pressure in the lung may be higher than what is shown on the monitor display. The key to preventing this problem is ensuring that expiratory time is sufficient to avoid gas trapping and a buildup of pressure.

With HFOV devices, the attenuation of the pressure signal can be significant, especially when a 1:2 I:E ratio is used.[34] In other words, the pressure (amplitude) signal sampled by the device at the patient connector may be much higher than the actual pressure (amplitude) in the lung.[9,35,36]

With an HFJV device (such as the Bunnell Life Pulse), the pressure signal is sampled at the hub of the triple-lumen adapter. The transducer is located in the patient box, close to the patient connector, rather than back in the ventilator. This arrangement allows for measurement of an undampened signal. Despite this, high gas velocity and the Venturi effect of the gas flow make accurate pressure monitoring difficult.[36]

General Patient Management Principles

General guiding principles for management of patients on HFV depend on the disease state and the device. Caregivers must (1) provide enough Paw to (2) stabilize optimal lung volumes while (3) avoiding gas trapping and cardiac impairment.[9,35]

Optimal lung volumes depend on the disease state. In general, there should be no significant atelectasis, no extraventilatory air, no hyperinflation, and good ventilation-to-perfusion matching. At optimal lung

FIGURE 12-8
Valve box.

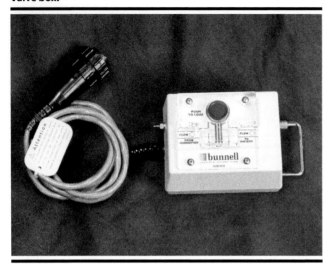

Bunnell Incorporated, 436 Lawndale Drive, Salt Lake City, UT 84115.
www.bunl.com/product-tabs2.html. Reprinted by permission.

FIGURE 12-9
LifePort endotracheal tube adapter.

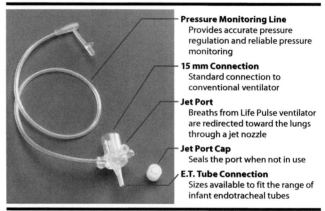

- **Pressure Monitoring Line**
  Provides accurate pressure
  regulation and reliable pressure
  monitoring
- **15 mm Connection**
  Standard connection to
  conventional ventilator
- **Jet Port**
  Breaths from Life Pulse ventilator
  are redirected toward the lungs
  through a jet nozzle
- **Jet Port Cap**
  Seals the port when not in use
- **E.T. Tube Connection**
  Sizes available to fit the range of
  infant endotracheal tubes

Bunnell Incorporated, 436 Lawndale Drive, Salt Lake City, UT 84115.
www.bunl.com/product-tabs2.html. Reprinted by permission.

volume, there will be appropriate oxygenation and ventilation and the least risk of lung injury.

The Paw required to achieve optimal lung volume depends on the disease state and the device. The Paw may be high or low, depending on what is to be accomplished. The optimal Paw provides an adequate lung volume with the fewest adverse side effects.[37] The challenge is the difficulty of monitoring lung volume (see Chapter 5). The most frequently used tool is the chest x-ray.[38] Others are physical examination, vital signs, and blood gas analysis. In addition, echocardiography may be used to evaluate pulmonary pressures, cardiac filling, and associated decrease in cardiac output during HFV.

OPTIMIZING LUNG VOLUMES

A key to successful treatment with HFV is maintaining adequate lung volumes and FRC.[38,39] Although there are device-specific issues, most strategies for optimizing lung volumes can be employed with either HFJV or HFOV devices. It may be necessary to use a Paw higher than for CMV to adequately inflate the lungs. This high-lung-volume strategy has been shown to improve gas exchange and reduce lung injury.[23,24,26,40–42] It also improves the efficacy of surfactant therapy.[43]

Some treatments and procedures that require the infant to be disconnected from the ventilator circuit, such as position or circuit changes, will result in some degree of lung deflation. Lung volume can be restored with either a sustained inflation (sigh) or a gradual increase in Paw on the HFV device until oxygenation or chest x-ray improves.[38] Caution must be used with both

sustained inflations and increased Paw because both can impede venous return, decrease cardiac output, decrease cerebral blood flow, and damage the airways.[9,24,44,45]

Surfactant and HFV may be synergistic in their effects.[43,46,] Surfactant can be used before and during HFV therapy.[47] It is usually administered with the infant off HFV because reflux of surfactant into the endotracheal tube can occur, as can tube obstruction, especially when small amplitudes are employed.

The clinical strategies focus on pulmonary management, but other patient needs must not be forgotten. The key to successful HFV is stable and effective hemodynamics. Frequently, intravascular volume and inotropic support are needed, especially when high Paw is required to resolve atelectasis. Attention to nutrition, pain control, and parent needs is also essential to provide a holistic approach to patient care.

HIGH-FREQUENCY JET VENTILATION

HFJV uses a jet injector to introduce a small volume of rapidly moving gas into the neonate's airway. Exhalation of gases occurs passively, as a result of the elastic recoil of the lung.[48] Tidal volumes, although difficult to measure accurately, are thought to be slightly greater than ADS.[27,28]

In the U.S., as noted earlier, HFJV is provided by the Bunnell Life Pulse, a microprocessor-controlled, positive pressure–limited, time-cycled, high-frequency ventilator. The jet pulses (breaths) are delivered from a valve box located close to the patient (Figure 12-8). The frequency range of these pulses is 240–600 breaths per minute.[49] This valve box also contains the transducer that monitors airway pressure. The valve box is connected to the patient through a specialized triple-lumen endotracheal tube adapter (LifePort endotracheal tube adapter, Bunnell, Inc., Salt Lake City, Utah) (Figure 12-9). One lumen in this adapter provides jet flow, the second one produces background gas flow, and the third lumen allows for pressure monitoring. To establish a patient on HFJV, it is necessary to change the endotracheal tube adapter, but reintubation of the patient is not required. The Life Pulse ventilator provides HFV in tandem with a CMV device. The CMV device provides the PEEP and background CMV breaths (sighs) as needed.

Ventilation (carbon dioxide removal) is mainly determined by the amplitude or size of the breath as measured by ΔP. The size of these jet pulses (tidal volume) is controlled by the jet PIP and length of inspiration. Inspiratory time is generally held at 20 milliseconds. Therefore, tidal volume is not affected by rate changes unless inspiratory time is specifically changed. Lower peak and mean airway pressures are needed for CO_2 removal with HFJV than with HFOV.[50–53]

Paw, a more complex calculation, is determined by the interrelationship of numerous factors, including jet PIP and frequency, and the rate, inspiratory time, and PEEP provided by the tandem conventional breaths.[6] The gas flow to create the jet impulses is governed by a microprocessor-controlled pressure regulator that adjusts to meet the operating conditions. This gas flow, or servopressure, changes in response to lung volume, respiratory compliance, or airway resistance. In the absence of an air leak in the system, rising servopressure usually indicates improved compliance. A drop may indicate increased airway resistance, decreased compliance, or tension pneumothorax.[54] The key concepts for HFJV use are as follows:

- Oxygenation is related to Paw, CO_2 removal, and tidal volume.
- Generally, HFJV allows use of a lower Paw and PIP than does CMV.
- The HFJV (Bunnell Life Pulse) requires use of a background CMV device to provide PEEP. The CMV device also sustains inflations (sighs) when recruitment of an atelectatic lung is needed.
- The HFJV can utilize an "elevated" or "high" Paw strategy to support oxygenation and optimal lung volumes.
- HFJV requires a specific type of endotracheal tube adapter.

Clinical Strategies

When dealing with an infant with restrictive lung disease and air leak syndromes such as pulmonary interstitial emphysema (PIE) and pneumothorax, the goal in using HFJV is to use less PIP and Paw, to allow the air leaks to heal. Starting with a PIP at the same level as that used for CMV is suggested. The Paw should be the same or 1–2 cmH_2O less to support oxygenation. The PEEP can be the same or greater by 1. The HFJV rate is usually started at 420 breaths per minute.[36]

As the infant is placed on HFJV, the CMV is weaned to a rate of 5 and, if possible, an HFJV PIP less than that used for CMV. To avoid further injury in patients with air leak injury, lower tandem CMV rates (down to 0), or use only continuous positive airway pressure (CPAP) when oxygenation is adequate.[36] The CPAP levels must be high enough to stabilize open alveoli, but not so high as to prevent healing. The risk of delayed air leak healing from the CPAP level needed to support oxygenation must be balanced against the trauma of the CMV rate (large tidal volume breaths).

Severe atelectatic disorders, such as respiratory distress syndrome (RDS), may also benefit from HFJV as a way to reduce airway injury. These atelectatic disorders require a different strategy than restrictive or obstructive lung diseases. The PIP may be slightly reduced or the same as the CMV setting. The PEEP setting is usually increased to the range of 6–8 cmH_2O pressure.[55] The HFJV rate will be 420 breaths per minute.

Again, the infant is weaned from background CMV support, but if oxygenation falls, the CMV PIP may need to be slightly higher than the HFJV PIP. This is to help recruit atelectatic air spaces. The CMV support, usually PIP, is reduced as rapidly as lung volume stabilization allows; then the HFJV PIP is reduced as tolerated. However, to prevent atelectasis, PEEP may need to remain elevated as PIP is decreased.

Obstructive disorders, such as meconium aspiration syndrome (MAS), can be treated with HFJV. The device is used to support gas exchange and also creates vibratory energy, which facilitates debris removal.[10] Until stabilized, the patient may require high HFJV and background settings. Often, once lung volume is restored, the infant can be effectively ventilated (or hyperventilated) with HFJV at a lower PIP.

It is essential to assess the patient constantly for gas trapping. Sufficient expiratory time is required to avoid significant gas trapping. Expiratory time can be gained by lowering the HFJV rate (to as low as the 240–360

TABLE 12-3
Matching Ventilator Strategy and Disease Process

Disease Process	Pathophysiology	Strategy/Goals	Initial Settings	Weaning
Air leak syndrome (PIE, pneumothorax)	PIE: gas interstitium compressing alveoli, airways, and pulmonary venules Pneumothorax: loss of V_T through chest tube	Minimize distending and peak pressure, accept lower PaO_2, higher FiO_2, and $PaCO_2$, target lower lung volume.	Drop PIP by 10–20% from value on DV; PEEP 4–6 cmH_2O; avoid background sigh if severe PIE	Lower PIP aggressively. Look for atelectasis, and increase PEEP as needed.
Severe uniform lung disease (RDS)	Atelectasis, hypoxemia, lungs highly susceptible to volutrauma and oxygen exposure	Recruit lung volume, achieve optimal expansion, avoid overventilation. Use frequent x-rays to guide management.	PIP initially same as CV, but must be dropped quickly; once lung volume is recruited, PEEP 6–9 cmH_2O, depending on FiO_2	Wean FiO_2 before Paw; (may need to increase PEEP to avoid drop in Paw when PIP is lowered).
Nonuniform disease (MAS)	Uneven aeration, risk of gas trapping, surfactant inactivation, inflammation, high risk of air leak (Atelectasis or gas trapping may predominate.)	Tailor strategy to predominant pathophysiology. Avoid gas trapping, optimize lung volume.	Lower frequency (300–360) PIP to achieve minimal acceptable PCO_2. Moderate PEEP 5–8 cmH_2O	Lower PIP and use PEEP to avoid loss of lung volume.
Chest wall restriction (severe NEC, repaired gastroschisis)	Restricted chest and/or diaphragmatic movement, atelectasis, hemodynamic impairment	Recruit lung volume, avoid atelectasis, minimize adverse hemodynamic effects.	Adjust PIP to achieve adequate chest wall movement. Sufficient PEEP to maintain FRC (usually 6–8 cmH_2O)	Wean PIP to avoid hypocarbia. Maintain Paw with PEEP.
Lung hypoplasia (CDH)	Small, atelectasis-prone lungs, susceptible to volutrauma, pulmonary hypertension	Gently recruit lung volume, avoid overexpansion, minimize adverse hemodynamic effects.	Set PIP at lowest level to achieve adequate ventilation. Fast rates okay as time constants are short. Sufficient PEEP to maintain FRC (usually 6–8 cmH_2O)	Wean carefully but fast enough to avoid overexpansion and air leak.
Obstructive disease (BPD)	Long time constants, risk of gas trapping, nonuniform inflation	Achieve adequate gas exchange with minimal pressures, optimize lung volume, improve uniformity of inflation.	Lower frequencies due to long time constants, moderate PEEP to optimize gas distribution and splint airways open	Wean slowly; rapid improvement is not anticipated.

Key: BPD = bronchopulmonary dysplasia; CDH = congenital diaphragmatic hernia; CV = conventional ventilation; FRC = functional residual capacity; Paw = mean airway pressure; MAS = meconium aspiration syndrome; NEC = necrotizing enterocolitis; PEEP = positive end-expiratory pressure; PIE = pulmonary interstitial emphysema; PIP = positive inspiratory pressure; RDS = respiratory distress syndrome; V_T = tidal volume.

Adapted from: Keszler M. 2005. High-frequency jet ventilation. In *Intensive Care of the Fetus and Neonate,* 2nd ed., Spitzer AR, ed. Philadelphia: Mosby, 664. Reprinted by permission.

breaths per minute range).[37] This is indicated by an increasing I:E ratio.

Weaning from HFJV has not been systematically studied. In general, the therapy is used during the acute phase of the disease. The air leaks, if present, should be resolved for one to two days before weaning. It is recommended that Paw not be decreased until the neonate is requiring less than 40 percent FiO_2. Methods of weaning vary, but they usually involve decreasing the tidal volume (PIP) in low birth weight infants to 12 cmH_2O pressure and Paw to 6–8 cmH_2O prior to extubation.[55] Table 12-3 presents additional suggestions for managing specific diseases with HFJV.

HIGH-FREQUENCY OSCILLATORY VENTILATION

The SensorMedics 3100A ventilator provides most of the HFOV in the U.S. This time-cycled, pressure-limited device uses an electromagnetically driven diaphragm to move bias gas flow. The resulting oscillations of gas are delivered to the patient via a traditional endotracheal tube. The diaphragm used in HFOV also pulls air from the lungs, creating an active exhalation rather than the passive exhalation provided by HFJV.[48]

Ventilation in HFOV is determined by the size of the oscillations, or amplitude. The amplitude of each cycle is controlled by the driving pressure (or stroke volume) generated by the diaphragm. It is measured at the hub of the endotracheal tube as ΔP, which is proportional to the volume of each breath. Decreasing the amplitude decreases chest wall movement and increases PCO_2 levels, whereas increasing the amplitude has the opposite effect.[36]

Paw in HFOV is governed by the rate of gas flow into the patient and the resistance to flow out of the circuit.[6] Unlike in HFJV, in HFOV, amplitude and Paw can each be adjusted separately.[38]

Inspiratory time is a percentage of the breath cycle. It is adjustable and is usually set between 30 and 50 percent of the respiratory cycle. This reduces the risk of gas trapping. Frequency is adjustable from 180 to 900 cycles/minute (3–15 Hz). It is usually set at between 600 and 900 cycles/minute (10–15 Hz).[36]

Tidal volumes are usually less than ADS and are adjusted by changing the amplitude of the cycle (breath). An adequate amplitude provides a tidal volume that causes minimal chest vibrations. However, tidal volume is also highly dependent upon inspiratory time. Because inspiratory time is a percentage of the time cycle, it changes when the frequency is altered. Reducing the frequency increases the inspiratory time and, therefore, the tidal volume. Conversely, increasing the frequency decreases inspiratory time and tidal volume.

In HFOV, oxygenation is determined by Paw, which is provided by PEEP. The PEEP is controlled by continuous fresh gas (bias flow) and the resistance of a low-pass filter. PEEP is usually adjusted by manipulating this low-pass filter. Initially, a Paw equal to that given by CMV is recommended.[36]

The basic concepts for HFOV use are as follows:

- Oxygenation is dependent upon Paw, and ventilation is dependent on tidal volume or amplitude.
- HFOV permits use of a higher Paw than CMV.
- HFOV allows for ventilation with very small (less than ADS) tidal volumes.
- HFOV requires stabilization of lung volumes. Adjusting support as lung volumes change is critical to success.
- HFOV requires close monitoring of cardiac output, which may be reduced as the lung volume stabilizes.
- HFOV uses a standard endotracheal tube.

Clinical Strategies

The approach to treating homogeneous processes such as RDS or diffuse atelectasis is one of increasing the Paw to open and stabilize the lung volume. The Paw is increased by 1–2 cmH_2O over CMV. If oxygenation is poor, the Paw is further increased in 1–2 cmH_2O steps.

The Paw needed to stabilize the lung volume may be as high as 25–30 cmH_2O. However, significant changes in lung volume can occur with small changes in Paw. The ventilatory rate is set at 600–900 breaths per minute (10–15 Hz) with an I:E ratio of 1:3 or 1:1, depending upon the device. The amplitude of the oscillations (tidal volume) is adjusted to move the chest.

For nonhomogeneous lung disease such as MAS or pneumonia, a Paw 1–2 cmH_2O less than that for CMV is suggested. The rate, I:E ratio, and amplitude are the same as for homogeneous disease. Because the HFOV oscillations are very small, their effectiveness may be reduced when the airways are full of secretions or meconium.

The approach to air leak syndrome depends on its severity and the predominant underlying pathology. If the lung volumes are low, a modified high lung volume strategy may be used. Rapid weaning is necessary once lung volumes are stabilized. If the air leak is severe, with gas trapping, then a lower lung volume strategy is employed. Risk for gas trapping increases when the airways are contaminated with debris. Airway collapse may occur if Paw is too low.

Weaning from HFOV is achieved by decreasing Paw if oxygenation is adequate and CO_2 levels are normal or decreasing ΔP if CO_2 levels are low. As Paw is decreased, a point may be reached where loss of lung volume occurs and respiratory acidosis or increased oxygen levels are required. This often occurs around a Paw of 8–10 cmH_2O and responds to an increase in Paw.[36]

Theoretically, patients could be extubated directly from HFOV. However, data to support this practice are limited. One study done by Clark and associates[56] demonstrated that neonates treated with HFOV had better outcomes than those who were switched back to CMV after 72 hours on HFOV.

Studies of HFV

Although HFV is a relatively recent technique in the treatment of infants and adults with respiratory failure, the idea is not new. In 1915, Henderson and colleagues noted that panting dogs maintained adequate gas exchange with tidal volumes less than ADS.[30] Brisco, Foster, and Comroe noted in 1954 that alveolar ventilation could be maintained with small tidal volumes.[57] In 1959, John H. Emerson, a pioneer in respiratory devices, built and patented an apparatus for vibrating the patient's airway. Although it was never used on patients, Emerson's device was the first true high-frequency oscillation (HFO) device.[58]

EARLY STUDIES

During the 1970s, interest in HFV increased. In 1972, Lunkenheimer and colleagues reported the ability to ventilate dogs with the use of HFO delivered by a loudspeaker unit.[59] HFJV was successfully used by Klain and Smith in 1977 and by Sjostrand in 1980 to support adults during bronchoscopy or airway surgery.[60,61] Early studies using animal models demonstrated clear advantages for HFV, especially HFOV, when compared with CMV.[40,42,52,62–66]

Clinical studies using HFV in neonates were mixed. Most of the early reports of HFV were either attempts to rescue infants failing conventional ventilation or short-term experiments.[67,68] In 1981, Marchak and associates reported the first successful short-term treatment of RDS with HFV using an oscillatory system.[69] Two years later, Pokora and coworkers described the successful short-term treatment of neonates with intractable respiratory failure and progressive pulmonary air leaks using HFJV.[50]

By 1984, Harris and Christensen had treated 22 infants with PIE who were unresponsive to conventional therapy. Sixteen of them had a favorable response to HFJV, requiring less ventilatory support; 11 infants survived.[70] Also in 1984, Carlo and colleagues showed the ability of HFJV to ventilate infants with RDS using less airway pressure than CMV.[71] This supported the earlier HFO work of Frantz and associates.[72] Thus, in the early 1980s, there was preliminary evidence showing that HFV was potentially effective in improving the survival of infants with severe RDS, pulmonary air leak, and intractable respiratory failure.

During the 1980s, HFV was also used to treat persistent pulmonary hypertension of the newborn (PPHN). Pauly and coworkers, in 1987, used HFJV to treat nine infants with PPHN who were failing CMV. Four responded. From their limited experience, they concluded that if the infant showed no improvement after three hours on HFV, alternative forms of support, such as extracorporeal membrane oxygenation (ECMO), should be considered.[73] However, Carlo and colleagues, in 1989, were not able to show improvement in a group of patients with PPHN who were treated with a different HFJV device.[74]

In 1988, Kohelet and associates reported their ability to rescue infants with PPHN using HFOV. Of 41 infants rescued, 83 percent survived.[75] Also using HFOV, Carter and coworkers were able to rescue about 46 percent of the patients with PPHN (and other diseases) referred to their nursery for ECMO therapy. They found that, of all patient groups, those with MAS or pulmonary hypoplasia were least likely to respond to HFOV.[76] During the mid- to late 1980s, studies continued to validate the efficacy of HFV in a variety of disease states with a variety of devices.

In 1986, Gonzalez and colleagues found decreased gas flow through pneumothoraces in neonates receiving HFJV (Life Pulse, Bunnell, Inc.) versus CMV. They found that gas flow rates out of chest tubes decreased from 227 ± 96 mL/minute during CMV to 104 ± 59 mL/minute on HFJV.[77]

Also in 1986, Clark and associates reported successful rescue of infants with PIE and air leak using HFOV.[44] In 1987, Mammel and coworkers reported improved survival rates in their seven-year experience with HFJV rescue for intractable pulmonary air leaks and very severe respiratory failure.[78]

In 1989, two significant papers were published. The first was a report of the large National Institutes of Health (NIH)–sponsored, randomized, comparison trial of HFOV versus CMV as the primary treatment for infants with RDS. More than 670 infants were enrolled and treated with either the "local" CMV device or a piston-driven, fixed-I:E-ratio HFOV device. The results showed no improvement in survival and no reduction in air leaks or BPD with HFOV. There was, however, a small but significant increase in Grades III and IV intraventricular hemorrhage (IVH) in the study group.[79] These findings led to much controversy concerning the study design and interpretation of the results.[22,80]

LATER STUDIES

During the 1990s, numerous randomized clinical studies using HFV to treat infants with RDS, PIE, and other air leaks were reported. Studies done during the 1990s until the present can be grouped by the underlying disease process being examined.

RDS

Several meta-analyses of HFV have been conducted. Cools and colleagues reviewed 17 randomized clinical trials, conducted between 1989 and 2009, that compared elective HFOV to CMV in preterm infants.[81] These 17 trials enrolled a total of 3,652 infants and used various types of devices to provide the high-frequency ventilation.[56,82–97]

Findings of this review demonstrated no evidence of effect on mortality rates at 28–30 days or at approximately term gestational age. A increased rate of pulmonary air leaks was demonstrated in the high frequency oscillatory ventilation group. Increased rates of Grade 3 or 4 intraventricular hemorrhage were found in the trial that did not use a high lung volume strategy.[82,88]

In another meta-analysis, Bhuta and colleagues examined the use of rescue HFOV for infants with severe RDS or PIE. Only one trial (81 subjects) met the inclusion criteria. That trial was conducted by the HiFO Study Group.[98] It demonstrated no difference in mortality at 28 days, days of ventilation, days in hospital, or days on oxygen.[99]

Bhuta and associates also reviewed HFJV for both elective[100] and rescue[101] treatment of preterm infants with RDS. In the case of elective HFJV, three studies were included in the review.[102–104] The incidence of CLD was no different with HFJV than with CMV at 28 days, but Keszler and coworkers did find a decrease in CLD at 36 weeks in infants receiving HFJV.[103] Wiswell and colleagues identified an increased risk of PVL with HFJV, but this increase was not significant in the overall analysis.[104] Again, trials that used a low lung volume strategy reported more adverse neurologic outcomes.[105]

The meta-analysis of rescue HFJV examined data from one trial of 144 infants with PIE.[106] It found no significant differences between infants on HFJV and CMV in the reported outcomes (CLD in survivors at 28 days of age, IVH, new air leaks, airway obstruction, and necrotizing tracheobronchitis).

In 2003, Bollen and associates[107] performed a cumulative meta-analysis of 14 published trials of HFV representing data on 3,260 infants.[56,82–85,87,88,90,91,102–104,108,109] They noted that there are no clinical studies comparing HFV with high lung volumes to HFV with low lung volumes. They concluded that HFV was shown to be optimal compared with CMV when a high lung volume strategy HFV was studied against a CMV strategy that did not use lung protective strategies.[56,84,87,103] In studies where high-volume HFV was compared with a lung-protective CMV strategy, there were no differences in CLD rates.[88,90,91,108] When Bollen and coworkers performed further statistical analysis on an updated number of HFV studies, they noted a further decrease in the differences in outcome between optimal lung volume HFV and optimal lung protection CMV.[110]

Other clinicians argue that the lack of significant benefits of HFV in some of these studies may come from the inclusion of infants with minimal lung disease or from ineffective lung recruitment strategies.[11]

Air Leaks

In examining the treatment of air leaks, Keszler and colleagues, in 1991, reported on 144 infants who were randomized to CMV or HFJV for treatment of PIE. The HFJV group had a better response than the CMV group and improved survival, but there were no differences between the groups in the incidence of BPD or IVH.[106]

In 1993, the HiFO Study Group, a multicenter research consortium, reported a randomized trial investigating the effect of HFOV on the development of air leak syndrome. They found fewer new air leaks in the HFOV group than in controls and no differences in BPD. IVH rates were much lower than those found in the NIH-sponsored HIFI Study Group, but there were methodologic differences.[79,98]

One of the advantages of HFV in treating infants with PIE is the ability of HFV, especially HFJV, to provide an I:E ratio of 1:6 or 1:10.[11] Traditional CMV has a ratio of 1:1 or 1:2.

Surgical Procedures

HFV has also been used to support infants undergoing various surgical procedures. For example, it has been used during and after surgery for congenital tracheal stenosis, tracheoesophageal fistula, and cardiac and abdominal defect repairs.[111,112] Davis and associates reported in 1994 that HFJV provided better gas exchange at lower Paw when compared with CMV in a group of nine infants undergoing Blalock-Taussig shunt placement.[113] Postoperative cardiac function was improved with HFJV in a small group of patients after they underwent the Fontan procedure.[114]

Congenital Diaphragmatic Hernia

The patients who have sparked the most interest are those with congenital diaphragmatic hernia. Early reports on the use of HFV in these patients were not encouraging. Although there was some clinical improvement, survival was poor.[51,115,116] Later studies demonstrated improved outcomes, especially with HFOV.[117,118] Regardless of the device used, treatment of infants with congenital diaphragmatic hernia remains challenging.

TABLE 12-4
Clinical Indications for HFV

PIP >25 cmH$_2$O

Tidal volume >6 mL

Conventional rates >60–80 breaths per minute

Air leak syndromes

Potential ECMO candidate

Extreme prematurity (<1,000 g)

Rescue of infants failing CMV

Adapted from: Courtney SE, and Asselin JM. 2006. High-frequency jet and oscillatory ventilation for neonates: Which strategy and when? *Respiratory Care Clinics of North America* 12(3): 453–467.

Meconium Aspiration

The efficacy of HFV treatment of infants with MAS has been described. In 1985, Trindale and coworkers compared HFJV (Bunnell device) with CMV in a MAS piglet model. They found that HFJV required a PIP 50 percent lower than that of CMV to keep the PCO$_2$ equal.[119] Keszler and colleagues studied combined jet ventilation in a MAS puppy model. In their study, combined HFJV/CMV (sighs) provided the best oxygenation and ventilation at less Paw and PIP than CMV alone.[120]

HFV has also been studied as a means to avoid ECMO in infants with MAS. By using HFJV, Baumgart and associates avoided ECMO in 38 percent of patients with MAS. They also noted that, in general, patients responded within one to six hours.[121] Carter's group avoided the use of ECMO in 50 percent of infants with MAS by using HFOV.[76] Varnholt and coworkers, in 1992, used HFOV to rescue 46 percent of infants referred for ECMO. Of their HFOV infants, 50 percent suffered air leak (either continued or new).[122]

ECMO Avoidance

In relation to HFV and ECMO avoidance, Clark and colleagues reported in 1994 a randomized crossover trial comparing HFOV and CMV. Although there was no ultimate difference in outcome or ECMO use because of crossover, HFOV was able to rescue 63 percent of those failing CMV, and CMV was able to rescue 23 percent of the patients. These investigators concluded that HFOV was a safe and effective device for avoiding ECMO therapy.[123] As part of Clark and associates' study and a larger retrospective review, Paranka and coworkers reported on predictors of HFOV failure. They found that the presence of congenital diaphragmatic hernia, lung hypoplasia, and an arterial-to-alveolar oxygen ratio of ≤0.05 at initiation or 0.08 after six hours of HFOV predicted the need for ECMO or death.[124] A single-center

study done by Engle and colleagues used either HFJV or CMV in near-ECMO patients and found that HFJV significantly improved blood gases and demonstrated a nonsignificant trend toward a reduction in infants needing ECMO.[125]

HFV and Specialized Therapies

HFV has also been used in conjunction with other specialized therapies. Davis and associates, in 1992, reported on the use of rescue treatment with a combination of HFJV and surfactant to avoid ECMO in infants with severe respiratory failure. Of the 28 patients, 25 survived.[126]

The use of nitric oxide and HFV has become common. Kinsella and coworkers mounted a large multicenter trial using HFOV combined with inhaled nitric oxide (iNO) and found that, in infants with significant lung disease, iNO delivered with HFOV was more effective than iNO given with CMV.[127] Dobyns and colleagues found similar results in pediatric patients with severe hypoxemic respiratory failure.[128] However, Schreiber and associates found no difference between HFV and CMV in infants less than 34 weeks receiving iNO.[94]

Reasons for Varied Research Findings on HFV

Clearly, significant volumes of research have examined the safety and efficacy of HFV. Despite this work, many questions remain. The early results of animal studies showing promising support for HFV have not been borne out in clinical studies. Given the clinical experience of clinicians across North America, Europe, and Australia suggesting that, for many infants, HFV is a life-saving therapy, the lack of clear support for HFV in the research literature remains an enigma.

Several reasons for the varied research findings have been suggested. Many of the inconsistencies may be explained by the numerous changes in clinical practice that have taken place since HFV was first introduced. Lung protective strategies such as the use of surfactant and earlier extubation to nasal CPAP have changed the outcomes of neonates receiving CMV.[11] Early use of HFV focused on the use of low airway pressures, which resulted in less than optimal lung volumes. Low lung volumes have been shown to increase the risk for lung injury.[129] Studies that used a low lung volume strategy reported more complications such as IVH and PVL.[107] Finally, differences in devices and protocols across HFV studies have made it impossible to compare results and combine studies into effective meta-analyses.[39,129]

INDICATIONS FOR HFV

Despite the lack of clear data supporting the use of HFV, clinical experience suggests that there are a number of infants who may benefit from its use. Courtney and Asselin suggest using the infant's severity of illness or requirement for high CMV settings as a guide for the use of HFV (Table 12-4).[129]

Certain disease conditions have also been shown to benefit from the use of HFV. In particular, HFV use has been well accepted for the treatment of air leak syndromes, including PIE and bronchopleural fistula.[11,107] It is also well accepted for treating conditions such as diaphragmatic hernia and pulmonary hypoplasia.[11] Aspiration syndromes have also been successfully treated with HFV.[130] HFJV has been shown to mobilize secretions, which may be of benefit in MAS.[10] Severe respiratory failure is another accepted indication for HFV, with trials demonstrating a reduction in the need for ECMO when HFV is used.[9,125]

The use of HFV in the management of infants with RDS remains more controversial. The provision of small tidal volumes may be of benefit to premature infants in preventing volutrauma, barotrauma, and subsequent alveolar injury. The availability of newer modes of conventional ventilation capable of synchronizing ventilatory efforts with those of the patient and able to target volumes along with concerns about the potential for hyperventilation and subsequent neurologic injury have lessened the appeal of HFV as an initial strategy for ventilating the premature infant with RDS.[11,131]

COMPLICATIONS

Although HFV appears to be efficacious in treating pulmonary air leak and respiratory failure, several serious complications have been reported. Most are similar to those seen with CMV and include air leaks, BPD, and IVH. Rates, incidences, and severity of complications vary according to the type of device and the ventilation strategy used. A key factor in the complications seen appears to be the learning curve of the care providers.

Complications can be either "chronic" (such as BPD) or acute (such as air leak syndromes, impaired cardiac output, or airway damage). Various complications have been attributed to certain machines and ventilation strategies, but few causal relationships have been identified, and generalizations are limited. The same ventilator used with different clinical strategies can produce different rates of complications or injury.[22,132,133]

INTRAVENTRICULAR HEMORRHAGE

IVH is a multifactorial complication that has been reported at varying rates in infants treated with HFV. Infants with severe IVH were excluded from the early experimental trials. However, there was no increased incidence of IVH in the survivors of rescue therapy.

In 1989, the HIFI study showed a significant increase in severe IVH in the HFOV-treated infants compared with the CMV-treated infants (26 percent versus 18 percent). There was also an increase in the incidence of PVL (12 percent versus 7 percent).[79] A review of this study focused on how differences among strategies, devices, and centers influenced results.[80] There was speculation that greater impairment of venous return might have resulted in the increase in IVH. This increase was not found in Japan by Ogawa and coworkers, who reported a small, randomized study with IVH rates of 15 percent in HFV-treated subjects and 13 percent for CMV subjects.[83]

In a study reported in 1993 involving HFO, there was no significant difference in the incidence of IVH between groups treated with HFO and CMV. Because of methodology issues, however, the authors concluded that the association between HFOV and IVH remains open.[98] In the HFJV study of PIE, there was no significant difference in IVH rates between the CMV and HFJV groups, but there was a trend toward a lower incidence in the HFJV group.[106] This is countered by the more recent experience of Wiswell and colleagues, reported in 1996. They found an increased incidence of IVH with use of HFJV.[104]

CARDIAC IMPAIRMENT/HYPOTENSION

HFV can cause impaired hemodynamics.[134] This complication is most commonly seen when lung overdistention occurs; therefore, using strategies to prevent lung overdistention should avoid significant cardiac impairment.[26]

Hypotension occurs in many infants treated with HFV; this may be related to primary pathology, cardiac impairment, or hyperventilation. Therapy is focused on avoiding or correcting the underlying cause and providing supportive care such as volume infusion and inotropic support. If no improvement occurs and the cardiac impairment remains severe, the ventilatory strategy or even the device may have to be changed.

AIRWAY DAMAGE

Airway damage can occur in any infant treated with mechanical ventilation. Airway damage spans a

TABLE 12-5
Assessment of Chest Vibration

Lack of or decreased chest wall motion can be caused by:

    Plugged, dislodged, or malpositioned endotracheal tube

    Massive pneumothorax

    Machine failure or gas leak

    Not enough PIP or amplitude

    Gas trapping

Excessive chest wall motion can be caused by:

    Excessive PIP or amplitude

    Improved compliance

    Machine failure

wide spectrum, but most attention has been focused on necrotizing tracheobronchitis, a condition of acute inflammation, extensive hemorrhage, tissue necrosis, erosion of tracheal epithelium, increased thick secretions, and mucus plugging.[36] Necrotic debris can slough off the trachea and, together with the thick secretions, lead to total or partial airway obstruction. Emergency intervention such as bronchoscopy may be required to remove airway debris.[135–137]

The cause of necrotizing tracheobronchitis is most likely multifactorial.[36] Lack of proper humidification of respiratory gases was originally considered to be the main etiologic factor.[138,141] Early models of HFV systems, especially HFJV, used various methods, both singly and in combination, to humidify respiratory gases. Current models provide extensive humidity, to the point of "rainout" in some cases.

Direct trauma has also been suggested as a factor for the etiology of necrotizing tracheobronchitis.[133] This trauma may result from a strategy of providing high Paw in an uninterrupted pattern or from direct shear forces.[140] Therapy is aimed at early recognition to minimize trauma, along with airway intervention. Bronchoscopy may be necessary for diagnosis and to clear the airway.

The incidence of necrotizing tracheobronchitis seems to have decreased, but it may occur on either a microscopic or a clinical level in 2–4 percent of patients on HFV.[138] A 1995 report by Nicklaus suggests that follow-up for airway injury should continue even after discharge. Manifestation of the injury (webs and scars) may not become symptomatic until years after therapy.[141]

Mechanical Problems

The ventilators used for HFV have evolved from crude devices to sophisticated, highly technical machines with many built-in safeguards. As with all devices, however, mechanical failures or problems can occur. Proper connection of pressure-monitoring devices and an accurate understanding of alarm states are imperative to protect the patient from high airway pressures.

Use of HFV may expose the patient to certain undefined risks such as silicone debris from the ventilator circuit.[142] Proper patient positioning is necessary to avoid risk of water intoxication from either the humidifier or breathing circuits. However, prolonged placement in any one position may lead to skin breakdown, especially in the occipital area.[143]

As with all methods of mechanical ventilation, HFV has adverse side effects and complications. These complications must be closely monitored and reported. Careful analysis of benefits versus risks is required prior to widespread use of any treatment modality.

Nursing Care

Nursing care of infants during HFV therapy is based on the nursing process and general standards of neonatal nursing. Most patients receiving HFV are critically ill, although HFV is now used increasingly in less acutely ill infants, particularly in extremely low birth weight infants. Some patients treated with HFV may be enrolled in research studies or may receive other highly technical treatments such as ECMO or concomitant therapies such as head cooling or nitric oxide. The clinical course for these infants may be one of worsening lung disease reflected in deteriorating blood gas values and chest x-ray films. Frequently, air trapping or air leaks have developed or worsened. Integrating HFV technology into the bedside care for these complex patients requires the adaptation, revision, and evaluation of various aspects of nursing practice.

Assessment

Assessment of patients on HFV is frequent and extensive, consisting mainly of inspection, auscultation, and palpation. Although the basic nursing methods for gathering data remain unchanged, the HFV technology affects interpretation of the information. Assessment is also influenced by underlying disease state and drug use.

Respiratory System

HFV dramatically affects assessment of the respiratory system. The high breath rates and small tidal volume of each cycle cause significant chest vibration. The amount of chest movement is directly related to the size or amplitude of the cycle and makes counting total respiratory rates impractical.

During normal ventilator operation, the vibrations are continuous, except when some type of sustained inflation is given. During HFJV, the chest vibrations will be interrupted when the CMV PIP or the infant's spontaneous breaths exceed the HFJV PIP. These pauses are very short and have no obvious adverse effect on most infants.

It is important to constantly monitor the amount of vibration because it appears to be related to tidal volume delivery. As HFOV amplitude or HFJV PIP is reduced, the amplitude of the vibrations decreases. Lack of vibration usually results from too small a tidal volume or airway obstruction and may precede an acute deterioration (Table 12-5). The status of chest vibration is assessed formally every 30 minutes and informally whenever the patient is observed.

Spontaneous respirations can occur provided the infant is not hypocapnic or receiving paralytic agents. These breaths are best assessed by inspection for retractions and other signs of distress.

The breath sounds created by HFV have a loud "jackhammer rumbling" quality with a high-pitched tone. Different than traditional breath sounds, these sounds provide much information, especially when monitored over time. Decreased tone of these sounds may indicate poor ventilation or pneumothorax.[144] Higher pitched tones, especially those of musical quality, seem to indicate mucus secretions, plugs, or bronchospasm. Decreasing or absent breath sounds may indicate airway obstruction, especially when accompanied by very small amplitude cycles. The chest should also be palpated to assess the symmetry and quality of vibrations. Excessive vibrations may signal improving lung compliance or excessive amplitude or PIP. Decreased vibrations may be noted in the presence of secretions in the endotracheal tube, poor lung compliance, air leak, or decreased lung compliance.

The patient should be assessed frequently for the presence of air leaks. Changes in the air leak rate or occurrence of new leaks will alter therapeutic plans. Constant vigilance for new air leaks, especially pneumopericardium, is vital. Although it is unclear if pneumopericardium is more frequent with HFV than with CMV, it does occur. In situations of acute deterioration, especially with cardiovascular compromise, pneumopericardium must be considered.

Assessment of tracheal secretions is very important during HFV. Changes in tracheal secretion consistency and color may be the first warning signs of developing airway damage or nosocomial pneumonia.

Cardiovascular System

Most infants requiring HFV therapy have concomitant cardiovascular compromise. It may be secondary to the underlying disease state, therapeutic maneuvers, or lung overinflation. Pulmonary hypertension and poor left ventricular output are the most common alterations seen. The high lung volumes and/or high Paw required to support these infants may hamper venous return and impair cardiac output. Cardiovascular assessment utilizes auscultation, inspection, and palpation as well as other information such as urine output and acid-base status.

Inability to hear heart sounds during HFV operation hampers physical assessment of the cardiovascular system. Murmurs usually cannot be heard unless they are very loud, and pulse rate cannot be counted unless the ventilator is on standby or disconnected. Evaluation for murmurs may require a temporary pause in HFV therapy. Ability to locate the point of maximal impulse (PMI) is greatly limited by chest vibration, except in infants with an extremely active precordium. The PMI is usually seen in the subxiphoid area. Assessment of peripheral pulses is hampered by total body vibration. The more peripheral pulses (radial and posterior tibial) are less affected than the central pulses (femoral and brachial) because of distance from the vibrating thorax.

During HFV operation, electrocardiogram and vascular pressure waveforms can show movement artifact. The degree of artifact appears to depend upon the vigor of body movement, pulmonary compliance, and transducer sensitivity.

Other Systems

The body vibrations and noise produced during HFV influence assessment of the gastrointestinal tract. Gross assessment can be performed, but fine assessments, such as listening for bowel sounds and liver evaluation, can be difficult. Abdominal distention and tenderness can be determined, and stooling is not impaired. Tolerance of feedings can be monitored as with CMV.

The genitourinary system is not affected by HFV. The use of paralytic or sedative agents in infants on HFV necessitates frequent evaluation for urinary retention.

Assessment for alterations in skin integrity should be done frequently. Body vibration does not seem to increase the incidence of skin breakdown. In fact, the

TABLE 12-6
Selected Nursing Interventions[12,13,149]

Intervention	HFJV	HFOV
Endotracheal suctioning	• Can perform with HFJV on or off. When HFJV is off, procedure is similar to that with CMV. • Place suction catheter down tube with continuous suction applied. • Avoid manual bagging. • Adjust HFJV or CMV setting to facilitate recovery.	• Perform with HFOV off. • Avoid procedure as much as possible to limit disconnection from HFOV. Actual procedure similar to CMV. • Avoid manual bagging. • Increase Paw if needed to facilitate recovery.
Positioning	• Patient can be placed in all positions. Limited by short, but flexible, length of "jet" tubing to patient box. • Patient box sits next to head. • Patient can be moved while connected to HFJV. • Patient can be held by parents to facilitate bonding.	• Generally no position changes during first 48 hours requiring disconnection of HFOV. • Changes while on HFOV limited by rigid tubing that delivers bias flow. Head-to-toe movement on either a horizontal or vertical axis can be employed. • Patient can be held by parents. • Infant must always remain elevated above the rigid tubing to prevent aspiration of condensed water from circuit humidity. • Side cuts may be placed in sidewalls of radiant warmer to facilitate positioning.

movement may help reduce impairment in those infants who are heavily sedated or paralyzed.

Assessment of neurologic status depends more upon the severity of the underlying disease state, any specific complications, and pharmacotherapy than it does on HFV therapy. Some infants are obtunded; others are active and alert. With adequate ventilation and oxygenation, infants do not appear distressed while on HFV, although in some infants excessive breathing may interfere with the delivery of HFV ventilation. Behavioral signs of distress are interpreted in their usual context. Developmental states and signs can also be assessed. Seizure activity can be observed. Fontanel, tone, and basic reflexes can be assessed within limitations of patient status.

Monitoring Needs and Equipment

Because patients receiving HFV are generally critically ill, constant assessment of vital signs and blood gas values is necessary. The noise and vibration produced by HFV precludes many normal assessment activities: Heart sounds cannot be heard, so continuous heart rate monitoring is vital. Chest movement artifact

may alter the electrocardiogram waveform, depending on electrode placement. When an arterial line is in place, it may be helpful to obtain the heart rate from the arterial waveform.

Frequent blood gas monitoring is required, as with any critically ill child. Carbon dioxide monitoring is mandatory because HFV may significantly alter blood levels in a very short period of time. Oxygen saturation and PO_2 monitors (internal or transcutaneous) can be used to assess the patient's oxygenation status. Bedside pulmonary mechanics monitoring may be helpful in assessing the adequacy of lung volumes and in adjusting ventilator settings (see Chapter 5). Frequent chest x-rays may also be needed to monitor lung volumes and detect hypo- or hyperinflation. Adequate lung inflation is defined as "the top margin of the dome of the right hemidiaphragm [being] located between the bottom of the eighth rib and no more than midway between the ninth and tenth ribs."[89]

For patient safety, the nurse must be familiar with the displays and alarms on the HFV monitoring device. As new ventilators or updated models of earlier devices are introduced, the bedside nurse must master new operating and troubleshooting procedures. Failure to keep up to date may put the patient at increased risk for harm. Physiologic and patient parameters to monitor include but are not limited to:

- Arterial blood gases
- O_2 saturation
- Transcutaneous CO_2
- Heart rate
- Respiratory rate
- Blood pressure
- Temperature
- Pulmonary function tests
- Specific ventilator parameters

Patient response to ventilator changes on HFV is somewhat unpredictable. As previously discussed, oxygenation is related to Paw and normal lung volumes, and ventilation is related to tidal volume (or amplitude/ΔP). Frequent blood gas analysis is required during the initiation of therapy, weaning after normal lung volumes are established, and periods of instability. Chest x-rays may also be taken as often as every four to six hours during these periods. Currently, chest x-rays are the most common means of evaluating lung volumes.

Many factors are considered before ventilator settings are changed. A team approach with frequent consultation is needed. Because much of the care for infants on HFV is based on anecdote and experience, tremendous flexibility in treatment plans is necessary.

INTERVENTIONS

Nursing care interventions are individualized according to acuity and patient need. Many general nursing interventions for infants on HFV are similar to those for infants requiring CMV (see Chapter 7).

Certain interventions are the result of the HFV technology and are device dependent. For infants receiving HFJV therapy, the first nursing activity is assistance with the placement of the special endotracheal tube adapter (LifePort ETT adapter, Bunnell, Inc., Salt Lake City, Utah) (see Figure 12-9). Where available, an inline suction system should also be added to the circuit if one is not already in use. Use of an inline system minimizes ventilation interruption during suctioning (see below).

For HFV, no change in the endotracheal tube is required to initiate therapy; however, a change to a tube of a different size can dramatically affect the tidal volume delivered for any given amplitude. The use of HFV can require modification of both suctioning and positioning procedures.[13,145,146] Table 12-6 lists these selected nursing interventions.

SUCTIONING

Suctioning of the endotracheal tube is associated with a number of complications including hypoxemia, increased intracranial pressure, and loss of lung volume.[147] Routine suctioning should be avoided in all ventilated infants, including those on HFV.[55] When suctioning is required in neonates on HFJV, it is important to suction with the ventilator in standby mode if tolerated. When the neonate doesn't tolerate interrupting jet ventilation, suctioning should be done with suction applied during both insertion and withdrawal of the catheter to avoid excessive pressure buildup in the system.[55]

In-line suctioning devices have been shown to reduce the loss of volume associated with disconnection of the ventilator during suctioning procedures.[148] Given the importance of maintaining lung volumes during HFO, the use of inline suction catheters should be considered.

PLAN EVALUATION AND REVISION

Evaluation of nursing care plans for patients receiving HFV occurs frequently because these patients' needs are complex. The evaluation process is ongoing, providing feedback into the various steps of the nursing process. Most of the evaluation activities occur on an informal level at the bedside among the staff nurse, primary care provider, attending physician, and family.

Evaluation must also occur on a formal level. Various mechanisms for formal evaluation can include but are not limited to (1) formal nursing care rounds, (2) patient care conferences, and (3) quality assessment meetings. In these conferences and meetings, parents and medical, social service, clergy, and nursing staff, as well as other family members and support people (where appropriate), review the case or pertinent issues. The information and decisions from these conferences are then integrated into the daily nursing care plan.

The steps of the nursing process require that the information obtained, goals established, interventions performed, and evaluations conducted be analyzed to provide the basis for revision of the care plan. Frequent revisions are required because of limited ability to predict patient responses to HFV and are dictated by progression or deterioration of the patient's condition.

Because most infants treated with HFV now survive, the degree of residual CLD is a prime factor in planning future care for them. If the degree of pulmonary hypertension or CLD is severe or air leaks persist, the infant may require prolonged HFV. If improvement does not occur, then plans must be made for the use of alternate technology (such as ECMO) or for care of the infant and family during the terminal portion of hospitalization. Usually, death results from progressive respiratory failure. The ability of HFV to support ventilation in infants with very diseased lungs can prolong the terminal period.

PARENT CARE

When an infant is born sick, the emotional stress on the parents is very great. The decision to place their baby on HFV may increase that stress. Not only are these infants generally extremely ill, but they are receiving a nonstandard therapy that may appear to the parents to be nonphysiologic. This may create additional parental stress. HFV technology is often offered in the hope of rescuing a child who has not responded to CMV and surfactant. Yet for some extremely ill infants, such as those with pulmonary hypoplasia, HFV may only delay, not prevent, death.

The HFV technology and the associated parental stress level require additional nursing care for family education and support. The infant's degree of illness or the sedation given to some neonates on HFV may limit the interaction between parent and infant. Explanations of the technology and the unconventional breathing pattern provide important reassurance to parents, who may question how the vibrations created by HFV can sustain ventilation. Parents may have misconceptions or misunderstandings regarding the effects of this breathing pattern on their infant's ability to "remember" how to breathe or to maintain strength in the respiratory muscles.

Parents should be encouraged to participate in their infant's care as much as is feasible, especially when use of HFV is expected to be long term. Infants on HFV can be held, although provisions need to be made for the additional equipment and special positioning requirements. For infants who are terminally ill, ongoing assessment of the infant and the family and frequent, open communication with the family can help to ensure appropriate support during this difficult period. The families of all patients undergoing HFV therapy should be provided specialized support.

SUMMARY

HFV has now become a standard therapy in the care of selected newborns. It has been shown to be useful for rescue ventilation with infants suffering severe respiratory failure and possibly useful as an early therapeutic device for infants not responding to CMV. However, despite the plethora of research studies examining the use of HFV in neonates, definitive evidence demonstrating its efficacy continues to elude us. Clear delineation of which device is optimal for which type of patient, when HFV should be considered, and when (or if) weaning to CMV should be undertaken are all questions that remain to be answered.

The impact of HFV on nursing care has also been thoroughly examined. Much of the care provided to infants on HFV is based on practices used in CMV. Nursing research addressing positioning, suctioning, sedation, and developmental care practices for infants on HFV is limited. Our current and future challenge is to answer these and other questions in a collaborative, multidisciplinary fashion based on research and enhanced by our art of caring.

REFERENCES

1. Henderson-Smart DJ, Wilkinson AR, and Raynes-Greenow CH. 2005. Mechanical ventilation for newborn infants with respiratory failure due to pulmonary disease. *Cochrane Database of Systematic Reviews* (2): CD002770.

2. Long W, ed. 1993. *Clinics in Perinatology*. Philadelphia: Saunders, 696–831.

3. Bhandari A, and Panitch HB. 2006. Pulmonary outcomes in bronchopulmonary dysplasia. *Seminars in Perinatology* 30(4): 219–226.

4. Dreyfuss D, Saumon G. 1998. Ventilator-induced lung injury: Lessons from experimental studies. *American Journal of Respiratory and Critical Care Medicine* 157:294–323.

5. Truog WE, and Golombek SG. 2005. Principles of management of respiratory problems. In *Avery's Neonatology: Pathophysiology and Management of the Newborn*, 6th ed., MacDonald MG, Mullett MD, and Seshia MMK, eds. Philadelphia: Lippincott Williams & Wilkins, 600–621.

6. Durand DJ, and Asselin JM. 2004. High-frequency ventilation. In *Fetal and Neonatal Physiology*, Polin RA, Fox WW, and Abman SH, eds. Philadelphia: Saunders, 979–984.

7. Van Kaam AH, and Rimesberger PC. 2007. Lung-protective ventilation strategies in neonatology: What do we know—What do we need to know? *Critical Care Medicine* 35(3): 925–931.

8. Horbar JD, Carpenter JH, and Kenny M, eds. Vermont Oxford Network annual database summaries 1997–2005. Burlington, Vermont: Vermont Oxford Network: 1998–2006.

9. Clark R. 1994. High-frequency ventilation. *Journal of Pediatrics* 5(1): 661–670.

10. Keszler M, and Durand DJ. 2001. Neonatal high-frequency ventilation: Past, present, and future. *Clinics in Perinatology* 28(3): 579–607.

11. Keszler M. 2006. High-frequency ventilation: Evidence-based practice and specific clinical indications. *NeoReviews* 7(5): e234–e248.

12. Karp TB, et al. 1986. High frequency jet ventilation: A neonatal nursing perspective. *Neonatal Network* 4(5): 42–50.

13. Avila K, Mazza LV, and Morgan-Trujillo L. 1994. High-frequency oscillatory ventilation: A nursing approach to bedside care. *Neonatal Network* 13(5): 23–30.

14. Karp T. 1997. High-frequency ventilation: The current challenge to neonatal nursing. In *Acute Respiratory Care of the Neonate*, 2nd ed., Askin DF, ed. Santa Rosa, California: NICU INK, 313–340.

15. Boros SJ. 1979. Variation in inspiratory:expiratory ratio and airway pressure wave form during mechanical ventilation: The significance of mean airway pressure. *Journal of Pediatrics* 94(1): 114–117.

16. Ciszek TA, et al. 1981. Mean airway pressure—Significance during mechanical ventilation in neonates. *Journal of Pediatrics* 99(1): 121–126.

17. Carlo WA, and Martin RJ. 1986. Principles of neonatal assisted ventilation. *Pediatric Clinics of North America* 33(2): 221–237.

18. Frantz I, and Close RH. 1985. Elevated lung volumes and alveolar pressure during jet ventilation of rabbits. *American Review of Respiratory Disease* 131(1): 134–138.

19. Bancalari A, et al. 1987. Gas trapping with high frequency ventilation: Jet versus oscillatory ventilation. *Journal of Pediatrics* 110(4): 617–622.

20. Chang HK. 1984. Mechanisms of gas transport during high frequency ventilation. *Journal of Applied Physiology* 56(3): 553–563.

21. Chan V, and Greenough A. 1993. Determinants of oxygenation during high frequency oscillation. *European Journal of Pediatrics* 152(4): 350–353.

22. Gerstmann DR, deLemos RA, and Clark RH. 1991. High frequency ventilation: Issues of strategy. *Clinics in Perinatology* 18(3): 563–580.

23. Kolton M, et al. 1982. Oxygenation during high-frequency ventilation compared with conventional mechanical ventilation in two models of lung injury. *Anesthesia and Analgesia* 61(4): 323–332.

24. Walsh MC, and Carlo WA. 1988. Sustained inflation during HFOV improves pulmonary mechanics and oxygenation. *Journal of Applied Physiology* 65(1): 368–372.

25. Froese AB.1989. Role of lung volume in lung injury: HFO in the atelectasis-prone lung. *Acta anaesthesiologica Scandinavica. Supplementum* 90: 126–130.

26. Kinsella JP, et al. 1991. High-frequency oscillatory ventilation versus intermittent mandatory ventilation: Early hemodynamic effects in the premature baboon with hyaline membrane disease. *Pediatric Research* 29(2): 160–166.

27. Weisberger SA, et al. 1986. Measurement of tidal volume during high-frequency jet ventilation. *Pediatric Research* 20(1): 45–48.

28. Weisberger SA, et al. 1986. Effects of varying inspiratory and expiratory times during high frequency jet ventilation. *Journal of Pediatrics* 108(4): 596–600.

29. Permutt S, Mitzner W, and Weinmonn G. 1985. Model of gas transport during high-frequency ventilation. *Journal of Applied Physiology* 58(6): 1956–1970.

30. Henderson Y, Chillingworth FP, and Whitney JL. 1915. The respiratory dead space. *American Journal of Physiology* 38(1): 1–19.

31. Haselton FR, and Scherer PW. 1980. Bronchial bifurcation of respiratory mass transport. *Science* 208(4): 69–71.

32. Taylor GI. 1954. Dispersion of matter in turbulent flow through a pipe. Proceedings of the Royal Society of London 223(1155): 446–468.

33. Jaegar MJ, Kursweg UH, and Banner MJ. 1984. Transport of gases in high frequency ventilation. *Critical Care Medicine* 12(9): 708–710.

34. Gerstmann DR, et al. 1990. Proximal, tracheal and alveolar pressures during high-frequency oscillatory ventilation in normal rabbit model. *Pediatric Research* 28(4): 367–373.

35. Venegas JG, and Fredberg JJ. 1994. Understanding the pressure cost of ventilation: Why does high-frequency ventilation work? *Critical Care Medicine* 22(9): S49–S57.

36. Mammel MC. 2003. High-frequency ventilation. In *Assisted Ventilation of the Neonate*, 4th ed., Goldsmith JP, and Karotkin EH, eds. Philadelphia. Saunders, 183–201.

37. Richards E, and Bunnell B. 1995. Fundamentals of patient management during high frequency jet ventilation. *Neonatal Intensive Care* 8(3): 22–27.

38. Cotton CM, and Clark RH. 2005. High-frequency oscillatory ventilation. In *Intensive Care of the Fetus and Neonate*, 2nd ed., Spitzer AR, ed. Philadelphia: Mosby 671–679.

39. Lampland AL, and Mammel MC. 2007. The role of high-frequency ventilation in neonates: Evidence-based recommendations. *Clinics in Perinatology* 34(1): 129–144.

40. Hamilton PP, et al. 1983. Comparison of conventional and high-frequency ventilation: Oxygenation and lung pathology. *Journal of Applied Physiology* 55(1 part 1): 131–138.

41. McCulloch PR, Forkert PG, and Froese AB. 1988. Lung volume maintenance prevents lung injury during high frequency oscillatory ventilation in surfactant-deficient rabbits. *The American Review of Respiratory Disease* 137(5): 1185–1192.

42. Meredith KS, et al. 1989. Role of lung injury in the pathogenesis of hyaline membrane disease in premature baboons. *Journal of Applied Physiology* 66(5): 2150–2158.

43. Froese AB, et al. 1993. Optimizing alveolar expansion prolongs the effectiveness of exogenous surfactant therapy in the adult rabbit. *The American Review of Respiratory Disease* 148(3): 569–577.

44. Clark RH, et al. 1986. Pulmonary interstitial emphysema treated by high frequency oscillatory ventilation. *Critical Care Medicine* 14(11): 926–930.

45. Walker AM, et al. 1992. High-frequency oscillatory ventilation compared with conventional mechanical ventilation in newborn lambs: Effects of increasing airway pressure on intracranial pressures. *Pediatric Pulmonology* 12(1): 11–16.

46. Jackson JC, et al. 1994. Reduction in lung injury after combined surfactant and high-frequency ventilation. *American Journal of Respiratory and Critical Care Medicine* 150(2): 534–539.

47. Patel CA, and Klein JM. 1995. Outcome of infants with birth weights less than 1,000 g with respiratory distress syndrome treated with high-frequency ventilation and surfactant replacement therapy. *Archives of Pediatric and Adolescent Medicine* 149(3): 317–321.

48. Donn SM, and Sinha SK. 2003. Invasive and noninvasive neonatal mechanical ventilation. *Respiratory Care* 48(4): 439–441.

49. Thome UH, and Carlo WA. 2008. High-frequency ventilation in neonatal respiratory failure. In *The Newborn Lung, Neonatal Questions and Controversies*, Bancalari E, and Polin RA, eds. Philadelphia: Saunders, 377–391.

50. Pokora T, et al. 1983. Neonatal high-frequency jet ventilation. *Pediatrics* 72(1): 27–32.

51. Boros SJ, et al. 1985. Neonatal high-frequency jet ventilation: Four years' experience. *Pediatrics* 75(4): 657–663.

52. Boros SJ, et al. 1989. Comparison of high-frequency oscillatory ventilation and high-frequency jet ventilation in cats with normal lungs. *Pediatric Pulmonology* 7(1): 35–41.

53. Mammel MC, et al. 1991. Acute airway injury during high-frequency jet ventilation and high-frequency oscillatory ventilation. *Critical Care Medicine* 19(3): 394–398.

54. Bunnell B. 1995. Personal communication concerning servo-pressure.

55. Keszler M. 2005. High-frequency jet ventilation. In *Intensive Care of the Fetus and Neonate*, 2nd ed., Spitzer AR, ed. Philadelphia: Mosby, 655–669.

56. Clark RH, et al. 1992. Prospective randomized comparison of high-frequency oscillatory and conventional ventilation in respiratory distress syndrome. *Pediatrics*. 89(1):5–12.

57. Brisco WR, Foster RE, and Comroe J Jr. 1954. Alveolar ventilation at very low tidal volumes. *Pediatric Research* 7(7): 27–30.

58. Emerson JH. 1959. Apparatus for vibrating portions of a patient's airway. U.S. patent no. 2,918,917.

59. Lunkenheimer PP, et al. 1972. Application of transtracheal pressure oscillations as a modification of "diffusion" respiration. *British Journal of Anaesthesia* 44(6): 627–631.

60. Klain M, and Smith RB. 1977. High frequency percutaneous transtracheal jet ventilation. *Critical Care Medicine* 5(6): 280–287.

61. Sjostrand U. 1980. High frequency positive pressure ventilation (HFPPV), a review. *Critical Care Medicine* 8(6): 345–364.

62. Thompson WK, et al. 1982. High frequency oscillation compared with standard ventilation in pulmonary injury model. *Journal of Applied Physiology* 52(3): 543–548.

63. Truog WE, et al. 1983. Effect of high-frequency oscillation on gas exchange and pulmonary phospholipids in experimental hyaline membrane disease. *The American Review of Respiratory Disease* 127(5): 585–589.

64. Bell RE, et al. 1984. High-frequency ventilation compared to conventional positive-pressure ventilation in the treatment of hyaline membrane disease. *Critical Care Medicine* 12(9): 764–768.

65. Ackerman NB Jr, et al. 1984. Pulmonary interstitial emphysema in the premature baboon with hyaline membrane disease. *Critical Care Medicine* 12(6): 512–516.

66. deLemos RA, et al. 1987. Ventilatory management of infant baboons with hyaline membrane disease: The use of high frequency ventilation. *Pediatric Research* 21(6): 594–602.

67. Butler WJ, et al. 1980. Ventilation by high frequency oscillation in humans. *Anesthesia and Analgesia* 59(8): 577–584.

68. Carlon GC, et al. 1981. Clinical experience with high frequency jet ventilation. *Critical Care Medicine* 9(1): 1–6.

69. Marchak BE, et al. 1981. Treatment of RDS by high-frequency oscillatory ventilation: A preliminary report. *Journal of Pediatrics* 99(2): 287–292.

70. Harris TR, and Christensen RD. 1984. High frequency jet ventilation of pulmonary interstitial emphysema. *Pediatric Research* 18(4): 326A.

71. Carlo WA, et al. 1984. Decrease in airway pressure during high-frequency jet ventilation in infants with respiratory distress syndrome. *Journal of Pediatrics* 104(1): 101–107.

72. Frantz I, Werthammer J, and Stark A. 1983. High frequency ventilation in premature infants with lung disease: Adequate gas exchange at low tracheal pressure. *Pediatrics* 71(4): 483–488.

73. Pauly TH, et al. 1987. Predictability of success of high-frequency jet ventilation in infants with persistent pulmonary hypertension. Ross Special Conference in Neonatology: Two Great Debates (program syllabus), 172A.

74. Carlo WA, et al. 1989. High frequency jet ventilation in neonatal pulmonary hypertension. *American Journal of Diseases of Children* 143(2): 233–238.

75. Kohelet D, et al. 1988. High frequency oscillation in the rescue of infants with persistent pulmonary hypertension. *Critical Care Medicine* 16(5): 510–516.

76. Carter J, et al. 1990. High frequency oscillatory ventilation and extracorporeal membrane oxygenation for the treatment of acute neonatal respiratory failure. *Pediatrics* 85(1): 159–164.

77. Gonzalez F, et al. 1986. Decreased gas flow through pneumothoraces in neonates receiving high-frequency jet ventilation versus conventional ventilation. *Journal of Pediatrics* 110(3): 464–466.

78. Mammel MC, et al. 1987. High frequency jet ventilation: The Children's Hospital of St. Paul experience and viewpoint. Ross Special Conference in Neonatology: Two Great Debates (program syllabus), 181–182.

79. High-Frequency Oscillatory Ventilation Study Group. 1989. High-frequency oscillatory ventilation compared with conventional mechanical ventilation in the treatment of respiratory failure in premature infants. *New England Journal of Medicine* 320(2): 88–93.

80. Bryan AC, and Froese AB. 1991. Reflections on the HIFI trial. *Pediatrics* 87(4): 565–567.

81. Cools F, et al. 2009. Elective high frequency oscillatory ventilation versus conventional ventilation for acute pulmonary dysfunction in preterm infants. *Cochrane Database of Systematic Reviews* (3): CD000104.

82. HIFI Study Group. 1989. High-frequency oscillatory ventilation compared with conventional mechanical ventilation in the treatment of respiratory failure in preterm infants. *New England Journal of Medicine* 320(2): 88–93.

83. Ogawa Y, et al. 1993. A multicenter randomized trial of high frequency oscillatory ventilation as compared with conventional mechanical ventilation in preterm infants with respiratory failure. *Early Human Development* 32(1): 1–10.

84. Gerstmann DR, et al. 1996. The Provo multicenter early high-frequency oscillatory ventilation trial: Improved pulmonary and clinical outcome in respiratory distress syndrome. *Pediatrics* 98(6 part 6): 1044–1057.

85. Rettwitz-Volk W, et al. 1998. A prospective, randomized, multicenter trial of high-frequency oscillatory ventilation compared with conventional ventilation in preterm infants with respiratory distress syndrome receiving surfactant. *Journal of Pediatrics* 132(2): 249–254.

86. Thome U, et al. 1998. High frequency oscillatory ventilation(HFOV) compared with high rate intermittent positive pressure ventilation (IPPV) as first line therapy for premature infants with respiratory insufficiency: A prospective randomized multicenter trial. *Pediatric Research* 43: 300A.

87. Plavka R, et al. 1999. A prospective randomized comparison of conventional mechanical ventilation and very early high frequency oscillatory ventilation in extremely premature newborns with respiratory distress syndrome. *Intensive Care Medicine* 25(1): 68–75.

88. Moriette G, et al. 2001. Prospective randomized multicenter comparison of high-frequency oscillatory ventilation and conventional ventilation in preterm infants of less than 30 weeks with respiratory distress syndrome. *Pediatrics* 107(2): 363–372.

89. Durand DJ, et al. 2001. Early high-frequency oscillatory ventilation versus synchronized intermittent mandatory ventilation in very low birth weight infants: a pilot study of two ventilation protocols. *Journal of Perinatology* 21(4): 221–229.

90. Courtney SE, et al. 2002. High-frequency oscillatory ventilation versus conventional mechanical ventilation for very-low-birth-weight Infants. *New England Journal of Medicine* 347(9): 643–652.

91. Johnson AH, et al. 2002. High-frequency oscillatory ventilation for the prevention of chronic lung disease of prematurity. *New England Journal of Medicine* 347(9): 633–642.

92. Van Reempts P, et al. 2003. Early use of high frequency ventilation in the premature neonate. *European Journal of Pediatrics* 162(4): 219–226.

93. Craft AP, Bhandari V, and Finer NN. 2003. The sy-fi study: A randomized prospective trial of synchronized intermittent mandatory ventilation versus a high-frequency flow interrupter in infants less than 1000 g. *Journal of Perinatology* 23(1):14–19.

94. Schreiber MD, et al. 2003. Inhaled nitric oxide in premature infants with the respiratory distress syndrome. *New England Journal of Medicine* 349(22): 2099–2107.

95. Vento G, et al. 2005. HFOV in premature neonates: Effects on pulmonary mechanics and epithelial lining fluid cytokines. A randomized controlled trial. *Intensive Care Medicine* 31(3): 463–470.

96. Dani C, et al. 2006. Effects of pressure support ventilation plus volume guarantee vs. high-frequency oscillatory ventilation on lung inflammation in preterm infants. *Pediatric Pulmonology* 41(3): 242–249.

97. Lista G, et al. 2008. Volume guarantee versus high-frequency ventilation: Lung inflammation in preterm infants. *Archives of Disease in Childhood. Fetal and Neonatal Edition* 93(4): F252–F256.

98. HiFO Study Group. 1993. Randomized study of high-frequency oscillatory ventilation in infants with severe respiratory distress syndrome. *Journal of Pediatrics* 122(4): 609–619.

99. Bhuta T, Clark RH, and Henderson-Smart DJ. 2001. Rescue high frequency oscillatory ventilation vs conventional ventilation for infants with severe pulmonary dysfunction born at or near term. *Cochrane Database of Systematic Reviews* (1): CD002974.

100. Bhuta T, and Henderson-Smart DJ. 2000. Elective high frequency jet ventilation versus conventional ventilation for respiratory distress syndrome in preterm infants. *Cochrane Database of Systematic Reviews* (4): CD000328.

101. Joshi VH, and Bhuta T. 2006. Rescue high frequency jet ventilation versus conventional ventilation for severe pulmonary dysfunction in preterm infants. *Cochrane Database of Systematic Reviews* (1): CD000437.

102. Carlo WA, et al. 1990. Early randomized intervention with high-frequency jet ventilation in respiratory distress syndrome. *Journal of Pediatrics* 117(5): 765–770.

103. Keszler M, et al. 1997. Multicenter controlled clinical trial of high-frequency jet ventilation in preterm infants with uncomplicated respiratory distress syndrome. *Pediatrics* 100(4): 593–599.

104. Wiswell TE, et al. 1996. High-frequency jet ventilation in the early management of respiratory distress syndrome is associated with a greater risk for adverse outcomes. *Pediatrics* 98(6 part 1): 1035–1043.

105. Soll RF. 2006. The clinical impact of high frequency ventilation: Review of the Cochrane meta-analyses. *Journal of Perinatology* 26(supplement 1): S38–S42.

106. Keszler M, et al. 1991. Multi-center controlled trial comparing high-frequency jet ventilation and conventional mechanical ventilation in newborn infants with pulmonary interstitial emphysema. *Journal of Pediatrics* 119(1): 85–93.

107. Bollen CW, Uiterwaal CS, and van Vught AJ. 2003. Cumulative metaanalysis of high-frequency versus conventional ventilation in premature neonates. *American Journal of Respiratory and Critical Care Medicine* 168(10): 1150–1155.

108. Thome U, et al. 1999. Randomized comparison of high-frequency ventilation with high-rate intermittent positive pressure ventilation in preterm infants with respiratory failure. *Journal of Pediatrics* 135(1): 39–46.

109. Froese AB, et al. 1987. High-frequency oscillatory ventilation in premature infants with respiratory failure: A preliminary report. *Anesthesia and Analgesia* 66(9): 814–824.

110. Bollen CW, Uiterwaal CS, van Vught AJ. 2007. Meta-regression analysis of high-frequency ventilation vs conventional ventilation in infant respiratory distress syndrome. *Intensive Care Medicine* 33(4): 680–688.

111. Schur MS, et al. 1988. High-frequency jet ventilation in the management of congenital tracheal stenosis. *Anesthesiology* 68(6): 952–955.

112. Donn SM, et al. 1990. Use of high-frequency jet ventilation in the management of congenital tracheoesophageal fistula associated with respiratory distress syndrome. *Journal of Pediatric Surgery* 25(12): 1219–1221.

113. Davis DA, et al. 1994. High-frequency jet versus conventional ventilation in infants undergoing Blalock-Taussig shunts. *Annals of Thoracic Surgery* 57(4): 846–849.

114. Meliones JN, et al. 1991. High-frequency jet ventilation improves cardiac function after the Fontan procedure. *Circulation* 84(5 supplement): 364–368.

115. Harris TR, et al. 1984. High frequency jet ventilation treatment of neonates with congenital left diaphragmatic hernia. *Clinical Research* 32(2): 123A.

116. Bohn D, Tamura M, and Bryan C. 1984. Respiratory failure in congenital diaphragmatic hernia: Ventilation by high frequency oscillation. *Pediatric Research* 18(4): 387A.

117. Stoddard R, et al. 1993. Treatment of congenital diaphragmatic hernia (CDH) with high frequency oscillatory ventilation (HFOV). *Pediatric Pulmonology* 15(6): 367.

118. Miguet D, et al. 1994. Preoperative stabilization using high frequency oscillatory ventilation in the management of congenital diaphragmatic hernia. *Critical Care Medicine* 22(9): S77–S82.

119. Trindale O, et al. 1985. Conventional versus high frequency jet ventilation in a piglet model of meconium aspiration: Comparison of pulmonary and hemodynamic effects. *Journal of Pediatrics* 107(1): 115–120.

120. Keszler M, et al. 1986. Combined high frequency jet ventilation in a meconium aspiration model. *Critical Care Medicine* 14(1): 34–37.

121. Baumgart S, et al. 1992. Diagnosis-related criteria in consideration of extracorporeal membrane oxygenation in neonates previously treated with high frequency jet ventilation. *Pediatrics* 89(3): 491–494.

122. Varnholt V, et al. 1992. High frequency oscillatory ventilation and extracorporeal membrane oxygenation in severe persistent pulmonary hypertension of the newborn. *European Journal of Pediatrics* 151(10): 769–774.

123. Clark RH, Yoder BA, and Sell MS. 1994. Prospective, randomized comparison of high frequency oscillation and conventional ventilation in candidates for extracorporeal membrane oxygenation. *Journal of Pediatrics* 124(3): 447–454.

124. Paranka MS, et al. 1995. Predictors of failure of high frequency oscillatory ventilation in term infants with severe respiratory failure. *Pediatrics* 95(3): 400–404.

125. Engle WA, et al. 1997. Controlled prospective randomized comparison of high frequency jet ventilation and conventional ventilation in neonates with respiratory failure and persistent pulmonary hypertension. *Journal of Perinatology* 17(1): 3–9.

126. Davis J, et al. 1992. High frequency jet ventilation and surfactant treatment of newborns with severe respiratory failure. *Pediatric Pulmonology* 13(1): 108–112.

127. Kinsella JP, et al. 1997. Randomized, multicenter trial of inhaled nitric oxide and high-frequency oscillatory ventilation in severe, persistent pulmonary hypertension of the newborn. *Journal of Pediatrics* 131(1 part 1): 55–62.

128. Dobyns EL, et al. 2002. Interactive effects of high-frequency oscillatory ventilation and inhaled nitric oxide in acute hypoxemic respiratory failure in pediatrics. *Critical Care Medicine* 30(1): 2425–2429.

129. Courtney SE, and Asselin JM. 2006. High-frequency jet and oscillatory ventilation for neonates: Which strategy and when? *Respiratory Care Clinics of North America* 12(3): 453–467.

130. Wiswell TE, et al. 1992. Management of a piglet model of meconium aspiration syndrome with high-frequency or conventional ventilation. *American Journal of Diseases of Children* 146(1): 1287–1293.

131. Henderson-Smart DJ, et al. 2007. Elective high frequency oscillatory ventilation versus conventional ventilation for acute pulmonary dysfunction in preterm infants. *Cochrane Database of Systematic Reviews* (3): CD000104.

132. Gaylord MS, Quissell BJ, and Lair ME. 1987. High frequency ventilation in the treatment of infants weighing less than 1,500 grams with pulmonary interstitial emphysema: A pilot study. *Pediatrics* 79(6): 915–921.

133. Wiswell TE, et al. 1988. Tracheal and bronchial injury in high-frequency oscillatory ventilation and high-frequency flow interruption compared with conventional positive-pressure ventilation. *Pediatrics* 112(2): 249–256.

134. Traverse JH, et al. 1988. Impairment of hemodynamics with increasing mean airway pressure during high frequency oscillatory ventilation. *Pediatric Research* 49(1): 21–28.

135. Pietsch JB, et al. 1985. Necrotizing tracheobronchitis: A new indication for emergency bronchoscopy in the neonate. *Journal of Pediatric Surgery* 20(4): 391–393.

136. Boros SJ, et al. 1986. Necrotizing tracheobronchitis: a complication of high-frequency ventilation. *Journal of Pediatrics* 109(1): 95–100.

137. Wilson KS, et al. 1987. Necrotizing tracheobronchitis: A newly recognized cause of acute obstruction in mechanically ventilated neonates. *Laryngoscope* 97(9): 1017–1019.

138. Ophoven JP, et al. 1984. Tracheobronchial histopathology associated with high-frequency jet ventilation. *Critical Care Medicine* 12(9): 829–832.

139. Kirpalani H, et al. 1985. Diagnosis and therapy of necrotizing tracheobronchitis in ventilated neonates. *Critical Care Medicine* 13(10): 792–797.

140. Wiswell TE, et al. 1990. Different high frequency strategies: Effect on the propagation of tracheobronchial histopathologic changes. *Pediatrics* 85(1): 70–78.

141. Nicklaus P. 1995. Airway complications of jet ventilation in neonates. *Annals of Otology, Rhinology, and Laryngology* 104(3): 24–29.

142. Minton S, et al. 1987. Silicone particulate debris in the Life Pulse high frequency jet ventilator. *Pediatric Pulmonology* 3(10): 375A.

143. Schmidt J, et al. 1995. Skin breakdown with high frequency oscillatory ventilation. Twelfth Annual Conference on High-Frequency Ventilation of Infants, Snowbird, Utah (abstract and presentation).

144. Haney C, and Allingham TM. 1992. Nursing care of the neonate receiving high-frequency jet ventilation. *JOGNN* 21(3): 187–195.

145. Olson DL, et al. 1986. High frequency jet ventilation: Endotracheal suction procedure. *Neonatal Network* 4(5): 66–68.

146. Guntupalli K, Sladen A, and Klain M. 1984. High-frequency jet ventilation and tracheobronchial suctioning. *Critical Care Medicine* 12(9): 791–792.

147. Hageman JR, et al. 2003. Pulmonary care. In *Assisted Ventilation of the Neonate*, 4th ed., Goldsmith JP, and Karotkin EH, eds. Philadelphia: Saunders, 91–105.

148. Choong K, et al. 2003. Comparison of loss in lung volume with open versus in-line catheter endotracheal suctioning. *Pediatric Critical Care Medicine* 4(1): 69–73.

149. Inwood S. 1991. High frequency oscillation. In *Acute Respiratory Care of the Neonate*, Nugent J, ed. Petaluma, California: NICU INK, 1–19.

NOTES

NOTES

13 Extracorporeal Membrane Oxygenation in the Newborn

Gerry Matranga, MN, APRN, NNP-BC
Kristine Strecker, APRN, NNP-BC

Advances in technology have challenged clinicians to consider alternative therapies for the small percentage of infants with severe pulmonary dysfunction who respond poorly to maximal ventilatory, medical, and surgical treatment.[1-3] Application of research in the management of neonatal pulmonary disease has led to the use of therapies including high-frequency ventilation, surfactant replacement, and inhaled nitric oxide. The use of these therapies has reduced but not eliminated the need for extracorporeal membrane oxygenation (ECMO).

After maximal standard therapy (conventional ventilator support, high-frequency ventilator support, surfactant replacement, and the use of inhaled nitric oxide) has been exhausted, ECMO can provide lifesaving cardiopulmonary support in some neonates with predictably fatal pulmonary/cardiac failure. Nurses caring for these infants need a basic understanding of the principles of ECMO perfusion as well as excellent physical assessment and psychosocial skills. The nurse's ability to provide this sophisticated level of care will have a direct and significant impact on the outcome of this mode of therapy.

VENTILATOR THERAPY

Despite significant advances in the care of infants with severe pulmonary dysfunction, respiratory failure remains a leading cause of neonatal death. Contributing respiratory pathologies include respiratory distress syndrome (RDS); meconium aspiration syndrome (MAS); persistent pulmonary hypertension of the newborn (PPHN), which may occur as a primary entity or as a secondary complication of respiratory failure;

and pulmonary hypoplasia associated with congenital diaphragmatic hernia (CDH).[3]

Varying methods of ventilator management exist. In addition to conventional ventilator therapy (pressure-limited, time-cycled, continuous-flow mechanical ventilation), the use of high frequency ventilation has proved to be beneficial in the treatment of hypoxic pulmonary disease. Adjuncts to ventilator therapy include the use of surfactant replacement therapy, inotropic agents (dopamine, dobutamine) to augment systemic circulation, and the use of inhaled nitric oxide as a selective pulmonary vasodilator. Sodium bicarbonate and THAM have also been utilized to induce alkalosis, thus dilating the pulmonary vasculature.[3-5] More recently, sildenafil has been used as an alternative therapy in pulmonary hypertension. Sildenafil selectively inhibits phosphodiesterase-type 5 (PDE-5), which is found in high concentrations in the lungs. The inhibition of PDE-5 enhances the vasodilatory effects of nitric oxide in pulmonary hypertension by preventing the breakdown of cyclic guanosine monophosphate (cGMP). cGMP promotes relaxation of vascular smooth muscle and thus increases blood flow through the pulmonary arteries.[6]

The aggressive management required to treat severe pulmonary dysfunction and PPHN can contribute significantly to acute parenchymal damage. This can lead to therapeutic failure and death or to chronic respiratory disease. A small percentage of infants who survive the acute stages of their disease may be chronically crippled by bronchopulmonary dysplasia from barotrauma and oxygen toxicity.[7] Recent trends in respiratory management include tolerance for permissive hypercarbia, oxygen targeting with lower oxygen saturation levels, and decreased ventilator pressures to reduce the incidence of barotrauma and the sequelae of chronic lung disease.[3] Despite these new management strategies, lung injury and chronic lung disease continue to occur.

A HISTORICAL PERSPECTIVE

The process of prolonged extracorporeal circulation (cardiopulmonary bypass) achieved by extrathoracic vascular cannulation provides cardiorespiratory support for infants in reversible, profound, respiratory, or cardiac failure.[7] Rashkind and associates were the first to report use of neonatal extracorporeal oxygenation via femoral arteriovenous shunt through a bulb oxygenator in 1965.[8] Initial work with an extracorporeal membrane oxygenator was reported by other investigators during the late 1960s and early 1970s.[9–11] There were no survivors reported in these early trials, but the work of these clinicians established the feasibility of ECMO as a treatment modality and demonstrated the need for further refinements in both apparatus and technique.

The chief problems the early investigators encountered were fairly daunting. The heart-lung machine required a large blood reservoir, which necessitated complete suppression of coagulation and a large priming volume. The oxygenator, which functioned by direct exposure of blood to oxygen, damaged blood cells and proteins if operated for more than a few hours. The blood pump hemolyzed red cells and caused significant leukopenia. Vascular access was a problem: Umbilical vessels or vessels in the leg were used to gain access to the infant's circulation, but these proved too small to provide extracorporeal flow sufficient for adequate respiratory support.

Extracorporeal therapy required that the patient be heparinized until coagulation ceased. This practice was safe for only a limited period of time because of the real potential of producing life-threatening hemorrhage when treatment was extended over a period of days. No simple laboratory procedure for instantaneous evaluation of clotting time existed. This made accurate titration of systemic anticoagulants impossible.[12]

Medical researchers, lured by the prospect of developing a clinical revolution in cardiopulmonary support, began extensive clinical trials supported by grants from the National Institutes of Health. Kolobow and coworkers began work on the roller pump and membrane lung in 1969, demonstrated the superior

blood compatibility of silicone in a membrane lung in 1974, and published data on long-term survivability of lambs perfused up to ten days in 1976.[13–16]

Concurrent clinical work on the technique of extracorporeal circulation via extrathoracic vascular access was begun by Bartlett and colleagues in 1971. They managed their first newborn patient in 1975. In 1982, they published data on the use of ECMO in 45 moribund infants who were unresponsive to maximal therapy with a reported success rate of 25 survivors. The retrospective study's conclusion was that ECMO decreased respiratory failure mortality and morbidity rates.[17]

Since the early 1980s, the survival rate has improved because of extensive experience with the technique, case selection, and earlier intervention. Bartlett and associates determined that ECMO was safe (the risks of the treatment itself were less than the risks of the disease) and effective in trials that included 55 moribund patients treated in three centers over a nine-year period. Of the 40 infants with birth weights >2 kg, 28 (70 percent) survived. Of the 15 infants with birth weights <2 kg, 3 (20 percent) survived.[17–19]

Encouraged by the reported overall survival rate of 56 percent, groups in several major medical centers evaluated the use of ECMO in neonates.[3,20,21] During this phase of clinical research, ECMO was used when all other therapy had failed and the infant was considered moribund. The moribund condition was quantified by objective criteria predictive of high mortality (>80 percent). Commonly used predictors of mortality rate were the Newborn Pulmonary Insufficiency Index (NPII) and the alveolar-arterial gradient (Table 13-1).[22–24] The NPII has since been eliminated as an effective tool because it was not accurately predictive in those infants who had alkalization as part of their treatment modality.[25]

Prompted by the successful outcome of this phase of research, Bartlett and coworkers designed and conducted a prospective, controlled, randomized study. From October 1982 until April 1984, a group of 12 infants with birth weights >2 kg who met the greater than 80 percent mortality risk criteria entered the study. One patient was randomly assigned to conventional therapy and later died. Then 11 patients were randomly chosen for ECMO and all survived.[19]

This study used the "randomized play-the-winner" technique, which assigns an infant to treatment based on the outcome of each previous patient in the study—that is, if one treatment is more successful, more patients

TABLE 13-1
Criteria Predictive of Potential Mortality

1. Newborn Pulmonary Insufficiency Index (NPII)

In the past, the NPII was used as a measure of high mortality risk (greater than 80 percent). The NPII score is a single-number cumulation of oxygen requirement, acidosis, and time. This score assesses the severity of an infant's respiratory distress in the first day of life. It is calculated by plotting the newborn's FiO_2 and pH on a graph over the first 24 hours of life. The NPII graph has 10 percent FiO_2 increments and one-tenth pH increments on the vertical axis and hourly time increments on the horizontal axis. The score is determined by the number of boxes outlined between the FiO_2 and pH lines when the plotted FiO_2 is greater than the plotted pH on the graph.[38,70] However, with the advent of induced alkalosis as a treatment for PPHN, the NPII will not accurately predict mortality.[18,70,71] The following predictors of mortality are the most widely used.

2. Alveolar-Arterial Gradient >605–620 for 4–12 Hours

Alveolar-arterial oxygen difference ($AaDO_2$) is a measure of alveolar efficiency in transporting oxygen to pulmonary capillaries. Use of this criterion assumes that the baby is ventilated with 1 FiO_2 and that the $PACO_2 = PaCO_2$. The following calculation is used:

$$AaDO_2 = (FiO_2) \times (713) - (PaO_2 - PaCO_2)$$

The numeric value 713 assumes an atmospheric pressure of 760 mmHg minus vapor pressure (47 mmHg); PaO_2 and $PaCO_2$ are measured by assaying arterial blood gases. Retrospective reviews demonstrate that an $AaDO_2$ >620 for 12 consecutive hours correlates with >80 percent mortality.[24,24,70] More recent resources utilize an $AaDO_2$ >605–620 for 4–12 hours as a selection criterion for ECMO.[3,28]

3. Oxygenation Index (OI) >40

The oxygenation index can be utilized to predict mortality and the incidence of bronchopulmonary dysplasia. The OI is calculated by dividing the product of the FiO_2 (%) and the mean airway pressure by the postductal PaO_2:

$$OI = \frac{Mean\ Airway\ Pressure\ (FiO_2 \times 100)}{Postductal\ PaO_2}$$

Retrospective data demonstrate that an oxygenation index ≥40 correlates with a predicted mortality risk of 80–90 percent; an index ≥25–40 correlates with a 50–60 percent risk of mortality.[7]

4. Presence of Acute Respiratory Failure/Deterioration

Evidence of a PaO_2 <40 torr for >2 hours as determined by arterial blood gas sampling once optimal response to conventional therapy has been achieved.

5. Acidosis and Shock

Persistent acidosis pH (<7.25 for >2 hours) and hypotension despite use of pharmacologic therapies.

6. Congenital Diaphragmatic Hernia with Respiratory Failure

ECMO may provide preoperative stabilization in infants with CDH to allow pulmonary bed vascular remodeling or may be used as a rescue modality in infants who are unresponsive to other medical and/or surgical management.[3,28]

Adapted from: Nugent J. 1986. Extracorporeal membrane oxygenation in the neonate. *Neonatal Network* 4(5): 29. Reprinted by permission.

are randomly assigned to it. The researchers utilized this methodology to address the scientific/ethical issue of withholding an unproved but potentially lifesaving treatment. Thus, some patients were saved from exposure to an inferior treatment. The research of this phase documented that survival is better with ECMO (90 percent) than with conventional ventilation.[19]

The research results, the small study size, and the statistical method used generated significant controversy.[24–26] This controversy compelled O'Rourke and colleagues to design a prospective clinical trial comparing ECMO with conventional mechanical ventilation (CMV). To limit the number of infants assigned to what might ultimately be a less effective therapy, the researchers used an adaptive design with both a randomized and a nonrandomized phase. If the therapies were proved to be of equal efficiency, all patients would be randomized. Enrolled in the study were 39 newborns (weight >3 kg, 39–40 weeks gestation) with severe PPHN and respiratory failure who

met the 85 percent mortality criteria. Randomization was halted after the fourth infant treated with CMV died, and the next 20 infants were treated with ECMO. The overall survival of ECMO-treated infants was 97 percent (28 of 29), compared with 60 percent (6 of 10) in the CMV group.[28,29]

In 1986, Bartlett and associates published a summary of their group's first 100 cases, which validated an overall survival rate of 72 percent. In infants weighing >2 kg, the survival rate was 83 percent. The study concluded that ECMO could be used as the treatment of choice for full-term infants with respiratory failure not responsive to conventional therapy.[30]

In 1989, Bartlett and coworkers completed a study addressing the use of ECMO earlier in the course of the disease, at a time of lower predicted mortality. Neonates who met criteria for 50 percent predicted mortality using an oxygen index (OI) >25 were randomized to either ECMO or CMV. Those in the CMV group either improved or were offered late ECMO after meeting

TABLE 13-2
Outcome Information for Infants on ECMO

Neonatal ECMO Cases	Total Patients	Survived Extracorporeal Life Support	Survived to Discharge or Transfer
Respiratory	24,770	20,951 (85%)	18,558 (75%)
Cardiac	4,375	2,649 (61%)	1,723 (39%)
Emergency cardiopulmonary resuscitation	694	438 (63%)	270 (39%)
Respiratory Runs by Diagnosis	**Total Runs**	**Survived**	**% Survived**
MAS	7,814	7,322	94
CDH	6,280	3,198	51
Persistent pulmonary hypertension of the newborn	4,129	3,200	78
Sepsis	2,646	1,974	75
RDS	1,508	1,269	84
Pneumonia	345	197	57
Air leak syndrome	117	87	74
Other	2,261	1,433	63

Adapted from: Extracorporeal Life Support Organization (ELSO). July 2011. International Summary. Ann Arbor, Michigan.

criteria for 80 percent predicted mortality. The study evaluated differences in length of hospital stay, length of mechanical ventilation, cost, and patient morbidity among groups receiving early ECMO, late ECMO, and CMV. Results suggested that the group with the least morbidity were those who were placed on ECMO early: There were 15 of 20 normal survivors in this group versus 6 of 11 normal survivors in the late ECMO group and 1 of 5 normal survivors in the CMV group, which did not receive ECMO. There was no statistical difference in cost.[31]

Through July 2011, the Extracorporeal Life Support Organization (ELSO), which publishes data from institutions in the U.S. and abroad, lists more than 24,000 infants treated with ECMO since 1975 (Table 13-2). These statistics include all participating medical institutions.[32]

CRITERIA FOR ECMO USE

ECMO is an extreme life-support procedure with significant inherent risks. Neonates are considered candidates only if their risk of mortality is estimated at greater than 80 percent, with failure to respond to maximum therapy.

ECMO acts as a temporary heart-lung substitute. A neonate's pulmonary or cardiac pathology must be acute and reversible within a variable amount of time to prevent significant lung injury. Ideally, an infant should be placed on ECMO when the risk of barotrauma from prolonged mechanical ventilation outweighs the risks of bypass. Reversible neonatal disease processes that may fit this criterion include RDS, MAS, PPHN, congenital diaphragmatic hernia with respiratory failure, pneumonia, and selected operable cardiac anomalies.

ECMO therapy places the neonate at risk of life-threatening and serious physiologic and mechanical complications. Selection criteria must identify infants destined to die even with maximum support while excluding hypoxic neonates who would survive without ECMO; therefore, the patient selection process must have a high degree of predictability and specificity. To achieve this specificity, each neonatal ECMO center must determine its own mortality indicators and criteria.[3,7,33]

In the early stages of the development of such an invasive and inherently risky technique as ECMO, it was appropriate to begin with patients who had failed conventional therapy and were moribund. As more patients survived and the efficacy of this treatment modality was validated, selection criteria underwent (and continue to undergo) a natural metamorphosis based on patient outcomes.

Today, final selection is based on objective criteria predictive of >80 percent mortality (see Table 13-1). However, not all of these infants will benefit from ECMO. Contraindications to ECMO include the following:
- Cyanotic congenital heart disease (uncorrectable anomalies)
- Irreversible pulmonary damage
- Any nonreversible condition incompatible with

normal quality of life (e.g., bilateral pulmonary hypoplasia, certain chromosomal abnormalities, or severe neurologic damage)

- Intracranial hemorrhage
- Birth weight of <2 kg
- Gestational age of <35 weeks

Before ECMO is initiated, each candidate has a pediatric cardiology evaluation, including an echocardiogram and a cranial ultrasound. An electroencephalogram (EEG) may be indicated to rule out irreversible neurologic impairment.

In the infant with congenital heart disease (which can mimic PPHN), the treatment of choice may be palliative surgery. An exception would be the infant who, because of cardiovascular crisis, requires stabilization and life support before or after cardiac surgery.[34–36] The use of ECMO before surgery can potentially improve patient survival and/or eliminate the need for emergency palliative procedures in favor of complete intracardiac repair.[35]

ECMO is not usually indicated in neonates who have received more than ten to 14 days of mechanical ventilation. Application of this criterion excludes infants with significant ventilator-induced lung disease.[3]

An abnormal EEG, although not in itself a contraindication to the use of ECMO, helps the pediatric neurologist determine if the infant has irreversible neurologic damage. An EEG is of particular importance if chemical paralysis hinders neurologic assessment.

Intracranial hemorrhage (bilateral Grade II or higher) is a contraindication for ECMO because the systemic heparinization of ECMO patients significantly increases the risk of extending the hemorrhage.[14,37,38] Infants with Grade I or higher intraventricular hemorrhage who are placed on ECMO should be followed with serial cranial ultrasounds, and ECMO should be discontinued in the event of an extending hemorrhage.[37,39]

A birth weight of <2 kg or a gestational age of <35 weeks has been considered a contraindication for treatment with ECMO because the incidence of intracranial hemorrhage occurring during ECMO among newborns with these characteristics is significant. Consequently, the survival rate of these tiny preterm infants is discouragingly low.[19,30] However, a study published in 2004 by Rozmiarek and colleagues has challenged that guideline. The investigators report that safe cannulation can be achieved in infants <2 kg and as small as 1.6 kg with an overall survival rate of 53 percent as long as anticoagulation therapy is managed carefully.[40]

FIGURE 13-1
Anteroposterior chest film demonstrates correct placement of (1) venous cannula (left arrow) in the right atrium via the right internal jugular vein and (2) the arterial cannula (right arrow) in the aortic arch via the right common carotid artery.

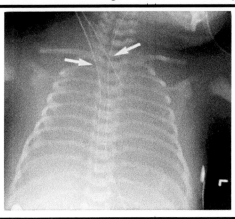

ROUTES OF PERFUSION

In the ECMO circuit, blood is drained from the venous system and diverted outside the body, where a membrane oxygenator removes carbon dioxide and adds oxygen. The oxygenated blood is then returned to the patient. This support achieves adequate gas exchange for the infant and permits ventilator settings to be reduced to low parameters, minimizing barotrauma and oxygen toxicity. The two most common methods of perfusing infants on ECMO are venoarterial (VA) bypass and venovenous (VV) bypass.

VENOARTERIAL BYPASS

The VA route, once the exclusive route of perfusion, is achieved by positioning a venous drainage cannula into the right atrium via the right internal jugular vein. An arterial cannula returns oxygen-enriched blood to the aortic arch via the right common carotid artery (Figure 13-1).[38,41] The carotid artery is the arterial vessel of choice because its diameter facilitates adequate blood flow to the aortic arch.

VA bypass is the access of choice when both respiratory support and cardiac support are required. VA bypass provides circulatory support for infants exhibiting cardiac failure by (1) decompressing the right ventricle and the pulmonary circulation, which in turn decreases pulmonary artery pressure, pulmonary capillary filtration pressure, and right heart pressures, and (2) supporting the pumping action of the heart and systemic circulation mechanically, via the roller head pump.[38]

FIGURE 13-2
Anteroposterior chest film demonstrating correct placement of VVDL catheter in right atrium via internal jugular vein.

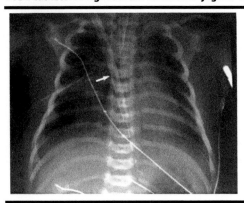

VA bypass offers several technical advantages over VV bypass: The lungs can be lavaged and suctioned without hazarding hypoxia; positive-pressure ventilation can be reduced to minimal parameters, giving the lungs a period of recovery; and stabilization and total respiratory support can be achieved in less time and at lower pump flow rates than with the venovenous route.[3,38,42]

Major risks inherent in VA bypass include the potential for infusing emboli (air or particulate) directly into the arterial circulation and disruption of usual cerebral perfusion as a result of ligation of the right common carotid artery. Walker and associates suggest that infants may maintain adequate cerebral blood flow via the adjacent vertebral circulation and the left carotid artery through the circle of Willis.[14,38]

Venovenous Bypass

Initially, the venovenous procedure necessitated two operative sites for cannulation: the internal jugular vein for blood drainage and the femoral vein for return of oxygenated blood. Technically, this form of VV bypass was more difficult to manage because these two surgical incisions and dissections were needed and stabilization required more time. VV bypass patients were at risk for groin wound infections and serious venous insufficiency in the leg because of the femoral vein ligation.[43] Despite these concerns, research documenting the efficacy of VV bypass contributed to Bartlett and coworkers' development of a single-site, double-lumen VV catheter (VVDL).[30] Reports continue to document the effectiveness of this technique and support this route as the approach if cardiac function is adequate.[44–46]

VV bypass involves cannulation of the right atrium via the internal jugular vein with a double-lumen

catheter (Figure 13-2). The venous blood is drained from the right atrium via the drainage lumen, circulated through a membrane oxygenator, and returned to the right atrium via the inflow lumen. Echocardiography can be used to aid in proper placement of the cannula: The goal is to direct the oxygenated blood toward the tricuspid valve and into the right ventricle to prevent "recirculation" of oxygenated blood back to the ECMO circuit.[14,39]

The VV route is advantageous because it does not require ligation and cannulation of the common carotid artery. Preload and afterload of the heart remain unchanged. Because the right atrium and ventricle are not decompressed, there is no change in cardiac output or pulmonary artery pressure. Oxygenated blood returns to the right side of the heart and lungs, minimizing the danger of arterial embolization. Perfusing the pulmonary artery system with oxygenated blood theoretically should increase pulmonary arteriolar dilation and reduce right ventricular afterload.[41,46]

Disadvantages to the VV route include the additional time required to stabilize the patient, possible need to continue inotropic therapy, and slower weaning of ventilator support than with VA ECMO. Because VV bypass does not provide direct circulatory support, this use has been limited to patients whose cardiac function is adequate to circulate oxygenated blood from the right atrium to the systemic circulation. Hence, evidence of left- or right-sided cardiac dysfunction via echocardiogram or clinical physiologic parameters (persistent metabolic acidosis, hypotension, or anuria despite maximal inotropic support) has been a relative contraindication to VV ECMO.[45]

However, studies have been performed to determine whether cardiac performance was impaired in infants with severe lung disease that required ECMO. Infants were divided into two groups: those who received CMV and those who received ECMO. The conclusion was that there was no difference in cardiac output.[47] Additionally, echocardiographic measurements of infants on VV bypass demonstrate normalization and no deterioration of cardiac performance, establishing that VV bypass can improve ventricular dysfunction.[41,48] Continued research is warranted to determine the specific degree of ventricular dysfunction that would limit the use of VV double-lumen bypass and dictate the need for VA bypass. A small percentage of patients require conversion to the VA route because of inadequate support.[32]

The physical limitation of VVDL ECMO is internal jugular vessel size. The double-lumen catheters used are #12, 14, and 15 French.[39]

Displacement of the mediastinum in patients with a diaphragmatic hernia, tension pneumothorax, or prominent first rib may also prevent atraumatic introduction of the cannula.[45] Larger dual-lumen catheters are available in Europe and Asia and may one day be available in the U.S. Percutaneous neck cannulation is also being evaluated.

THE ECMO CIRCUIT

Components of the ECMO circuit include cannulas, a system of polyvinylchloride (PVC) tubing with Luer-Lok connectors and stopcocks, a bladder box assembly or pressure monitoring system, a roller or centrifugal pump, a membrane oxygenator, and a heat exchanger. Additionally, in-line oxygen saturation and/or blood gas monitors may be utilized (Figure 13-3). A detailed description of the development of the ECMO circuit is available in the literature.[49,50]

The size and position of the venous drainage catheter determine venous drainage volume. The venous catheter must be capable of delivering the total cardiac output (120–150 mL/kg/minute) and should be positioned to drain blood from the superior and inferior vena cava.[12]

The internal diameter of the cannulas has the greatest impact on resistance to flow. Because the ECMO system must be capable of providing total heart-lung support, cannulas of the largest possible internal diameter are inserted. This ensures adequate venous drainage to support required bypass flow rates.[49]

After the patient has received local anesthesia and analgesia, the surgeon carefully isolates and dissects the right internal jugular vein and the carotid artery. Both vessels are dissected regardless of the route of perfusion. When the VV route is used, the carotid artery is dissected as well to permit rapid conversion to the VA route if needed. Extensive manipulation of the vessels can produce vasospasm, prohibiting cannulation with a catheter of adequate size. Application of topical papaverine promotes venodilation to permit insertion of the venous catheter.[45]

The patient is systemically heparinized just before the cannulas are introduced. Before administering a heparin loading dose of 50–100 units/kg, the nurse assesses all invasive sites for adequate hemostasis.[45] Once the patient's ACT has reached 250 seconds and before introduction of the catheter into the internal

FIGURE 13-3
Components of the ECMO circuit: (a) PVC tubing with stopcocks, (b) silicone rubber bladder with infusion sites, (c) bladder box assembly, (d) roller pump, (e & f) membrane oxygenator and gas sources, (g & h) heat exchanger and water bath, (j) ACT machine, and (k) heparin infusion.

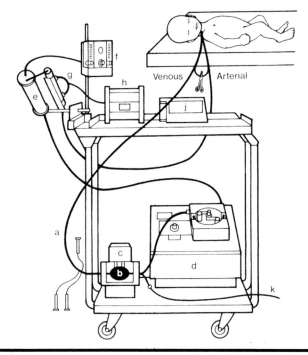

Adapted from: Nugent J. 1986. Extracorporeal membrane oxygenation in the neonate. *Neonatal Network* 4(5): 36. Reprinted by permission.

jugular vein, chemical muscle relaxants are given to prevent respiratory movement and air embolism.

To initiate VA bypass, the carotid artery and the internal jugular vein are ligated distally before introduction of the cannulas. Collateral circulation through the external carotid artery, the circle of Willis, and the ophthalmic artery maintains brain perfusion.[51]

The arterial cannula is advanced so that the catheter tip reaches just to the aortic arch. The venous cannula is positioned so that the tip lies in the right atrium with the side holes draining the right atrium and the superior vena cava.[52] The cannulas are flushed with a retrograde blood flow from the right atrium and aortic arch, sutured to the skin of the upper neck, and connected to the ECMO circuit tubing. The position of the cannulas is immediately determined by chest x-ray examination.

To initiate VVDL catheter bypass, the caregiver ligates the distal portion of the internal jugular vein. A venotomy is created in the proximal jugular vein, and a lubricated double-lumen catheter is inserted and advanced into the right atrium.

The catheter is placed so that the tip is in the right atrium and the most proximal venous drainage hole is within the superior vena cava. The arterial "angled Y" portion of the catheter should be oriented anteriorly on the infant's head. This positioning directs oxygenated blood from the arterial lumen of the catheter toward the tricuspid valve. The "angled Y" of the catheter is sutured to the skin behind the ear to prevent catheter rotation.[45] Correct catheter placement is assessed via chest radiograph and/or echocardiography.

The PVC tubing, with its system of connectors, ports with stopcocks, and silicone bladder, provides for circulation of blood from the infant through the components of the circuit as well as for removal of blood and administration of fluids, medications, and blood products. This system has a volume of approximately 400–800 mL for neonatal circulation.

Before cannulation, the circuit is primed. It is flushed with carbon dioxide, which helps to remove microbubbles by making them more soluble, and is then filled with a crystalloid solution. Albumin, 25 percent, is added to precondition and coat the surface area of the circuit, minimizing fibrinogen adherence and platelet destruction. The albumin solution is displaced with citrated packed red blood cells to which calcium and heparin have been added. The pH of the blood is corrected with THAM, and 25 percent albumin is added to equalize oncotic pressure. It is essential to verify that the electrolytes, blood gases, and acid-base balance of the priming solution are physiologic before instituting bypass. Platelets are added to the priming solution once bypass is begun and the activated clotting time is within the desired range.

The system of ports with stopcocks on the PVC tubing and the infusion sites on the bladder provide access to the circuit. Each of the ports is designed for a singular purpose. The port closest to the patient is used to remove blood samples; the second, third, and fourth ports are for administering blood products, medications, and alimentation solutions. The number of stopcocks and their positions vary with each institution's protocol.

Fluid can stagnate in the bladder, so it is preferable to infuse heparin, alimentation solutions, and medications through the ports rather than through the infusion sites on the bladder. These sites are suitable for administering blood products and, in emergencies, for removing air. To avoid contamination, use sampling sites for blood withdrawal only, and infusion sites for infusion only.

Because all ECMO patients are heparinized, institutional protocols may recommend that all intravenous infusion sites be discontinued before cannulation. This reduces the possibility of bleeding from puncture sites. All medications, fluids, and blood products except platelets are given through the venous side of the ECMO circuit. The only exceptions are fluids infused via umbilical catheters or peripheral arterial lines. When medications are given via syringe, care must be taken to aspirate each syringe gently for air bubbles because there is no in-line air filter.

Precautions and guidelines for safe administration of medications and blood into the ECMO circuit are the same as those for infusion of medications and blood directly into patients. Platelets are infused on the arterial side of the circuit between the membrane oxygenator and the heat exchanger. This prevents inadvertent filtration of platelets by the membrane oxygenator.

The bladder box assembly is a fail-safe alarm system. The collapsible silicone bladder distends with returning venous blood. If the flow into the ECMO circuit is not adequate, the bladder collapses, causing a servoswitch to sound an audible alarm and stop the roller pump. Upon reexpansion of the bladder, the servoswitch reengages the pump, and normal pump operation continues.[38] This servoregulation feature prevents the pump flow rate from exceeding venous return.

Transducer-based technology allows for servoregulation of extracorporeal flow, independent of bladder volume. Transducers placed in-line in the circuit monitor premembrane (venous) and postmembrane (arterial) pressures. This advance in servoregulation technique allows for early detection of flow problems and timely intervention.

A decrease in premembrane pressure signals decreased venous return before collapse of the silicone bladder. Causes of decreased or inadequate venous return are hypovolemia, kinked venous catheter, incorrect positioning of the venous catheter in the right atrium, inadequate catheter diameter, and pneumothorax. Adequate venous return is critical to achieving the pump flow needed for cardiopulmonary support. Persistent decreased venous return causes hemodynamic instability in the patient. It is therefore essential to recognize and immediately correct the cause of the decreased return. A rise in postmembrane pressure could indicate kinking of the arterial catheter, accidental clamping of the catheter, a clot in the membrane oxygenator or heat exchanger, or impending oxygenator failure.

One type of ECMO blood pump is a double-roller device that compresses and displaces the blood in the PVC tubing that is positioned in the pump raceway. The action of the pump pushes fluid forward, creating suction within the venous catheter. The pump is electrically powered, but can be hand cranked or attached to a battery power source if a power failure occurs. A digital display indicating circuit flow in liters/minute appears on the face of the pump. Some ECMO centers are now using centrifugal pumps, which operate like a vortex. Blood enters the centrifugal pump in an area of low pressure (at the center) and then exits in a high pressure area on the outside of the pump. This area of high pressure is transformed into flow and is measured in RPMs. Centrifugal pumps may also be hand-cranked in the event of a power failure.[74]

The membrane oxygenator, which functions as the lung of the ECMO circuit, provides a large surface for the exchange of oxygen and carbon dioxide. One type of oxygenator has a thin silicone layer that separates the infant's blood from the gas source. Oxygen flows through the inside of the membrane in a direction countercurrent to the flow of blood. The oxygen diffuses across the silicone membrane into the blood as carbon dioxide is removed. The oxygenator is more efficient in carbon dioxide removal, so a small amount of carbon dioxide may be added to prevent severe respiratory alkalosis.[28,39] A new polymethyl pentene (PMP) hollow fiber oxygenator (Quadrox-iD Pediatric Oxygenator) was recently approved for use by the FDA. The benefits of this type of oxygenator include a high gas (O_2/CO_2) transfer rate with a high volume efficiency index; elimination of plasma leaks, thus reducing the need for circuit changes; prevention of bubble formation; and preservation of platelet function, thus reducing clot and thrombus formation.[75]

A heat exchanger is located downstream from the oxygenator to warm the blood, to keep it normothermic.[38] The blood loses heat during ECMO because of the cooling effect of ventilating gases inside the oxygenator and exposure of the circuit to ambient air temperature. The infant requires heat from a radiant heat source to maintain normal body temperature during the ECMO procedure.

Fiberoptic technology continuously monitors arterial and venous blood gases. These monitoring devices, which are integral parts of the arterial and venous sides of the PVC circuit, provide digital readouts of arterial pH, PaO_2, PCO_2, base excess/bicarbonate and venous pH, PvO_2, $PvCO_2$, and venous oxygen saturation (SvO_2). Arterial monitoring allows for assessment of membrane oxygenator function. Venous monitoring provides the clinician with data to assess the adequacy of extracorporeal perfusion and the efficiency of the extracorporeal circulation in meeting the infant's metabolic needs.

An ACT machine is used to intermittently monitor the patient's whole-blood activated clotting time. It is essential to use whole-blood ACT, rather than plasma partial thromboplastin time because of the interactions between platelets, white cells, and heparin.[53] ACT is checked every 30–60 minutes. A loading dose of heparin is given at the time of cannulation. The ACT is maintained at 180–250 seconds. Heparin at a low dose of approximately 30–60 units/kg/hour is continuously infused via pump into the circuit, titrated to keep the clotting time within the desired range.

To control the amount of heparin administered, none is added to any other medications or fluids. An exception may be fluids infusing through umbilical catheters or peripheral arterial lines. Factors that influence heparin requirements are thrombocytopenia and abnormal coagulation studies.[38]

PHYSIOLOGY OF EXTRACORPOREAL CIRCULATION

Physiologic function during prolonged cardiopulmonary bypass differs considerably from normal physiology. The normal functions of blood flow, gas exchange, blood surface interface interactions, and reticuloendothelial functions are replaced in various degrees by the extracorporeal device.[53]

VA bypass drains blood from the right ventricle and returns oxygenated blood to the aortic arch. These flow dynamics significantly reduce preload and increase afterload. After initiation of VA bypass, left ventricular performance decreases. The changes in preload and afterload potentially increase the workload of the left ventricle, resulting in a transient decrease in left ventricular function. This decrease typically resolves in 48–72 hours.[54]

During VA ECMO, the venous catheter only partially drains venous return from the right atrium. Hence, total systemic blood flow is the sum of residual left ventricular output and the ECMO pump flow rate. Calculations from a flow partition model demonstrate that, in VA bypass, blood flow from the arterial catheter in the aortic arch is preferentially directed to the upper body.

TABLE 13-3
ECMO Complications

Electrolyte/glucose/fluid imbalance	Sodium requirements decrease to 1–2 mEq/kg/day. Potassium requirements increase to 4 mEq/kg/day secondary to the action of aldosterone.
	Calcium replacement may be required if citrate is a component of prime blood anticoagulant.
	Hyperglycemia may occur if citrate-phosphate-dextrose anticoagulated blood is used: Reduce dextrose concentration of maintenance and heparin infusions.
	Maintain total fluid intake 100–150 mL/kg/day.
	Fluid intake should balance output; furosemide may be required if positive fluid balance occurs.[39]
Central nervous system deterioration: cerebral edema, intracranial hemorrhage, seizures	This significant complication of ECMO can be related to pre-ECMO hypoxia, acidosis, hypercapnia, or vessel ligation.
	The drug of choice for seizures is phenobarbital.
	Serial electroencephalograms and cranial ultrasounds may be required.
Generalized edema	Extracellular space is enlarged by distribution of crystalloid solution from the prime fluid, action of aldosterone and antidiuretic hormone, or tissue injury from hypoxia or sepsis.
	Furosemide or hemofiltration may be indicated if edema causes brain or lung dysfunction.
	Restrict fluid (80 mL/kg/day) until diuresis is established.
Renal failure	Acute tubular necrosis results from pre-ECMO hypotension and hypoxia.
	Monitor output and indicators of renal failure: blood urea nitrogen and creatinine.
	Increase renal perfusion by increasing pump flow and using pressor support.
	Hemodialysis may be added to the circuit if necessary.[39]
Bleeding/thrombocytopenia	This is the most frequent cause of death.
	This is most common in infants requiring surgery or chest tubes.
	The large foreign surface of the ECMO circuit lowers platelet function and count.
	Minimize with good control of ACT (180–220 seconds) and judicious use of platelets and fresh frozen plasma.
	All surgical procedures must be done with electrocautery.
	Amicar (100 mg/kg IV infused over 1 hour, then 30/mg/kg/hour continuous infusion) decreases bleeding at the surgical site and decreases intracranial and extracranial hemorrhage.[59]
Decreased venous return and/ or hypovolemia	Infant must have adequate circulating volume to obtain adequate flow rates.
	Manifested by collapsing silicone bladder triggering bladder box alarm, decrease in extracorporeal flow rate, arterial pressure, and arterial pulse amplitude.
	Blood sampling, wound drainage, or peripheral vessel dilation may account for hypovolemia.
	Check for pneumothorax, partial venous catheter occlusion, or malposition, which may decrease venous drainage and return.
	Replace volume with packed cells, fresh frozen plasma.
	Treat pneumothorax with chest tube placement.
	Raise level of bed to enhance gravity drainage of venous blood.

(continued on next page)

Coronary artery and abdominal blood flows are derived predominantly from the left ventricle. Oxygen delivery to the heart is therefore more closely related to pulmonary status and pulmonary venous saturation than to the ECMO pump arterial oxygen content. These findings have implications when ECMO is instituted for postoperative management of compromised cardiac performance and may also contribute to the etiology of cardiac stun syndrome (Table 13-3) seen in some infants following initiation of ECMO.[55] Cardiac stun (hypotension, poor perfusion, decreased PaO_2) is the transient loss of ventricular contractility usually lasting one to three days. The stun is believed to be caused by the mismatch between the afterload and ventricular contractility during ECMO.[56]

In VVDL bypass, blood is drained from the right atrium, and oxygenated blood is returned to the right atrium. Hence, systemic perfusion is dependent on the infant's native cardiac output. The heart's preload and afterload are unchanged, and there is no selective distribution of systemic blood flow. Theoretically, because the coronary arteries are perfused by blood from the left ventricle, the increased oxygen content of the blood coming from the ECMO circuit via the left ventricle should improve oxygen delivery to the coronary arteries if the infant is hemodynamically stable.[48,57]

TABLE 13-3
ECMO Complications *(continued)*

Hypertension	This is caused by hypervolemia due to overinfusion of blood products, which causes a larger percentage of blood to flow through malfunctioning lungs.
	Hypertension can also be caused by renal ischemia and excretion of rennin/angiotensin.
	Hypertension, secondary to hypervolemia, is manifested by widening pulse amplitude and decreasing systemic oxygenation at a fixed extracorporeal flow rate.
	Treat overinfusion by removing blood from the circuit. Renal hypertension may dictate use of captopril or labetalol.
Patent ductus arteriosus	Left-to-right shunting may occur, causing increased blood flow to the lungs, necessitating high pump flow without expected increase in PaO_2.
	Ligation may be indicated because weaning from ECMO will not be successful.
Cardiac stun	Transient loss (1–3 days) of ventricular contractility.
	Manifested by hypotension, marked decrease in aortic pulse pressure, poor peripheral perfusion, and decrease in PaO_2.
	Possibly due to mismatch between afterload and ventricular contractility during ECMO.
	Adjust pump flow to provide circulatory support, and maintain inotropic therapy.[72]
Mechanical	**Rationale and Treatment**
Tubing rupture, air in circuit, oxygenator malfunction	Increase ventilator to pre-ECMO parameters. Take patient off bypass. Repair circuit, aspirate air, and replace oxygenator. Be prepared to resuscitate infant.
Power failure	Always plug pump into hospital's emergency power supply. Hand crank until emergency power is available.
Decannulation	Apply firm pressure. Come off bypass; increase ventilator parameters. Repair vessel; replace blood volume. Be prepared to resuscitate infant.

Adapted from: Nugent J. 1986. Extracorporeal membrane oxygenation in the neonate. *Neonatal Network* 4(5): 33. Reprinted by permission.

VA bypass is instituted by draining venous blood by siphon into the extracorporeal circuit; a like amount of arterialized blood is returned to the arterial circulation. As bypass flow is gradually increased, flow through the pulmonary artery decreases at a faster rate than bypass flow, reducing total flow in the systemic circulation. Peripheral and pulmonary hypotension may occur.

In VVDL bypass, total systemic flow dynamics are not changed (there is no alteration in preload or afterload). However, peripheral hypotension occurs with this route of perfusion. Though the exact mechanisms causing hypotension are not well understood, reduction in blood viscosity and the release of vasoactive substances may contribute to this phenomenon.[53] Blood volume replacement is required to correct hypotension, optimize tissue perfusion, and prevent metabolic acidosis.

Hypotension after initiation of ECMO by either route is associated with decreased ionized calcium levels. The citrate in the priming blood may bind with ionized calcium, causing functional hypocalcemia and depressed cardiac performance.[57] Calcium should be added to the priming solution, normalizing ionized calcium in the circuit. Additionally, the infant's serum calcium levels should be monitored closely and corrected when indicated.

In VVDL perfusion, hypotension may also be caused by removal of inotropic drugs when the catheter drains the right atrium. An extension tube may be attached to the arterial side of the double-lumen catheter to allow additional infusion of inotropes when bypass is begun. As the infant's blood pressure stabilizes, this infusion may be weaned and the extension tube capped off.[45]

ECMO via the VA route is nonpulsatile, meaning that pulse contour decreases as VA flow rate increases, and systemic perfusion is dependent on circuit flow and cardiac output. The precise nature of the physiologic effects of nonpulsatile flow during extracorporeal circulation has been the subject of controversy. Experts agree, however, that the kidney interprets the nonpulsatile flow as inadequate, resulting in renin and aldosterone production and antidiuresis.[53] VV bypass perfusion is pulsatile. The pulse contour does not change or dampen, and systemic perfusion depends only on the infant's native cardiac output.[58]

The total flow to the patient during ECMO is a function of blood volume and the diameter of the venous catheter. An increase in blood volume at a stable ECMO flow increases pulmonary-artery–to–left-atrial flow, decreasing the relative percentage of cardiopulmonary bypass. Conversely, a reduction in patient blood volume can inadvertently increase extracorporeal flow and decrease pulmonary-artery–to–left-atrial flow.

Total patient flow is the sum of extracorporeal flow plus pulmonary blood flow. Adequate flow in ECMO bypass is reached when oxygen delivery and tissue perfusion result in normoxia, normal pH, normal SvO_2, and normal organ function. Normal cardiac output in an infant is 120–150 mL/kg/minute. Total gas exchange and support are usually achieved at this flow rate.

Gas exchange is accomplished via the membrane lung. The lung consists of two compartments divided by a semipermeable membrane: Ventilating gas is on one side of the membrane; blood is on the other. As the blood flows past the membrane, oxygen diffuses into the blood because of a pressure gradient between the 100 percent oxygen in the ventilating gas and the low oxygen pressure in the mixed venous blood. The chemical binding of oxygen to hemoglobin proceeds very rapidly. The oxygen transfer capacity of a membrane oxygenator is related to the rate of blood flow through the membrane and the degree of oxyhemoglobin desaturation of the blood entering the oxygenator. The flow rate at which venous blood leaves the oxygenator at 95 percent saturation is called "rated flow."

The limiting factor in oxygenation of flowing blood is the rate of oxygen diffusion through plasma. As blood flow through the membrane oxygenator is increased, a point is reached when the thickness of the blood film limits the rate at which oxygen can diffuse into the blood. At this point, the outflow blood exits at less than 95 percent saturation. The rated flow for a membrane oxygenator is that at which this limitation is reached.

Simultaneously, carbon dioxide diffuses from the blood compartment, responding to a pressure gradient between the venous carbon dioxide pressure and the ventilating gas. The rate of carbon dioxide transfer is greater than that of oxygen; hence, a carbon dioxide–enriched mixture is usually necessary for ventilating the oxygenator. This prevents inadvertent hypocapnia, respiratory alkalosis, and cessation of the infant's spontaneous respirations.

The carbon dioxide pressure is controlled by gas flow through the membrane oxygenator. To remove excess carbon dioxide, the sweep flow (the total liter flow of oxygen, carbon dioxide, and compressed air to the oxygenator) may be increased. The manufacturer's recommended limit for sweep flow should not be exceeded. If the pressure on the gas side of the membrane exceeds that on the blood side, gas embolization could occur.

The rated oxygen delivery is the amount of oxygen that can be taken up by the blood at the rated flow. Oxygen delivery is related to the flow and to the amount of unsaturated hemoglobin presented to the oxygenator per minute. Thus, decreasing flow will conversely decrease oxygen delivery.

In selecting an oxygenator, the clinician must be sure that the rated flow is greater than cardiac output—that is, the infant's oxygen requirement should not exceed the oxygenating performance of the membrane lung.

Other factors may influence systemic oxygenation during ECMO. Total oxygen delivery to tissues is equal to extracorporeal oxygen plus pulmonary oxygen. Increasing extracorporeal flow and decreasing patient lung flow will increase the infant's PaO_2. Decreasing extracorporeal flow and increasing patient lung flow will decrease the infant's PaO_2 as long as the infant's lung function is not adequate.

In VVDL bypass, higher pump flows and a larger membrane oxygenator (0.6 m^2 or 0.8 m^2) may be required to compensate for the problem of pump recirculation. Pump recirculation refers to drainage of oxygenated blood from the right atrium and return of that blood to the ECMO circuit. As a consequence of pump recirculation, less oxygenated blood is available for the infant's circulation because a portion of the oxygenated circulating blood volume goes into the drainage cannula.

Recirculation can range from 5 to 29 percent of blood flow; hence, higher flows may be required to maintain oxygenation. Typical blood flow for optimal gas exchange in VV bypass is 100–120 mL/kg/minute; in VA bypass, it is 80–100 mL/kg/minute.[31,45]

Because of recirculation, VV bypass does not result in as great a degree of oxygenation as does VA bypass. Oxygen tensions of 50–60 torr and oxygen saturations of 85–90 percent are accepted.[45] Increasing flow in VV bypass may increase recirculation and decrease patient oxygenation.

In situations where the patient is hypoxic and no additional recirculation is desired, an increase in extracorporeal flow is not indicated. Oxygenation may be improved by optimizing the infant's cardiac output and hemoglobin level. Cardiac output may be improved by increasing venous return to the heart. This can be accomplished by reducing positive inspiratory pressure and positive end-expiratory pressure (PEEP), thereby decreasing mean airway pressure and allowing increased venous return.[55]

A less than optimal hemoglobin (less than 15 g/dL [150 g/liter]) decreases oxygen-carrying capacity.[39] Rapid infusion or overinfusion of blood products decreases oxygenation because a larger percentage of blood flow is shifted to the pulmonary artery to left atrial flow, decreasing the relative percentage of cardiopulmonary bypass. Care must be taken to recognize and avoid this problem.[38]

During ECMO, at least 80 percent of the cardiac output is exposed to a large artificial surface each minute. All blood cellular components and protein molecules come into contact with a foreign surface hourly. Flow patterns in the circuit include areas of stagnation and turbulence.[38] All these factors stimulate both the protein and the platelet arms of the clotting system.

Within seconds of blood's exposure to this foreign surface, a molecular layer of proteins would adhere to the surface. One of these proteins is fibrinogen, which is converted into fibrin. This causes clot formation to occur within a few minutes. Other protein clotting factors are absorbed to some extent by the foreign surface, decreasing the clotting factors in the blood when bypass begins. Concurrently, the liver and spleen increase synthesis of fibrinogen and other clotting factors, returning their serum concentrations to prebypass levels within a period of hours.[53]

Exposing the circuit's inner surface to albumin before initiating bypass appears to minimize fibrin surface adherence and platelet destruction.[38] In the presence of heparin, fibrinogen is not converted to fibrin, and clotting does not occur.

Platelets show the greatest effect from exposure to a foreign surface, as evidenced by continuous platelet aggregate formation and decreasing platelet count and function. The concentration of platelets drops abruptly with the onset of extracorporeal circulation and continues to fall as long as bypass continues. The thrombocytopenia results in part from platelets adhering directly to the foreign surface. To a greater extent, however, it results from platelets adhering to each other and to white cells, forming platelet aggregates of 2–200 microunits, which are infused into the patient. These aggregates are picked up by the liver, the spleen, and to a lesser extent the lung, where they are bound, or phagocytized. Platelet aggregate formation is not detrimental to microcirculation, as is evidenced by lack of microembolic tissue damage even in prolonged bypass.[37,38,58]

Because a large number of platelet aggregates are generated continuously, it can be estimated that all circulating platelets are incorporated into aggregates every few hours. The platelet count plateaus at 30,000–60,000/mm^3 when a balance between aggregation, regeneration from bone marrow, disaggregation, and recirculation is achieved.[38] This chronic thrombocytopenia requires frequent platelet transfusions.

Platelet transfusions are necessary when the platelet level drops below 100,000/mm^3. If the patient is experiencing abnormal amounts of bleeding, the platelet count is maintained at >100,000/mm^3, and the ACT is restricted to 180–220 seconds. Use of concentrated platelets is recommended to minimize the increase in fluid volume. Platelet transfusions do increase heparin consumption; to compensate, the heparin infusion may need to be increased briefly during the transfusion.[39]

When extracorporeal circulation is discontinued, clotting factors and platelets return to normal or above-normal levels.[31,53] However, thrombocytopenia can occur up to four days after the cessation of ECMO. Platelet counts must be monitored during this critical period. Infants at highest risk for prolonged thrombocytopenia are those with MAS or sepsis and those whose ECMO course was marked by mechanical complications (tubing rupture, oxygenator malfunction; see Table 13-3).[59–61]

Physiologic changes occur as a result of systemic heparinization. Heparin inhibits several of the steps between activation of the surface factor (Factor XII) and fibrin formation.[53] These actions result in prolonged clotting times. Heparin has an almost immediate onset of action following intravenous administration and is inactivated by the liver and excreted by the kidney. Clotting times return to normal within two to six hours after the drug is discontinued.

The effects of prolonged extracorporeal circulation on blood cell survival and function demonstrate that hemolysis is negligible and the survival of red blood cells is not altered by continuous exposure to the ECMO circuit. All the various types of white cells decrease in concentration because of the combined effects of dilution and aggregation.

Studies of phagocytosis and bacterial killing of circulating leukocytes during extracorporeal circulation demonstrate significantly decreased phagocytic activity in the circulating white cells. It is postulated that the mechanical or chemical effects of the ECMO circuit on blood cause these changes. It is thought that the phagocytes may become saturated with platelet aggregates, reducing their ability to further phagocytize

Figure 13-4
Example of an arterial pressure waveform and bypass flow rates. On venoarterial bypass, conduction and contraction continue even thought little blood is flowing through the heart. The EKG pattern will remain normal. The normal peaked pattern of the arterial pressure waveform will flatten as bypass flow increases. Total bypass (70–80 percent of cardiac output) is reached when the arterial pressure tracing flattens and no peaked contours are evident during positive pressure inflation.

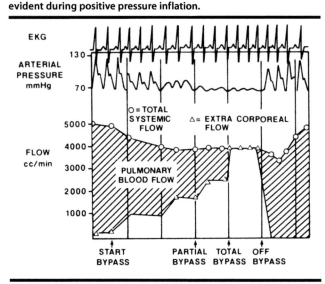

From: Chapman R, Toomasian J, and Bartlett R. 1988. *Extracorporeal Membrane Oxygenation Technical Specialist Manual,* 9th ed. Ann Arbor: University of Michigan, 8. Reprinted by permission.

bacteria. White cell concentration rebounds after ECMO is stopped.[53]

Fluid and electrolyte changes occur frequently during extracorporeal circulation. Sodium retention, expanded extracellular fluid, and decreased total body potassium are characteristic changes. These conditions are thought to be attributable to (1) third spacing of albumin, the source of which is the circuit priming fluid; (2) the action of aldosterone, which causes sodium retention, expansion of extracellular fluid, and kaliuresis; and (3) fluid and electrolyte shifts from the intravascular to the extravascular space caused by hypoxic-ischemic injury or sepsis.[62]

The goal of fluid management is to promote diuresis while maintaining adequate circulatory volume.[62] Potassium replacement is required, and excessive extracellular fluid can be removed through use of furosemide or continuous hemofiltration.[31] Calcium and magnesium levels can remain low throughout the ECMO run; correction is achieved with moderate supplementation via parenteral fluids.[53]

CARE OF THE INFANT UNDERGOING ECMO

Cannulation and the initiation of bypass usually occur in the NICU under local anesthesia and with operating room staff in attendance. This avoids the risks inherent in moving a critically ill newborn to and from the operating room with bypass in progress. The operating room team provides an ECMO surgical case cart, an electrocautery unit, and a fiberoptic headlight. While the team is readying the surgical equipment, the ECMO specialist assembles and primes the circuit.

An indwelling arterial line is essential for arterial sampling as well as for continuous blood pressure monitoring. The site of choice is the umbilical artery. If this is not feasible, a postductal site such as the left radial or posterior tibialis artery will be utilized. An umbilical venous catheter or a peripheral venous line is inserted for infusion of parenteral fluids and medications during the surgical procedure. Necessary lines are kept to a minimum and are inserted prior to heparinization.

During the surgical procedure, NICU nursing staff continuously monitor the infant's cardiopulmonary status and administer necessary medications. Blood products and emergency drugs are available for administration as needed. Initiation of bypass frequently causes hypotension, which is generally corrected using volume replacement. Care must be taken not to dislodge the infant's endotracheal tube or arterial or venous lines during the cannulation.

Following cannulation, bypass is gradually instituted until approximately 80 percent of the infant's cardiac output is diverted through the ECMO circuit. This usually requires flow rates of 80–120 mL/kg/minute (Figure 13-4). At maximum flow, hypoxia, hypercarbia, and acidosis will be reversed. The infant will become normotensive, and vasoactive drugs and muscle relaxants can be discontinued. During VV bypass, continued inotropic pressor support may be indicated because the infant is totally dependent on native cardiac output for blood pressure.[45]

Ventilator parameters are reduced to minimal settings to "rest" the lungs. VV bypass may require higher resting parameters. The extracorporeal flow is adjusted to maintain systemic arterial PaO_2 at 60–80 torr on VA and 50 torr on VV bypass, $PaCO_2$ at 35–45 torr, pH at 7.35–7.45, SvO_2 at >70 percent, and arterial saturation at >90 percent on VA or 85–90 percent on VV bypass.

In the infant on VA bypass, SvO_2 is considered an excellent indicator of adequate flow because it is a measure of tissue perfusion and oxygen delivery. A decrease in SvO_2 indicates tissue hypoxia. The best end-point indicator for VV bypass is the PaO_2, or oxyhemoglobin saturation, measured by pulse oximetry.[45] Continuous monitoring of venous and arterial oxyhemoglobin saturation via fiberoptic technology allows for optimal management of bypass flow.

Total blood flow to the infant on bypass is the sum of extracorporeal flow and pulmonary blood flow. Total oxygen delivery is the combination of extracorporeal oxygen delivery and pulmonary oxygen delivery. The resultant systemic arterial blood gases reflect the sum of these relative oxygen contents.

Maintaining the hematocrit at 35–45 percent maximizes oxygen delivery. Blood products are also given to correct hypovolemia, excessive bleeding, and thrombocytopenia. Maintenance and alimentation fluids are administered at 80–120 mL/kg/day. The usual sodium requirement is 1–2 mEq/kg/day, with a potassium requirement of 4 mEq/kg/day. Gastric feedings may be initiated if bowel function is normal.

Significant insensible water loss can occur secondary to the radiant warmer and the membrane lung. Daily weights are the best indicator of fluid balance, although weighing may not be feasible. A weight gain will occur during the first 24–48 hours, followed by diuresis and weight loss.

Prophylactic antibiotic therapy with therapeutic levels monitored are usually ordered. Serial cultures of blood, urine, and tracheal aspirates are followed. Daily chest x-rays are evaluated for endotracheal tube and cannula placement as well as for lung pathology. Endotracheal suctioning should be provided based on assessment of the infant's need. Vital signs, intake and output, neurologic evaluation, and arterial blood gases should be documented based on patient status and unit policy.

Oozing at the cannulation site may require frequent dressing changes. The amount of blood loss must be quantified and replaced.

Frequent infant repositioning is warranted. Use of an air mattress may eliminate circulatory complications from immobilization. Catheter dislodgement is a fatal complication; for that reason, caution must be used to avoid inadvertent decannulation when changing the infant's position. The ECMO specialist should assist the nurse in all position changes.

TABLE 13-4
Circuit Emergency Procedures

Circuit Emergencies	
Air embolism (arterial)	Power failure
Tubing rupture	Gas source failure
Oxygenator malfunction	
Decannulation	
Pump failure	
↓	
Come off bypass	

Procedures	
Nurse	ECMO specialist
Ventilation	Clamp catheters
Anticoagulation	Open bridge
Chemical resuscitation	Remove gas source
Replace blood loss	Repair circuit

Because of the thin-walled polyurethane construction of the VV double-lumen catheter, cannula kinking remains a concern and can contribute to interruption in blood flow that can be a major problem. The infant's head and neck are often kept immobilized to prevent kinking. Occupational therapists can help develop individualized nursing care plans to address this immobility concern.

Wedges and blanket rolls can be useful when repositioning the infant. To provide greater stability for the catheter, place a protective "sleeve," fashioned from a large-diameter endotracheal tube, around the catheter proximal to the "angled Y."

COMPLICATIONS

Complications associated with ECMO are both physiologic and mechanical. Mechanical complications most commonly reported to the ELSO data registry include clots in the circuit (52 percent), followed by cannula problems (11 percent).[32] Although these complications rarely affect morbidity and mortality, catastrophic events such as raceway rupture and inadvertent decannulation create emergency situations that require immediate recognition and resolution.[3] Tables 13-3 and 13-4 outline these complications with their rationale and corrective actions.

Data collected from members of ELSO document that physiologic complications include, but are not limited to, neurologic complications (seizures, cerebral infarction), hemorrhagic complications (bleeding, hemolysis), cardiopulmonary complications (cardiac arrest, hypo/hypertension, pulmonary hypertension, pneumothorax,

TABLE 13-5
ECMO Specialist Responsibilities and Interventions

Responsibility	Intervention
Maintain and monitor ECMO circuit	Check circuit carefully for air, dots, tightness of connectors, stopcocks.
	Check bladder box alarm function.
	Monitor pump arterial and venous blood gases each shift to assess oxygenator function. (Pump arterial PO_2 <100 mmHg, CO_2 retention, or leaking membrane indicates oxygenator failure.)
Assess infant	Check cannula placement and stability.
	Assess breath sounds, neurologic status.
	Observe volume of fluid and blood drainage.
	Monitor vital signs and laboratory values.
Maintain prescribed parameters: pH 7.35–7.45 PaO_2 60–80 mmHg (VA) PaO_2 50 mmHg (VV) $PaCO_2$ 35–45 mmHg Paw 45–55 mmHg Hct 45–55% Platelets 70–100,000/mm³ SvO_2 >70% SaO_2 >90% (VA) SaO_2 >85% (VV) ACT 180–250 seconds	Maintain infant's systemic arterial blood gases by adjusting sweep gas and pump flow.
	Maintain mean arterial blood pressure, hematocrit, and adequate platelet count by infusing appropriate blood products. Assess ACT hourly or as needed; titrate heparin infusion to maintain parameters.
Assist nurse in care	Draw *all* blood samples from circuit except systemic arterial blood gases.
	Coordinate recording of intake and output with nurse.
	Assist in all position changes.
	Administer and monitor all medications, blood products, and fluids placed into the pump circuit.
Be prepared to deal with pump emergencies	See Tables 13-3 and 13-4.

Adapted from: Nugent J. 1986. Extracorporeal membrane oxygenation in the neonate. *Neonatal Network* 4(5): 36. Reprinted by permission.

arrhythmias), renal complications (creatinine >1.5 mg/dL [114 micromols/liter], use of dialysis/hemofiltration), and metabolic complications (electrolyte imbalances, pH derangement).[32]

In comparing data from VV ECMO with that from VA ECMO, researchers found the incidence of neurologic complications to be greater in the VA group than in the VVDL group, as was the incidence of symptomatic patent ductus arteriosus. Hemorrhage and mechanical complications were similar. Catheter kinking was limited to use of the double-lumen catheter. The increased rate of complications in the VA group reflects the fact that patients treated with VA bypass are more unstable at the outset of ECMO than those who receive VV bypass.[55]

THE ECMO TEAM

The complex and challenging care of infants on ECMO requires a highly trained and skilled team of professionals that includes a physician (neonatologist and/or pediatric surgeon), perfusionist, neonatal intensive care nurse, respiratory therapist, and ECMO specialist. The most important factor in maintaining

ECMO for days or weeks is the ability of all team members to work collaboratively.

Providing this mode of care is not feasible for many hospitals because of the expense and commitment involved in training personnel. The training of an ECMO specialist alone requires a minimum of 50–80 hours of class and laboratory work.

Both a nurse and an ECMO specialist are assigned to care for the ECMO patient each shift. The nurse is responsible for ongoing assessment, hemodynamic monitoring, data collection, administration of fluids and medications, and pulmonary care, in conjunction with the respiratory therapist. The ECMO specialist is responsible for checking and monitoring the circuit, adjusting gas and pump flow, maintaining heparinization, administering appropriate blood products, drawing blood specimens, and documenting data.

The nurse practice acts in many states do not allow nurses to delegate administration of medications and blood products to nonlicensed personnel; hence, this responsibility rests with the nurse if the ECMO specialist

TABLE 13-6
Nursing Responsibilities and Interventions for ECMO

Prior to Cannulation	
Responsibility	**Intervention**
Obtain and document baseline physiologic data	Record weight, length, head circumference.
	Draw blood samples for CBC, electrolytes, calcium, glucose, BUN, creatinine, PT/PTT, platelets, and arterial blood gases.
	Record vital signs: heart rate; respiratory rate; systolic, diastolic, mean blood pressure; temperature.
Assure adequate supply of blood products for replacement	Draw type and cross-match samples for 2 units of packed red cells, fresh frozen plasma.
	Keep 1 unit of packed red cells and fresh frozen plasma always available in the blood bank.
Maintain prescribed pulmonary support	Maintain ventilator parameters.
	Administer muscle relaxants if indicated.
Assemble and prepare equipment	Prepare infusion pumps to maintain arterial lines and infusion of parenteral fluids and medications into the ECMO circuit.
	Place the infant on a radiant warmer with the head positioned at the foot of the bed to provide thermoregulation and access for cannulation.
	Attach infant to physiologic monitoring devices to monitor heart rate, intra-arterial blood pressure, transcutaneous oxygen, and other parameters.
	Insert urinary catheter and nasogastric tube; place to gravity drainage.
	Remove intravenous lines just prior to heparinization (optional).
	Prepare loading dose of heparin (50–100 units/kg).
	Prepare heparin solution for continuous infusion (100 units/mL/D_5W).
	Prepare paralyzing drug (pancuronium bromide, 0.1 mg/kg or succinylcholine, 1–4 mg/kg).
	Assist in insertion of arterial line (umbilical or peripheral).
	Administer prophylactic antibiotics.

During Cannulation	
Monitor cardiopulmonary status during procedure	Monitor heart rate and intra-arterial blood pressure continuously.
	Obtain blood gases after paralysis and during cannulation, as indicated by the infant's response to the procedure.
Be prepared to administer cardiopulmonary support	Have medications and blood products available to correct hypovolemia, bradycardia, acidosis, cardiac arrest.
Administer medications	Give loading dose of heparin systemically when vessels are dissected free and are ready to be cannulated.
	Give paralyzing drug systemically just prior to cannulation of internal jugular vein if infant has not been previously paralyzed.
Reduce ventilator parameters to minimal settings	Once adequate bypass is achieved, reduce peak inspiratory pressure to 16–20 cmH$_2$O, PEEP to 4 cmH$_2$O, ventilator rate to 10–20 breaths per minute, and FiO$_2$ to 21–30%. Venovenous bypass patients may require greater respiratory support.

During ECMO Run	
Responsibility	**Intervention**
Monitor and document physiologic parameters	Record hourly: heart rate, blood pressure (systolic, diastolic, mean), respirations, temperature, transcutaneous PO$_2$, CO$_2$, oxygen saturation, ACT, ECMO flow.
	Measure hourly: accurate intake and output of all body fluids (urine, gastric contents, blood). Measure every 4 hours: urine pH, protein, glucose, specific gravity; Hematest all stools.
	Assess hourly: color, breath sounds, heart tones, murmurs, cardiac rhythm, arterial pressure waveform (Figure 13-4), peripheral perfusion.
	Perform hourly: neurologic check, including fontanel tension, pupil size and reaction, level of consciousness, reflexes, tone, and movement of extremities.
	Record ventilator parameters hourly.
	Assess weight and head circumference daily.
Monitor and document biochemical parameters	Draw arterial blood gases from umbilical or peripheral line as indicated.
	All other blood specimens are drawn from the ECMO circuit by the ECMO specialist: electrolytes, calcium, platelets, Chemstrip, hematocrit every 4–8 hours, CBC, PT/PTT, BUN, creatinine, total and direct bilirubin, plasma hemoglobin, fibrinogen, fibrin split products, and blood culture as indicated.

(continued on next page)

TABLE 13-6
Nursing Responsibilities and Interventions for ECMO *(continued)*

Prior to Cannulation

Responsibility	Intervention
Administer medications	Remove air bubbles and double-check dosages before infusion.
	Administer no medications intramuscularly or by venipuncture.
	Place all medications and fluids into the venous side of the ECMO circuit.
	Prepare and administer the arterial line (umbilical or peripheral) infusion.
	Administer parenteral alimentation.
Provide pulmonary support	Perform endotracheal suctioning based on individual assessment and need.
	Maintain patent airway; be alert to extubation or plugging.
	Obtain daily chest films and tracheal aspirate cultures as indicated.
	Maintain ventilator parameters.
Prevent bleeding	Avoid all of the following: rectal probes, injections, venipunctures, heelsticks, cuff blood pressures, chest tube stripping, restraints, chest percussion.
	Avoid invasive procedures: Do not change nasogastric tube, urinary catheters, or endotracheal tube unless absolutely necessary; use premeasured endotracheal tube suction technique.
	Observe for blood in the urine, stools, endotracheal or nasogastric tubes.
Maintain excellent infection control	Change all fluids and tubing daily.
	Change dressings daily and as needed.
	Clean urinary catheter site daily.
	Maintain strict aseptic and hand washing techniques.
	Use universal barrier precautions.
Provide physical care	Keep skin dry, clean, and free from pressure points.
	Give mouth care as needed.
	Provide range of motion exercises as indicated.
	Turn side to side every 1–2 hours.
Provide pain management, sedation, stress reduction	Minimize noise level.
	Group patient care to maximize sleep period.
	Administer analgesia: fentanyl 9–18 mcg/kg/hour (increased dosage due to fentanyl binding to membrane oxygenator).
	Manage iatrogenic physical dependency by following a dose reduction regime (reduce dose 10% every 4 hours).[73]
Be alert to complications and emergencies	See Tables 13-3 and 13-4.

Key: CBC = complete blood count; BUN = blood urea nitrogen; PT = prothrombin time; PTT = partial thromboplastin time; PEEP = positive end expiratory pressure; ACT = activated clotting time; FiO_2 = fraction of inspired oxygen; PO_2 = partial pressure of oxygen.

is not a registered nurse. Tables 13-5 and 13-6 outline ECMO specialist and nursing responsibilities and interventions.

WEANING AND DECANNULATION

ECMO is a palliative measure that allows the body time to recover from various underlying pathologic processes. As the body heals, certain indicators signal that the infant is ready to be weaned from bypass. Infants placed on bypass for MAS and/or pneumonia may demonstrate improvement in lung fields as seen on chest x-rays. Initially, lung fields may appear opaque on radiographic studies, indicating volume loss; but

as diuresis occurs, either naturally or with use of a loop diuretic, lung-field clearing becomes evident. It is important to keep in mind, however, that signs of clinical improvement typically precede radiographic changes.[63] Frequent weights, as permissible, may demonstrate diuresis of excess extracellular fluid, which in turn heralds improving pulmonary function.

Echocardiography is useful when assessing resolution of PPHN. As the primary pathology of PPHN resolves and pulmonary function improves, oxygenation in the fraction of cardiac output traversing the lungs improves. This is indicated by a rise in systemic PaO_2. Research has shown that changes in lung compliance can be a sensitive indicator of a neonate's lung improvement while on ECMO. Lotze and colleagues suggest that lung compliance measurements can be used to monitor the infant's clinical course and improvement as well as to predict whether the patient can be successfully removed from bypass.[64] Employment of sensitive measures of lung function, such as lung compliance, can be very useful in the weaning process and can potentially shorten total time on bypass. This is of particular importance when the infant's condition (e.g., excessive bleeding) warrants immediate cessation of bypass, but arterial blood gas measurements are marginal.

Once improvement in pulmonary gas exchange has been ascertained, weaning from VA ECMO may proceed by decreasing the flow rate of the pump in small increments. The flow is decreased in this manner, usually over a period of days, until extracorporeal support is no longer needed to maintain adequate gas exchange. Decreasing the flow of the pump diverts less blood into the extracorporeal circuit and increases blood flow to the infant's lungs. Concurrently, ventilator settings are increased to maintain adequate gas exchange. Weaning from VV bypass may be accomplished by decreasing the FiO_2 of the sweep gas, or the membrane lung can be capped off so no gas flow occurs.

During VA bypass, when the flow rate is decreased to 30–50 mL/kg/minute, a state of "idling" is achieved. The infant is kept at this lowest possible flow rate for four to eight hours. Heparinization must be maintained for as long as the catheters are in place. During the idling period, the heparin infusion may need to be switched to the patient to maintain appropriate activated clotting time levels.[39] If the infant's condition deteriorates, extracorporeal flow is increased, and support is resumed.

If gas exchange remains adequate and stable at low ventilator settings during idling, a test period with the infant removed from ECMO is attempted. The cannulas are clamped, and the circuit is slowly recirculated via the bridge to prevent stagnation. If the heparin infusion has not already been switched to the patient during idling, it is switched now. The gas flow into the oxygenator is discontinued, the heat exchanger temperature is decreased, and all infusions into the ECMO circuit are switched to the patient.[40]

Decannulation may proceed if blood gas values remain satisfactory. Preparation, equipment, and staff needs are the same as for cannulation. Decannulation is performed as a sterile surgical procedure. Muscle relaxants and sedation are administered to the infant before decannulation to prevent air embolization.

Ventilator settings are increased to compensate for the loss of spontaneous ventilation caused by drug-induced paralysis.[39]

As the cannulas are removed, the internal jugular vein (and carotid artery with VA ECMO) are ligated. Debate remains as to the efficacy of carotid reconstruction because of the significant risk of thrombus formation and embolization at the cannulation site.[64] Some studies argue that reconstruction can be performed safely with no significant morbidity or mortality in select ECMO patients.[65-67] Long-term follow-up of patients who have undergone carotid repair is needed to determine the efficacy of this procedure.

After decannulation, the infant is weaned as tolerated from mechanical ventilation. Heparin reversal is usually not warranted because heparin is metabolized in a few hours. Once the infant's ACT is within normal limits, routine NICU care can resume. Transfusions to correct anemia are frequently required during the first 24 hours after ECMO. Platelet counts should be followed closely because thrombocytopenia may persist for up to four days following cessation of bypass.[60]

SUPPORT FOR PARENTS

Support of the family of the infant undergoing ECMO presents some unique challenges. Parents are usually in crisis: Their infant has been critically ill since birth, and they are aware that the baby's chances for survival are poor. Parents are informed that the ECMO procedure itself is a method of last resort, with no guarantee of a positive outcome. The technical environment is overwhelming. It is not unusual for the parents to be grieving and in a state of withdrawal.

Listening, communicating, educating, and providing various types of support are all staff responsibilities. Parents need continuous communication of concise, accurate information about their child's condition and the required procedures. The staff should be empathetic and as reassuring as the situation allows. Parents should be allowed access to their infant to facilitate parent-infant bonding, and nurses should make every effort to encourage parental involvement and bonding with the infant.

Parent-to-parent support from parents whose infants have experienced ECMO is efficacious, and it is a positive experience for all families involved. Parent support groups have been established both locally and nationally to educate and assist parents of infants on ECMO.

FOLLOW-UP AND OUTCOME

The survival rate for infants treated with ECMO varies, depending on the primary disease. In centers that provide ECMO, it is a feasible lifesaving measure for neonates who might otherwise die. Overall survival of infants treated with ECMO remains at approximately 76 percent.[32] Survival rates for ECMO-treated infants with various pathologies are as follows: MAS, 94 percent; RDS, 84 percent; PPHN, 78 percent; sepsis, 75 percent; pneumonia, 59 percent; CDH, 52 percent; and other, 64 percent (see Table 13-2).[32]

Differentiating between preexisting deficits and those secondary to ECMO manipulation can be difficult. Critical scrutiny of survivors is essential to properly assess the efficacy and continued safety of this mode of treatment. Neonatal ECMO survivors are followed closely for possible complications caused by hypoxia and acidosis occurring both before and during the procedure. Survivors are systematically and periodically evaluated for the following parameters: growth and development, cardiorespiratory development, cerebrovascular status, and neurologic and psychological functioning. Prompt identification of deficits or disabilities makes early intervention and remediation possible.[3,39]

Approximately 15 percent of ECMO survivors are oxygen dependent at 28 days of life; this may contribute to the high rate of rehospitalization for pulmonary conditions after discharge.[3,39] In addition, continued medical management and pharmacotherapy may be indicated for those infants with chronic lung disease. Consistent parental teaching and support are critical in promoting growth and development and optimal wellness.[68]

Continued monitoring by the American Academy of Pediatrics as well as by ECMO centers is warranted to monitor morbidity data as they relate to quality of survival. Regionalization of ECMO centers is recommended to accommodate patient bed needs and to provide a milieu of safe and effective EMCO care.[69]

SUMMARY

Despite improvements in mechanical ventilation and the introduction of adjunct therapies such as iNO, ECMO remains a life-saving treatment for select groups of critically ill neonates. The success of ECMO is dependent on the expertise of the ECMO team and the exquisite attention to detail demanded by this mode of therapy. Well-established selection criteria determine which neonates are optimal candidates for ECMO. While the success of ECMO has been demonstrated through on-going evaluation, this mode of treatment carries a significant risk for morbidity, and infants undergoing ECMO must be monitored closely by experienced health care providers. Parent support and ongoing follow-up are also an important part of an ECMO program.

REFERENCES

1. Chatburn R. 1984. High frequency ventilation: A report on a state of the art symposium. *Respiratory Care* 29: 839.
2. Bancalari E, and Goldberg RN. 1987. High-frequency ventilation in the neonate. *Clinics in Perinatology* 14(3): 581–597.
3. Cook LN. 2004. Update on extracorporeal membrane oxygenation. *Paediatric Respiratory Reviews* 5 (supplement A): S329–S337.
4. Kinsella J, et al. 1992. Low-dose inhalational nitric oxide in persistent pulmonary hypertension of the newborn. *Lancet* 340(8823): 819–820.
5. Kinsella J, et al. 1993. Clinical response to prolonged treatment of persistent pulmonary hypertension of the newborn with low doses of inhaled nitric oxide. *Journal of Pediatrics* 123(1): 103–108.
6. Buck ML. 2004. Sildenafil for the treatment of pulmonary hypertension in children. *Pediatric Pharmacotherapy* 10(2): 1–8.
7. Ortiz RM, Cillery RE, and Bartlett RH. 1987. Extracorporeal membrane oxygenation in pediatric respiratory failure. *Pediatric Clinics of North America* 34(1): 39–46.
8. Rashkind W, et al. 1965. Evaluation of a disposable plastic low flow volume pumpless oxygenator as a lung substitute. *Journal of Pediatrics* 66(1): 94–102.
9. Dorson W, et al. 1969. A perfusion system for infants. *Transactions—American Society for Artificial Internal Organs* 15: 155–160.
10. White J, et al. 1971. Prolonged respiratory support in newborn infants with a membrane oxygenator. *Surgery* 70(2): 288–296.
11. Pyle R, et al. 1975. Clinical use of the membrane oxygenator. *Archives of Surgery* 110(8): 966–970.
12. Bartlett R. 1984. Extracorporeal oxygenation in neonates. *Hospital Practice* 19(4): 139–151.
13. Kolobow T, Zapol W, and Pierce J. 1969. High survival and minimal blood damage in lambs exposed to long term (1 week) veno-venous pumping with a polyurethane chamber roller pump with and without a membrane blood oxygenator. *Transactions—American Society for Artificial Internal Organs* 15(3): 172–174.
14. Walker G, et al. 2003. Extracorporeal life support—State of the art. *Paediatric Respiratory Reviews* 4(2): 147–152.
15. Kolobow T, et al. 1974. Superior blood compatibility of silicone rubber free of silica filler in the membrane lung. *Transactions—American Society for Artificial Internal Organs* 20: 269A–276A.
16. Kolobow T, Stool E, and Pierce J. 1976. Long-term perfusion with the membrane lung in lambs. In *Artificial Lungs for Acute Respiratory Failure: Theory and Practice*, Zapol WM, and Qvist J, eds. New York: Academic Press, 234–242.
17. Bartlett R, et al. 1982. Extracorporeal membrane oxygenation for newborn respiratory failure: Forty-five cases. *Surgery* 92(2): 425–433.
18. Bartlett RH, et al. 1976. Extracorporeal membrane oxygenation (ECMO) cardiopulmonary support in infancy. *Transactions—American Society for Artificial Internal Organs* 22: 80–93.
19. Bartlett R, et al. 1985. Extracorporeal circulation in neonatal respiratory failure: A prospective randomized study. *Pediatrics* 76(4): 479–487.
20. Krummel T, et al. 1982. Extracorporeal membrane oxygenation in neonatal pulmonary failure. *Pediatric Annals* 11(11): 905–908.
21. Hardesty R, et al. 1981. Extracorporeal membrane oxygenation: Successful treatment of persistent fetal circulation following repair of congenital diaphragmatic hernia. *Journal of Thoracic and Cardiovascular Surgery* 81(4): 556–569.
22. Wetmore N, et al. 1979. Defining indications for artificial organ support in respiratory failure. *Transactions—American Society for Artificial Internal Organs* 25: 459–461.
23. Kirkpatrick B, et al. 1983. Use of extracorporeal membrane oxygenation for respiratory failure in term infants. *Pediatrics* 72(6): 872–876.
24. Raphaely R, and Downes J. 1973. Congenital diaphragmatic hernia: Prediction of survival. *Journal of Pediatric Surgery* 8(5): 815–818.
25. Krummel TM, et al. 1984. Alveolar-arterial oxygen gradients versus the Neonatal Pulmonary Insufficiency Index for prediction of mortality in ECMO candidates. *Journal of Pediatric Surgery* 19(4): 380–384.
26. Paneth N, and Wallenstein S. 1985. Extracorporeal membrane oxygenation and the play the winner rule. *Pediatrics* 76(4): 622–623.

27. Ware J, and Epstein M. 1985. Extracorporeal circulation in respiratory failure: A prospective randomized study. *Pediatrics* 76(5): 849–851.

28. Singh AR. 2002. Neonatal and pediatric extracorporeal membrane oxygenation. *Heart Disease* 4(1): 40–46.

29. O'Rourke P, et al. 1989. Extracorporeal membrane oxygenation and conventional medical therapy in neonates with persistent pulmonary hypertension of the newborn: A prospective randomized study. *Pediatrics* 84(6): 957–963.

30. Bartlett R, et al. 1986. Extracorporeal membrane oxygenation (ECMO) in neonatal respiratory failure. *Annals of Surgery* 204(3): 236–245.

31. Bartlett R, et al. 1989. Prospective randomized study of cost effectiveness of neonatal ECMO. Ann Arbor, Michigan: ELSO chapter meeting, October. 32. Extracorporeal Life Support Organization (ELSO). July 2011. International summary. Ann Arbor, Michigan.

33. Marsh D, Wilkerson S, and Cook L. 1988. Extracorporeal membrane oxygenation selection criteria: Partial pressure of arterial oxygenation versus alveolar-arterial oxygen gradient. *Pediatrics* 82(2): 162–166.

34. Klein M, et al. 1990. Extracorporeal membrane oxygenation for the circulatory support of children after repair of congenital heart disease. *Journal of Thoracic and Cardiovascular Surgery* 100(4): 498–505.

35. Hunkeler NM, et al. 1992. Extracorporeal life support in cyanotic congenital heart disease before cardiovascular operation. *American Journal of Cardiology* 69(8): 790–793.

36. von Alleman D, and Ryckman FC. 1991. Cardiac arrest in the ECMO candidate. *Journal of Pediatric Surgery* 26(2): 143–146.

37. O'Rourke PP. 1993. ECMO: Current status. *Neonatal Respiratory Diseases* 3(3): 1–11.

38. Chapman R, Toomasian J, and Bartlett R. 1988. *Extracorporeal Membrane Oxygenation Technical Specialist Manual*, 9th ed. Ann Arbor: University of Michigan Press.

39. Kim E. 2000. ECMO in the newborn. *American Journal of Perinatology* 17(7): 345–355.

40. Rozmiarek AJ, et al. 2004. How low can you go? Effectiveness and safety of extracorporeal membrane oxygenation in low-birth-weight neonates. *Journal of Pediatric Surgery* 39(5): 845–847.

41. Kugelman A, et al. 2003. Venovenous versus venoarterial extracorporeal membrane oxygenation in congenital diaphragmatic hernia. *Journal of Pediatric Surgery* 38(8): 1131–1136.

42. Klein MD, et al. 1985. Venovenous perfusion in ECMO for newborn respiratory insufficiency: A clinical comparison with venoarterial perfusion. *Annals of Surgery* 201(4): 520–526.

43. Andrews A, et al. 1983. Venovenous extracorporeal membrane oxygenation in neonates with respiratory failure. *Journal of Pediatric Surgery* 18(4): 339–346.

44. Skarsgard ED, et al. 2004. Venovenous extracorporeal membrane oxygenation in neonatal respiratory failure: Does routine, cephalad jugular drainage improve outcome? *Journal of Pediatric Surgery* 39(5): 672–676.

45. Anderson HL, et al. 1989. Venovenous extracorporeal life support in neonates using a double lumen catheter. *Transactions—American Society for Artificial Internal Organs* 35(3): 650–653.

46. Cornish JD, et al. 1993. Extracorporeal membrane oxygenation service at Egleston: Two year's experience. *Journal of the Medical Association of Georgia* 82(9): 471–476.

47. Karr SS, Martin GR, and Short BL. 1991. Cardiac performance in infants referred for extracorporeal membrane oxygenation. *Journal of Pediatrics* 118(3): 437–442.

48. Strieper MJ, et al. 1993. Effects of venovenous extracorporeal membrane oxygenation on cardiac performance as determined by echocardiographic measurements. *Journal of Pediatrics* 122(6): 950–955.

49. Bartlett RH, and Gazzaniga AB. 1978. Extracorporeal circulation for cardiopulmonary failure. *Current Problems in Surgery* 15(5): 1–96.

50. Lawson DS, et al. 2004. North American neonatal extracorporeal membrane oxygenation (ECMO) devices: 2002 survey results. *Journal of the American Society of ExtraCorporeal Technology* 36(1): 16–21.

51. Krummel T, et al. 1984. The early evaluation of survivors after extracorporeal membrane oxygenation for neonatal pulmonary failure. *Journal of Pediatric Surgery* 19(5): 585–589.

52. German J, et al. 1980. Technical aspects in the management of the meconium aspiration syndrome with extracorporeal circulation. *Journal of Pediatric Surgery* 15(4): 378–383.

53. Bartlett R, and Gazzaniga A. 1980. Physiology and pathophysiology of extracorporeal membrane circulation. In *Techniques in Extracorporeal Circulation*, Ionescu M, ed. Boston: Butterworth, 1–43.

54. Hirschl RB, Heiss KF, and Bartlett RH. 1992. Severe myocardial dysfunction during extracorporeal membrane oxygenation. *Journal of Pediatric Surgery* 27(1): 48–53.

55. Anderson HL, et al. 1993. Multicenter comparison of conventional venoarterial access versus venovenous double-lumen catheter access in newborn infants undergoing extracorporeal membrane oxygenation. *Journal of Pediatric Surgery* 28(4): 530–535.

56. Chung DH, and Zwischenberger JB. 2000. Emergencies during extracorporeal membrane oxygenation and their management. In *ECMO: Extracorporeal Cardiopulmonary Support in Critical Care*, 2nd ed., Zwischenberger JB, Steinhorn RH, and Bartlett R, eds. Ann Arbor, Michigan: Extracorporeal Life Support Organization, 357–362.

57. Kinsella JP, Gerstmann DR, and Rosenberg AA. 1992. The effect of extracorporeal membrane oxygenation on coronary perfusion and regional blood flow distribution. *Pediatric Research* 31(1): 80–83.

58. Meliones JN, et al. 1991. Hemodynamic instability after the initiation of extracorporeal membrane oxygenation: Role of ionized calcium. *Critical Care Medicine* 19(10): 1247–1251.

59. Downard CD, et al. 2003. Impact of Amicar on hemorrhagic complications of ECMO: A ten year review. *Journal of Pediatric Surgery* 38(8): 1212–1216.

60. Anderson H, et al. 1986. Thrombocytopenia in neonates after extracorporeal membrane oxygenation. *Transactions—American Society for Artificial Internal Organs* 32(1): 534–537.

61. Anderson KD. 1993. Extracorporeal membrane oxygenation. In *Pediatric Surgery*, 2nd ed., Ashcraft KW, and Holder TM, eds. Philadelphia: Saunders, 956–968.

62. Heiss K, et al. 1987. Renal insufficiency and volume overload in neonatal ECMO managed by continuous ultrafiltration. *Transactions—American Society for Artificial Internal Organs* 33(3): 557–560.

63. Lewis FC, Reynolds M, and Arensman RM. 2003. Extracorporeal membrane oxygenation. In *Assisted Ventilation of the Neonate*, 4th ed., Goldsmith JP, and Karotkin EH, eds. Philadelphia: Saunders, 261–277.

64. Lotze A, Short B, and Taylor G. 1987. Lung compliance as a measure of lung function in newborns with respiratory failure requiring extracorporeal membrane oxygenation. *Critical Care Medicine* 15(3): 226–229.

65. Spector ML, et al. 1991. Carotid artery reconstruction in the neonate: Discharge data and eighteen month follow-up (abstract). Seventh Annual Children's Hospital–National Medical Center–ECMO Symposium, February.

66. Moulton SL, et al. 1991. Carotid artery reconstruction following neonatal extracorporeal membrane oxygenation. *Journal of Pediatric Surgery* 26(7): 794–799.

67. Riggs P, et al. 1991. Repair following ECMO: Colorflow Doppler studies (abstract). Seventh Annual Children's Hospital–National Medical Center–ECMO Symposium, February.

68. Tulenko DR. 2004. An update on ECMO. *Neonatal Network* 23(4): 11–18.

69. Glass P, Miller M, and Short B. 1989. Morbidity for survivors of extracorporeal membrane oxygenation: Neurodevelopmental outcome at 1 year of age. *Pediatrics* 83(1): 72–78.

70. Andrews A, Bartlett R, and Roloff D. 1982. Mortality risk graphs for neonates with respiratory distress. *Pediatric Respiration* 16: 275A.

71. Beck R, Anderson KD, and Pearson GD. 1986. Criteria for extracorporeal membrane oxygenation in a population of infants with persistent pulmonary hypertension of the newborn. *Journal of Pediatric Surgery* 21(4): 297–302.

72. Martin G. 1993. Cardiac changes during prolonged extracorporeal membrane oxygenation. In *Extracorporeal Life Support*, Arensmen RM, and Cornish JD, eds. Boston: Blackwell Scientific, 136.

73. Caron E, and Maguire DP. 1990. Current management of pain, sedation and narcotic physical dependency of the infant on ECMO. *Journal of Perinatal and Neonatal Nursing* 4(1): 63–74.

74. Short BL, and Williams L. 2010. *ECMO Specialist Training Manual*, 3rd ed. Ann Arbor, Michigan: Extracorporeal Life Support Organization, 83–84.

75. Manufacturer's product literature. Quadrox-iD Pediatric Oxygenator. Wayne, New Jersey: Maquet.

NOTES

Appendix A
Siggaard-Andersen Alignment Nomogram

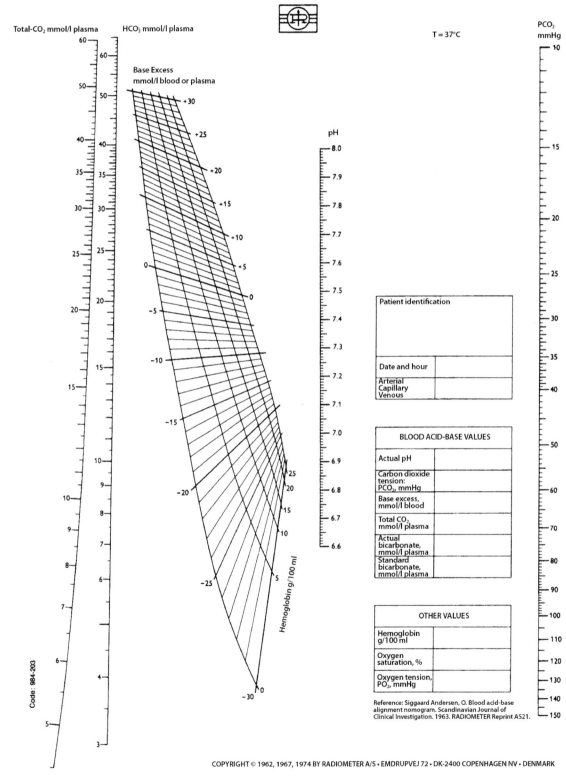

Glossary

Acidemia: An increase in the hydrogen ion concentration of the blood or a fall in pH below normal.

Acidosis: A state characterized by actual or relative decrease of alkali in body fluids in proportion to the acid content; the pH of body fluid may be normal or decreased.

Acinus, pulmonary: Respiratory bronchiole and all of its branches.

Air bronchogram: The outline of the bronchus on x-ray, visible because of diminished air in the alveolus.

Alkalemia: A decrease in hydrogen ion concentration of the blood, or a rise in pH, irrespective of alterations in the level of bicarbonate ion.

Alkalosis: A pathophysiologic disorder characterized by hydrogen ion loss or base excess in body fluids (metabolic alkalosis), or caused by CO_2 loss due to hyperventilation (respiratory alkalosis).

Alveolar minute ventilation: The volume of gas moved into the alveolus per unit of time.

Alveolar-arterial oxygen gradient ($AaDO_2$): A measure of the alveolar efficiency in transporting oxygen to the pulmonary capillaries.

Amplitude: In high-frequency ventilation, the size of the ventilator breath or oscillation, also referred to as *delta p* (PIP – PEEP).

Anemometry: A technique for monitoring airway flow that consists of a heated filament that senses temperature changes that correspond to the airway flow.

Apnea: Cessation of breathing for >20 seconds accompanied by changes in color or heart rate.

Atelectasis: A collapsed or airless state in the lung.

B-line: The B-line is a comet-tail artifact seen on ultrasound. The presence of this artifact is usually related to pathologic findings, but it may be seen in healthy term newborns.

Ball-valve effect: The free flow of gas or fluid in one direction, coupled with the partial or complete obstruction to flow in the opposite direction.

Barotrauma: Injury to lung tissue resulting from pressure.

Base deficit: A reflection of the concentration of buffer or base available in the blood. A base deficit reflects an excess of acid or a diminished amount of base available and is expressed as a negative number.

Base excess: Refers to either a deficit in the amount of acid present in the blood or an increased amount of base. Base excess is expressed as a positive number.

Capnogram: A graph demonstrating the concentrations of inspired and expired carbon dioxide.

Closing capacity: The lung volume at which dependent regions of the lung collapse or close to the main bronchi.

Compensation: An attempt to maintain a normal blood pH by altering the component of the blood gas that is not primarily responsible for the abnormality.

Compliance: A measurement of the elastic properties of the lung opposing a change in volume per unit of change in pressure.

Correction: An attempt to maintain a normal blood pH by altering the component of the blood gas responsible for the abnormality.

De novo: Latin expression meaning "from the beginning" or "anew."

Double lung point: Point of division seen on a lung ultrasound of an infant with transient tachypnea of the newborn; more widely spaced "A lines" in the upper lung meet more compactly spaced "B lines" in the inferior lung fields.

Dynamic mechanics: In a pulmonary function profile, testing during active, uninterrupted breathing.

Elastic recoil: The tendency of stretched objects to return to their resting state.

Emphysematous: A condition of the lung marked by an abnormal increase in the size of the lung's air sacs (alveoli), making breathing difficult.

Energetics: A component of the pulmonary function profile that includes work of breathing.

Frequency: Breaths or cycles per minute.

Functional residual capacity (FRC): The volume of air remaining in the lung at the end of expiration.

Glycosaminoglycans: One type of a variety of polysaccharides, the most abundant one in the body, with high molecular weight that contains amino sugars. Highly negatively charged, they often form complexes with proteins.

Hertz (Hz): A unit of frequency equal to one cycle per second (60 cycles per minute).

High-frequency ventilation (HFV): Ventilation provided at least four times the normal neonatal respiratory rate and at a tidal volume close to or less than anatomic dead space.

I:E ratio: The ratio of the time (in seconds) spent in inspiration compared to the time allowed for expiration.

Intrapleural pressure: Pressure within the pleural space.

Knockout of a gene: A genetic technique in which one of an organism's genes is made inoperative.

Lamellar bodies: The site of surfactant synthesis and storage, lamellar bodies are located in Type II pneumocytes in the alveoli.

Laplace relationship: Describes the relationship between pressure, surface tension, and the radius of a structure. According to Laplace, the pressure needed to stabilize an alveolus is directly proportional to twice the surface tension and inversely proportional to the radius of that alveolus.

Mean airway pressure (Paw): The average pressure transmitted to the airways over a series of breaths.

Metaplasia: Benign process of change in tissue from one type to another due to a type of stress.

Necrotizing tracheobronchitis: A process causing cellular death and tissue sloughing in the trachea and bronchi. Pathogenesis is most likely multifactorial.

Nitric oxide: An endogenous pulmonary vasodilator.

Osmiophilic: Having an affinity for, or easily stained with, osmium tetroxide.

Oxyhemoglobin dissociation curve: A graphic representation of the relationship between oxygen and hemoglobin.

Parturition: The process of giving birth.

Patient-triggered ventilation: A system of assisted ventilation which recognizes and supports patient-initiated breaths.

Pendelluft: Transient movement of gas out of some alveoli and into others when flow has just stopped at the end of inspiration, or such movement in the opposite direction just at the end of expiration; occurs when regions of the lung differ in compliance, airway resistance, or inertance so that the time constants of their filling (or emptying) in response to a change of transpulmonary pressure are not the same.

Perfluorochemicals: Inert liquids derived by replacing carbon-bound hydrogen atoms on organic compounds with fluorine.

pH: The negative logarithm of hydrogen ion concentration used to determine the relative acidity or alkalinity of a solution.

Phosphatidylcholine (PC): A phospholipid that comprises two-thirds of the lipid component of surfactant and is responsible for surfactant's ability to reduce lung surface tension.

Phosphatidylglycerol (PG): A phospholipid comprising eight percent of the lipid in surfactant. PG is unique to the pulmonary cells, making it a good marker for the presence of surfactant.

Pneumomediastinum: Air in the mediastinal space.

Pneumopericardium: Air in the pericardial space.

Pneumoperitoneum: Air in the peritoneum.

Pneumotachograph: A device that measures breath flow by detecting pressure drops across a fixed flow resistance.

Pneumothorax: Air in the pleural space.

Postductal: Distal to the ductus arteriosus.

Preacinar: Conducting airways of the lungs above the alveoli.

Preductal: Blood flow from the aorta between the left ventricle and the ductus arteriosus.

Pulmonary insufficiency index: A scoring system used to calculate mortality risk based on oxygen requirement, acidosis, and time.

Pulmonary mechanics: A component of the pulmonary function profile that includes measurement of flow and pressure.

Pulse oximetry: A device utilizing a light source and photosensor to measure the amount of saturated hemoglobin in arterial blood.

Rales: An abnormal, nonmusical sound usually heard during inspiration, also referred to as *coarse crackles*.

Resistance: Opposition to airflow resulting from friction. Resistance is proportional to the length of the airway or endotracheal tube and inversely proportional to the radius of the tube.

Respiratory dead space: The volume of the anatomic passages between the external environment and the alveoli, which do not function in gas exchange.

Retraction: A drawing in of the chest wall resulting from noncompliant lungs and a compliant chest wall.

Rhonchi: Deep, coarse, snoring or rattling sounds resulting from mucus plugs or debris in the bronchi.

Sail sign: A sail-shaped thymic outline seen on x-ray as the result of free air in the mediastinum.

Static mechanics: In a pulmonary function profile, testing done while briefly occluding the airway at one or more points in the respiratory cycle.

Stroke volume: The driving pressure of the piston in high-frequency ventilation.

Surface tension: The attractive force exerted upon the surface molecules of a liquid by the molecules beneath that tends to draw the surface molecules into the bulk of the liquid and makes the liquid assume the shape having the least surface area.

Surfactant: A surface-active substance which reduces surface tension in the alveolus.

Tidal volume: The volume of gas inspired with each breath.

Time constant: A measure of how quickly pressure generated in the proximal airway results in a 64 percent pressure change in the alveoli.

Tracheobronchomalacia: Softening of the tissues in the trachea and bronchi.

Transpulmonary pressure: Pressure across the lung from airway opening to the pleural space.

Ventilation:perfusion ratio: Expresses the relationship between alveolar ventilation and blood flow in the pulmonary capillaries.

Waveform: The shape of the delivered breath.

BIBLIOGRAPHY

Lexicus, lexic.us.

McDonough JT Jr. 1994. *Stedman's Concise Medical Dictionary*, 2nd ed. Philadelphia: Lippincott Williams & Wilkins.

Merriam-Webster, merriam-webster.com/medical.

O'Toole M. 1992. *Miller-Keane Encyclopedia, and Dictionary of Medicine, Nursing, and Allied Health*, 5th ed. Philadelphia: Saunders.

The Free Medical Dictionary, medical-dictionary.thefreedictionary.com. Accessed 5/2/2012.

Abbreviations

ΔP	Airway pressure gradient		IMV	Intermittent mandatory ventilation
AaDO$_2$	Alveolar-arterial gradient		IPPV	Intermittent positive pressure ventilation
A/C	Assist/Control ventilation		IWL	Insensible water loss
ACD	Alveolar capillary dysplasia		LAP	Left atrial pressure
ADS	Anatomic dead space		LBW	Low brith weight
BAL	Bronchoalveolar lavage		MABP	Mean arterial blood pressure
BAT	Brown adipose tissue		MAS	Meconium aspiration syndrome
BPD	Bronchopulmonary dysplasia		mCBFv	Mean cerebral blood flow velocity
C$_L$	Lung compliance		NAVA	Neurally adjusted ventilation assist
CLD	Chronic lung disease		NC	Nasal cannula
cmH$_2$O	Centimeters of water		NCPAP	Nasal continuous positive airway pressure
CMV	Conventional mechanical ventilation		NIPPV	Nasal intermittent positive pressure ventilation
CP	Cerebral palsy			
CPAP	Continuous positive airway pressure		NIV	Noninvasive ventilation
CVP	Central venous pressure		OI	Oxygen index
DPPC	Dipalmitoylphosphatidylcholine		PaCO$_2$	Partial pressure of CO$_2$ in arterial blood
FiO$_2$	Fraction of inspired oxygen		PaO$_2$	Partial pressure of O$_2$ in arterial blood
FRC	Functional residual capacity		PAP	Pulmonary artery pressure
GER	Gastroesophageal reflux		PAV	Proportional assist ventilation
Hb	Hemoglobin		Paw	Mean airway pressure
HbF	Fetal hemoglobin		PC	Phosphatidylcholine
HFJV	High-frequency jet ventilation		PDE	Phosphodiesterase
HFNC	High-flow nasal cannula		PEEP	Positive end-expiratory pressure
HFO	High-frequency oscillation		PG	Phosphatidylglycerol
HFOV	High-frequency oscillatory ventilation		PIE	Pulmonary interstitial emphysema
HFV	High-frequency ventilation		PIP	Peak inspiratory pressure
HMD	Hyaline membrane disease		PMI	Point of maximal impulse
HNF-3β	Hepatocyte nuclear transcription factor			
IGF-1	Insulin-like growth factor			

Ppl	Pleural pressure	SOD:	Superoxide dismutase
PRVC	Pressure-regulated volume control	ST	Surface tension
PSV	Pressure support ventilation	SvO_2	Venous oxygen saturation
PVR	Pulmonary vascular resistance	SVR	Systemic vascular resistance
Paw	Mean airway pressure	SVRI	Systemic vascular resistance index
PTXF	Pentoxifylline	T_3	Triiodothyronine
$\dot{Q}_C$	Volume of blood per unit of time (perfusion)	T_4	Thyroxine
RDS	Respiratory distress syndrome	TAPVR	Total anomalous pulmonary venous return
SaO_2	Oxygen saturation of arterial blood	T_I	Inspiratory time
SAP	Systemic arterial pressure	T_E	Expiratory time
SEM	Standard error of the mean	$\dot{V}_A$	Gas volume per unit time (ventilation)
SIMV	Synchronized intermittent mandatory ventilation	VAPS	Volume-assured pressure support
SNIPPV	Synchronized nasal intermittent positive pressure ventilation	$\dot{V}_A/\dot{Q}_C$	Ventilation-to-perfusion ratio
		VEGF	Vascular endothelial growth factor
SNP	Sodium nitroprusside	VG	Volume guarantee
		V_T	Tidal volume

NOTES

Index

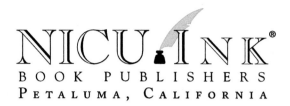

Continuing Education Program

The continuing education test based on this text, that can be taken for CNE credit is located at www.NICUInk.net. Click on the Continuing Education link and follow the instructions.

Cost for the course:

$90.00   30 contact hours

VISA and Mastercard are accepted for payment on our secure website.